MEMBRANE PROTEIN STRUCTURE

THE AMERICAN PHYSIOLOGICAL SOCIETY
METHODS IN PHYSIOLOGY SERIES

MEMBRANE PROTEIN STRUCTURE

Experimental Approaches

Edited by

Stephen H. White, Ph.D.

Professor of Physiology and Biophysics
University of California, Irvine,
College of Medicine

New York   Oxford
OXFORD UNIVERSITY PRESS
1994

Oxford University Press

Oxford   New York   Toronto
Delhi   Bombay   Calcutta   Madras   Karachi
Kuala Lumpur   Singapore   Hong Kong   Tokyo
Nairobi   Dar es Salaam   Cape Town
Melbourne   Auckland   Madrid

and associated companies in
Berlin   Ibadan

Copyright © 1994 by the American Physiological Society

Published by Oxford University Press, Inc.,
200 Madison Avenue, New York, New York 10016

Oxford is a registered trademark of Oxford University Press

Library of Congress Cataloging-in-Publication Data
Membrane protein structure : experimental approaches
edited by Stephen H. White
p. cm.   (Methods in physiology series ; 1)
Includes bibliographical references and index.
ISBN 0-19-607112-3
1. Membrane proteins. I. White, Stephen H, II. Series.
[DNLM: 1. Membrane Proteins—ultrastructure.
2. Protein Conformation. QU 55 M513 1994]
QP552.M44M435   1994
574.87'5—dc20   DNLM/DLC
for Library of Congress   93-26101

1 3 5 7 9 8 6 4 2

Printed in the United States of America
on acid-free paper

Preface

The structures of membrane proteins are of vital interest to researchers in physiology, cell biology, and biochemistry. Their determination, however, constitutes one of the most challenging problems of structural biology. During the 18 years that have elapsed since Henderson and Unwin (1975) reported the first low-resolution three-dimensional structure of bacteriorhodopsin, the structures of only two types of trans-membrane proteins have been determined to high resolution with three-dimensional crystals. During the same time, hundreds, if not thousands, of amino acid sequences for membrane proteins have been reported because studies of receptors, channels, and transporters have come to the fore as major activities of the biological research community. The creation of hypothetical protein structural models to serve as guides for these studies is crucially important but problematic, because our knowledge of protein folding in membrane environments is limited. The development of suitable model structures requires an understanding of protein structure and structure-prediction methods as well as membrane biophysics and lipid physical chemistry. Because the literature for each of these fields is expanding rapidly and can be daunting even for the experts, I have attempted to assemble into a single compact volume the experiences of some of the experts in these areas that I hope will be helpful to researchers who need to know about the critical issues of membrane protein structure.

My goal was not to provide an exhaustive compendium of information relevant to the membrane protein problem but rather to plant some signposts. However, there are several important destinations that the serious student of membrane protein structure should consider but which are not explicitly posted as chapters: stability and folding of globular proteins, sequence analysis, protein structure prediction, and lipid physical chemistry. These subjects have been covered nicely by others. A very readable and informative account of protein stability is given in the recent review of Ken Dill (1990). Thomas Creighton (1992) has assembled an excellent volume on various aspects of the protein folding problem and Russell Doolittle (1990) one on the analysis of protein and nucleic acid sequences. Authoritative discussions of the principles of protein conformation and structure prediction are provided in the volume edited by Gerald Fasman (1989). The unique feature of membrane proteins is that they are embedded in a lipid bilayer, and one cannot therefore ignore the physical chemistry of lipids. A comprehensive account of this area is provided by Donald Small (1986).

This volume would not have come into existence without the interest and enthusiasm of Oxford University Press and the Publications and Technical Book Committees of the American Physiological Society. In addition to the authors who contributed to the volume despite many other pressing obligations, I thank Brenda Rauner, Directer of Publications for the American Physiological Society, and Jeffrey House, Vice President of Oxford University Press, for their patience and understanding during the prolonged birth of this project.

References

Creighton, T. E. (1992) *Protein Folding.* New York: W. H. Freeman.

Dill, K. A. (1990) Dominant forces in protein folding. *Biochemistry* 29: 7133–7155.

Doolittle, R. F. (1990) *Methods in Enzymology, Vol. 183, Molecular Evolution: Computer Analysis of Protein and Nucleic Acid Sequences.* San Diego: Academic Press.

Fasman, G. D. (1989) *Prediction of Protein Structure and the Principles of Protein Conformation.* New York: Plenum Press.

Henderson, R., and Unwin, P.N.T. (1975) Three-dimensional model of purple membrane obtained by electron microscopy. *Nature* 257: 28–32.

Small, D. M. (1986) *The Physical Chemistry of Lipids.* New York: Plenum Press.

Contents

Contributors

Christian Altenbach
Jules Stein Eye Institute
and Department of Chemistry & Biochemistry
University of California
Los Angeles, California

L. Mario Amzel
Department of Biological Chemistry
and Department of Biophysics and Biophysical
Chemistry
Johns Hopkins University
School of Medicine
Baltimore, Maryland

Ariane Atteia
Institut de Biologie Physico-Chimique
Collège de France
Paris, France

Mario A. Bianchet
Department of Biological Chemistry
and Department of Biophysics and Biophysical
Chemistry
Johns Hopkins University
School of Medicine
Baltimore, Maryland

J. Kent Blasie
Department of Chemistry
University of Pennsylvania
Philadelphia, Pennsylvania

Dana Boyd
Department of Microbiology and Molecular
Genetics
Harvard Medical School
Boston, Massachusetts

David S. Cafiso
Department of Chemistry and Biophysics
University of Virginia
Charlottesville, Virginia

A. J. Chirino
Division of Chemistry and Chemical
Engineering
California Institute of Technology
Pasadena, California

W. F. DeGrado
DuPont Merck Pharmaceutical Company
Wilmington, Delaware

Gunnar von Heijne
Department of Molecular Biology
Karolinska Institute Center for Structural
Biochemistry
Huddinge, Sweden

Wayne L. Hubbell
Jules Stein Eye Institute
and Department of Chemistry & Biochemistry
University of California
Los Angeles, California

Isabella L. Karle
Laboratory for the Structure of Matter
Naval Research Laboratory
Washington, D.C.

K.-H. Kim
Division of Chemistry and Chemical
Engineering
California Institute of Technology
Pasadena, California

H. Komiya
Division of Chemistry and Chemical
Engineering
California Institute of Technology
Pasadena, California

Werner Kühlbrandt
European Molecular Biology Laboratory
Heidelberg, Germany

x   Contributors

J. D. Lear
Department of Biochemistry
University of Pennsylvania
Philadelphia, Pennsylvania

Stanely J. Opella
Department of Chemistry
University of Pennsylvania
Philadelphia, Pennsylvania

Peter L. Pedersen
Department of Biological Chemistry
and Department of Biophysics and Biophysical
Chemistry
Johns Hopkins University
School of Medicine
Baltimore, Maryland

Jean-Luc Popot
Institut de Biologie Physico-Chemique
Collège de France
Paris, France

D. C. Rees
Division of Chemistry and Chemical
Engineering
California Institute of Technology
Pasadena, California

Lukas K. Tamm
Department of Molecular Physiology
and Biological Physics
University of Virginia
School of Medicine
Charlottesville, Virginia

Catherine de Vitry
Institut de Biologie Physico-Chimique
Collège de France
Paris, France

B. A. Wallace
Department of Crystallography
Birkbeck College, University of London
London, United Kingdom

Z. R. Wasserman
DuPont Merck Pharmaceutical Company
Wilmington, Delaware

Stephen H. White (Editor)
Department of Physiology and Biophysics
University of California
Irvine, California

Robert W. Williams
Department of Biochemistry
Uniformed Services University of the Health
Sciences
Bethesda, Maryland

G. Andrew Woolley
Department of Chemistry
University of Toronto
Toronto, Ontario
Canada

I. The Nature of the Membrane Protein Structure Problem

The quest for three-dimensional structure is one of the main driving forces of protein science. Before the structure of a protein is known from crystallographic measurements, we urgently seek approximate structures by means of spectroscopy, secondary structure algorithms, homology modeling, and other methods. We can be reasonably optimistic these days that in many cases, for globular proteins, the approximations can be replaced relatively quickly by real structures due to advances in crystallization and crystallographic technology. The outlook for membrane proteins is more pessimistic, because there are still no general and reliable methods for forming three-dimensional crystals suitable for crystallographic analysis. The prediction of three-dimensional structures from amino acid sequences is thus a problem of exceptional importance for membrane proteins. However, the absence of a large (or even modest) database of membrane proteins of known structures complicates progress toward successful structure prediction.

Looking on the bright side, there is a possibility that the special features of membrane proteins may simplify structure prediction. The lipid bilayer of the membrane, for example, imposes strong physicochemical constraints that may limit the number of structural motifs possible. The aqueous insolubility of membrane proteins seems to demand special cell machinery for managing their transport from ribosomes to the membrane and possibly for regulating their membrane insertion and folding. Studies of the physical chemistry of membranes, bilayers, and peptide–lipid interactions and investigations of the biology of transport, folding, and targeting may reveal an array of constraints that lead to serviceable model structures.

The four chapters in this section are concerned with the features of membrane proteins that may form a starting point for successful structure prediction. Douglas Rees and his colleagues summarize the general characteristics of membrane proteins revealed by cyrstallographic structures of the photosynthetic reaction centers and compare and contrast them with those of globular proteins. Gunnar von Heijne considers "signals" embedded in membrane protein sequences that are important for their transport and assembly, while Jean-Luc Popot and colleagues provide a broad overview of folding and assembly. Finally, I consider the inevitable starting algorithm for structure prediction, the hydropathy plot, in the context of recent advances in our understanding of the structure of fluid bilayer membranes.

1

Membrane Protein Structure and Stability: Implications of the First Crystallographic Analyses

D. C. REES, A. J. CHIRINO, K.-H. KIM, and H. KOMIYA

Beyond their diverse and essential biological functions, membrane proteins provide an important opportunity for examining the structural and energetic basis of protein folding and stability. In contrast to water-soluble proteins, the tertiary structures of integral membrane proteins are adopted in the predominantly nonaqueous and apolar environment of the lipid bilayer. Consequently, hydrophobic interactions, believed to contribute substantially to the stability of water-soluble proteins (Kauzmann, 1959; Tanford, 1980; Dill, 1990a), should play a less significant role in the stabilization of integral membrane proteins (Engelman, 1982). Nevertheless, membrane proteins do adopt stable tertiary structures and maintain their biological functions under the same cellular growth conditions as water-soluble proteins. To rationalize the apparent contradiction that membrane proteins can fold stably despite the diminished significance of hydrophobic interactions, speculation has arisen that "there is something basically different about how membrane proteins fold relative to most other proteins" (Zubay, 1983). This chapter will survey the structural characteristics of membrane proteins of known three-dimensional structures, with emphasis on a comparison of general structural features observed in both water-soluble and membrane proteins. The purpose of this comparison is to assess whether membrane proteins and water-soluble proteins actually do exhibit fundamentally different types of structural organization. As the following discussion indicates, it appears that this is not the case. Despite the difference in polarity of the surrounding environment, membrane proteins and water-soluble proteins seem to represent variations on common structural themes, differing primarily in the polarity of the residues on the protein surface (Rees et al., 1989a,b).

This chapter focuses on structural analyses of globular, integral membrane proteins, defined as "having peptide chains with substantial tertiary structure within the nonpolar region of the lipid bilayer" (Engelman, 1982). Particular emphasis is placed on analyses of the *Rhodobacter sphaeroides* photosynthetic reaction center studied in the authors' laboratory. Integral membrane proteins with toroidal topology, such as water-filled channels or pores, are dealt with only peripherally. The fascinating issues of membrane protein insertion and folding are not addressed

(Popot and Engelman [1990] and Singer [1990] should be consulted for more physically oriented reviews of these topics). Due to space constraints, the chapter is necessarily selective in scope and depends heavily on references (appearing before the
end of 1991) for more detailed discussions.

General Structural Features of Water-Soluble Proteins

Given the large number of available structures of water-soluble proteins (at least,
relative to membrane proteins), an appropriate starting point for this discussion is a
brief review of some general features observed in the structures of water-soluble proteins. Given the diversity of structural motifs adopted by water-soluble proteins, it is
desirable to focus on general structural features that are independent of the local folding patterns of the polypeptide chain. One approach to this problem utilizes the concepts of molecular surface area and volume introduced and implemented for the analysis of macromolecular structures by Richards (1977). Two classes of amino acid
residues in proteins may be naturally identified and characterized by these methods:
surface residues, which are in contact with the surrounding solvent; and **buried
residues,** which are in the protein interior and are shielded from contact with solvent
by the surface residues. Characteristic trends in the general properties of surface and
buried residues of water-soluble proteins have been identified, including (*1*) residue
polarity; (*2*) surface area and interior volume; and (*3*) sequence conservation. These
are briefly discussed in turn.

Residue Polarity

Prior to the first protein structure determination, Kauzmann (1959) proposed that
water-soluble proteins would be organized such that apolar amino acid residues
would be buried in the protein interior, while polar residues would tend to be exposed
on the protein surface. The first structures of myoglobin and hemoglobin strikingly
confirmed this prediction (Perutz et al., 1965). These early observations have since
been repeatedly quantified and extended; recent analyses of the amino acid compositions of buried and surface residues of water-soluble proteins may be found, for
example, in Miller et al. (1987) and Janin et al. (1988). While the tendency for buried and surface residues in water-soluble proteins to be either apolar or polar, respectively, is clearly demonstrated in these studies, it should be emphasized that these are
trends and not an absolute distinction between buried and surface residues. There
are numerous examples of apolar, surface residues and polar, buried residues, so that
the above-stated generalization (as well as the below-stated generalizations) should
not be interpreted as an inviolable distinction between surface and buried residues.

Interior Volume/Surface Area

The packing of buried residues in the interior of water-soluble proteins is relatively
efficient; there are typically few interior cavities in proteins, and the overall atomic
packing density approaches that observed in amino acid crystals (Richards, 1977).
This general impression of the compactness of water-soluble proteins is also rein-

forced by an examination of the molecular surface. Quantification of the accessible surface area of water-soluble proteins indicates that, on average, water-soluble proteins have about twice the surface area of a perfectly spherical protein enclosing the same molecular volume (Richards, 1977). Since proteins are constructed from irregularly shaped amino acids, a surface area to volume ratio comparable with that of spheres implies (at least qualitatively) that both the protein surface is relatively smooth and the overall structure is relatively compact and globular. Again, it should be emphasized that this statement is a generalization; examples of nonspherical water-soluble proteins certainly exist, such as the dumbbell-shaped troponin and fibrous molecules such as tropomyosin.

Sequence Conservation

Buried and surface residues exhibit characteristic patterns of sequence conservation within families of homologous water-soluble proteins. In particular, surface residues are generally less well-conserved relative to buried residues (Perutz et al., 1965; Smith, 1967; Chothia and Lesk, 1986).

Overall, a general picture of water-soluble proteins emerges that emphasizes (*1*) the polar protein surface that minimizes the surface area exposed to water and (*2*) the efficiently packed, relatively nonpolar protein interior. These characteristics are believed to reflect directly a significant role for water and hydrophobic interactions in protein folding and stability. The tendency of protein surfaces to be polar and interiors to be apolar, for example, is precisely the distribution that Kauzmann (1959) predicted on the basis of thermodynamic considerations of hydrophobic interactions. The relatively smooth protein surface and the compact nature of water-soluble proteins should minimize the energetic cost of creating the cavity needed to accommodate a protein molecule in an aqueous solution of high surface tension. Maintaining the compact nature of proteins also imposes significant restrictions on the types of amino acid substitutions that may be tolerated in the protein interior. In contrast, similar constraints are not present on surface residues, providing the general polarity of the protein surface can be maintained.

Membrane Protein Structures

What Is Expected?

An important distinction between membrane proteins and water-soluble proteins involves the different solvent environments in which the three-dimensional structures are adopted and maintained. As discussed in the previous section, many of the general structural features of water-soluble proteins reflect the apparent significance of hydrophobic interactions. While hydrophobic effects provide the thermodynamic driving force for insertion of membrane proteins into the lipid bilayer, once the protein is embedded in the membrane, hydrophobic interactions should play a less significant role in stabilizing the tertiary structure fold of the protein in this essentially nonaqueous environment (Engelman, 1982). In the absence of hydrophobic interactions that may significantly stabilize water-soluble proteins, it could be (and was) anticipated that alternative modes of structural organization might be exhibited by membrane proteins. Models for membrane protein structure were proposed that reflected a less significant contribution of hydrophobic interactions to membrane protein stability (Engelman and Zaccai, 1980; Engelman, 1982; Burres and Dunker, 1982). Among the general structural features of these models were:

1. *Apolar surface:* The membrane protein surface should be relatively apolar to interact favorably with the hydrocarbon chains of the bilayer phospholipids (Lenard and Singer, 1966; Wallach and Zahler, 1966).
2. *Polar interior:* The role of hydrophobic interactions in stabilizing the three-dimensional structures of water-soluble proteins could be replaced in membrane proteins by polar interactions (hydrogen bonds and salt bridges) occurring within the protein interior.
3. *Less compact structure; more irregular surface:* Since the surface tension of hydrocarbon liquids (~ 30 cal/Å^2), is much smaller than water (105 cal/Å^2), it might also be expected that membrane proteins would have a less compact interior and a more irregular surface relative to water-soluble proteins, since the energetic penalty for creating larger molecular cavities in apolar environments would be less severe than for water.

Collectively, the first two features were termed an "inside-out" model for membrane protein structure, since the hydrophobic organization would be "inside-out" with respect to that of water-soluble proteins. It should be noted that the general features of this model were based to a significant extent on considerations of the proton-pumping bacteriorhodopsin (BR) molecule (Engelman and Zaccai, 1980), where internal polar residues are functionally required.

What Is Observed?

Three central developments in the structural analysis of membrane proteins have been (*1*) the low resolution (7 Å) structure of BR, determined by Henderson and Unwin (1975) using electron diffraction methodology; (*2*) the high resolution (2.3 Å) structure of the photosynthetic reaction center (RC) from *Rhodopseudomonas viridis,* determined by Deisenhofer et al. (1984, 1985) and Deisenhofer and Michel (1989), followed by structure determinations of the homologous RC from *Rhodob. sphaeroides* (Allen et al., 1986, 1987a,b,1988; Yeates et al., 1987, 1988; Komiya et al., 1988; Chang et al., 1986, 1991); and (*3*) the high resolution (1.8 Å) structure of the membrane-channel-forming protein porin, determined by Weiss et al. (1990, 1991).

Bacteriorhodopsin.
BR is a light-driven proton pump found in the membrane of *Halobacterium halobium.* A striking feature of the initial BR structure was the arrangement of the membrane-spanning region of the protein into seven rod-like features identified as α-helices. The structure indicated that α-helical conformations could be adopted by integral membrane proteins, as was suggested by the formation of α-helical structures by polypeptides in nonaqueous solvents (Lenard and Singer, 1966; Wallach and Zahler, 1966). Although the initial BR structure was not at atomic resolution, this work catalyzed extensive efforts in understanding membrane protein folding, especially in the development of sequence analysis methods for the

identification of potential membrane-spanning sequences (Kyte and Doolittle, 1982; Eisenberg, 1984; Engelman et al., 1986).

Many of the general features described in the initial BR structure have been confirmed by the recent high resolution structural analysis (Henderson et al., 1990). The seven rod-like features observed in the low resolution electron density maps were indeed established to be α-helices, each containing 20–25 predominantly hydrophobic residues. The helices are arranged in two layers that are packed together like a sandwich, with the layers containing either three or four α-helices. The α-helices are ordered in a simple up-and-down fashion so that helical regions adjacent in the sequence are also nearest neighbors in the structure. Remarkably, this folding pattern had been proposed as the most probable arrangement, based on the low resolution structure analysis and other considerations (Engelman et al., 1980). The retinal cofactor involved in proton pumping is located in the interior of the protein, between the two layers. Stereoviews of the membrane-spanning helices in BR are depicted in Figure 1.1.

Photosynthetic Reaction Center. The first description of a membrane protein structure with atomic-level resolution was achieved for the *Rhodop. viridis* RC (Deisenhofer et al., 1984, 1985). RCs are integral membrane protein–pigment complexes that carry out the initial electron transfer steps in photosynthesis (reviewed in Feher et al., 1989). The *Rhodop. viridis* RC structure unambiguously demonstrated that α-helices could serve as bilayer-spanning motifs in membrane proteins, detailed the folding pattern and molecular interactions of the RC, and provided a structural model for the spatial organization of the cofactors participating in the light-driven electron transfer reactions.

The RCs from *Rhodop. viridis* and *Rhodob. sphaeroides* are composed of three integral membrane bound subunits, designated L, M, and H. A central feature of the RC structure is the presence of 11 hydrophobic α-helices, each containing approximately 20–30 residues. Five membrane-spanning helices are present in both the L and M subunits, while a single helix is present in the H subunit. Helices in the L and M subunits are designated A, B, C, D, and E, in the order of sequence appearance, and are prefixed with either L or M to designate the particular subunit. The single transmembrane helix in the H subunit is termed HA. The folds of the L and M subunits are similar, consistent with significant sequence similarity between the two polypeptide chains. α-Helices in the L or M subunits are arranged in a single layer, with a strong tendency for helices adjacent in the structure to be adjacent in the sequence (helix order A, B, C, E, D). The photosynthetic cofactors are predominantly positioned between the helices. Stereoviews of the α-helical arrangement in the transmembrane region of the RC are presented in Figure 1.2.

Porin. Although the structures of the first water-soluble proteins to be crystallographically determined (globins) consisted principally of α-helical secondary structures, subsequent analyses revealed that a diversity of folding patterns are exhibited by this class of proteins. Similarly, the α-helical nature of the first integral membrane proteins to be established (RCs and BR) does not imply that all integral membrane proteins will be composed of α-helices. The ability of other types of folding motifs to span lipid bilayers has been dramatically illustrated by the recent high resolution

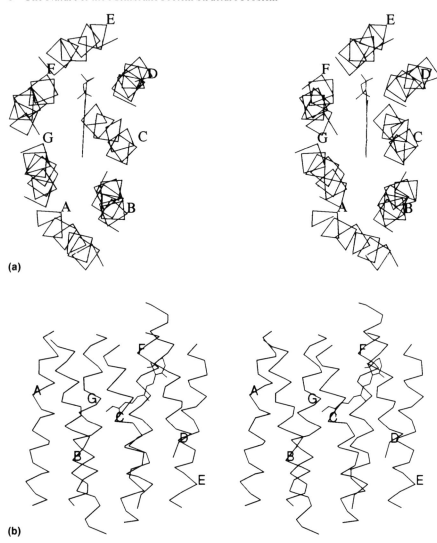

Fig. 1.1. Stereoview of the Cα trace of the polypeptide chain in the membrane-spanning helices of bacteriorhodopsin. The views are approximately along (*a*) and perpendicular to (*b*) the
membrane normal. (This figure was prepared from coordinate set 1BRD of the Brookhaven
Protein Data Base.)

structural analysis of the porin from *Rhodobacter capsulatus* (Weiss et al., 1990,
1991). Porins are channels that permit small hydrophilic molecules to pass through
the outer membrane of gram-negative bacteria, mitochondria, and chloroplasts.
Spectroscopic (Nabedryk et al., 1988) and crystallographic analyses reveal that
porins consist predominantly of β-pleated sheet structure. The *Rhodob. capsulatus*
porin is a trimer of three identical subunits. Each subunit contains a 16 strand antiparallel β-sheet folded into a barrel that creates a channel (the β-barrel interior) of
approximate dimensions 6 × 10 Å. Individual β-strands are between 6 and 17 residues in length and are organized into the barrel in a simple up-and-down fashion

such that strand regions are adjacent in both the sequence and the structure. Amino acids lining the channel interior are polar, while the residues surrounding the membrane-spanning circumference of the trimer are nonpolar. As the presently published descriptions of the porin structure have focused primarily on the protein fold, further details of the channel and membrane-spanning regions of this β-sheet protein are eagerly awaited (for further details, see Weiss et al., 1991; Weiss and Schulz, 1992; Cowan et al., 1992).

Definition of the Bilayer-Spanning Region of Membrane Proteins

Any detailed discussion of the structural features characterizing membrane-spanning proteins requires a definition of the interaction region between protein and membrane. From the perspective of this chapter, such assignments are essential for the identification of surface and buried residues in the membrane-spanning region. Unfortunately, precise identification of the bilayer-spanning zone of a membrane

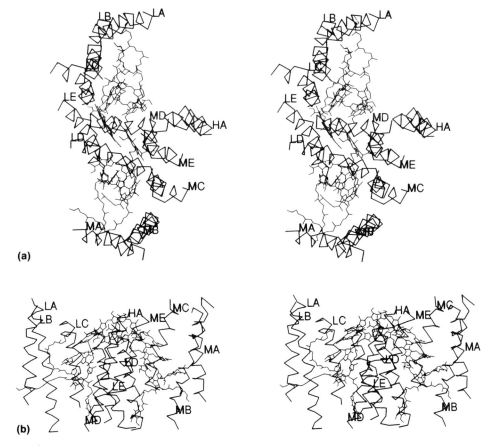

Fig. 1.2. Stereoview of the Cα trace of the polypeptide chain in the membrane-spanning helices of the *Rhodob. sphaeroides* RC. The views are approximately along (a) and perpendicular to (b) the membrane normal. (This figure was prepared from coordinate set 4RCR of the Brookhaven Protein Data Bank.)

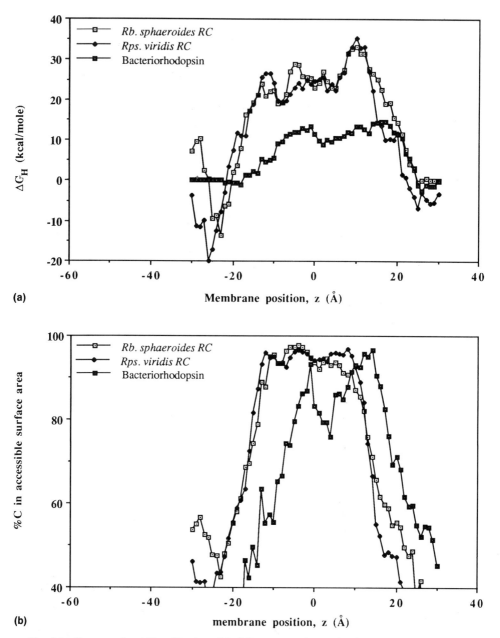

Fig. 1.3. Computational identification of the bilayer-spanning region for membrane proteins. The molecular position is measured along the z-axis, which is perpendicular to the assumed plane of the membrane, with the origin approximately at the bilayer center. Symbols designating the curves for the *Rhodob. sphaeroides* RC (Protein Data Bank set 4RCR), *Rhodop. viridis* RC (set 1PRC), and bacteriorhodopsin (1BRD) are indicated. Possible contributions of internal cavities to the calculated surface area have not been eliminated. *a*: The energy, ΔG_H, estimated (Eisenberg and McLachlan, 1986) for the transfer of 5 Å thick section of a membrane protein from the bilayer to water, calculated as a function of the position in the membrane, z. *b*: The percentage of the accessible surface area contributed by carbon atoms in a 1 Å thick section of a membrane protein, calculated as a function of the position in the membrane, z.

10

protein is difficult to accomplish experimentally. Many of the phospholipids in the BR samples (Henderson et al., 1990) and essentially all the detergents used to sol-ubilize the RC samples (Deisenhofer and Michel, 1989; Yeates et al., 1988) are dis-ordered and therefore not observed in high resolution diffraction studies. The general location of the disordered detergent surrounding the *Rhodop. viridis* RC was deter-mined by low resolution (15 Å) neutron diffraction studies (Roth et al., 1989). In these studies, the detergent was observed to surround the 11 hydrophobic α-helices of the RC, but a more precise mapping of the boundary of the detergent binding site was not possible.

In the absence of detailed experimental evidence, two related computational meth-ods have been used to characterize the interaction region between bilayer and mem-brane protein. Both methods attempt to identify the position and extent of the most hydrophobic surface surrounding the membrane protein and consequently make the (hopefully) reasonable assumption that the membrane-spanning region coincides with the most hydrophobic surface region.

In the first approach (Yeates et al., 1987; Rees et al., 1989a), the free energy of transfer from membrane to water, ΔG_H, for surface atoms contained within a 5 Å thick section of a protein is estimated by an energetic expression developed by Eisen-berg and McLachlan (1986). The region exhibiting the most unfavorable transfer energy from the membrane to water can be identified from the dependence of ΔG_H on the position of the section as it is moved through the protein. Results of this cal-culation for the RC and BR structures are presented in Figure 1.3a. These calcu-lations reveal a hydrophobic region for the RCs of approximately 35–40 Å width, which should represent the interaction region of the membrane protein with the bilayer. The narrower hydrophobic region observed for BR may reflect the absence of residues in the interhelical loops from the present model (Henderson et al., 1990). Integration of the areas under these curves (correcting for the 5 Å slab width and the number of helices in the structure) yields a value for ΔG_H of about 15–20 kcal/mol/ helix. This is consistent with an estimated 30 kcal/mol for the transfer of a single transmembrane α-helix from the bilayer to water (Engelman et al., 1986).

A second method for assigning the bilayer-spanning region of membrane proteins identifies nonpolar protein surfaces from the fraction of the accessible surface area contributed by carbon atoms (Deisenhofer and Michel, 1989). Surface regions con-taining a high proportion of carbon atoms are taken to represent nonpolar surfaces, since they necessarily have a low proportion of polar oxygen and nitrogen atoms. The surface area contribution of carbon atoms is calculated for thin sections (1–3 Å) through the membrane protein as a function of the section position. Results of this calculation are presented in Figure 1.3b for the RC and BR structures. Over 90% of the surface area in the membrane-spanning region of these proteins is contributed by carbon atoms compared with about 60% of the surface area for the water-soluble regions. The nonpolar surface covers a slab ~ 35 Å wide around the RC and BR structures, which is similar to the width of the membrane-spanning region estimated by the ΔG_H calculations.

General Structural Features of Membrane Proteins

Once the bilayer-spanning region of a membrane protein has been identified, amino acid residues may be assigned to either surface or buried categories. Following the analyses described for water-soluble proteins, characteristic properties of surface and buried residues of membrane proteins may be assessed in terms of residue polarity, interior volume/surface area, and sequence conservation. The following discussion draws heavily on published analyses of the *Rhodob. sphaeroides* RC structure (Rees et al., 1989a,b).

Residue Polarity. Surface residues in the membrane-spanning region of the *Rhodob. sphaeroides* RC tend to be more apolar than buried residues (Rees et al., 1989b). There is not, however, a simple reversal of polarity for buried and surface residues of water-soluble and membrane proteins. Significantly, the average hydrophobicity of buried residues in both water-soluble and membrane proteins are nearly identical. Consequently, there is no evidence for significant numbers of polar residues or interactions in the interior of the RC. Surface residues of water-soluble proteins are more polar than the buried residues, while surface residues in the RC tend to be more apolar (Fig. 1.4). While this analysis has not yet been performed for the *Rhodop. viridis* RC or BR structures, the general conclusions were consistent with sequence analyses of a more extensive database of transmembrane helical sequences from different membrane protein families (Rees et al., 1989b).

Interior Volume/Surface Area. The packing volume of buried residues in the *Rhodob. sphaeroides* RC is very similar to that observed in water-soluble proteins (Yeates et al., 1987). Furthermore, there is no significant difference in the accessible surface area of the *Rhodob. sphaeroides* RC and oligomeric, water-soluble proteins of comparable size (Rees et al., 1989a).

Sequence Conservation. Comparison of sequence alignments for the L and M subunits of the RCs from four different bacteria revealed that 35% of the residues at a given position in the membrane-spanning region were identical in all four sequences (Komiya et al., 1988; Rees et al., 1989b). There were significant differ-

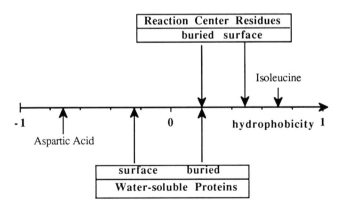

Fig. 1.4. Average hydrophobicities for the surface and buried residues observed in water-soluble, globular proteins (Miller et al., 1987) and the *Rhodob. sphaeroides* RC (Rees, et al., 1989a). Hydrophobicities were calculated using the Eisenberg consensus scale (Eisenberg et al., 1982). For reference, the hydrophobicities of isoleucine and aspartic acid are indicated.

ences in the conservation of buried and surface residues, however, since 46% of the buried residues were identical in all four sequences, compared with only 10% of the surface residues. More frequent substitution of surface residues, relative to buried residues, was also indicated by sequence analysis of residue variability and polarity in transmembrane-spanning regions of membrane protein families of unknown structure (Rees et al., 1989b). The increased variability of surface residues in the membrane-spanning region indicates that there are few specific interactions between proteins and lipid that place severe restrictions on residue substitution.

With the exception of surface residue polarity, membrane proteins and water-soluble proteins share strong similarities in such general features as hydrophobicity of buried residues, surface area, interior packing efficiency, and the relative sequence conservation of buried and surface residues. The implications of these observations for protein folding and stability, and the role of hydrophobic interactions in these processes, will be discussed in the concluding section of this chapter.

Helix–Helix Packing in Water-Soluble and Membrane Proteins

Although the emphasis in this chapter has been on general structural characteristics of proteins that are independent of the precise folding details, given the significance of helix–helix packing for the structures of both water-soluble and membrane proteins, this specific type of interaction will be examined in more detail. Helix-to-helix packing in water-soluble, globular proteins has been extensively analyzed by Chothia et al. (1981). These authors developed a model for helix packing picturesquely termed "ridges in grooves." Ridges along a helix are formed by rows of residue side chains separated in the sequence by either 3 ($i,i + 3$) or 4 ($i,i + 4$) residues or, more rarely, by 1 ($i,i + 1$) residue. Ridges on one helix can pack into the grooves created by ridges on a second helix. In the water-soluble, globular proteins surveyed, 50% of the helix–helix contacts involved the $i,i + 4$ ridges on both helices (class 4–4), resulting in an interaxial angle of about $-50°$ between the two helices. The next most abundant type of helix packing (16% of contacts) involved the $i,i + 3$ ridge on one helix with the $i,i + 4$ ridge on the second (class 3–4). The interaxial angle between the helices in the 3–4 class, $+23°$, reflects a more nearly parallel arrangement of the two helices. This type of interaction, which is similar to the "knobs in holes" packing described by Crick (1953), characterizes the helix-to-helix packing found in coiled-coiled structures, such as leucine zippers (O'Shea et al., 1991).

For the *Rhodob. sphaeroides* RC, the dominant helix–helix interactions are of the 3–4 class (Table 1.1). Of the 15 helix-to-helix contacts in the RC, 8 (53%) are of the 3–4 class, while an additional 3 (20%) involve a crossover interaction between these two ridge types (designated class 3×4). These latter contacts primarily involve the α-helices at the core of the RC that interact extensively with the photosynthetic cofactors. The remaining four helix contacts involve too few residues to determine the interaction type accurately. The predominance of 3–4 type helix-to-helix contacts in the RC structure almost certainly reflects the necessity of forming a compactly folded structure from the helical interactions. Due to the more nearly parallel alignment of the helix axes, 3–4 contacts can generate a more extensive interface between helices than is possible with the 4–4 contacts crossing at $-50°$. Consistent with this expla-

Table 1.1. Helix–Helix Contacts in the Membrane-Spanning
Region of the *Rhodob. sphaeroides* RC

Helix Pairs	Residues in Contact	Interhelical Angle (Degrees)	Contact Type
LA/LB	10–10	24	3–4
LB/LC	10–8	22	3–4
LC/LE	9–8	38	3–4
LE/LD	9–9	21	3–4
MA/MB	12–14	25	3–4
MB/MC	10–8	2	3–4
MC/ME	7–7	7	3–4
MD/ME	11–13	18	3–4
LD/ME	5–7	54	3×4
LE/MD	6–6	53	3×4
LD/MD	7–5	67	3×4
LC/MD	3–1	18	Uncertain
LD/MC	1–3	51	Uncertain
MD/HA	2–4	17	Uncertain
ME/HA	9–7	4	Uncertain

Residues in contact are the numbers of residues in each member of the helical pair
that are assigned to the contact region by visual inspection of the structure on a graphics
terminal. The interhelical angle between the axes of two interacting helices is calculated as described by Allen et al. (1987b). The contact types are classified according to
Chothia et al. (1981).

nation, many water-soluble proteins containing compactly folded, predominantly α-helical domains, such as the four helical bundles (Weber and Salemme, 1988) and the helical domains of an insect toxin (Li et al., 1991) and colicin A (Parker et al., 1989), are based almost exclusively on 3–4 contacts, although some 4–4 contacts between helices are observed in interferon-γ (Ealick et al., 1991) and annexin (Huber et al., 1990).

The distribution of amino acid residues found in the *Rhodob. sphaeroides* RC transmembrane helices and at the helix–helix interfaces can be compared (Fig. 1.5) to the distributions observed for water-soluble proteins (Chothia et al., 1981). In terms of overall amino acid distribution in the helical regions, the RC, not surprisingly, has more hydrophobic and less polar/charged residues than water-soluble proteins. Residues forming the helix–helix contacts in the RC tend to follow the overall residue distribution for the transmembrane region. In water-soluble proteins, hydrophobic residues contribute proportionally more residues to the contact region than do polar/charged residues. While the amino acid composition of the contact residues is roughly comparable between RC and water-soluble proteins, there are some noticeable differences. Among amino acids comprising over 5% of the contacts, the RC exhibits a greater proportional abundance of Phe, Trp, and Ala, and a deficiency of Val, with respect to water-soluble proteins.

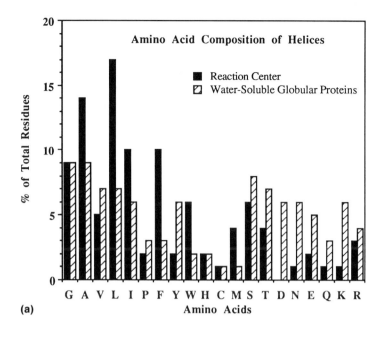

(a)

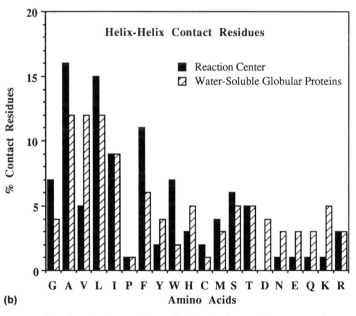

(b)

Fig. 1.5. *a*: Overall amino acid composition of helices in the membrane-spanning region of the *Rhodob. sphaeroides* RC and water-soluble, globular proteins (Chothia et al., 1981). *b*: Amino acid composition of residues forming the contacts between helices in the membrane-spanning region of the *Rhodob. sphaeroides* RC and water-soluble, globular proteins.

Stability of Water-Soluble and Membrane Proteins

Questions of protein stability are fundamentally thermodynamic in nature. Calorimetric techniques provide a critical experimental approach for obtaining accurate thermodynamic measurements of protein stability. The following general observations have emerged from calorimetric studies of the stability of small, water-soluble, globular proteins (reviewed by Privalov, 1979, 1990; and Privalov and Gill, 1988).

Two-State Behavior

Thermodynamically, the unfolding of proteins can be characterized in terms of a transition between two states, the native form (N) and an unfolded, denatured form (D). While intermediates between the N and D states can exist, and may be significant for folding kinetics and pathways, their populations are typically too low to contribute to the overall unfolding thermodynamics of small, globular, water-soluble proteins.

Positive ΔC_p of Unfolding

The unfolding of water-soluble proteins is associated with a large, positive heat capacity change (ΔC_p) of unfolding. To a reasonable approximation, ΔC_p is temperature independent. Thermodynamic studies of hydrophobic interactions demonstrate that the exposure of apolar groups to water is characterized by a large, positive ΔC_p. Accordingly, observation of a large, positive ΔC_p during protein denaturation is widely interpreted as reflecting the involvement of hydrophobic interactions in protein stability. Consistent with this interpretation, the magnitude of ΔC_p has been shown to be proportional to the number of hydrophobic residues in a protein sequence.

Water-Soluble Proteins Are Stable by About 10–15 kcal/mol

Energetically, the stabilizing and destabilizing interactions involved in protein folding are rather closely balanced, with a net difference of about 10–15 kcal/mol favoring protein folding under optimal conditions. Similar stabilizing energies have been observed for a variety of small, water-soluble, globular proteins.

   For a two-state process with constant ΔC_p, the free energy of unfolding (ΔG_{ND}) may be expressed (Privalov and Gill, 1988):

$$\Delta G_{ND} = \Delta H_m \left[\frac{T_m - T}{T_m} \right] - \Delta C_p \left\{ T_m - T \left[1 - \ln \left(\frac{T}{T_m} \right) \right] \right\} \quad (1)$$

where T_m is the transition temperature for unfolding during heat denaturation (the temperature at which $\Delta G_{ND} = 0$); and ΔH_m is the enthalpy change at T_m. The entropy change at T_m is given by $\Delta S_m = \Delta H_m / T_m$. Provided ΔC_p is temperature independent, ΔG_{ND} is completely specified by the three parameters T_m, ΔH_m, and ΔC_p. The dependence of ΔG_{ND} on T for a given set of solution conditions (pH, μ, and so forth) defines the stability curve for a protein (Becktel and Schellman, 1987).

   In the physiological temperature range, to a good approximation, the logarithm term in Eq. 1 may be expanded to second order in $[(T - T_m)/T_m]$, yielding an expression for ΔG_{ND} with a quadratic dependence on T (Day et al., 1992):

$$\Delta G_{ND} \cong \left[\Delta H_m - \frac{(\Delta C_p)T_m}{2} \right] + T \left[\Delta C_p - \frac{\Delta H_m}{T_m} \right] - T^2 \left[\frac{\Delta C_p}{2T_m} \right] \quad (2)$$

Parenthetically, this quadratic form implies (for $\Delta C_p > 0$) that there are, in general, two temperatures for which $\Delta G_{ND} = 0$: one at $T = T_m$ (heat denaturation), characterized by $\Delta H_m, \Delta S_m > 0$, and a lower temperature $T = T_m'$ (cold denaturation), characterized by $\Delta H_m, \Delta S_m < 0$. The process of cold denaturation has been experimentally observed (reviewed by Privalov, 1990) and has the intriguing property that the system (protein plus solvent) becomes more ordered ($\Delta S_m < 0$) upon denaturation.

From Eq. 2, the temperature of greatest protein stability, T^*, occurs when (Zipp and Kauzmann, 1973)

$$T^* \cong T_m - \left[\frac{\Delta H_m}{\Delta C_p} \right] \quad (3)$$

with the free energy of maximal stability given by

$$\Delta G_{ND}(T^*) \cong \left[\frac{\Delta H_m^2}{2T_m \Delta C_p} \right] = \left[\frac{\Delta H_m \Delta S_m}{2\Delta C_p} \right] \quad (4)$$

For the hypothetical "typical" water-soluble protein, $\Delta H_m = 100$ kcal/mol, $T_m = 340$K and $\Delta C_p = 2$ kcal/mol/K, giving $T^* = 290°$ K and $\Delta G_{ND}(T^*) = 7.4$ kcal/mol.

From Eq. 4, the maximal stability of a protein increases as ΔH_m increases, which is intuitively reasonable since the enthalpy term should be dominated by energetic interactions that stabilize the protein structure. Somewhat surprisingly, perhaps, is the decrease in $\Delta G_{ND}(T^*)$ as either T_m or ΔC_p increases, for fixed values of the other parameters. Since ΔC_p is generally believed to reflect hydrophobic effects associated with the exposure of apolar residues to water upon denaturation, the inverse dependence of ΔG_{ND} on ΔC_p supports Privalov and Gill's interpretation (1988) that hydrophobic effects actually destabilize the native structure, ultimately leading to cold denaturation (Privalov and Gill, 1988; Murphy et al., 1990). Needless to say, this particular conclusion of Privalov and Gill has been controversial (see, for example, Baldwin, 1986; Dill, 1990a,b), since it contradicts the fundamental tenet that hydrophobic interactions are an integral contributor to protein stability. Given this controversy, and the significantly nonaqueous folding environment of lipid bilayer, the thermodynamics of membrane protein stability could provide an important system for assessing the contributions of hydrophobic interactions to protein stability.

If the magnitude of ΔC_p exclusively reflects the exposure of apolar groups to water during the unfolding process, then one would expect that the ΔC_p observed for membrane protein denaturation should be smaller than that observed for water-soluble proteins. Furthermore, since a decrease in ΔC_p will tend to increase $\Delta G_{ND}(T^*)$ (Eq. 4), then it is possible that the maximal stability of membrane proteins might generally be higher than that observed for water-soluble proteins. Unfortunately, calorimetric analyses of membrane protein folding are rather scarce, no doubt reflecting serious difficulties in analyzing the thermal behavior of irreversible systems containing multiple components (protein and membrane) that can undergo structural transitions. The most detailed calorimetric studies of membrane protein stability have been performed for BR (Jackson and Sturtevant, 1978; Brouillette et al., 1987, 1989; Kahn et al., 1992). While a complete determination of the three parameters required to specify ΔG_{ND} has not yet been reported, intriguing glimpses are available. Around pH 7, BR denatures at $T_m \sim 100°$ C, with $\Delta H_m \sim 100$ kcal/mol. An accurate value of ΔC_p has not been directly determined from the calorimetric studies, but from the variation in ΔH_m with T_m (measured as a function of pH), ΔC_p for BR denaturation has been estimated as 0.046 cal/K/g ~ 1.2 kcal/K/mol (Brouillette et al., 1987). As the authors note, on a per gram basis, the value of ΔC_p for BR is about one-third that observed for one of the most hydrophobic water-soluble proteins that has been studied, myoglobin. This trend is consistent with the proposal that ΔC_p reflects the exposure of apolar groups to water during unfolding. Using values for T_m, ΔH_m, and ΔC_p of 373° K, 100 kcal/mol, and 1.2 kcal/K/mol, respectively, the maximal stability of BR estimated from Eq. 4 is $\Delta G_{ND}(T^*) \sim 11$ kcal/mol and is obtained at the temperature $T^* \sim 290°$ K. Although extremely preliminary, this analysis for BR hints that membrane proteins are likely to be at least as stable as water-soluble proteins.

In addition to the relevance for biological systems, the dependence of protein stability on solvent polarity may provide a useful approach for modifying the thermostability of proteins in nonbiological systems. Volkin et al. (1991) have demonstrated that the stability of water-soluble proteins can be markedly enhanced in anhydrous organic solvents compared with aqueous solutions. Ribonuclease, for example, denatures at 61° C in aqueous solution, while a T_m of 124° C is observed for suspensions of ribonuclease in nonane. The mechanism of thermostability in these anhydrous organic solvents was suggested to originate from the"conformational rigidity" of proteins in the dehydrated state and the resistance of proteins to many of the modification reactions (e.g., deamidation) that cause irreversible thermoinactivation in aqueous solutions (Volkin et al., 1991). Additionally, the nonpolar environment of proteins in these solutions should decrease ΔC_p for unfolding, which by Eq. 4 will tend to stabilize the protein. As with membrane proteins, more detailed thermodynamic analyses of protein stability in these nonaqueous and nonbiological systems could provide critical insights into the role of the solvent in protein stability.

Conclusions

Similarities Between Water-Soluble and Membrane Proteins: The Crystal Morphology Analogy

At the present stage of analysis, water-soluble and membrane proteins seem quite similar in terms of various structural (surface area, interior packing, interior hydrophobicity, and sequence conservation of buried residues) and energetic (protein stability) criteria. The most striking and characteristic difference between these two classes of proteins is the chemical nature of the exposed surface groups. To minimize surface energies, water-soluble proteins fold to generate a polar surface, while membrane proteins require an apolar surface. This behavior is similar to the effect of solvent conditions on the morphology of small molecule crystals. Gibbs (1928) demonstrated that the equilibrium morphology of a crystal will have the minimum sur-face free energy. Since different crystal faces have different exposed chemical groups, changing solvent conditions will alter the crystal morphology so as to maintain the state with lowest surface energy. For example, polar crystal faces with exposed car-boxyl groups dominate the morphology of succinic acid crystals grown from water, whereas more apolar crystal faces with exposed methylene carbons are prominent in crystals grown from apolar solvents or by sublimation (Berkovitch-Yellin, 1985). The interior packing of succinic acid molecules remains, however, unchanged under these different solvent conditions. Thus crystal morphology may be viewed as being analogous to the"morphologies" of water-soluble and membrane proteins; i.e., while the surface composition of proteins is sensitive to solvent (water or bilayer) condi-tions, the same types of interior interactions are utilized by both protein classes (Rees et al., 1989b).

Role of Hydrophobic Interactions in Protein Stability

Adopting an extreme and overly simplistic viewpoint, three alternate conclusions fol-low from the observations that water-soluble and membrane proteins exhibit strong similarities in structure and stability, despite the apparently reduced role played by hydrophobic interactions in membrane protein stability:

1. Hydrophobic interactions are actually critical for the stability of both water-soluble and membrane proteins.
2. Hydrophobic interactions are critical for the stability of water-soluble pro-teins, but not for the stability of membrane proteins.
3. Hydrophobic interactions are not essential for the stability of either water-soluble or membrane proteins.

Brief discussions of these three possibilities follow.

Possibility 1.   Hydrophobic interactions are critical for the stability of both water-soluble and membrane proteins. While integral membrane proteins adopt their ter-tiary structure within the apolar region lipid bilayer, membrane proteins are not completely surrounded by the membrane. Membrane proteins such as RC, BR, and porin have significant regions of the protein surface that protrude from the bilayer and interact with water. Consequently, it is possible that hydrophobic interactions involving these regions of the protein might play a major role in protein stability. While this possibility cannot be dismissed, it seems unlikely. The magnitude of the hydrophobic effect is often considered to be proportional to the apolar surface area buried from exposure to water (Chothia, 1974). Inside the membrane, however, there should be little energetic penalty for the exposure of buried, apolar residues to the bilayer. This statement assumes that unfolding of a membrane protein does not involve the creation of extensive contacts between buried residues and water. Since a significant fraction of the surface of an integral membrane protein (such as RC or BR) is in contact with the membrane, it seems intuitively unlikely that the positions of buried and surface residues in the bilayer could be restricted by hydrophobic inter-actions occurring in the aqueous exposed regions of the protein. This line of reasoning therefore suggests that hydrophobic interactions should not contribute significantly to the stability of integral membrane proteins (Engelman, 1982).

Possibility 2. Nonhydrophobic interactions are critical for membrane protein stability. It is possible that hydrophobic interactions are critical for the stability of water-soluble proteins, but not for membrane proteins, if there are nonhydrophobic interactions that can compensate for the loss of this stabilizing interaction in membrane proteins. Possible candidates would be (*1*) interior polar interactions, (*2*) entropic effects, and (*3*) general "solvophobic interactions":

1. Interior polar interactions: As indicated by the similar hydrophobicities of interior residues in both membrane proteins and water-soluble proteins (based on analyses of the RC structure and membrane protein sequences), there does not appear to be a general tendency for increased numbers of polar interactions inside membrane proteins.

2. Entropic stabilization: Special entropic considerations arise in the stability of membrane proteins, since to a first approximation membrane proteins exist in a two-dimensional system. Consequently, the number of degrees of freedom that are available to the denatured form of a membrane protein should be significantly reduced relative to a three-dimensionally denatured form of a water-soluble protein (see Dill, 1990a, for a relevant discussion). In this view, membrane proteins would be stabilized not so much by special interactions in the native form (corresponding to the role of hydrophobic interactions in water-soluble protein stability), but rather by a destabilization of the denatured form. The observation that proteolytic fragments of BR can reassemble to form the native protein (Popot et al., 1987; Kahn et al., 1992) suggests, however, that these entropic considerations are not dominant, since otherwise the various fragments would diffuse independently through the bilayer and not associate to form the native structure.

3. Solvophobic interactions: Similarities in surface areas between the RC and water-soluble proteins of similar size suggest that the surface energies of these proteins must be similar, despite the differences in surface tensions between hydrocarbon liquids ($\sim$30 cal/Å^2) and water ($\sim$100 cal/Å^2). The surface tension of a liquid provides only one component to the surface energy associated with the interaction between a surface and a solution, however (Israelachvili, 1985). The surface energy associated with the interface between a liquid and a preformed surface is given by the difference between the liquid-liquid interaction energy (i.e., the solvent surface tension) and the compensating adhesion energy between the surface and liquid. While the solvent surface tension is much higher for water than for hydrocarbons, it is also likely that the protein–water adhesion energies are higher than membrane protein–hydrocarbon adhesion energies. Protein–water interactions will typically include relatively strong hydrogen bond interactions between polar groups and water, while the protein–bilayer interaction will be dominated by weaker van der Waals interactions. As a consequence of these compensating effects, the net result could be comparable surface energies for the interaction of the relevant solvents with either water-soluble or membrane proteins, so that the

work associated with placing a protein in a solvent could be, to first order, independent of the solvent. By analogy to the term *hydrophobic,* this more general type of effect could be termed *solvophobic.* Like hydrophobic effects, solvophobic effects will also tend to minimize the exposed surface area and create compactly folded structures.

Possibility 3. Hydrophobic interactions are not essential for the stability of either water-soluble or membrane proteins. Compactly folded structures could, in principle, arise primarily from van der Waals interactions between interior atoms, without the need for hydrophobic interactions. The packing density of water-soluble proteins is efficient, which should maximize the contributions of van der Waals interaction energies to protein stability. Since the packing density of the RC is comparable to water-soluble proteins, the contribution of van der Waals interactions to protein stability should also be comparable. If the van der Waals interactions between buried atoms are sufficiently strong, then the folded state of a protein could be stabilized, irrespective of the solvent environment. The sufficiency of van der Waals interactions to drive molecular assembly has been recently demonstrated in model systems. Bryant et al. (1990) have synthesized molecules that dimerize in nonaqueous solvents in the absence of hydrophobic, hydrogen bonding and ion-pair interactions, demonstrating the sufficiency of van der Waals interactions to stabilize molecular assemblies.

Discussion

The relative importance of these various possibilities cannot be quantitatively assessed at present. In our opinion, the most significant effects are likely to be solvophobic interactions and packing (van der Waals) interactions.

An important lesson from the study of membrane proteins is that water is not absolutely indispensable for the ability of proteins to adopt stable three-dimensional structures; nonaqueous solvents (whether in the membrane bilayer or in nonbiological systems) can also facilitate protein folding. By definition, then, hydrophobic interactions are not essential for protein folding, since proteins can fold in nonaqueous solvents. The formation of compact structures may be driven in a solvent-independent fashion by van der Waals interactions. While weak, van der Waals interactions have the important properties that they occur between all atom types and are nondirectional. The properties of van der Waals interactions are thus quite different from hydrogen bonding and other types of polar interactions, which are stronger, occur only between specific atom types, and are highly directional. One might speculate that the apolar nature of protein interiors arises from the nondirectional nature of van der Waals interactions; if large numbers of polar side chain atoms were to be buried in the protein interior, severe restrictions might be placed on the course of the polypeptide chain so that all polar interactions could be fulfilled. A great advantage of apolar atoms is that they can be packed together, without additional orientational restrictions imposed on their location to permit van der Waals interactions with neighboring atoms. Perhaps it is too difficult to fold a protein containing large numbers of polar residues, such that the hydrogen-bonding requirements of both main chain and side chain atoms are simultaneously satisfied. Hence, the relative apolarity of protein interiors may be less a consequence of hydrophobic interactions than a reflection of the difficulty in creating alternative types of interiors based on polar interactions between amino acid side chains.

Future Outlook

Recent advances in the structure and molecular biology of membrane proteins have heralded a new era in understanding the folding and properties of membrane proteins. Based on these developments, several areas for future progress may be identified:

1. The structures of more membrane proteins must be determined, to address such fundamental structural questions as What types of folding motifs are observed for membrane proteins? Are mixed α-helical and β-sheet structures observed in integral membrane proteins, as proposed for Na channels (Guy and Seetharamulu, 1986)? Do the folding patterns of membrane proteins tend to be simpler than those seen with water-soluble proteins (Weiss et al., 1991)? Structures of membrane proteins such as receptors, redox protein complexes, ion pumps, ATPases, and channels are central to understanding the functional details of these biologically critical molecules.

2. Experimental studies of membrane protein stability must be actively pursued, as they will have important consequences for understanding the structural basis of protein stability. Of special interest is the value of the heat capacity change, ΔC_p, associated with membrane protein unfolding. As ΔC_p appears to reflect the exposure of apolar groups to water, it would be expected that ΔC_p will be smaller for membrane protein unfolding than for the unfolding of water-soluble proteins, although this expectation needs experimental attention. A useful approach for experimentally characterizing the roles of ΔC_p and hydrophobic interactions in protein stability might be to study protein unfolding calorimetrically in D_2O. Hydrophobic interactions should be stronger in D_2O than in H_2O (Kresheck et al., 1965) so that, if ΔC_p does arise from exposure of apolar groups to water, then ΔC_p for unfolding in D_2O should be larger than for unfolding in H_2O.

3. If water-soluble proteins can really be considered as modified membrane proteins containing built-in detergent (Rees et al., 1989a), then it should be possible to design water-soluble forms of membrane proteins by substitution of apolar surface residues with polar residues. Successful accomplishment of this conversion (as well as the reverse process) would demonstrate that membrane proteins and water-soluble proteins are based on the same types of design principles.

4. Certain proteins can adopt both water-soluble and membrane-bound forms. The structures of two proteins in this category, colicin A and an insect toxin, have been crystallographically determined in the water-soluble forms (Parker et al., 1989; Li et al., 1991). These proteins share a common general structural theme of a predominantly α-helical domain consisting of one or two central α-helices surrounded by an outer layer of additional α-helices. It is believed that these central helices somehow penetrate the bilayer in the membrane-associated form. Structural and mechanistic studies of the conversion of these

proteins from the water-soluble to the membrane-bound forms should provide a fascinating example of the adaptability of protein structures to different environments.

Acknowledgments

Our collaboration with G. Feher and J. P. Allen on the *Rhodob. sphaeroides* RC crystallographic analyses is gratefully acknowledged. This work was supported by USPHS grant GM45162.

References

Allen, J. P., Feher, G., Yeates, T. O., Komiya, H., and Rees, D. C. (1987a) Structure of the reaction center from *Rhodopseudomonas sphaeroides* R-26: the protein subunits. *Proc. Natl. Acad. Sci. USA* 84: 6162–6166.

Allen, J. P., Feher, G., Yeates, T. O., Komiya, H., and Rees, D. C. (1987b) Structure of the reaction center from *Rhodopseudomonas sphaeroides* R-26: the cofactors. *Proc. Natl. Acad. Sci. USA* 84: 5730–5734.

Allen, J. P., Feher, G., Yeates, T. O., Komiya, H., and Rees, D. C. (1988) Structure of the reaction center from *Rhodopseudomonas sphaeroides* R-26: protein-cofactor (quinones and Fe^{2+}) interactions. *Proc. Natl. Acad. Sci. USA* 85: 8487–8491.

Allen, J. P., Feher, G., Yeates, T. O., Rees, D. C., Deisenhofer, J., Michel, H., and Huber, R. (1986) Structural homology of reaction centers from *Rhodopseudomonas sphaeroides* and *Rhodopseudomonas viridis* as determined by x-ray diffraction. *Proc. Natl. Acad. Sci. USA* 83: 8589–8593.

Baldwin, R. L. (1986) "Temperature dependence of the hydrophobic interaction in protein folding. *Proc. Natl. Acad. Sci. USA* 83: 8069–8072.

Becktel, W. J., and Schellman, J. A. (1987) Protein stability curves. *Biopolymers* 26: 1859–1877.

Berkovitch-Yellin, Z. (1985) Toward an *ab initio* derivation of crystal morphology. *J. Am. Chem. Soc.* 107: 8239–8253.

Brouillette, C. G., McMichens, R. B., Stern, L. J., and Khorana, H. G. (1989) Structure and thermal stability of monomeric bacteriorhodpsin in mixed phospholipid/detergent micelles. *Proteins Struct. Funct. Gen.* 5: 38–46.

Brouillette, C. G., Muccio, D. D., and Finney, T. K. (1987) pH dependence of bacteriorhodpsin thermal unfolding. *Biochemistry* 26: 7431–7438.

Bryant, J. A., Knobler, C. B., and Cram, D. J. (1990) Organic molecules dimerize with high structural recognition when each possesses a large lipophilic surface containing two preorganized and complementary host and guest regions. *J. Am. Chem. Soc.* 112: 1254–1255.

Burres, N., and Dunker, A. K. (1980) Membrane transport through α-helical bundles. IV. Preliminary model building investigation of helix-helix interactions. *J. Theor. Biol.* 87: 723–736.

Chang, C.-H., El-Kabbani, O., Tiede, D., Norris, J., and Schiffer, M. (1991) Structure of the membrane-bound protein photosynthetic reaction center from *Rhodobacter sphaeroides*. *Biochemistry* 30: 5352–5360.

Chang, C.-H., Tiede, D., Tang, J., Smith, U., Norris, J. R., and Schiffer, M. (1986) Structure of *Rhodopseudomonas sphaeroides* R-26 reaction center. *FEBS Lett.* 205: 82–86.

Chothia, C. (1974) Hydrophobic bonding and accessible surface area in proteins. *Nature* 248: 338–339.

Chothia, C., and Lesk, A. M. (1986) The relation between the divergence of sequence and structure in proteins. *EMBO J.* 5: 823–826.

Chothia, C., Levitt, M., and Richardson, D. (1981) Helix to helix packing in proteins. *J. Mol. Biol.* 145: 215–250.

Cowan, S. W., Schirmer, T., Rummel, G., Steiert, M., Ghosh, R., Pauptit, R. A., Jansonius, J. N., and Rosenbusch, J. P. (1992) Crystal structures explain functional properties of two *E. coli* porins. *Nature* 358: 727–733.

Crick, F.H.C. (1953) The packing of α-helices: simple coiled-coils. *Acta Crystallogr.* 6: 689–697.

Day, M. W., Hsu, B. T., Joshua-Tor, L., Park, J.-B., Zhou, Z. H., Adams, M.W.W., and Rees, D. C. (1992) X-ray crystal structures of the oxidized and reduced forms of the rubredoxin from the marine hyperthermophilic archaebacterium *Pyrococcus furiosus. Protein Sci.* 1: 1494–1507.

Deisenhofer, J., Epp, O., Miki, K., Huber, R., and Michel, H. (1984) X-ray structure analysis of a membrane–protein complex: electron-density map at 3 Å resolution and a model of the chromophores of the photosynthetic reaction center from *Rhodopseudomonas viridis. J. Mol. Biol.* 180: 385–398.

Deisenhofer, J., Epp, O., Miki, K., Huber, R., and Michel, H. (1985) Structure of the protein subunits in the photosynthetic reaction center of *Rhodopseudomonas viridis* at 3 Å resolution. *Nature* 318: 618–624.

Deisenhofer, J., and Michel, H. (1989) The photosynthetic reaction center from the purple bacterium *Rhodopseudomonas viridis. EMBO J.* 8: 2149–2170.

Dill, K. A. (1990a) Dominant forces in protein folding. *Biochemistry* 29: 7133–7155.

Dill, K. A. (1990b) The meaning of hydrophobicity. *Science* 250: 297.

Ealick, S. E., Cook, W. J., Vijay-Kumar, S., Carson, M., Nagabhushan, T. L., Trotta, P. P., and Bugg, C. E. (1991) Three-dimensional structure of recombinant human interferon-γ. *Science* 252: 698–702.

Eisenberg, D. (1984) Three-dimensional structure of membrane and surface proteins. *Annu. Rev. Biochem.* 53: 595–623.

Eisenberg, D., and McLachlan, A. D. (1986) Solvation energy in protein folding and binding. *Nature* 319: 199–203.

Eisenberg, D., Weiss, R. M., Terwilliger, T. C., and Wilcox, W. (1982) Hydrophobic moments and protein structure. *Faraday Symp. Chem. Soc.* 17: 109–120.

Engelman, D. M. (1982) An implication of the structure of bacteriorhodopsin: globular membrane proteins are stabilized by polar interactions. *Biophys. J.* 37: 187–188.

Engelman, D. M., Henderson, R., McLachlan, A. D., and Wallace, B. A. (1980) Path of the polypeptide in bacteriorhodopsin. *Proc. Natl. Acad. Sci. USA* 77: 2023–2027.

Engelman, D. M., Steitz, T. A., and Goldman, A. (1986) Identifying nonpolar transbilayer helices in amino-acid sequences of membrane-proteins. *Annu. Rev. Biophys. Biophys. Chem.* 15: 321–353.

Engelman, D. M., and Zaccai, G. (1980) Bacteriorhodopsin is an inside-out protein. *Proc. Natl. Acad. Sci. USA* 77: 5894–5898.

Feher, G., Allen, J. P., Okamura, M. Y., and Rees, D. C. (1989) Structure and function of bacterial photosynthetic reaction centres. *Nature* 339: 111–116.

Gibbs, J. W. (1928) *Collected Works of J. W. Gibbs.* New York: Longmans.

Guy, H. R., and Seetharamulu, P. (1986) Molecular model of the action potential sodium channel. *Proc. Natl. Acad. Sci. U.S.A.* 83: 508–512.

Henderson, R., Baldwin, J. M., Ceska, T. A., Zemlin, F., Beckmann, E., and Downing, K. H. (1990) Model for the structure of bacteriorhodopsin based on high-resolution electron cryomicroscopy. *J. Mol. Biol.* 213: 899–929.

Henderson, R., and Unwin, P.N.T. (1975) Three-dimensional model of purple membrane obtained by electron microscopy. *Nature* 257: 28–32.

Huber, R., Romisch, J., and Paques, E. P. (1990) The crystal and molecular structure of human annexin V, an anticoagulant protein that binds to calcium and membranes. *EMBO J.* 9: 3867–3874.

Israelachvili, J. N. (1985) *Intermolecular and Surface Forces.* London: Academic Press.

Jackson, M. B., and Sturtevant, J. M. (1978) Phase transitions of the purple membranes of *Halobacterium halobium. Biochemistry* 17: 911–915.

Janin, J., Miller, S., and Chothia, C. (1988) Surface, subunit interfaces and interior of oligomeric proteins. *J. Mol. Biol.* 204: 155–164.

Kahn, T. W., Sturtevant, J. M., and Engelman, D. M. (1992) Thermodynamic measurements of the contributions of helix-connecting loops and of retinal to the stability of bacteriorhodopsin. *Biochemistry* 31: 8829–8839.

Kauzmann, W. (1959) Some factors in the interpretation of protein denaturation. *Adv. Prot. Chem.* 14: 1–63.

Komiya, H., Yeates, T. O., Rees, D. C., Allen, J. P., and Feher, G. (1988) Structure of the reaction center from *Rhodopseudomonas sphaeroides* R-26 and 2.4.1: symmetry relations and sequence comparisons between different species. *Proc. Natl. Acad. Sci. U.S.A.* 85: 8487–8491.

Kresheck, G. C., Schneider, H., and Scheraga, H. A. (1965) The effect of D₂O on the thermal stability of proteins. Thermodynamic parameters for the transfer of model compounds from H_2O to D_2O. *J. Phys. Chem.* 69: 3132–3144.

Kyte, J., and Doolittle, R. F. (1982) A simple method for displaying the hydropathic character of a protein. *J. Mol. Biol.* 157: 105–132.

Lenard, J., and Singer, S. J. (1966) Protein conformation in cell membrane preparations as studied by optical rotatory dispersion and circular dichroism. *Proc. Natl. Acad. Sci. USA* 56: 1828–1835.

Li, J., Carroll, J., and Ellar, D. J. (1991) Crystal structure of insecticidal δ-endotoxin from *Bacillus thuringiensis* at 2.5 Å resolution. *Nature* 353: 815–821.

Miller, S., Lesk, A. M., Janin, J., and Chothia, C. (1987) Interior and surface of monomeric proteins. *J. Mol. Biol.* 196: 641–656.

Murphy, K. P., Privalov, P. L., and Gill, S. J. (1990) Common features of protein unfolding and dissolution of hydrophobic compounds. *Science* 560: 559–561.

Nabedryk, E., Garavito, R. M., and Breton, J. (1988) "The orientation of beta sheets in porin—a polarized Fourier transform infrared spectroscopic investigation. *Biophys. J.* 53: 671–676.

O'Shea, E. K., Klemm, J. D., Kim, P. S., and Alber, T. (1991) X-ray structure of the GCN4 lecuine zipper, a two-stranded, parallel coiled coil. *Science* 254: 539–544.

Parker, M. W., Pattus, F., Tucker, A. D., and Tsernoglou, D. (1989) Structure of the membrane-pore-forming fragment of colicin A. *Nature* 337: 93–96.

Perutz, M. F., Kendrew, J. C., and Watson, H. C. (1965) Structure and function of haemoglobin. II. Some relationships between polypeptide chain configuration and amino acid sequence. *J. Mol. Biol.* 13: 669–678.

Popot, J.-L., and Engelman, D. M. (1990) Membrane protein folding and oligomerization: the two-stage model. *Biochemistry* 29: 4031–4037.

Popot, J.-L., Gerchman, S.-E., and Engelman, D. M. (1987) Refolding of bacteriorhodopsin in lipid bilayers—a thermodynamically controlled two stage process. *J. Mol. Biol.* 198: 655–676.

Privalov, P. L. (1979) Stability of proteins: small globular proteins. *Adv. Prot. Chem.* 33: 167–241.

Privalov, P. L. (1990) Cold denaturation of proteins. *Crit. Rev. Biochem. Mol. Biol.* 25: 281–305.

Privalov, P. L., and Gill, S. J. (1988) Stability of protein structure and hydrophobic interaction. *Adv. Prot. Chem.* 39: 191–234.

Rees, D. C., DeAntonio, L., and Eisenberg, D. (1989a) Hydrophobic organization of membrane proteins. *Science* 245: 510–513.

Rees, D. C., Komiya, H., Yeates, T. O., Allen J. P., and Feher, G. (1989b) The bacterial photosynthetic reaction center as a model for membrane proteins. *Annu. Rev. Biochem.* 58: 607–633.

Richards, F. M. (1977) Areas, volumes, packing and protein structure. *Annu. Rev. Biophys. Bioeng.* 6: 151–176.

Roth, M., Lewit-Bentley, A., Michel, H., Deisenhofer, J., Huber, R., and Oesterhelt, D. (1989) Detergent structure in crystals of a bacterial photosynthetic reaction center. *Nature* 340: 659–662.

Singer, S. J. (1990) The structure and insertion of integral proteins in membranes. *Annu. Rev. Cell Biol.* 6: 247–296.

Smith, E. L. (1967) The evolution of proteins. *Harvey Lect.* 62: 231–256.

Tanford, C. (1980) *The Hydrophobic Effect.* 2nd Ed. New York: Wiley.

Volkin, D. B., Staubli, A., Langer, R., and Klibanov, A. M. (1991) Enzyme thermoinactivation in anhydrous organic solvents. *Biotech. Bioengin.* 37: 843–853.

Wallach, D.F.H., and Zahler, P. H. (1966) Protein conformations in cellular membranes. *Proc. Natl. Acad. Sci. U.S.A.* 56: 1552–1559.

Weber, P. C., and Salemme, F. R. (1980) Structural and functional diversity in 4-α-helical proteins. *Nature* 287: 82–84.

Weiss, M. S., Abele, U., Weckesser, J., Welte, W., Schiltz, E., and Schulz, G. E. (1991) Molecular architecture and electrostatic properties of a bacterial porin. *Science* 254: 1627–1630.

Weiss, M. S., Kreusch, A., Schiltz, E., Nestel, U., Welte, W., Weckesser, J., and Schulz, G. E. (1991) The structure of porin from *Rhodobacter capsulatus* at 1.8 Å resolution. *FEBS Lett.* 280: 379–382.

Weiss, M. S., Wacker, T., Weckesser, J., Welte, W., and Schulz, G. E. (1990) The three-dimensional structure of porin from *Rhodobacter capsulatus* at 3 Å resolution. *FEBS Lett.* 267: 268–272.

Weiss, M. S., and Schulz, G. E. (1992) Structure of porin refined at 1.8Å resolution. *J. Mol. Biol.* 227: 493–509.

Yeates, T. O., Komiya, H., Chirino, A., Rees, D. C., Allen, J. P., and Feher, G. (1988) Structure of the reaction center from *Rhodopseudomonas sphaeroides* R-26 and 2.4.1: protein–cofactor (bacteriochlorophyll, bacteriopheophytin, and carotenoid) interactions. *Proc. Natl. Acad. Sci. U.S.A.* 85: 7993–7997.

Yeates, T. O., Komiya, H., Rees, D. C., Allen, J. P., and Feher, G. (1987) Structure of the reaction center from *Rhodopseudomonas sphaeroides* R-26: membrane–protein interactions. *Proc. Natl. Acad. Scie. U.S.A.* 84: 6438–6442.

Zipp, A., and Kauzmann, W. (1973) Pressure denaturation of myoglobin. *Biochemistry* 12: 4217–4228.

Zubay, G. (1983) *Biochemistry.* 1st Ed. Reading, MA: Addison-Wesley, p. 104.

2

Decoding the Signals
of Membrane Protein Sequences

GUNNAR VON HEIJNE

In order to understand membrane protein structure in a general sense, one needs an efficient conceptual framework. When discussing globular proteins, we tend to use hierarchical descriptions and distinguish what we think are semi-independent levels of increasing structural complexity (Brändén and Tooze, 1991): the amino acid sequence (primary structure); local structural elements such as helices, β-strands, and turns (secondary structure); structural units (β-α-β units, β-strand hairpins); larger folding domains (Rossman fold, TIM barrel); globular single-chain structures (tertiary structure); and oligomeric assemblies (quaternary structure). In addition to being a purely descriptive scheme, it is often assumed that the unidirectional path leading from simple, locally determined structural elements to complex, global structures also in some way approximates the real *in vivo* folding process, although this is still very much a controversial point (Dill, 1990).

A similar scheme based on a "top-down" analysis of known three-dimensional structures can of course be devised to describe integral membrane proteins (see Chapters 1 and 3), but I will argue that a more fruitful way to understand their structure is in terms of how they are synthesized, targeted to the appropriate membrane, inserted into this membrane, and finally form their full three-dimensional-structure within the confines of a lipid bilayer. Thus we need to widen our conceptual universe to include not only the static picture of the final structure but also the dynamics of the biosynthetic pathway leading to this structure. In fact, since many important aspects of membrane protein biosynthesis seem to rely on rather well-defined "signals" encoded in the protein chain (targeting signals, topological signals, packing signals), the resulting logic is a rather simple one of successive "decoding" of these signals, ultimately giving rise to the correctly folded, functional molecule in its proper location.

This chapter is organized around three main sections. First, I will give a brief introduction to the general problem of intracellular protein sorting. Then follows a discussion of how proteins insert into membranes and how their transmembrane topology is determined, and finally I try to derive some implications for membrane protein structure prediction. Throughout, the focus is on the so-called helical bundle integral membrane proteins, i.e., proteins with transmembrane segments formed by long hydrophobic α-helices. Typical examples of this structural class are bacterio-

27

rhodopsin (Henderson et al., 1990) and the bacterial photosynthetic reaction center (Deisenhofer and Michel, 1991); in general, all bacterial inner membrane proteins, all eukaryotic membrane proteins initially inserted into the endoplasmic reticular (ER) membrane, all mitochondrial inner membrane proteins, and all chloroplast thylakoid membrane proteins most likely are of this type. The second well-characterized class of integral membrane proteins is the "β-barrel" variety, in which the transmembrane segments are amphiphilic β-strands that together form a closed β-sheet barrel with a hydrophobic outside facing the lipids and a more polar inside lining a central pore. Such structures are known to atomic resolution (e.g. Weiss et al., 1991), but relatively little information on the membrane insertion of such molecules is available (Bosch et al., 1988, 1989; Struyve et al., 1991), and they will not be discussed further here.

Targeting Signals

All cells need to be able to sort proteins between a number of subcellular compartments. In *Escherichia coli*, there are at least five well-defined compartments: the cytoplasm, the inner and outer membranes, the periplasm, and the extracellular medium. A membrane protein must thus somehow "know" that it should not remain in the cytoplasm and further whether it is supposed to go to the inner or outer membrane. The highly complex subcellular structure of eukaryotic cells makes protein sorting a very complicated business, in which proteins must not only be routed into the correct organelle but further sorted to the correct intraorganellar compartment.

In all cases known, the targeting information is encoded within the nascent polypeptide, often as an N-terminal extension that is removed by appropriately located proteases once the correct compartment has been reached (von Heijne, 1990a). The targeting signal in the nascent protein is recognized by receptors in the cytoplasm or on the surface of the organelle, and the protein is translocated across one or more membranes and finally delivered to its site of action.

Sorting Between Organelles

Major recipients of cytoplasmically synthesized proteins are mitochondria, chloroplasts, the nucleus, peroxisomes, and the organelles in the secretory pathway. Targeting signals specific for each of these organelles have been defined by, for example, gene fusion studies, and their basic designs have been elucidated by a combination of experimental and statistical techniques.

Mitochondrial targeting peptides are in most cases found as N-terminal extensions that are cleaved by a mitochondrial matrix protease. They are rich in positively charged (Arg in particular) and hydroxylated (Ser, Thr) amino acids, but lack negatively charged residues (Asp, Glu). An apparently very important property is their ability to form amphiphilic α-helices with one highly charged and one hydrophobic face (von Heijne, 1986b; Gavel and von Heijne, 1990a) (Fig. 2.1).

Chloroplast transit peptides from higher plants are also N-terminal extensions and are removed in the chloroplast by a stromal processing peptidase. They are characterized by an extremely high content of hydroxylated amino acids ($\sim$30% Ser + Thr) and contain few if any negatively charged residues (von Heijne et al., 1989;

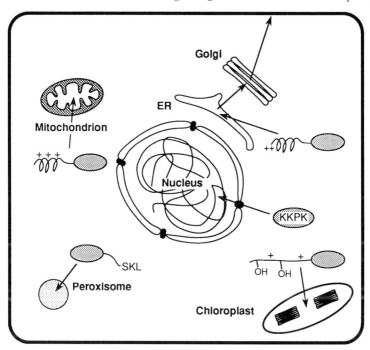

Fig. 2.1. Protein sorting pathways.

Gavel and von Heijne, 1990b). It is not clear if they are designed to have any partic-ular conformational preferences (von Heijne and Nishikawa, 1991). Transit pep-tides from the green algae *Chlamydomonas reinhardtii*, in contrast, are strikingly similar to mitochondrial targeting peptides and probably form amphiphilic α-helices (Franzén et al., 1990), raising the question of how the specificity of proteins sorting between mitochondria and chloroplasts is maintained in this organism.

Nuclear location signals are not removed from the mature protein and are gener-ally found in internal positions (Silver, 1991). Clusters of positively charged residues presumably exposed on the surface of the folded molecule signal nuclear import, and the presence of multiple copies of an import signal in a protein chain often lead to enhanced levels of import.

Peroxisomal targeting signals are less well understood, but a C-terminal tripeptide Ser-Lys-Leu (SKL) has been shown to promote peroxisomal import in a number of cases (Gould et al., 1989, 1990; Miyazawa et al., 1989). Many peroxisomal proteins lacking this signal are known, however.

Secretory signal peptides, finally, have a tripartite design, with an N-terminal pos-itively charged region, a central hydrophobic region, and a C-terminal region that specifies the cleavage site (von Heijne, 1985, 1990b; Gierasch, 1989). This basic structure is similar throughout nature, from bacteria to man.

Sorting Within Organelles

Sorting within the mitochondrion is believed to follow a "conservative" sorting path-way (Hartl et al., 1989), i.e., proteins destined for the inner membrane or the inter-

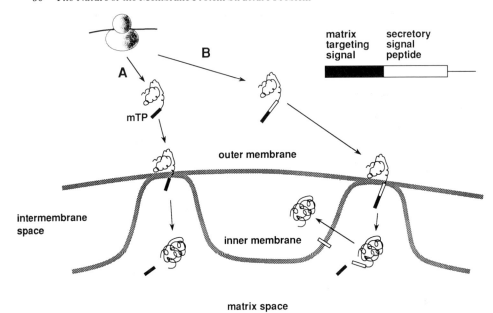

Fig. 2.2. Intramitochondrial protein sorting. Matrix-targeting signals (mTP) allow entry into the matrix space *(path A)*. Signals composed of a matrix-targeting part and a signal peptide-like part allow transport into the intermembrane space via a "conservative sorting" pathway (*B*).

membrane space are first imported all the way into the matrix and subsequently re-exported across or inserted into the inner membrane (Fig. 2.2). This two-step process is neatly mirrored in the design of the targeting peptides (von Heijne et al., 1989): an N-terminal matrix-targeting signal (positively charged amphiphilic α-helix) is immediately followed by a second cleavable targeting signal that has all the characteristics of a secretory signal peptide. It is thus thought that the mitochondrial inner membrane has a machinery for protein translocation similar to that found in bacteria.

Thylakoid lumen proteins, as well as some of the thylakoid membrane proteins, also have composite targeting peptides of this kind, but with the N-terminal part now being a chloroplast transit peptide (von Heijne et al., 1989). The analogy with secretory signal peptides goes even further in this case, since the substrate specificity of the so-called thylakoid processing peptidase responsible for removing the signal peptide-like thylakoid transfer domain is nearly identical to that of the corresponding *E. coli* enzyme (Halpin et al., 1989; Shackleton and Robinson, 1991).

Sorting in the Secretory Pathway

The secretory pathway comprises a number of subcompartments that are traversed in sequel from the ER through the Golgi stacks and the trans-Golgi network to the plasma membrane or to the lysosome (Breitfeld et al., 1989; Pugsley, 1989). Each subcompartment has its own specific complement of resident proteins that are thought to be actively retained in or recycled to that compartment in response to retention signals present in their amino acid sequence. Thus, lumenal ER proteins have a C-terminal tetrapeptide retention signal (Lys-Asp-Glu-Leu or -KDEL) (Pelham, 1990). Resident ER membrane proteins seem to have a retention signal located in their cytoplasmically exposed parts; one or two lysines in their cytoplasmic tails have been implicated in retention, but this is still a somewhat controversial point (Gabathuler and Kvist, 1990; Jackson et al., 1990).

Transmembrane proteins can also be specifically degraded in the ER. This "quality control" feature may enable the cell to remove, for example, subunits of multichain complexes that have failed to associate properly with their partners (Klausner and Sitia, 1990). Isolated charged residues present in a transmembrane segment seem to signal ER degradation (Bonifacino et al., 1990); presumably, such degradation signals become masked when subunits associate with each other.

Some resident Golgi membrane proteins apparently have a retention signal located in their transmembrane segment(s) (Machamer and Rose, 1987; Colley et al., 1989); other Golgi-specific retention signals have not yet been defined. Lumenal lysosomal proteins carry a mannose-6-phosphate modification that serves as the targeting signal and ensures routing to the lysosome from the trans-Golgi network (Kornfeld and Mellman, 1989; Baranski et al., 1990); lysosomal membrane proteins, on the other hand, carry no such modification, and targeting information is believed to be present in their cytoplasmic domains (Peters et al., 1990).

A final aspect of membrane protein sorting is that of endocytosis. Many plasma membrane receptors continually cycle back and forth between the plasma membrane and the trans-Golgi network via endocytosis through coated pits. A critical tyrosine placed in the cytoplasmic tail near the membrane has been implicated as being part of the endocytosis signal (Jing et al., 1990; Ktistakis et al., 1990; Bansal and Gierasch, 1991; Eberle et al., 1991).

Topological Signals

Once a protein has reached its target membrane, it needs to insert into that membrane in its correct orientation. Once inserted, changes in the orientation of the whole protein or of individual transmembrane segments (flip-flop) would seem to be impossible on energetic grounds and has never been observed experimentally. It is during the insertion process that the number of transmembrane segments in the final structure as well as their orientation are decided. For a multispanning (polytopic) protein with most of its chain embedded in the membrane, the membrane insertion event is thus the most important step on the folding pathway; what remains after this step has been completed is only the final packing of the transmembrane segments against each other.

Topological Signals: An Overview

Most membrane proteins use one of the machineries normally used to translocate proteins across membranes for their insertion. From this point of view, a membrane protein can be regarded as a partially translocated protein—a molecule that, in addition to the normal targeting signal(s), contains additional signals that cannot be

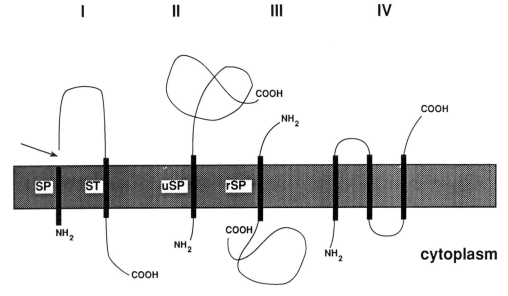

Fig. 2.3. Classification of integral membrane proteins. *SP*, signal peptide; *ST*, stop-transfer sequence; *uSP*, uncleaved signal peptide; *rSP*, reverse signal peptide.

translocated across the membrane but rather get stuck and provide a permanent transmembrane anchoring.

One useful classification based on the kinds of signals present in a protein is shown in Figure 2.3 (von Heijne, 1988). Class I proteins have a cleavable signal peptide and a second hydrophobic stop-transfer sequence; the orientation of the mature protein is N_{out}–C_{in}. Class II proteins have an uncleavable signal peptide, i.e., a signal peptide lacking the C-terminal cleavage domain, and hence get anchored to the membrane in the N_{in}–C_{out} orientation. Class III proteins also lack a cleavable signal peptide and have a hydrophobic transmembrane segment close to the N terminus (a "reverse signal peptide" [Dalbey, 1990]), but this segment is now oriented N_{out}–C_{in}, i.e., opposite to the class II proteins. Class IV proteins have multiple transmembrane segments, and examples are known with all possible combinations of N_{in}, N_{out}, C_{in}, and C_{out} orientations.

Statistical Studies: The "Positive Inside" Rule

Proteins with a cleavable signal peptide (class I) are always oriented N_{out}, but it is not immediately clear what feature(s) of the nascent chain determine the orientation of the other classes. Early statistical studies of both single-spanning (classes II and III) and multispanning proteins gave the first hint that topological determinants should be sought in the polar tail and loop regions flanking the transmembrane segments and that the distributions of positively charged residues (Arg, Lys) seemed to be particularly well correlated with the topology (von Heijne, 1986a,d). In a sample of bacterial inner membrane proteins, a fourfold higher frequency of Arg + Lys was found in the cytoplasmic than in the periplasmic flanking regions, and similar, though less extreme, biases have since been found in proteins from other membrane systems as well (see below). Thus a "positive inside" rule (von Heijne and Gavel, 1988) was proposed to account for the topology of most integral membrane proteins.

Membrane Protein Topogenesis in Escherichia coli

Translocation of proteins across the inner membrane of *E. coli* normally requires the participation of the *sec* machinery (Schatz and Beckwith, 1990; Wickner et al., 1991). The nascent precursor protein first binds to a cytoplasmic chaperone such as SecB, is then transferred to SecA (a large peripheral membrane protein with ATPase activity), is translocated across the membrane in a process involving the integral membrane components SecY and SecE (and possibly the late-acting factors SecD and SecF), and is finally released from the membrane after the signal peptide has been cleaved by the Lep protease.

   Many inner membrane proteins also need the *sec* machinery for translocation of their periplasmic domain(s), but some do not (notably those with only short periplasmic domains; see below). Obviously, the topology may be determined in different ways during *sec*-dependent and *sec*-independent membrane insertion, although it appears from the data at hand that positively charged amino acids are important in both contexts.

   Most of what is known about membrane protein insertion in *E. coli* comes from studies on three proteins: phage M13 coat protein, leader peptidase (Lep), and MalF (Fig. 2.4). M13 coat is made with a cleavable signal peptide, spans the membrane once, and inserts independently of the *sec* machinery (Wickner, 1988). Lep has no cleavable signal peptide and two transmembrane segments, and translocation of the C-terminal but not the N-terminal periplasmic domain is *sec* dependent (Wolfe et al., 1985; R. Dalbey, personal communication). MalF, finally, has eight transmembrane segments, and it is not clear which periplasmic parts, if any, are *sec* dependent (McGovern and Beckwith, 1991).

   The importance of cytoplasmically located positively charged residues for proper insertion of the M13 coat protein was established quite early (Kuhn et al., 1986a,b), although it could not be determined whether the molecules that failed to insert in

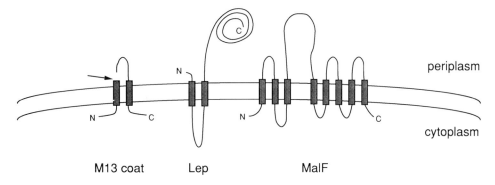

Fig. 2.4. Topology of the phage M13 coat, leader peptidase *(Lep)*, and the MalF proteins in the inner membrane of *E. coli*. The *arrow* marks the cleavage-site in the M13 coat protein signal peptide.

their normal orientation simply did not insert at all or inserted in some other orientation.

Studies of various MalF–PhoA fusion proteins have also shown that positively charged residues in cytoplasmic loops are important for preserving the transmembrane orientation (Boyd and Beckwith, 1989; Ehrmann and Beckwith, 1991; McGovern et al., 1991), but the most direct evidence for the role of positively charged residues as topological determinants has been obtained from studies of Lep-derived constructs in which it has been possible to "invert" the orientation of the molecule by redistribution of lysines and arginines. Both single-spanning and double-spanning Lep derivatives can be reoriented by the simultaneous removal of positively charged residues from their cytoplasmic regions and addition of such residues to the periplasmic regions (von Heijne et al., 1988; von Heijne, 1989; Andersson et al., 1992). Negatively charged residues have little effect on the topology by themselves (Nilsson and von Heijne, 1990), but apparently can, when suitably positioned, "neutralize" the effect of a nearby positively charged residue (Andersson and von Heijne, 1993a). Furthermore, insertion of the "inverted" double-spanning Lep constructs is *sec*-independent, in contrast to insertion of the wild-type molecule (von Heijne, 1989).

It is thus clear that positively charged amino acids are the most important topological determinants in *E. coli* (Boyd and Beckwith, 1990; Dalbey, 1990; von Heijne and Manoil, 1990; Yamane et al., 1990). However, one could still argue that they would act only to determine the orientation of the first one or two transmembrane segments in a multispanning protein such as MalF and that the more downstream segments would simply follow the dictates of their upstream neighbors, i.e., that the insertion process would progress sequentially from the N terminus toward the C terminus. The other extreme would be a locally determined insertion process, where individual "helical hairpins" (DiRienzo et al., 1978; von Heijne and Blomberg, 1979; Engelman and Steitz, 1981) composed of two neighboring transmembrane segments and the periplasmic loop in between insert independently of the rest of the chain. The statistical studies discussed above would favor the latter model, since the charge bias between periplasmic and cytoplasmic loops is equally strong in the early and late parts of multispanning proteins (von Heijne, 1992). Indeed, it has recently been reported both for MalF and LacY (which has 12 transmembrane segments) that deletions of single transmembrane segments at different positions often have no effects on the orientation of the downstream parts of the molecule (Bibi et al., 1991; Ehrmann and Beckwith, 1991; McGovern et al., 1991). This result cannot be explained on the basis of a sequential model (according to which the orientation of the downstream parts would be inverted) and strongly suggests that the topology is a local property of each helical hairpin.

Finally, why do some proteins apparently insert independently of the *sec* machinery, whereas others absolutely depend on it? First, the low frequency of positively charged residues in the periplasmic parts is only observed for relatively short loops, whereas loops longer than 60–80 residues have frequencies similar to what is found in soluble periplasmic proteins (von Heijne and Gavel, 1988). This might suggest that short loops for some reason cannot engage the *sec* machinery and hence have greater restrictions on the kinds of sequences that can be efficiently translocated. In agreement with this idea, it has been found that the insertion of the normally *sec*-independent M13 coat protein is *sec*-dependent in a construct in which the periplasmic domain has been increased in length from some 20 to about 100 residues (Kuhn, 1988). Also, translocation of the outer membrane protein OmpA through the inner membrane (a *sec*-dependent process) requires a chain length of at least 75 residues (Freudl et al., 1989); shorter chains are not translocated at all. We have successively lengthened the periplasmic loop in the"inverted" Lep construct; so far, we have found that a 50 residue long loop is still translocated independently of the *sec* machinery (Andersson and von Heijne, 1993b).

These observations all seem to support the idea that the length of the translocated domain is an important factor that would distinguish *sec*-dependent and *sec*-independent translocation; yet recent results from an analysis of MalF–PhoA fusion proteins seem to suggest that length cannot be the only factor (McGovern and Beckwith, 1991), since translocation of the large PhoA moiety in these fusions apparently does not require the *sec* machinery (PhoA is *sec*-dependent when targeted for secretion by its own signal peptide).

Membrane Protein Topogenesis in the ER

von Heijne and Gavel (1988) have shown that the positive inside rule holds also for membrane proteins that inset into the ER membrane and traverse the secretory pathway, although the bias in the distribution of Arg and Lys residues is less extreme than in bacterial proteins. A more detailed statistical study has suggested that the charge bias across the first transmembrane segment is an even better predictor of the topology than the total charge bias over the entire molecule (Hartmann et al., 1989). This would be consistent with the fact that protein translocation across the ER membrane is obligatory cotranslational (as opposed to the situation in *E. coli*), which makes it more likely that insertion proceeds according to the sequential model discussed above, with the topology being determined by the first transmembrane segment(s).

There is as yet no good experimental data on this point, since the topological role of charged residues has only been tested on single-spanning proteins so far. For these proteins, however, it has been shown that positively charged residues play a similar role as in *E. coli* (von Heijne and Manoil, 1990). The role of negatively charged amino acids has not been systematically studied, but they do seem to have some effects, at least in particular contexts (Haeuptle et al., 1989; Parks and Lamb, 1991).

Membrane Protein Topogenesis in Chloroplasts and Mitochondria

Thylakoid membrane proteins follow the positive inside rule (Gavel et al., 1991), with the more highly charged loops facing the stromal compartment (i.e., not being translocated). Likewise, mitochondrial inner membrane proteins have a strong charge bias, with the matrix-facing parts having a high content of positively charged residues (Gavel and von Heijne, 1992). Considering the evolutionary relationships between chloroplasts, mitochondria, and bacterial cells, it thus seems highly likely that the mechanism of organellar membrane protein insertion is similar to that in *E. coli*. As far as insertion into the outer membranes of mitochondria and chloroplasts and into the inner envelope chloroplast membrane are concerned, there are very few data available, either from known sequences or from biochemical studies.

Conclusion: The Structure Prediction Problem

One important goal of research on membrane protein biogenesis is to improve our abilities to predict three-dimensional structures directly from sequence. Today, one can often make a good guess as to where the transmembrane segments are based on hydrophobicity analysis, and once these segments have been identified one can predict the orientation in the membrane with high confidence from the positive inside rule. A major difficulty, however, is that one often finds peaks on a hydrophobicity plot that cannot be unambiguously assigned as transmembrane (see Chapter 4); they fall in the "twilight zone" (von Heijne, 1986c). In such cases, it might be possible to proceed by constructing all possible models that either include or exclude each one of the "twilight" peaks and rank these according to how well they conform to the positive inside rule. From preliminary studies, it seems that such a strategy works reasonably well and can be used to improve the raw results from the hydrophobicity analysis. Another means to the same end would be to study experimentally the putative transmembrane segments that fall in the twilight zone to gain a better understanding of how stop-transfer function relates to amino acid sequence characteristics (Davis et al., 1985; Davis and Model, 1985; Doyle et al., 1986; Kuroiwa et al., 1991).

As discussed elsewhere in this volume (Chapters 1 and 3), the final step in membrane protein structure prediction would be to develop algorithms that can pack transmembrane α-helices together in some optimal way. This may well be within reach of our present-day modeling capabilities, provided we had a sufficiently large database of known structures to calibrate against and reasonably simple experimental methods for testing our predictions. This is clearly not the case, and few remedies are seen on the horizon.

I would like to end on this note, with a plea for efforts to develop new techniques, e.g., for mapping the relative orientations of transmembrane helices or for determining distances between selected residues in different parts of a multispanning protein. These new techniques need not be high resolution: Since we know that we are dealing with α-helices that are oriented within some rather small angle of the membrane normal, already a few rough distances between helices or measures of relative helix orientations should suffice to give us the constraints we need for successful modeling. Thus we might be able to further our understanding of how transmembrane helices pack together to the point where we can finally solve the membrane protein folding problem: to go from sequence to structure at the touch of a button.

Acknowledgments

This work was supported by grants from the Swedish Natural Sciences Research Council and the Swedish Board for Technical Development.

References

Andersson, H., Bakker, E. and von Heijne, G. (1992) Different positively charged amino acids have similar effects on the topology of a polytopic transmembrane protein in *Escherichia coli. J. Biol. Chem.* 267: 1491–1495.

Andersson, H., and von Heijne, G. (1993a). Position-specific Asp-Lys pairing can affect signal sequence function and membrane protein topology. *J. Biol. Chem.* 268: 21398–21393.

Andersson, H., and von Heijne, G. (1993b). *Sec*-Dependent and *sec*-Independent Assembly of *E. coli* Inner Membrane Proteins—The Topological Rules Depend on Chain Length. *EMBO J.* 12: 683–691.

Bansal, A., and Gierasch, L. M. (1991) The NPXY internalization signal of the LDL receptor adopts a reverse-turn conformation. *Cell* 67: 1195–1201.

Baranski, T. J., Faust, P. L., and Kornfeld, S. (1990) Generation of a lysosomal enzyme targeting signal in the secretory protein pepsinogen. *Cell* 63: 281–291.

Bibi, E., Verner, G., Chang, C. Y., and Kaback, H. R. (1991) Organization and stability of a polytopic membrane protein—deletion analysis of the lactose permease of *Escherichia coli. Proc. Natl. Acad. Sci. USA* 88: 7271–7275.

Bonifacino, J. S., Cosson, P., and Klausner, R. D. (1990) Colocalized transmembrane determinants for ER degradation and subunit assembly explain the intracellular fate of TCR chains. *Cell* 63: 503–513.

Bosch, D., Scholten, M., Verhagen, C., and Tommassen, J. (1989) The role of the carboxy-terminal membrane-spanning fragment in the biogenesis of *Escherichia coli* K12 outer membrane protein PhoE. *Mol. Gen. Genet.* 216: 144–148.

Bosch, D., Voorhout, W., and Tommassen, J. (1988) Export and localization of N-terminally truncated derivatives of *Escherichia coli* K-12 outer membrane protein PhoE. *J. Biol. Chem.* 263: 9952–9957.

Boyd, D., and Beckwith, J. (1989) Positively charged amino acid residues can act as topogenic determinants in membrane proteins. *Proc. Natl. Acad. Sci. USA* 86: 9446–9450.

Boyd, D., and Beckwith, J. (1990) The role of charged amino acids in the localization of secreted and membrane proteins. *Cell* 62: 1031–1033.

Brändén, C., and Tooze, J. (1991) Introduction to Protein Structure. New York: Garland Publishing.

Breitfeld, P. P., Casanova, J. E., Simister, N. E.. Ross, S. A., McKinnon, W. C., and Mostov, K. E. (1989) Sorting signals, *Curr. Opin. Cell Biol.* 1: 617–623.

Colley, K. J., Lee, E. U., Adler, B., Browne, J. K., and Paulson, J. C. (1989) Conversion of a Golgi apparatus sialyltransferase to a secretory protein by replacement of the NH2-terminal signal anchor with a signal peptide. *J. Biol. Chem.* 264: 17619–17622.

Dalbey, R. E. (1990) Positively charged residues are important determinants of membrane protein topology. *Trends Biochem. Sci.* 15: 253–257.

Davis, N. G., Boeke, J. D., and Model, P. (1985) Fine structure of a membrane anchor domain. *J. Mol. Biol.* 181: 111–121.

Davis, N. G., and Model, P. (1985) An artificial anchor domain: hydrophobicity suffices to stop transfer. *Cell* 41: 607–614.

Deisenhofer, J., and Michel, H. (1991) High-resolution structures of photosynthetic reaction centers. *Annu. Rev. Biophys. Biophys. Chem.* 20: 247–266.

Dill, K. A. (1990) Dominant forces in protein folding. *Biochemistry* 29: 7133–7155.

DiRienzo, J. M., Nakamura, K., and Inouye, M. (1978) The outer membrane proteins of Gram-negative bacteria: biosynthesis, assembly, and function. *Annu. Rev. Biochem.* 47: 481–532.

Doyle, C., Sambrook, J., and Gething, M. J. (1986) Analysis of progressive deletions of the transmembrane and cytoplasmic domains of influenza hemagglutinin. *J. Cell. Biol.* 103: 1193–204.

Eberle, W., Sander, C., Klaus, W., Schmidt, B., von Figura, K., and Peters, C. (1991) The essential tyrosine of the internalization signal in lysosomal acid phosphatase is part of a β-turn. *Cell* 67: 1203–1209.

Ehrmann, M., and Beckwith, J. (1991) Proper insertion of a complex membrane protein in the absence of its amino-terminal export signal. *J. Biol. Chem.* 266: 16530–16533.

Engelman, D. M., and Steitz, T. A. (1981) The spontaneous insertion of proteins into and across membranes: the helical hairpin hypothesis. *Cell* 23: 411–422.

Fourel, D., Mizushima, S., and Pages, J. M. (1992) Dynamics of the exposure of epitopes on OmpF, an outer membrane protein of *Escherichia coli. Eur. J. Biochem.* 206: 109–114.

Franzén, L. G., Rochaix, J. D., and von Heijne, G. (1990) Chloroplast transit peptides from the green alga *Chlamydomonas reinhardtii* share features with both mitochondrial and higher plant chloroplast presequences. *FEBS Lett.* 260: 165–168.

Freudl, R., Schwarz, H., Degen, M., and Henning, U. (1989) A lower size limit exists for export of fragments of an outer membrane protein (OpmA) of *Escherichia coli* K-12. *J. Mol. Biol.* 205: 771–775.

Gabathuler, R., and Kvist, S. (1990) The endoplasmic reticulum retention signal of the E3/19K protein of adenovirus type-2 consists of 3 separate amino acid segments at the carboxy terminus. *J. Cell. Biol.* 111: 1803–1810.

Gavel, Y., Steppuhn, J., Herrmann, R., and von Heijne, G. (1991) The positive-inside rule applies to thylakoid membrane proteins. *FEBS Lett.* 282: 41–46.

Gavel, Y., and von Heijne, G. (1990a) Cleavage-site motifs in mitochondrial targeting peptides. *Prot. Eng* 4: 33–37.

Gavel, Y., and von Heijne, G. (1990b) A conserved cleavage-site motif in chloroplast transit peptides. *FEBS Lett.* 261: 455–458.

Gavel, Y., and von Heijne, G. (1992) The distribution of charged amino acids in mitochondrial inner membrane proteins suggests different modes of membrane integration for nuclearly and mitochondrially encoded proteins. *Eur. J. Biochem.* 205: 1207–1215.

Gierasch, L. M. (1989) Signal sequences. *Biochemistry* 28: 923–930.

Gould, S. J., Keller, G.-A., Hosken, N., Wilkinson, J., and Subramani, S. (1989) A conserved tripeptide sorts proteins to peroxisomes. *J. Cell. Biol.* 108: 1657–1664.

Gould, S. J., Krisans, S., Keller, G. A., and Subramani, S. (1990) Antibodies directed against the peroxisomal targeting signal of firefly luciferase recognize multiple mammalian peroxisomal proteins. *J. Cell. Biol.* 110: 27–34.

Haeuptle, M. T., Flint, N., Gough, N. M., and Dobberstein, B. (1989) A tripartite structure of the signals that determine protein insertion into the endoplasmic reticulum membrane. *J. Cell. Biol.* 108: 1227–1236.

Halpin, C., Elderfield, P. D., James, H. E., Zimmermann, R., Dunbar, B., and Robinson, C. (1989) The reaction specificities of the thylakoidal processing peptidase and *Escherichia coli* leader peptidase are identical. *EMBO J.* 8: 3917–3921.

Hartl, F. U., Pfanner, N., Nicholson, D. W., and Neupert, W. (1989) Mitochondrial protein import. *Biochim. Biophys. Acta* 988: 1–45.

Hartmann, E., Rapoport, T. A., and Lodish, H. F. (1989) Predicting the orientation of eukaryotic membrane proteins. *Proc. Natl. Acad. Sci. USA* 86: 5786–5790.

Henderson, R., Baldwin, J. M., Ceska, T. A., Zemlin, F., Beckmann, E., and Downing, K. H. (1990) A model for the structure of bacteriorhodopsin based on high resolution electron cryo-microscopy. *J. Mol. Biol.* 213: 899–929.

Jackson, M. R., Nilsson, T., and Peterson, P. A. (1990) Identification of a consensus motif for retention of transmembrane proteins in the endoplasmic reticulum. *EMBO J.* 9: 3153–3162.

Jing, S. Q., Spencer, T., Miller, K., Hopkins, C., and Trowbridge, I. S. (1990) Role of the human transferrin receptor cytoplasmic domain in endocytosis—localization of a specific signal sequence for internalization. *J. Cell. Biol.* 110: 283–294.

Klausner, R. D., and Sitia, R. (1990) Protein degradation in the endoplasmic reticulum. *Cell* 62: 611–614.

Kornfeld, S., and Mellman, I. (1989) The biogenesis of lysosomes. *Annu. Rev. Cell. Biol.* 5: 483–525.

Ktistakis, N. T., Thomas, D., and Roth, M. G. (1990) Characteristics of the tyrosine recognition signal for internalization of transmembrane surface glycoproteins. *J. Cell. Biol.* 111: 1393–1407.

Kuhn, A. (1988) Alterations in the extracellular domain of M13 procoat protein make its membrane insertion dependent on *secA* and *secY*. *Eur. J. Biochem.* 177: 267–271.

Kuhn, A., Kreil, G., and Wickner, W. (1986a) Both hydrophobic domains of M13 procoat are required to initiate membrane insertion. *EMBO J.* 5: 3681–3685.

Kuhn, A., Wickner, W., and Kreil, G. (1986b) The cytoplasmic carboxy terminus of M13 procoat is required for the membrane insertion of its central domain. *Nature* 322: 335–339.

Kuroiwa, T., Sakaguchi, M., Mihara, K., and Omura, T. (1991) Systematic analysis of stop-transfer sequence for microsomal membrane. *J. Biol. Chem.* 266: 9251–9255.

Machamer, C. E., and Rose, J. K. (1987) A specific transmembrane domain of a coronavirus E1 glycoprotein is required for its retention in the Golgi region. *J. Cell. Biol.* 105: 1205–1214.

McGovern, K., and Beckwith, J. (1991) Membrane insertion of the *Escherichia coli* MalF protein in cells with impaired secretion machinery. *J. Biol. Chem.* 266: 20870–20876.

McGovern, K., Ehrmann, M., and Beckwith, J. (1991) Decoding signals for membrane protein assembly using alkaline phosphatase fusions. *EMBO J.* 10: 2773–2782.

Miyazawa, S., Osumi, T., Hashimoto, T., Ohno, K., Miura, S., and Fujiki, Y. (1989) Peroxisome targeting signal of rat liver acyl-coenzyme A oxidase resides at the carboxy terminus. *Mol. Cell. Biol.* 9: 83–91.

Nilsson, I. M., and von Heijne, G. (1990) Fine-tuning the topology of a polytopic membrane protein. Role of positively and negatively charged residues. *Cell* 62: 1135–1141.

Parks, G. D., and Lamb, R. A. (1991) Topology of eukaryotic type-II membrane proteins—importance of N-terminal positively charged residues flanking the hydrophobic domain. *Cell* 64: 777–787.

Pelham, H.R.B. (1990) The retention signal for soluble proteins of the endoplasmic reticulum. *Trends Biochem. Sci.* 15: 483–486.

Peters, C., Braun, M., Weber, B., Wendland, M., Schmidt, B., Pohlmann, R., Waheed, A., and von Figura, K. (1990) Targeting of a lysosomal membrane protein—a tyrosine-containing endocytosis signal in the cytoplasmic tail of lysosomal acid phosphatase is necessary and sufficient for targeting to lysosomes. *EMBO J.* 9: 3497–3506.

Pugsley, A. P. (1989) Protein Targeting. San Diego: Academic Press.

Schatz, P. J., and Beckwith, J. (1990) Genetic analysis of protein export in *Escherichia coli. Annu. Rev. Genet.* 24: 215–248.

Shackleton, J. B., and Robinson, C. (1991) Transport of proteins into chloroplasts—the thylakoidal processing peptidase is a signal-type peptidase with stringent substrate requirements at the –3-position and –1-position. *J. Biol. Chem.* 266: 12152–12156.

Silver, P. A. (1991) How proteins enter the nucleus. *Cell* 64: 489–497.

Struyve, M., Moons, M., and Tommassen, J. (1991) Carboxy-terminal phenylalanine is essential for the correct assembly of a bacterial outer membrane protein. *J. Mol. Biol.* 218: 141–148.

von Heijne, G. (1985) Signal sequences. The limits of variation. *J. Mol. Biol.* 184: 99–105.

von Heijne, G. (1986a) The distribution of positively charged residues in bacterial inner membrane proteins correlates with the transmembrane topology. *EMBO J.* 5: 3021–3027.

von Heijne, G. (1986b) Mitochondrial targeting sequences may form amphiphilic helices. *EMBO J.* 5: 1335–1342.

von Heijne, G. (1986c) Net N-C charge imbalance may be important for signal sequence function in bacteria. *J. Mol. Biol.* 192: 287–290.

von Heijne, G. (1986d) Towards a comparative anatomy of N-terminal topogenic protein sequences. *J. Mol. Biol.* 189: 239–242.

von Heijne, G. (1988) Transcending the impenetrable: how proteins come to terms with membranes. *Biochim. Biophys. Acta* 947: 307–333.

von Heijne, G. (1989) Control of topology and mode of assembly of a polytopic membrane protein by positively charged residues. *Nature* 341: 456–458.

von Heijne, G. (1990a) Protein targeting signals. *Curr. Opin. Cell. Biol.* 2: 604–608.

von Heijne, G. (1990b) The signal peptide. *J. Membrane Biol.* 115: 195–201.

von Heijne, G. (1992) Membrane protein structure prediction—hydrophobicity analysis and the positive-inside rule. *J. Mol. Biol.* 225: 487–494.

von Heijne, G., and Blomberg, C. (1979) Trans-membrane translocation of proteins: the direct transfer model. *Eur. J. Biochem.* 97: 175–181.

von Heijne, G., and Gavel, Y. (1988) Topogenic signals in integral membrane proteins. *Eur. J. Biochem.* 174: 671–678.

von Heijne, G., and Manoil, C. (1990) Membrane proteins—from sequence to structure. *Prot. Eng.* 4: 109–112.

von Heijne, G., and Nishikawa, K. (1991) Chloroplast transit peptides—the perfect random coil? *FEBS Lett.* 278: 1–3.

von Heijne, G., Steppuhn, J., and Herrmann, R. G. (1989) Domain structure of mitochondrial and chloroplast targeting peptides. *Eur. J. Biochem.* 180: 535–545.

von Heijne, G., Wickner, W., and Dalbey, R. E. (1988) The cytoplasmic domain of *Escherichia coli* leader peptidase is a "translocation poison: sequence. *Proc. Natl. Acad. Sci. USA* 85: 3363–3366.

Weiss, M. S., Kreusch, A., Schiltz, E., Nestel, U., Welte, W., Weckesser, J., and Schulz, G. E. (1991) The structure of porin from *Rhodobacter capsulata* at 1.8 Å resolution. *FEBS Lett.* 280: 379–382.

Wickner, W. (1988) Mechanisms of membrane assembly: general lessons from the study of M13 coat protein and *Escherichia coli* leader peptidase. *Biochemistry* 27: 1081–1086.

Wickner, W., Driessen, A.J.M., and Hartl, F. U. (1991) The enzymology of protein translocation across the *Escherichia coli* plasma membrane. *Annu. Rev. Biochem.* 60: 101–124.

Wolfe, P. B., Rice, M., and Wickner, W. (1985) Effects of two *sec* genes on protein assembly into the plasma membrane of *Escherichia coli. J. Biol. Chem.* 260: 1836–1841.

Yamane, K., Akiyama, Y., Ito, K., and Mizushima, S. (1990) A positively charged region is a determinant of the orientation of cytoplasmic membrane proteins in *Escherichia coli. J. Biol. Chem.* 265: 21166–21171.

3

Folding and Assembly
of Integral Membrane Proteins:
An Introduction

JEAN-LUC POPOT, CATHERINE DE VITRY, and ARIANE ATTEIA

"That's right," shouted Vroomfondel, "we demand rigidly defined areas of doubt
and uncertainty!"

> Douglas Adams, *The Hitchhiker's Guide to the Galaxy*

As recently as 1980, the structure of integral membrane proteins was largely *terra
incognita*. None of them had yielded three-dimensional crystals, and determination
of the amino acid sequence of bacteriorhodopsin (BR) by the groups of Yu. A.
Ovchinnikov (Ovchinnikov et al., 1979) and H. G. Khorana (Khorana et al., 1979)
had been a biochemical *tour de force*. The most detailed three-dimensional information available was—and was to remain until 1985—the medium-resolution structure of BR that R. Henderson and N. Unwin (1975) had established by electron
microscopy. The electron density map showed the bulk of BR to be made up of a
bundle of transmembrane α-helices. Since spectroscopic data on bacterial outer
membrane porins (Rosenbusch, 1974) indicated that these integral proteins were
primarily made up of β-sheets, it was clear that the model offered by BR was not
universally transposable.

Two developments of the early 1980s were to change prospects radically, albeit at
quite different paces. Introduction of molecular genetic methods resulted in the determination of hundreds of coding sequences (for an overview of eukaryotic integral
proteins, see Popot and de Vitry, 1990). Development of procedures to grow three-
dimensional crystals of detergent-solubilized proteins, initiated by H. Michel and R.
M. Garavito (Michel and Oesterhelt, 1980; Garavito and Rosenbusch, 1980), led to
the atomic structures of photosynthetic reaction centers (Deisenhofer et al., 1985)
and of bacterial porins (Weiss et al., 1991; Cowan et al., 1992). However, growing
well-ordered crystals of membrane proteins has remained a rare exploit (for reviews,
see Kühlbrandt, 1988; Garavito and Picot, 1990; Michel, 1991; Reiss-Husson,
1992). A huge gap now exists between the number of proteins for which sequence
information is available and the prospects of access to their three-dimensional structure.

In addition to its intrinsic interest, understanding the folding of integral membrane proteins (IMPs) is a step toward deriving predictions from sequences in order to make for scarce crystallographic data. It will be apparent from this text and from other chapters in this volume that thermodynamic constraints on IMP folding are particularly strong. Up to a point, predicting the three-dimensional structure of an unknown IMP therefore appears easier than predicting that of a totally unknown soluble protein. Care should be exercised, however. The amount of hard structural information on which to base generalizations is presently limited, and we are far from fully understanding what, in the final structure of a membrane protein, is dictated by thermodynamics and what by biosynthesis.

The aim of this chapter is to present, in a necessarily sketchy way, a number of observations that bear on the problem of membrane protein folding and assembly—both questions being closely linked. Focus is on *integral* (also called *intrinsic*) membrane proteins, more specifically on those proteins whose polypeptide chain spans the membrane at least once, as opposed to *peripheral* (or *extrinsic*) membrane proteins. We first recall some basic facts about folding of soluble proteins and about the energetics of polypeptide insertion into membranes. We then summarize the salient features of the few IMPs whose structures are known and the main conclusions to be drawn from in vitro refolding experiments and genetic engineering of IMPs. We then propose that hydrophobic α-helices, which probably make up the transmembrane region of most IMPs, can be considered as autonomous folding domains, discuss some implications of this autonomy for IMP assembly and evolution, and summarize current data on the nature of topogenic determinants. Next, we describe some examples of IMP biosynthesis and assembly in various cell compartments and discuss the correlations existing between subcellular localization, structure, and assembly. Finally, we touch rapidly on the role that chaperones and other proteins may play in the folding and assembly of IMPs.

Throughout this chapter, the aim is not to provide exhaustive coverage, but to identify dominant trends and possible reasons for apparent exceptions. References are limited to a few key articles on each topic.

General Background

In this section we offer some background information on the folding of soluble proteins and on the particular problems raised by the insertion of polypeptides into lipid bilayers.

Folding of Soluble Proteins

Since much more is known about the structure and folding of soluble proteins than of IMPs, it is very useful, in the effort to understand the particular constraints that apply to IMPs, to consider first what is known about soluble proteins (see also Chapter 1). The present summary is highly schematic, and the reader is referred to recent reviews as a starting point for further reading (see, e.g., Ghélis and Yon, 1982; Finkelstein and Ptitsyn, 1987; Kim and Baldwin, 1990; Jaenicke, 1991).

According to the framework model, folding of soluble proteins starts with the formation of elements of secondary structure. These elements then assemble, with the hydrophobic effect playing a major role by driving burial of hydrophobic residues away from water. An intermediate stage is reached, called *molten globule,* in which the protein has essentially acquired all of its secondary structure. However, the molten globule is less compact than the native state, and its hydrophobic interior is more accessible and fluid-like. A final, rate-limiting step leads from the molten globule to the native state, in which precise packing of the internal side chains is achieved.

Examination of high-resolution structures of soluble proteins shows that almost all ionizable side chains and most polar residues have segregated to the surface of the protein. The rare buried ionizable groups are stabilized by multiple polar interactions, particularly hydrogen bonds. Main chain peptide bonds not in contact with water are engaged into periodic secondary structure elements, α-helices and β-sheets, that permit hydrogen bonding of the NH and CO groups. α-Helices and β-sheets organize into a relatively limited number of types of motifs, e.g., the four-helix bundle or the various β-barrels, in which there is optimal packing of side chains against one another. One or more motifs constitute a domain, i.e., a compact region with independent stability, generally comprising some 70–150 residues. Denaturation and renaturation experiments indeed often show that regions of a protein that have been defined as domains on the basis of compactness can unfold and refold independently from one another. One or several domains constitute a protein or a subunit. Function(s) can be carried by individual domains or be dependent on their association. Domains can often be separated one from another by proteolytic cleavage. If their surfaces of interaction show sufficient affinity, they may remain noncovalently associated and the protein may retain full activity. In the present discussion, the word *domains,* which tends to be used loosely to denote any region of a protein, will be used exclusively with the sense of "the smallest regions of a protein that are able to acquire a stable three-dimensional structure similar to the native one in the absence of the rest of the molecule."

In many cases, it has been shown than renaturation and subunit assembly in vitro lead to fully active proteins, implying that the native state lies at the (or at least a) free energy minimum and can be reached independently of the biosynthetic history of the protein. In vivo, however, folding and assembly are assisted by molecular chaperones. The possible roles of chaperones and other proteins in the folding and assembly of IMPs will be discussed later (see Insertion, Folding, and Assembly as Assisted Processes, below).

Insertion of Polypeptides into Lipid Bilayers

The energetics of protein insertion and folding into lipid membranes have been discussed in a number of reviews, and only the major conclusions will be summarized here. For further reading, see Chapters 1 and 4.

Because of its low dielectric constant and inability to establish hydrogen bonds, the fatty acyl region of a lipid bilayer is a very poor solvent for polar groups. A low dielectric constant means that burying charges or polarized groups will be energetically costly. It has been estimated that if an ionizable side chain is to be buried, it is energetically more favorable first to neutralize the charge, e.g., by protonating an acidic side chain, and to bury the polar but electrically neutral group. Neutralization away from the pK, however, is itself energetically costly. Various estimates have been made of the cost of burying ionizable side chains that have been incorporated into *hydrophobicity scales*. To give a numerical example, it is estimated that burying a lysine residue inserted into an otherwise hydrophobic α-helix costs about 8.8 kcal/mol (Engelman et al., 1986). This means that, at 25°C, inclusion of the lysine would shift the partition coefficient of the helix by a factor of about 3.10^6 in favor of the aqueous phase.

The inability of the fatty acyl chains to establish hydrogen bonds means that transferring hydrogen bonding groups from water to lipids will require breaking hydrogen bonds (or dragging water in, which only compounds the difficulty). Two issues should be distinguished here, main chain atoms and side chains.

Main chain hydrogen bonding groups (NH and CO), if they are dragged into a membrane, will behave as they do in the hydrophobic core of soluble proteins. Namely, hydrogen bonds will form between the main chain groups, which induces the formation of periodic secondary structures, α-helices or β-sheets. These structures will be immensely more stable than they would be in aqueous solution, where bonds broken upon unfolding can be reformed with water. It is estimated that breaking a single hydrogen bond without reforming it costs around 5 kcal/mol (corresponding to an equilibrium constant of about 2.4×10^{-4}) and that the free energy of stabilization of a 20 residue transmembrane α-helix against complete unfolding is about 60 kcal/mol (Engelman and Steitz, 1981). By comparison, the total free energy of stabilization of a soluble protein rarely exceeds 10 kcal/mol. Satisfaction of (most) main chain hydrogen bonds is expected to be a major constraint on polypeptides traversing a hydrophobic phase, and this constraint indeed is very well obeyed in known membrane protein structures. Individual α-helices can achieve the completion of hydrogen bonds within a single sequence segment, while β-strands must associate into sheets. For the hydrogen bonds at the edges of the sheet to be satisfied, the sheet must close upon itself to form a cylinder (β-barrel). Because of constraints on hydrogen bond linearity and on packing of internal side chains, regular β-barrels (in soluble proteins) comprise at least six strands, and generally more (Richardson, 1981). Since turns do not satisfy hydrogen bonds within the main chain, one should expect the rims of β-barrels or the connecting loops between α-helices to lie outside the fatty acyl chain region.

Burying a hydrogen-bonding side chain into lipids can be easy (e.g., tryptophan or threonine) or very costly (e.g., glutamine or asparagine), depending on the number of hydrogen bonds to be broken, on the ability of the side chain to bind to other buried atoms, and on the hydrophobicity of the rest of the side chain. Conversely, totally or largely hydrophobic side chains perturb the hydrogen bond network of water and tend to be expelled from it (hydrophobic effect). Given access to a nonpolar phase, hydrophobic side chains will partition favorably into it. The propensity of a given stretch of residues to partition into a lipid phase will thus depend on the balance between hydrophobic and polar side chains in the segment, an otherwise hydrophobic segment being able to drag into the lipid a very polar residue, and vice versa. Polar interactions between buried groups are expected to be very strong. It has been estimated that a single hydrogen bond would be sufficient to bring about a stable association between two transmembrane α-helices (Popot and Engelman, 1990). Interaction of buried basic and acidic residues has been shown experimentally to be responsible for oligomerization of subunits TCR-α and CD3-δ of the T-cell-receptor complex (Cosson et al., 1991).

While the above considerations must be borne in mind when evaluating transmembrane folding models and possible pathways for folding and assembly, one should not overlook the extreme simplification of the picture just drawn. A major shortcoming, discussed elsewhere in this volume by S. H. White (Chapter 4), is due to treating the water–lipid interface as a sharp barrier between a slab of highly hydrophobic solvent, the thickness of the fatty acyl chain region, and a water-like phase encompassing both lipid polar heads and the bulk solution. Changes in properties, including the effective dielectric constant, are continuous and complex, and this interfacial region is far from isotropic. Experimental data indicate that small hydrophobic peptides binding to the interfacial region of a lipid bilayer have already spent more than half the free energy of transfer due to the hydrophobic effect (Jacobs and White, 1989). Reasoning in terms of an all-or-none equilibrium between bulk aqueous solution and bulk hydrophobic phase is often convenient but should not lead to overlooking interfacial phenomena.

Known Structures

Detailed three-dimensional structures of four kinds of IMPs are presently available. They will not be described in detail here. Some of them are discussed in Chapters 1 and 9. Only major features will be recalled, particularly those that are needed for subsequent discussion.

Resolution Achieved

Photosynthetic reaction centers (RC) from two genuses of purple bacteria, *Rhodopseudomonas viridis* and *Rhodobacter sphaeroides,* and from three bacterial **porins** have yielded well-ordered three-dimensional crystals of protein–detergent complexes, whose structures have been studied at atomic resolutions (1.8–2.3 Å) by x-ray diffraction (see Deisenhofer and Michel, 1989; Rees et al., 1989; Weiss et al., 1991; Cowan et al., 1992; and references therein). Subsequent neutron diffraction studies have established the position in the RC crystals of the detergent that has been substituted for the lipids, i.e., by implication, that occupied in situ by the bilayer (Roth et al., 1989, 1991). Of some 200 molecules of bound water that have been resolved, only 5 lie in this region (Deisenhofer and Michel, 1989). **Bacteriorhodopsin** (BR) yields highly ordered two-dimensional crystals, which have been used by Henderson and colleagues to develop the methodology of high-resolution electron crystallography. In their 1975 study, Henderson and Unwin established that the transmembrane region of BR is made up of seven α-helices, whose connectivity, however, was to remain undecided for the next 15 years. Medium-resolution studies using neutron diffraction established the position and orientation of the chromophore retinal, which lies in the middle of the α-helix bundle (Jubb et al., 1984; Heyn et al., 1988), and of some specific transmembrane sequence segments (Popot et al., 1989). This information has facilitated the interpretation of a 3.5–10 Å resolution electron density map (Henderson et al., 1990). (For technical reasons, the resolution of maps calculated from electron microscopic [EM] data collected on planar 2D crystals is lower in the direction perpendicular to the membrane plane.) While uncertainties persist about some features of the resulting model, e.g., the exact arrangement of the extramembrane loops, there are no ambiguities about the secondary and tertiary structures of BR. Finally, electron crystallographic study of artificial two-dimensional crystals has recently yielded a three-dimensional map, at a similar resolution, of pea **light harvesting complex II** (LHCII), a chlorophyll–protein complex (Kühlbrandt and Wang, 1991; Kühlbrandt et al., 1994). While the extramembrane loops are not resolved and the connectivity of the transmembrane segments remains speculative, the general arrangement of the transmembrane region is clear (see chapter by W. Kühlbrandt, this volume).

Lower-resolution data, generally obtained by crystallographic analysis of EM images, are available on a number of other membrane proteins, e.g. rhodopsin, photosystem I reaction centers, the nicotinic acetylcholine receptor, cytochrome-c oxidase, gap junctions, as well as on a number of other porins. High-resolution x-ray data have been obtained on two pore-forming proteins in their soluble form, the C-terminal fragment of colicin A (Parker et al., 1989) and a δ-endotoxin (Li et al., 1991), leading to suggestions about their mode of membrane insertion. A number of membrane proteins anchored by one or a couple of transmembrane segment(s) have been crystallized after the anchor was proteolytically removed. This approach has led to high-resolution x-ray structures for hemagglutinin (Wilson et al., 1981; cf. Assembly of Hemagglutinin, below), neuraminidase (Varghese et al., 1983), histocompatibility antigen HLA-A2 (Bjorkman et al., 1987), and the bacterial aspartate receptor (Milburn et al., 1991). Finally, the structure of prostaglandin synthase, a non-spanning integral membrane protein, has recently been reported by Picot et al. (1994). Each of these studies offers numerous interesting insights, but they seldom permit definite conclusions to be drawn regarding the nature and arrangement of transmembrane segments, the main topic in this chapter.

Functions

Functionally, BR, RCs, LHCII, and porins belong to different classes. LHCII and RCs are solid-state electronic devices, which collect and transfer excitons (LHCII) and use their energy to drive an electron pump (RC). Both proteins contain a large number of prosthetic groups. The chemistry of energy conversion is done mainly (but not solely) by the chromophores. The main role of the polypeptides is to provide binding pockets to hold the chromophores in the proper geometrical arrangement. BR is a light-driven proton pump, in which limited but critical movements of the retinal and the protein couple proton transfer to retinal isomerization. RC and BR are located in the bacterial plasma membrane and LHCII in its topological equivalent, the chloroplast thylakoid membrane. Porins may also be considered as solid-state devices, although not electronic ones. Located in the outer membrane of gram-negative bacteria, porins form permanent pores, which ensure its permeability to small solutes (whether this function is regulated in vivo is a matter of debate; cf. Jap and Walian, 1990; Schirmer and Rosenbusch, 1991).

Quaternary Structures.

All four proteins mentioned above crystallize as oligomers. Porins (molecular mass = 32 kDa) form very tough homotrimers that resist denaturation in sodium dodecyl sulfate (SDS) at room temperature and certainly represent the native state of association of the protein in vivo (see Porin Folding and Assembly, below). LHCII (molecular mass of the protein part ≈25 kDa, plus 15 chlorophylls) and BR (≈27 kDa, plus 1 retinal) also organize in the plane of the membrane as homotrimers, those of LHCII resisting to some extent solubilization with nondenaturing detergents. Trimers are probably the natural state of LHCII in vivo. Trimerization of BR and the organization of trimers into a hexagonal lattice occur spontaneously in vivo (forming the so-called purple membrane), but are not required for BR function.

RCs have a much more complicated quaternary structure (see Rees et al., this volume). The core of the transmembrane region is formed by the quasisymmetrical association of two homologous but not identical subunits, L and M (with molecular masses of approximately 31 and 36 kDa, respectively), which together ligand four bacteriochorophylls, two pheophytins, two quinones, and a non-heme atom of iron. A third protein, H (≈28 kDa), is located mainly in the cytosol but spans the membrane with a single transmembrane segment. In *Rhodop. viridis*, the extremity of this segment (the N terminus of the protein) associates in the periplasmic space with a peripheral protein, a four-heme cytochrome that is bound noncovalently to the extramembrane loops of L and M and covalently (via its N terminus) to a lipid anchor. The cytochrome subunit is missing in the *Rhodob. sphaeroides* RC. In vivo, RCs further associate laterally with LHC–protein complexes.

Secondary Structures and Transmembrane Topologies.

The transmembrane region of BR consists, as already mentioned, of seven α-helices 20–27 residues long and 30–40 Å in length (Fig. 3.1*e*) (see Henderson et al., 1990). Three of them are nearly normal to the plane of the membrane, while the other four are tilted by up to 20° (see Chapter 1). Three helices contain proline residues and are slightly bent. The seven helices are arranged in a somewhat flattened, bean-shaped cylinder around the retinal. Helices follow each other in their order in the sequence, without interweaving. Although largely hydrophobic (Table 3.1), their transmembrane section nevertheless includes four aspartic acid residues, a lysine (to which the retinal is bound as a Schiff base), and a number of hydrogen-bonding residues (Fig. 3.1*e*). The most hydrophobic face of each helix is turned toward the lipids, while most of the polar residues face inside. BR molecules contact their neighbors in the trimer by the small ends of the bean, thereby forming a cylinder, two α-helices thick, in the middle of which six molecules of lipids are trapped (three in each monolayer). One remarkable feature of the 2D crystal is that trimers do not contact each other directly (at least at the bilayer level), but are separated by a layer of lipids, one molecule thick.

RCs follow the same general transmembrane organization as BR (Fig. 3.1*a–c*). Subunits L and M each comprise five transmembrane α-helices, which form a sort of cage around the chromophores, with the single transmembrane helix of subunit H

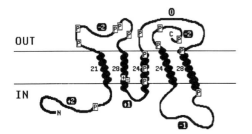

(a) Reaction center subunit L

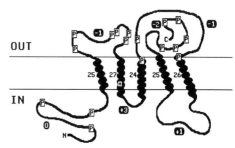

(b) Reaction center subunit M

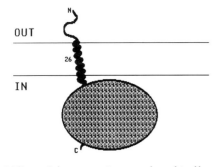

(c) Reaction center subunit H

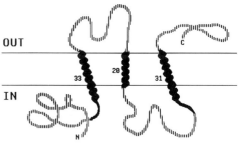

(d) LHC-II

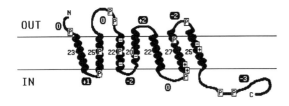

(e) Bacteriorhodopsin

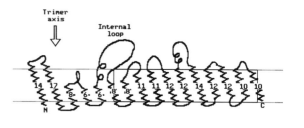

(f) Porin

lying on the outside of this core. (According to the nomenclature introduced by G. Blobel [1980], subunit H is a *bitopic* protein [possessing a single transmembrane segment that spans both halves of the bilayer] while subunits L and M, as well as BR, LHC, and porins, are *polytopic* [multispanning] proteins.) Homologous helices of L and M are arranged symmetrically with respect to a pseudo twofold axis normal to the plane of the membrane. A limited interweaving is present within each subunit, the last helix in each sequence, helix E, being located in the structure between helices C and D. Helices comprise from 24 to 28 residues, reaching about 42 Å, which means that in situ helices extend beyond the fatty acyl chain region (in most bilayers about 30 Å thick, corresponding to 20 residues in α-helical configuration). Tilt angles between the normal and the membrane plane are 22° on average and up to $\approx 38°$. The helices are very hydrophobic (Table 3.1), and the region that presumably lies at the level of the fatty acyl chains does not contain a single arginine, lysine, glutamate, or aspartate residue. Hydrogen-bonding residues tend to face inside, as in BR. Nevertheless, the inside of the bundle cannot be described as hydrophilic, since it is just as hydrophobic as the inside of a soluble, globular protein (Rees et al., 1989). Rather, it is the outside surface of the transmembrane region that is comparatively more hydrophobic.

LHCII does not depart from this scheme (Fig. 3.1*d*). The three α-helices in each protomer, two of which are tilted with respect to the membrane normal by up to 30

Fig. 3.1 *(opposite)*. A schematic representation of the transmembrane arrangement of integral membrane proteins of known three-dimensional structure. For the sake of homogeneity, all proteins have been represented with the same orientation, i.e., with the outside of the cell (or the lumen of the thylakoid) on top. They may therefore be inverted with respect to original representations. The schemes refer to *Rhodob. viridis* photosynthetic reaction center subunits L (*a*), M (*b*), and H (*c*) (see Michel and Deisenhofer, 1989), pea light harvesting complex II (*d*) (Kühlbrandt and Wang, 1991), bacteriorhodopsin (*e*) (Henderson et al., 1990), and *Rhodob. capsulatus* porin (*f*) (Weiss et al., 1991). *Helical proteins:* The number of residues in each helix, indicated next to it, is taken as defined by the authors. Note that helix limits do not necessarily correspond to the limits of the fatty acyl region of the bilayer, the position of which is not directly established. Orientation with respect to the membrane is indicated qualitatively, as is the approximate length of the extramembrane loops. Net charges of the loops (white-on-black figures) are calculated by assuming strongly acidic or basic residues (Asp, Glu, Lys, Arg) to be charged. It is generally ambiguous as to what extent residues close to the extremity of helices are buried. When not taken into account in the loops, these residues have been indicated by *plus* and *minus signs*, even though they may not carry an actual charge. Prolines are indicated by *P*. Prolines and charged residues are not indicated for subunit H nor for LHCII. In the latter case, the exact pathway of the polypeptide chain in the electron density map was not definitely established at the time the figure was prepared; the tentative connectivity shown has been confirmed since at high resolution (W. Kühlbrandt, personal communication). *Porin:* The number of residues in each β-strand is taken as defined by Weiss et al. (1991). Their actual inclination with respect to the membrane plane is not uniform. It varies from about 60° near the trimer axis to about 30° on the opposite, lipid-facing side of the barrel (cf. Fig. 3.2*a*). The exact position of the membrane is not known, and the orientation of the model with respect to the periplasm and external medium is tentative. The *solid rectangle* defines approximately the region of the barrel that faces the lipids. The largest extramembrane loop, which protrudes from the rim of the barrel close to the point where the rim is lowest, folds inside and lines the internal surface of the lipid-exposed wall (cf. Fig. 3.2*b*).

Table 3.1. Number and Hydrophobicity of Known and Putative Transmembrane α-Helices in Nine Integral Membrane Proteins

Protein	Helix (ΔG, kcal/residue)											
	A / I	B / II	C / III	D / IV	E / V	F / VI	G / VII	H / VIII	I / IX	J / X	K / XI	L / XII
Known 3D structure:												
Reaction center												
Subunit H	1.63											
Subunit L	2.60	1.86	2.11	1.70	1.89							
Subunit M	2.31	2.15	2.02	1.71	1.86							
Bacteriorhodopsin	2.02	2.01	0.94	1.50	2.13	1.74	1.25					
LHCII	0.89	1.46	2.09									
Unknown 3D structure:												
lac Permease	2.77	2.08	2.75	1.68	2.22	2.38	1.21	1.38	1.28	0.97	1.69	2.29
MalF	2.14	2.06	2.44	2.56	2.08	1.66	1.40	2.33				
β_2-AR	2.54	1.91	0.91	2.23	2.08	2.37	0.79					
AChR δ-subunit	2.06	1.91	2.01	2.59								

Helices are named alphabetically and numbered (roman numerals) according to their order in the sequence. Sequences are from the following organisms (except when otherwise indicated, sources of sequences are given in Popot and de Vitry [1990]): reaction center (RC), *Rhodob. viridis;* bacteriorhodopsin, *Halobacterium salinarium* (Khorana et al., 1979); LHCII, pea; *lac* permease, *Escherichia coli* (Büchel et al., 1980); MalF protein, *E. coli* (Froshauer and Beckwith, 1984); β_2-adrenergic receptor (β_2-AR), hamster; nicotinic acetylcholine receptor (AChR), *Torpedo californica.* The ΔG per residue indicated corresponds to the free energy penalty for transferring from lipids to water the most hydrophobic 17-residue segment overlapping the transmembrane α-helix, estimated using the GES scale (Engelman et al., 1986). Positive values indicate that transfer is unfavorable. For a comparison with other proteins, see Popot and de Vitry (1990).

degrees, form a scaffold on which chlorophyll molecules attach. Two helices are quite long (almost 50 Å) and the third particularly short (30 Å). At the current degree of resolution, the exact position of individual side chains cannot be ascertained.

Porins radically depart from the α-helix bundle scheme (Figs. 3.1f and 3.2) (Weiss et al., 1991), as was inferred long ago from secondary structure measurements (reviewed by Schirmer and Rosenbusch, 1991). Each protomer forms an antiparallel 16-strand β-barrel oriented with its axis normal to the membrane plane. The height of the rim varies from 40 to 20 Å, i.e., in the latter case, less than the $\approx$30 Å required to cross the fatty acyl chain region. The strands follow each other without interweaving, in their order in the sequence (Fig. 3.1f). Their length varies from 6 to 17 residues, and their tilt angle with respect to the normal varies from 30 degrees to 60 degrees (Fig. 3.2a). The outside of the barrel is hydrophobic, except where the rim is shortest. The interior of the barrel is partially filled by a loop that hangs from the rim and delimits the actual size of the pore (Fig. 3.2b). Protomers associate by juxtaposing the regions where the rim of the barrel is shortest and more polar, masking it from contact with the lipids.

Experimental Studies of Membrane Protein Folding

Refolding Full-Length Membrane Proteins

A key issue when considering protein folding is whether the native state is the most stable one, i.e. the one corresponding to the lowest free energy. There is no a priori

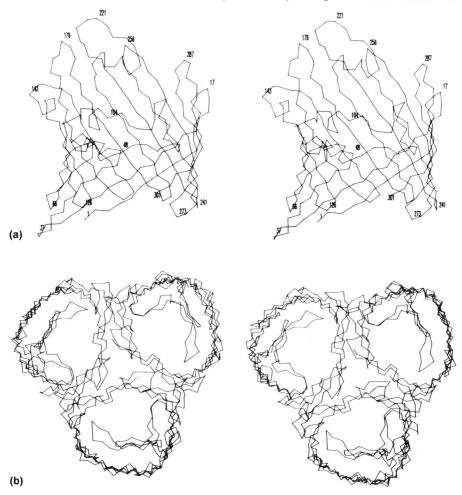

Fig. 3.2. Stereoviews of the structure of porin from *Rhodob. capsulatus. a:* A monomer viewed from a point inside the membrane, close to the trimer axis of symmetry. (From Weiss et al., 1991.) *b:* A trimer seen from a point lying outside the membrane on the trimer axis. (From Weiss et al., 1990.)

answer to this question. Since the pathway followed by a protein during folding does not involve equilibration among all possible conformational states, it is in principle possible for the protein to become trapped into a conformation that corresponds to a local minimum and has been determined by the particular pathway followed during folding. This possibility is particularly obvious for IMPs, given the barrier the membrane presents to extensive reorganization. The issue is of considerable interest from the point of view of cell biology and from that of the energetics of protein folding. Furthermore, a positive answer to this question makes it possible, at least theoretically, to deduce a protein's three-dimensional structure from its sequence.

The possibility that the native state corresponds to the global free energy minimum can be tested by examining whether a protein, which has lost all structural information except for its primary structure, can refold to the native state under non-physiological conditions. Note that (*1*) such a demonstration cannot be absolute; the true global minimum may be out of reach in each situation for kinetic reasons; and (2) as for enzymatic reactions, successful refolding in vitro does not exclude that, in vivo, the same final state is reached in a catalyzed manner.

For soluble proteins, the demonstration that the final state of a protein does not depend on its life history was first provided by the renaturation experiments of Anfinsen et al. (1961), and this line of research has been intensely pursued ever since (see, e.g., Jaenicke, 1991, and references therein). For IMPs, pioneering experiments were done by H. G. Khorana's group, with BR as the test protein. Huang et al. (1981) first demonstrated that bacterio-opsin (BO, i.e., the protein without the retinal) could be fully denatured (as ascertained by nuclear magnetic resonance [NMR]) in organic solvents, transferred to an SDS solution, and renatured by addition of a large excess of lipid/bile salt–mixed micelles, in which the SDS became diluted. The refolded protein bound retinal, regenerating the spectrum of BR, and, when transferred to lipid vesicles by dialyzing out the detergents, pumped protons. It was later shown, with a modification of this protocol, that refolded BR could form native-like two-dimensional crystals, whose x-ray and neutron diffraction patterns were identical to those of native purple membrane (Popot et al., 1986, 1987). Similar experiments have been reported with OmpF porin (Eiselé and Rosenbusch, 1990). To our knowledge, no other IMP has been fully renatured from a completely denatured state yet, although promising experiments have been reported using light-harvesting complexes (see Paulsen et al., 1990; Cammarata and Schmidt, 1992; and references therein).

Refolding of Membrane Proteins from Fragments In Vitro

As discussed earlier under Folding of Soluble Proteins, domains in soluble proteins can be separately denatured and renatured. In other words, they behave as structurally autonomous entities. Similar experiments can be done with fragments of BO. Liao et al. (1983) showed that two fragments of BO, obtained by a single proteolytic cleavage between the second and third of the seven transmembrane helices, could be separately refolded into lipid/detergent–mixed micelles. Due to the presence of detergent, the refolded fragments were unstable, but, if mixed rapidly together, they would reassociate to regenerate cleaved BO.

A variant of the Liao et al. protocol, which permitted direct transfer from the SDS solution to lipids rather than to mixed micelles, yielded lipid vesicles in which each fragment had been separately reinserted. Circular dichroism spectra indicated that each fragment contained the amount of α-helix expected if it had reformed the same number of transmembrane α-helices as it contained in the native protein. When the vesicles were fused, in the absence of any detergent, the fragments reassociated to yield BO and, if retinal was added, BR (Popot et al., 1987). The structure of (cleaved) BR renatured from fragments has been studied crystallographically and found, once again, to be indistinguishable from that of native BR (Popot et al., 1986). Helix rotational orientations in such reconstituted samples, determined by neutron crystallography (Popot et al., 1989; Samatey et al., 1992, 1993), are within experimental error (about 20 degrees) from those determined on native BR by electron crystallography (Henderson et al., 1990), a further confirmation of accurate renaturation.

These experiments show that BO fragments contain all of the information that is needed in order for them to refold properly under conditions that have very little to do with those prevailing during biosynthesis. By "properly," we mean that the refolded fragments must have reformed the correct number of transmembrane helices at approximately their correct position in the sequence. As mentioned, this is borne out by direct measurements of the amount of α-helical structure present in each preparation. This behavior is most simply explained by assuming that each transmembrane segment, given proper conditions, is able to form by itself a transmembrane helix, without assistance from other parts of the sequence. This conclusion is further supported by similar experiments using BO fragments encompassing other parts of the sequence (see Table 3.2 and later under Microassembly In Vitro). There are no

Table 3.2. Integral Membrane Proteins Assembled from Fragments That Had Been Either Refolded or Synthesized Independently

Origin of Fragments	Medium Where Assembly Takes Place	Protein	N. of Trans- membrane Helices	Hydrophobic Helices per Fragment	References
Proteolysis	Mixed micelles	Bacteriorhodopsin	7	2+5	a,b
Protolysis	Mixed micelles	Bacteriorhodopsin		5+2	c,d
Proteolysis	Lipid vesicles	Bacteriorhodopsin		2+5	e,f
Proteolysis	Lipid vesicles	Bacteriorhodopsin		5+2	g,h
Proteolysis plus synthesis	Lipid vesicles	Bacteriorhodopsin		1+1+5	h,i
Engineered mRNA	*Xenopus* oocyte (ER?)	β_2-Adrenergic receptor	7	5+2	j
Engineered plamids	*E. coli* plasma membrane	*lac* permease	12	2+10	k
		lac permease		6+6	l
		lac permease		1+11	m
Natural	Thylakoid	Cytochrome *b*	8	4+3+Δ	n,o
Natural	*E. coli* plasma membrane	Nicotinamide nucleotide transhydrogenase	14	4+Δ+9	p

The number of putative hydrophobic transmembrane helices is indicated for each fragment, in the order of the fragments in the sequence. For *lac* permease, we have followed the topology initially proposed by Foster et al. (1983), recently supported by gene fusion experiments (Calamia and Manoil, 1990). In addition to those listed, a number of complementation experiments have been reported in which some of the putative transmembrane segments are redundant (see under Helix Duplication and Shuffling), as well as experiments on integral proteins containing internal repeats (see under Biosynthesis by Fragments). Natural cases of split proteins correspond to integral proteins that are made up of one polypeptide chain in one type of membrane and two complementary, nonhomologous integral subunits in another. Cytochrome b_6 and subunit IV from the chloroplast $b_6 f$ complex are homologous to the N-terminal and C-terminal parts of cytochrome *b* from the mitochondrial bc_1 complex, respectively. A segment homologous to the last of the eight putative hydrophobic transmembrane α-helices in cytochrome *b* is missing in the chloroplast complex (indicated by Δ). The α- and β-subunits of *E. coli* nicotinamide nucleotide transhydrogenase (NNT) are homologous to the N- and C-terminal parts of beef NNT, respectively. The number of putative hydrophobic transmembrane segments in NNT has been corrected as suggested by M. Yamaguchi, in keeping with the revision of the bacterial sequence (cf. Yamaguchi and Hatefi, 1991). Helix 5 of beef NNT is missing from the bacterial α/β-complex (Δ). Updated from Popot and de Vitry (1990). References: a, Huang et al. (1981); b, Liao et al., (1983); c, Liao et al. (1984); d, Sigrist et al. (1988); e, Popot et al. (1986); f, Popot et al. (1987); g, Engelman et al. (1990); h, Kahn (1991); i, Kahn and Engelman (1992); j, Kobilka et al. (1988); k, Wrubel et al. (1990); l, Bibi and Kaback (1990); m, Kaback (1992); n, Heinemeyer et al. (1984); o, Cramer and Trebst, 1991; p, Yamaguchi et al. (1988).

direct observations on the arrangement of helices within each refolded fragment. However, retinal does not form a native-like chromophore with the five-helix fragment renatured in mixed micelles (Liao et al., 1983) or in vesicles (Popot et al., 1987), even though the five helices encompassed by this fragment form the quasitotality of the retinal-binding pocket in native BR (Popot et al., 1989; Henderson et al., 1990). This would suggest that, upon binding to the two-helix fragment, a native-like three-dimensional arrangement of helices in the five-helix fragment is acquired or at least that it becomes more stable. Another conclusion from these experiments is that the integrity of at least some of the extramembrane loops, while it will confer additional stability to the protein, is not essential to correct folding of the transmembrane region.

Assembly of Membrane Proteins from Fragments Synthesized Independently In Vivo

Using a different methodology, association of fragments of IMPs translated from separate mRNAs has been demonstrated with *lac* permease and with the β_2-adrenergic receptor (Table 3.2).

lac Permease is a lactose/proton symporter located in the plasma membrane of *E. coli* (for review, Kaback, 1992). According to its currently accepted topology (see Calamia and Manoil, 1990), its single polypeptide chain ($\approx$46 kDa) forms 12 transmembrane α-helices, most of which are very hydrophobic (cf. Table 3.1). Plasmids were constructed encompassing the regions coding for helices I–II or III–XII (Wrubel et al., 1990), I–VI or VII–XII (Bibi and Kaback, 1990), and I or II–XII (quoted in Kaback, 1992). In each case, expression of a single plasmid did not result in stable accumulation of the corresponding fragment or in any *lac* permease activity. Coexpression of two complementary fragments, on the other hand, resulted in the accumulation of cleaved but active permease. It seems highly likely that the two fragments were translated and inserted into the membrane independently and subsequently associated with each other, although the set-up of the experiments strictly does not permit one to rule out more complicated hypotheses. It is worth noting that the 11-helix C-terminal fragment started with an extramembrane segment that, in the natural situation, is part of the first periplasmic loop of the full-length protein. Functional complementation with the one-helix N-terminal fragment implies that at least a fraction of each fragment inserted with the correct vectoriality. This point is further discussed later under Determinants of Transmembrane Topology).

β_2-Adrenergic receptor ($\approx$47 kDa) is a member of the very large family of G-protein–coupled receptors (reviewed by Hargrave, 1991). As with all members of this family, it is thought to comprise seven transmembrane α-helices (cf. Schertler et al., 1993; Baldwin, 1993), some very hydrophobic and some only moderately so (cf. Table 3.1). Kobilka et al. (1988) constructed plasmids encoding either the first five or the last two of the putative helices, synthesized the corresponding mRNAs in COS-7 cells, and injected them either separately or simultaneously into *Xenopus* oocytes. Functional expression was tested by measuring ligand binding and adenylyl cyclase activation. As with *lac* permease, activity was observed upon simultaneous expression of both fragments.

Similar experiments have been described for proteins that contain internal repeats, in which the extramembrane region linking repeats was genetically cleaved and functionality recovered by simultaneous expression of the two fragments. These experiments do not bear directly on the folding autonomy of individual helices (repeats might be expected to be stable by themselves if they correspond to ancestral proteins) and are described later under α-Helix Autonomy and the Evolution of Integral Membrane Proteins.

Probing Transmembrane Topologies with Fusion Proteins

A powerful technique for probing the transmembrane topology of IMPs in *E. coli*, developed by J. Beckwith and colleagues (see Manoil and Beckwith, 1986; Manoil et al., 1990; D. Boyd, Chapter 6, this volume), is based on the observation that alkaline phosphatase, an enzyme encoded by the *phoA* gene, does not mature to its active form unless exported to the periplasm (critical disulfide bridges do not form in the cytosol). When the *phoA* gene (minus the region coding for the signal peptide) is fused in frame at the 3' extremity of the structural gene of an integral protein, high phosphatase activity is observed only if the enzyme has been exported to to the periplasm, which by inference indicates whether the C terminus of the integral protein normally faces the periplasm or the cytosol. Fusion to the *blaM* gene, which codes for β-lactamase and confers ampicillin resistance, can be used in much the same way (Broome-Smith et al., 1990).

Gene fusions can be used to probe the entire transmembrane topology by fusing *phoA* or *blaM* to truncated genes coding for an N-terminal fragment of the protein under study. This approach has been applied most extensively to MalF, a protein from *E. coli* plasma membrane that is involved in sugar import and contains eight putative transmembrane α-helices (Froshauer et al., 1988) (cf. Table 3.1). Presence and absence of phosphatase activity correlate well with fusion within predicted periplasmic and cytosolic loops, respectively. Less clear-cut results are obtained when fusions are made in the middle of a predicted transmembrane segment, or very close to its cytosolic end. In the latter case, there is evidence that lysine or arginine residues prevent flipping of the end of the helix through the membrane: in the absence of these residues, the phosphatase moiety of the fusion protein ultimately crosses to the periplasm (Boyd and Beckwith, 1989; Traxler et al., 1992) (see later under Determinants of Transmembrane Topology). The approach has been refined by introducing a positive test for cytosolic loops (see Manoil, 1990) and a method that permits insertion of *phoA* into the target sequence without deletion of the C-terminal end of the protein (Ehrmann et al., 1990). It has been further validated by applying it to a protein, subunit L of *Rhodob. sphaeroides* RC, whose topology has been definitely established by crystallography (Yun et al., 1991).

These observations show that, as a rule, the N-terminal part of an IMP is able to take up its correct transmembrane topology in the absence of the C-terminal part. Furthermore, truncated versions of *lac* permease (see earlier under Biosynthesis of Fragments) or the MalF protein (Ehrmann and Beckwith, 1991) that lack the first transmembrane α-helix have been shown to insert with the correct vectoriality and topology. These experiments again point to some structural autonomy between the various regions of a polytopic protein. They also indicate that its transmembrane orientation and topology are not determined solely by the vectoriality of insertion of its first transmembrane segment, followed blindly by insertion in alternating orientations of the hydrophobic segments downstream of it (cf. Hartmann et al., 1989). Topogenic signals, the nature of which is further discussed later under Determinants of Transmembrane Topology, are present throughout the sequence.

The Transmembrane Hydrophobic α-Helix as an Autonomous Folding Domain

Two-Stage Model of Polytopic Protein Folding

In the previous sections, we have summarized thermodynamic arguments, observations, and experiments indicating that a polytopic protein comprising several transmembrane α-helices can be considered as a "collegial" structure. In other words, the helices that make up the transmembrane region, together with a few residues from the extramembrane loops, are able to take up a correct transmembrane position and three-dimensional structure in the absence of information from the rest of the sequence. Folding of such proteins can be seen as a two-stage process in which the final structure results from the accretion of preformed transmembrane α-helices, with minimal rearrangement (Popot et al., 1987; Popot and Engelman, 1990; Popot, 1993) The model does not necessarily imply that, at some time during biosynthesis, the protein exists as a full collection of unassembled helices, but that each helix considered individually first folds and then packs. Forces that can concur in determining the three-dimensional geometry of the α-helix bundle include polar interactions between helices, the balance of van der Waals forces resulting from helix–helix, helix–lipid, and lipid–lipid packing, constraints due to the length or conformation of extramembrane loops, interactions with prosthetic groups or with other proteins, and so forth. By *minimal rearrangement* we mean that the transmembrane topology will not change: helices may bend, tilt, slide somewhat along the sequence, extend, or shorten, and so forth upon assembling, but no new segment will be inserted in transmembrane position at this step. As a result, no transmembrane segment should be found in the final structure that would not form a stable transmembrane helix by itself. This is actually the situation observed in the structures of BR and RCs (Table 3.1).

Many experiments indicate that integrity of all of the extramembrane loops connecting helices is not necessarily required for proper folding (see earlier under Experimental Studies of Membrane Protein Folding). This does not mean that extramembrane regions have no influence on assembly. Loops limit the diffusion of helices away from one another, which stabilizes the protein (see Kahn et al., 1992) and should favor interaction between helices connected by short loops. Site-directed mutagenesis work indicates that the formation of the retinal binding pocket between rhodopsin helices depends on the conformation of intradiscal loops (Khorana, 1992).

From the point of view of structure prediction, it is important to note that two-stage folding does not imply that any sequence segment that is long enough and hydrophobic enough to form a stable transmembrane α-helix will necessarily do so. Actually, hydrophobicity distributions for transmembrane and extramembrane segments overlap (see Popot and de Vitry, 1990, and references therein). Furthermore, the model does not address the vectoriality of helix insertion, a subject that is discussed later under Determinants of Transmembrane Topology.

There are obviously possible departures from the hydrophobic α-helix bundle scheme. One extreme case is that of porins, which is further discussed later under Integral Proteins of Bacterial Outer Membranes. Another possibility derives from the postulate that during biosynthesis pairs of transmembrane segments insert simultaneously (the "helical hairpin" hypothesis; see DiRienzo et al., 1978; von Heijne and Blomberg, 1979; Engelman and Steitz, 1981). If the overall hydrophobicity of the pair is the criterion for insertion, a very hydrophobic helix could drag into the membrane a segment that would not be expected to partition spontaneously into lipids by itself and that would become part of the final transmembrane region. Presently, there exists no well-characterized example of this happening, although something similar may occur during the folding of voltage-gated channels (see later under Voltage-Gated Cation Channels).

Several lines of reasoning can be used to try and rationalize the apparent rarity of transmembrane regions incorporating hydrophilic segments. One frequent view is that the sample of proteins whose transmembrane topology is known with reasonable certainty is just too small and that such polar transmembrane segments will be found in the future. Another, exemplified by Singer (1990), holds that putative transmembrane segments are individually probed for hydrophobicity by the insertion machinery. A third argument is that strongly polar transmembrane segments, assuming they can be inserted at all, would unnecessarily destabilize the protein. As noted above, the interior of proteins, whether soluble or integral, is essentially apolar. Burying polar groups is energetically costly. Most IMPs are synthesized in a compartment that is directly in contact with the membrane the proteins will be inserted into; they do not need to be stable in aqueous solution for extended periods of time, nor do they have to cross other membranes to reach their destination. It is difficult then to see what the selective pressure would be in favor of their transmembrane segments carrying more polar residues than strictly needed to stabilize helix packing and ensure function. Since hydrophobic α-helices (cf. Table 3.1) apparently suffice to line the water-filled channel of the nicotinic acetylcholine receptor (see later under Assembly of the Nicotinic Acetylcholine Receptor), and to make up the transmembrane region of *lac* permease, a sugar/proton symporter (see earlier under Biosynthesis by Fragments), the number of functions requiring the insertion of overall hydrophilic transmembrane segments may be limited. As a rule, therefore, it may be deemed safe to subject to particular scrutiny topological models that place strongly hydrophilic segments or helix ends in the middle of the bilayer (see, e.g., McCrea et al., 1988; Popot et al., 1991).

On the other hand, there are some well-characterized cases in which specific constraints may bear on the nature of transmembrane segments. Biosynthetic limitations on protein export toward the bacterial outer membrane may explain why porins do not contain extended hydrophobic segments (see below under Integral Proteins of Bacterial Outer Membranes). The β-barrel structure of porins neatly eludes the problem of burying polar residues: the protein has no core to speak of, but is shaped as a wide water-filled channel, the lumen of which a priori can accommodate polypeptide segments of any composition and secondary structure. Particular functional constraints also apply to Fregoli proteins like colicins, whose mode of action implies that they diffuse in free form under a water-soluble conformation before insertion into their target membrane (cf. Parker et al., 1989; van der Goot et al., 1991). Voltage-gated channels offer a case in which strongly charged segments may have to be buried for functional reasons (see later under Voltage-Gated Cation Channels).

It should be noted that an α-helix bundle is not necessarily a solid hydrophobic block. The center of the bundle may be more or less accessible from the aqueous space. For example, BR is thought to incorporate a small number of water molecules (Papadopoulos et al., 1990; Henderson et al., 1990) that contribute to the proton path. The binding site for catecholamines on adrenergic receptors is thought to be located not at the surface of the bundle, but between helices, suggesting that part of the bundle core is accessible to water (reviewed by Hargrave, 1991). It may not be coincidental that some of the purported transmembrane helices in this receptor family tend to be less hydrophobic than usual (see Table 4 in Popot and de Vitry, 1990). A continuum may thus exist between proteins whose transmembrane region is totally devoid of water, like the photosynthetic reaction centers, and proteins whose cores are more or less accessible to hydrophilic molecules, as must be the case for many carriers (cf. the cleft observed in *lac* permease by electron microscopy; see Costello et al., 1987; Li and Tooth, 1987). However, the examples of *lac* permease and the nicotinic acetylcholine receptor suggest that the water-exposed surfaces need not be strongly hydrophilic. (Hydrophobic clefts or tunnels exposed to water do occur in soluble proteins; see, e.g., Hyde et al., 1988; Sussman et al., 1991).

The degree of generality of the two-stage model will be further discussed below under Oligomerization and the Relationship Between Structure, Function, and Cellular Localization, in connection with subunit assembly. For the time being, we turn to another consequence of the folding autonomy of individual helices, namely, the existence of extremely small subunits made up of a single transmembrane α-helix.

Microassembly In Vivo

The two-stage model assumes that even a very short peptide (30 residues or less) may adopt a stable three-dimensional conformation as a transmembrane α-helix. This in principle endows it with the ability to interact specifically with other membrane proteins or with ligands, making it akin to the larger domains evidenced in soluble proteins. This property is responsible for the process of "microassembly" that takes place in the inner membranes of organelles. By this term, we mean to convey the idea that a covalent link between transmembrane α-helices is not a prerequisite to assembly and that individual helices can behave as full-fledged subunits.

Mitochondrial and chloroplast complexes comprise a large number of very small subunits, many of them shorter than 50 amino acid residues. Examination of their sequence indicates that each of these subunits could form a single hydrophobic transmembrane α-helix (for review, see Popot and de Vitry, 1990). The reaction center of photosystem II (PSII) purified from the unicellular green alga *Chlamydomonas reinhardtii*, for instance, comprises at least 10 such one-helix subunits, the shortest one only 34 residues long (de Vitry et al., 1991). Many such putative subunits are encoded in chloroplast open reading frames (ORFs), most of which probably correspond to yet unidentified subunits of photosynthetic complexes. Because of their small size and poor staining, many of these small polypeptides may have been overlooked during the biochemical characterization of purified complexes. A case in point is one of the 4 kDa subunits of cytochrome b_6f, identified in maize (Haley and Bogorad, 1989) and in *C. reinhardtii* (Pierre and Popot, 1993) by the use of antisera directed against synthetic peptides corresponding to the sequence of a chloroplast ORF (1 putative transmembrane α-helix, 37 residues). In most cases, the functional role of these small subunits is not established. Intramembrane light harvesting antennae of purple and green bacteria consist of pigments bound to small one-helix polypeptides 50–60 residues long (Zuber, 1986). In PSII reaction centers, two one-helix subunits comprising 39 and 83 residues, respectively, are proposed to cooperate in binding the heme of cytochrome b_{559}. Two histidine residues, one on each helix, would be involved in liganding the heme iron (Herrmann et al., 1984; Widger et al., 1985).

Examples of small one-helix subunits in membranes derived from the endoplasmic reticulum (ER) include the γ-subunit of the high-affinity IgE receptor (62 residues; Blank et al., 1989) and phospholamban (52 residues; Fujii et al., 1986). In eukaryotic cells, however, microassembly appears essentially restricted to organelle complexes, an observation that will be discussed below in the context of the relationship between IMP structure, function, and subcellular localization.

Microassembly In Vitro

Early refolding experiments with BR fragments strongly argued in favor of two-stage folding (see earlier under Refolding From Fragments). More recent experiments bear directly on the question of the stability of individual transmembrane α-helices. Engelman and coworkers synthesized peptides corresponding to each of the first two transmembrane helices of BR (helices A and B; cf Table 3.1) and showed by spectroscopic methods that upon insertion into lipid vesicles each peptide formed a transmembrane α-helix. The two populations of vesicles were then mixed with vesicles in which the proteolytic fragment encompassing the last five helices had been refolded. Upon fusion of the vesicles, the two synthetic helices reassociated with the five-helix fragment to regenerate BR (Kahn and Engelman, 1992) (Table 3.2).

Accumulating evidence suggests that transmembrane helices in bitopic proteins should not be considered as mere hydrophobic anchors but may in fact play a specific role in oligomerization, e.g., in the *neu* receptor (see Sternberg and Gullick, 1989), in the T-cell receptor complex (Manolios et al., 1990; Cosson et al., 1991), or in glycophorin (Bormann et al., 1989; for reviews, see Green, 1991; Bormann and Engelman, 1992; Lemmon and Engelman, 1992; Popot, 1993). In the latter case, it has been shown that a synthetic peptide mimicking the transmembrane helix is able to compete with the full-length protein for dimer formation. Competition is sequence specific and is not observed with a peptide mimicking the transmembrane helix of other bitopic proteins such as glycophorin C (Bormann et al., 1989). Using fusion proteins expressed in *E. coli,* the influence of each transmembrane residue on dimerization can be studied in a systematic manner (Lemmon et al., 1992a,b).

α-Helix Autonomy and the Evolution of Integral Membrane Proteins

Because transmembrane α-helices are able to fold autonomously, the formation of transmembrane regions in IMPs does not require necessarily that helices be covalently linked to one another. In support for this assertion, we have described several examples of functional IMPs assembling from fragments obtained by genetic or proteolytic cuts into interhelical loops. In this section, we review further experimental and natural cases of cleavage, fusion, duplication, deletion, and shuffling. They suggest that these phenomena play a role in the evolution of IMPs.

Gene Duplication and Fusion.   Internal repeats within the sequence of some integral protein families are a testimony to gene duplication and fusion. The members of the eye lens major integral protein family, for instance, probably comprise six transmembrane hydrophobic α-helices, generated by duplication of a three-helix module (Wistow et al., 1991; Pao et al., 1991, and references therein). An intriguing aspect of the model is that, given the odd number of putative transmembrane segments in each module, the second module must insert in the membrane with a vectoriality opposite to the first one. Gene triplication generated the family of mitochondrial carriers comprising the ADP/ATP carrier, the brown fat uncoupling protein, and the phosphate carrier, whose transmembrane topology is not definitely established (see Klingenberg, 1990).

At variance with these two families, in which no ancestral protein is known (a protein whose sequence would comprise a single module), voltage-gated channels can exist either as tetrameric proteins (the K^+-specific channels of the *Shaker* family) or as monomers with a fourfold repeat, each repeat homologous to a K^+-channel monomer (Na^+ and Ca^{2+} channels). The putative transmembrane topology of voltage-gated channels is discussed later under Voltage-Gated Cation Channels. Not too surprisingly, it is possible to introduce cuts into some of the linkers between Na^+-channel repeats without losing functionality (Stühmer et al., 1989). Conversely, functional, presumably dimeric K^+ channels are formed by fusion proteins in which two K^+ channels have been fused to one another (Isacoff et al., 1991).

A similar situation is found in the family of the bacterial plasma membrane carriers dependent on periplasmic binding proteins. Most of these carriers comprise two polytopic subunits (MalF and MalG in the maltose system) associated to a peripheral, cytosolic protein, presumably present in two copies (MalK) (see later under Oligomerization in the Bacterial Plasma Membrane: the MalF/MalG Heterodimer). Evidence has been presented for a distant homology between the two integral proteins (Dassa and Hofnung, 1985; Köster, 1991; Saurin and Dassa, 1994). In the Fe(III) hydroxamate transport system, these two subunits are fused into a single one, FhuB. FhuB can be split genetically in the linker region to generate two fragments, whose simultaneous expression in an *fhuB⁻* strain restores functionality (Köster and Braun, 1990). A similar experiment has been recently described with the tetracycline resistance (Tet) protein, which is made up of two homologous six-helix modules (Rubin et al., 1990; Rubin and Levy, 1991).

Naturally Split Integral Proteins.   More interestingly, polypeptides that do not present internal repeats may exist in one case as a single polypeptide and in another case as two separately encoded subunits (Table 3.2):

1. The N-terminal part of mitochondrial cytochrome b, comprising the first four of eight transmembrane helices, is homologous to chloroplast cytochrome b_6. Helices five to seven of cytochrome b are homologous to subunit IV of chlo-

roplast b_6f complex, which is encoded by a separate gene. Helix 8 of cytochrome b does not seem to have its counterpart in the chloroplast.

2. Mitochondrial NNT most likely features 14 transmembrane α-helices.[1] Its $E.$ $coli$ equivalent is made up of two subunits, one of which encompasses the first four helices and the other one the last nine. Helix 5 appears to be missing in the bacterial enzyme. The subunit structure of $Rhodobacter\ capsulatus$ NNT resembles that of $E.\ coli$ NNT (Lever et al., 1991).

Helix Duplication and Shuffling. One can easily conceive that duplication events may result in a protein with extra transmembrane α-helices, which, as far as they do not interfere with folding of the functional part of the protein, may well be tolerated. There are several precedents for this situation:

1. Functional BR has been reconstituted in vitro by mixing two overlapping proteolytic fragments, comprising the first five (A–E) and the last five (C–G) of its seven transmembrane α-helices (Liao et al., 1984). Each fragment certainly inserted with the correct topology, since in separate experiments it could complement its two-helix mate (Liao et al., 1983) (cf. Table 3.2). Upon assembly, three redundant helices must have remained dangling out of the way on the side of the renatured seven-helix molecule.

2. In lac permease (12 transmembrane helices), functional complementation has been reported between pairs of molecules, one of which carries a deletion of two or four helices in the N-terminal region and the other a deletion of two helices in the C-terminal one. Again, the complexes thus formed most likely comprise an excess of transmembrane helices. Interestingly, molecules that are less severely affected, e.g., carrying a single missense mutation, do *not* complement with molecules carrying different point mutations, suggesting that at least one of the mutated helix bundles is not destabilized enough to permit bimolecular assembly to take precedence over intramolecular assembly (Bibi and Kaback, 1992).

3. A similar case is that of the Tet protein, in which a fragment corresponding to one of the two internal repeats can functionally complement a full-length protein carrying a mutation in that repeat (Curiale and Levy, 1982).

4. Even more demonstrative is an experiment on the FhuB protein of the iron hydroxamate transport system, a protein thought to feature altogether 20 transmembrane helices in two ten-helix repeats (cf. earlier under Gene Duplication and Fusion). Expression in an fhuB⁻ strain of an elongated FhuB protein, created by internal duplication of a segment comprising putative helices 7 to 14, was found to restore growth on Fe^{3+} hydroxamate and albomycin sensitivity (Köster and Braun, 1990). This suggests that at least some of the molecules managed to fold correctly, presumably by expelling the eight redundant transmembrane segments to the side of the α-helix bundle.

---

1. A proposal that mitochondrial NNT comprises only 12 transmembrane helices [Popot and de Vitry, 1990] was put forward on the basis of a comparison with the bacterial enzyme. The latter sequence, however, has turned out to be partially erroneous. The revised sequence, together with additional proteolysis data, is in favor of the 14-helix topology [see Yamaguchi and Hatefi, 1991].

It is conceivable that such duplications of helices, were they to occur naturally, could create, e.g., redundant binding sites for lipophilic or hydrophilic ligands and serve as a starting point for subsequent evolution. In this context, it is to be noted that introns present in the structural genes encoding polytopic proteins tend to be located in regions coding for extramembrane loops (Jennings, 1989). As with soluble proteins, it is a matter of discussion whether this betrays exon shuffling or positional restrictions on intron insertion (for a recent discussion, see Patthy, 1991). Given the brevity of transmembrane segments and the limited set of residues they contain, establishing the reality of α-helix shuffling between IMPs by sequence comparison may be a difficult task.

The possibility that an ancestral structure has been altered by addition, deletion, internal duplication, and so forth, of transmembrane helices implies that evolutionarily related IMPs may present partially different topologies, even though it is likely that in most cases the three-dimensional arrangement of those helices that are homologous will be essentially the same.

For example, in mitochondrial-type oxidases, subunits I and III are predicted to feature 12 and 7 transmembrane hydrophobic α-helices, respectively (reviewed by Saraste, 1990; Capaldi, 1990). In aa_3-type oxidases from *Bacillus subtilis* and the thermophilic bacterium *Bacillus PS3*, as well as in *E. coli bo* complex, subunits I and III are clearly homologous to their mitochondrial equivalents but differ by the number of putative transmembrane helices: subunit I is larger, with a C terminus extended by two putative helices, while two helices are lacking at the N-terminus of subunit III (Ishizuka et al., 1990; Chepuri et al., 1990; Saraste et al., 1991). In the three bacteria, the two genes are part of the same operon and follow each other in the order COI–COIII, separated by a stop codon. This arrangement suggests that the two helices may have moved from one subunit to the other in the course of evolution. If such an event occurred, however, no trace at the level of sequence similarities remains. Even helix 12 of subunit I, which is particularly variable, shows some conservation throughout the whole family, while no such similarity is detectable between helices 13 and 14 of the elongated subunit I, on the one hand, and helices 1 and 2 of the full length subunit III, on the other.

As another example, bacterial and higher plant photosynthetic reaction centers present many common structural features. Even though higher plant photosystem I RC subunits contain more transmembrane helices than RC subunits from purple bacteria (see Krauss et al., 1993) they are considered to have evolved from a common ancestor (see Nitschke and Rutherford, 1991).

Determinants of Transmembrane Topology

We have argued up till now that all (or at least most) of the hydrophobic transmembrane helices encountered in integral protein are likely to behave as autonomous folding domains. In other words, each of these segments is presumed to be able to insert into a lipid bilayer and to take up an α-helical conformation independently from the presence of other regions of the protein. What about the vectoriality of its insertion? Is it somehow encoded within the sequence of each individual helix? Is it determined by surrounding elements of sequence? Or are there regions in a protein that contain vectorial information that determines how distant regions will insert?

A host of observations and experiments indicate that vectoriality of insertion during biosynthesis is controlled by signals distributed along the sequence, as originally suggested by Blobel (1980) (see von Heijne, Chapter 2). Transmembrane topology, however, is not obtained by the simple device of determining the vectoriality of the first transmembrane segment and inserting the following ones alternatively in one and the other direction. While transmembrane helices per se apparently contain little or no information about their orientation in the membrane, the primary determinant is the distribution of positively charged residues in the vicinity of helix ends. Specifically, helices tend to insert in the membrane in such a way that the extremity carrying the most positively charged residues will remain in the cytosol. In this respect, cleavable signal sequences appear as specialized variations on a more general theme (von Heijne, 1990). The so-called positive-inside rule statistically applies to prokaryotic (von Heijne, 1986a) (cf. Fig. 3.1a,b) and eukaryotic (von Heijne and Gavel, 1988; Hartmann et al., 1989) plasma membrane proteins, as well as those of chloroplast thylakoids (Gavel et al., 1991). Genetic manipulation of the distribution of lysine and arginine residues can cause a transmembrane segment to insert with inverted vectoriality (von Heijne et al., 1988; Yamane et al., 1990; McGovern et al., 1991; and references therein). This influence of positive charges depends on their being located relatively close to helix ends (Andersson and von Heijne, 1991).

The propensity of MalF transmembrane segments to insert with a given vectoriality depends on the density of positive charges in the cytosolic loop flanking them: when deletions are introduced such that the orientation of the N-terminal region of MalF will be inverted, some of the downstream segments may follow suit and insert with an inside-out orientation, but the C-terminal region contains strong vectoriality signals and will not invert. In the constructs thus obtained, it seems that the topologies of the two ends of the protein do not match, the N-terminal region being inside-out and the C-terminal region right-side-out (McGovern et al., 1991). This would imply either that a segment that is not transmembrane in the natural protein has been forced to insert or that one of the naturally transmembrane segments has been prevented from inserting or has been bent into a transmembrane hairpin. Similar observations have been made on *lac* permease (Bibi et al., 1991). The topological control exerted by positive charges at helix ends probably accounts at least in part for the fact that the hydrophobicity distributions of extramembrane and transmembrane segments in IMPs overlap, an indication that insertion is not determined by hydrophobicity alone (see Popot and de Vitry, 1990, and references therein).

Cytosolic positive charges prevent transmembrane α-helices from flipping through the membrane (Boyd and Beckwith, 1989; Traxler et al., 1991). These charges may thus contribute to stabilizing the native state of the protein. On the other hand, it is possible that their major role is merely to orient or prevent the insertion of some segments during biosynthesis. Thereby, they would impose a topology that may not be the most frequently realized if segments inserted independently from the composition of the loops. In thermodynamic terms, basic residues would impose such kinetic limitations on the process of insertion that the protein would become trapped into a local free energy minimum. It is conceivable that in the absence of this constraint some moderately hydrophobic segments would tend to distribute differently between trans-, juxta-, and extramembrane positions. Experimentally, such a kinetic role could be reflected in poorly effective folding under conditions in which the controlling effect of positive charges would be lost. From this point of view, it is unfortunate that, of the two integral proteins that have been refolded in vitro (see earlier under Refolding Full-Length Membrane Proteins), one, OmpF porin, is not an α-helix bundle and inserts according to a totally different mechanism (see later under Porin Folding and Assembly), and the other, BR, does not obey the positive-inside rule well (possibly because of the shielding afforded by the saturated-salt medium in which the bacterium thrives; cf. Fig. 3.1e).

The physical basis of topological control by basic residues is not understood. Interaction with negatively charged lipid headgroups on the cytosolic face of the membrane, the direction of the transmembrane electric field (negative inside, at least in bacteria), the great cost of burying lysine and arginine polar groups in lipids, and specific recognition machineries have been invoked (for discussions, see von Heijne and Gavel, 1988; Boyd and Beckwith, 1990; Dalbey, 1990; Singer, 1990; and von Heijne, this volume). The rules that govern the distribution of basic residues in extramembrane regions of polytopic IMPs are complex, which probably reflects the fact that different insertion mechanisms operate (for a discussion, see von Heijne, 1988; Andersson and von Heijne, 1993; see also chapter 2 in this book). While basic residues appear to be the major determinants of transmembrane vectoriality, the asymmetrical distribution of hydrogen bonding residues in reaction center proteins has prompted the suggestion that transient main chain–side chain hydrogen bonds play a role in lowering the free energy cost of burying helix ends into the membrane upon insertion of an α-helical hairpin (White and Jacobs, 1990).

Oligomerization and the Relationship between Structure, Function, and Cellular Localization

In this section, we discuss in parallel three questions:

1. What is the mechanism of oligomerization of IMPs? To what extent do folding, oligomerization, and membrane integration depend on one another?
2. What is the nature and organization of transmembrane segments in proteins that depart from the hydrophobic α-helix bundle scheme?
3. Are there structural constraints imposed upon IMPs by their localization in the cell?

These three questions are linked because cellular localization or function may impose or forbid the presence of certain types of transmembrane segments, which in turn will reflect on possible schemes for folding and oligomerization.

Oligomerization of IMPs may involve interactions within as well as outside of the membrane. Intramembrane interactions are illustrated by helix–helix interactions in the glycophorin or *neu* receptor homodimers and in the T-cell receptor heteroheptamer (see earlier under Microassembly In Vitro). They also play an essential role in the formation of the porin trimer (see later under Porin Folding and Assembly). Extramembrane interactions are exemplified by the fact that hemagglutinin (Wilson et al., 1981) and neuraminidase (Varghese et al., 1983), as well as many other bitopic proteins, remain oligomeric following resection of their transmembrane anchors. It is likely that in many cases both kinds of interactions contribute to the formation and stability of the oligomer, as in the cases of bacterial reaction centers (see earlier under

Quaternary Structures) and hemagglutinin (see later under Assembly of Hemagglutinin).

We summarize below the main features of a few particularly well-studied cases of oligomerization, taken in various cell compartments. As elsewhere in this review, emphasis is not on exhaustivity, but on illustrating what may be relatively general mechanisms.

Oligomerization in the Endoplasmic Reticulum

Plasma membrane proteins in eukaryotic cells are synthesized in the rough ER, where they undergo a number of covalent modifications, such as cleavage of the signal sequence, glycosylation, and formation of disulfide bridges. Generally, although not always, they fold and assemble while still in the ER and only then are transported to and through the Golgi apparatus and from there to the plasma membrane. Rapid and efficient folding and assembly depend on the presence in the lumen of the ER of numerous enzymes, including signal peptidase, oligosaccharide transferase, protein disulfide isomerase (PDI), cis–trans proline isomerase, and immunoglobulin heavy chain–binding protein (BiP, a molecular chaperone) (see later under Insertion, Folding, and Assembly as Assisted Processes). A considerable body of information exists regarding the various steps in this process, many of which have been elucidated by studying proteins expressed in cell culture (reviewed by Hurtley and Helenius, 1989; Klausner, 1989). We cursorily describe the assembly of two proteins that represent widely different classes of oligomers, hemagglutinin, a homotrimer of bitopic proteins, and the nicotinic acetylcholine receptor, a channel-forming heteropentamer of polytopic subunits. The folding of another family of plasma membrane IMPs, the voltage-gated channels, raises original problems that will be discussed later under Voltage-Gated Cation Channels.

Assembly of Hemagglutinin.

Hemagglutinin (HA) is one of the two major membrane proteins of the influenza virus (the second being neuraminidase) (reviewed by Wiley and Skehel, 1987). It follows the same biosynthetic pathway as endogenous plasma membrane proteins and reaches the plasma membrane, where the coat is assembled and viral particles bud.

HA is a homotrimer. In its unactivated form (HA0), each subunit is a bitopic protein 549 residues long. It is anchored to the membrane by a C-terminal hydrophobic sequence segment, presumably a transmembrane α-helix, leaving only the last ten residues or so exposed to the cytosol. Activation, a late process in the biosynthetic pathway, results from proteolytic cleavage of each HA0 subunit into two fragments, HA1 and HA2, which remain associated to one another and bound to the membrane by the C-terminal anchor (now a part of HA2). Subsequent acidification of the medium, which occurs when viral particles are endocytosed, triggers a transconformation of HA that confers it fusogenic properties. Fusion of the viral coat to the membrane of the endocytotic vesicle releases the viral RNA into the cytosol of the target cell (reviewed by Stegmann et al., 1989; White, 1990).

The C-terminal anchor of each HA1/HA2 subunit can be clipped off by bromelain, releasing the extracellular region of the trimer from the membrane. This extracellular fragment has been crystallized and its structure determined by x-ray crystallography (Wilson et al., 1981; Weis et al., 1988). It forms an elongated cylinder

(135 Å long) with a threefold axis of symmetry. The three subunits (each of them actually an HA1–HA2 heterodimer) associate primarily by contributing a long α-helix to a triple-stranded coiled coil that extends for almost 80 Å along the trimer axis. The quaternary structure is further stabilized by buried intersubunit salt bridges. Five of the six disulfide bridges in each subunit are intrachain, the sixth one connecting HA1 to HA2. Each subunit carries seven N-glycosylated sites, some of the sugars contacting a nearby subunit. Since the association between subunits is very intimate and involves interactions between large hydrophobic surfaces, it is doubtful that isolated subunits could have the same tertiary structure as in the trimer. It seems more likely that some reorganization occurs upon assembly (Wilson et al., 1981).

Biosynthesis of hemagglutinin has been studied in cell culture and in *Xenopus* oocytes (see Gething et al., 1986; Copeland et al., 1986; Hurtley and Helenius, 1989; Braakman et al., 1991; and references therein). The various steps of folding and assembly of HA0 have been followed by monitoring cleavage of the signal sequence, glycosylation, disulfide bridge formation, appearance or disappearance of specific epitopes, formation of detergent-resistant trimers, sugar modification, and so forth. The kinetics of the process vary from one cell line or virus strain to another and depend on experimental conditions. For example, 6 h after infection of Chinese hamster ovary cells at 37° C (where synthesis and cotranslational insertion and glycosylation take an average of 2 min), typical half-times are 3.2 min for disulfide bond formation, 8 min for trimerization, and 19 min for transport of the assembled trimers to the Golgi (Braakman et al., 1991). Metabolic energy is required for correct disulfide bonds to form (Braakman et al., 1992a). Under normal circumstances, disulfide bond formation starts before synthesis is completed, which sets restrictions on which cysteyl residues may pair. However, this is not a requirement for correct folding to be achieved, since correct bonds form when HA0 is synthesized in the presence of dithiothreitol and only subsequently allowed to oxidize (Braakman et al., 1992b). Most abnormal proteins are not transported to the Golgi: underglycosylated proteins, many engineered proteins carrying mutations either in the luminal or in the cytosolic regions, as well as properly folded but unassembled monomers, accumulate in the ER and are degraded. Among those, proteins with a misfolded or unglycosylated luminal region aggregate and associate with BiP (Gething et al., 1986; Hurtley et al., 1989).

Kinetic studies, therefore, indicate that folding of the HA0 monomers is a largely separate step from assembly: as tested by disulfide formation and epitope recognition, folding occurs prior to trimerization. In keeping with this, folding of HA0 is a first-order process whose rate does not depend on the level of expression, i.e., on the concentration of neosynthesized HA0 monomers in the ER membrane.

Trimerization, on the other hand, resembles a diffusion-controlled phenomenon: it is slower at low expression level (Ceriotti and Colman, 1990; Braakman et al., 1991). When distinct but compatible variants of HA0 are synthesized simultaneously, they assemble at random (Boulay et al., 1988). At low expression level, however, complete mixing becomes slower than folding, and preferential association of subunits synthesized from the same polysome is observed. These observations suggest that assembly rates of complex hetero-oligomers in the ER may depend on the level of expression of each subunit, the number of different subunits in the oligomer, and the number of distinct mRNAs they are translated from.

During the first few minutes after synthesis, therefore, newly completed HA0 subunits diffuse in the plane of the membrane away from their site of synthesis and mix up randomly. Assembly must await completion of the folding of the luminal region, which generates subunit–subunit interaction surfaces. It is interesting to note that, although the transmembrane anchor is not required for trimerization (Gething and Sambrook, 1982; Singh et al., 1990), it probably contributes to the stability of the trimer (Doms and Helenius, 1986). The transmembrane segment must adopt its presumed α-helical conformation immediately upon insertion. The existence of a lag between the completion of synthesis and trimerization implies that helix–helix interactions in the lipid phase are insufficient to drive HA0 assembly, or that they are hindered, due, e.g., to the presence of the much larger, improperly folded luminal region. It would be interesting to know whether the same situation holds, e.g., for glycophorin, for which direct experimental evidence indicates that helix–helix interactions suffice to ensure dimerization (see earlier under Microassembly In Vitro).

Another, particularly demonstrative case of independence between synthesis and oligomerization has been reported for the Uukuniemi virus coat protein heterodimer. The two bitopic glycoproteins (G1 and G2) that form the viral spikes are cotranslationally cleaved in the ER from a common 110 kDa precursor. However, because G1 folds in 10 min while G2 requires up to 60 min, dimers form between newly synthesized G1 and mature G2 originating from an older precursor (Persson and Pettersson, 1991).

Assembly of the Nicotinic Acetylcholine Receptor. The nicotinic acetylcholine receptor (AChR) is a cation-specific channel gated by the neurotransmitter acetylcholine (ACh) (for reviews, see Guy and Hucho, 1987; Changeux, 1990; Karlin, 1991; Changeux et al., 1992). AChR is present in the plasma membrane of muscle cells and neurons and is the prototype of a whole family of chemically gated channels. The AChR of the vertebrate neuromuscular junction is the best studied, and this discussion will be restricted to it.

The general structural organization of AChR has many differences compared with hemagglutinin, among which are the following:

1. AChR is made up of polytopic subunits. Each subunit is generally thought to comprise, from the N terminus on, (*a*) a large (≈220 residue) extracellular region, (*b*) a first transmembrane region made up of three closely spaced hydrophobic α-helices that contribute to forming the channel, (*c*) a large cytosolic region (≈100 residues), which contains phosphorylation sites, and (*d*) a last transmembrane hydrophobic α-helix that brings the short C-terminus back into the extracellular space.[2]

2. **Note added in proof.** Recent experiments have questioned the validity of the four-helix topology on which some aspects of the following discussion are based (see also D. S. Cafiso, Chapter 5). According to one proposal, the channel is lined by β-strands, not by α-helices (Akabas et al., 1992). According to another report (Unwin, 1993), the channel is indeed lined by hydrophobic α-helices, but these are surrounded by a wide β-barrel to which each of the five subunits would contribute 5 or 7 strands. Experimental data are difficult to reconcile with any single model. However, if either of these two models is correct, particularly the second one, the processes of insertion, folding, and assembly of the AChR subunits become mechanistically more complex than in the case of the 4-helix topology, where the transmembrane region of unassembled subunits is presumed to present a hydrophobic surface to the lipids and association by lateral aggregation without rearrangement of the transmembrane topology can account for the final structure of the complex. Some of the points raised below in connection with the folding and assembly of porins and of voltage-gated channels would become pertinent. For a brief discussion, see Popot (1993).

2. AChR is a hetero-oligomer, with the stoichiometry $\alpha_2\beta\gamma\delta$. The four types of subunits, close to 40% similar to one another, are translated separately from distinct mRNAs. In the course of calf embryonic development, transcription of the gene coding for the γ-subunit is inactivated and that of a gene coding for another subunit, ε, is turned on, resulting in the formation of $\alpha_2\beta\varepsilon\delta$-oligomers with different electrophysiological properties. All subunits feature a cleaved signal sequence, intrachain disulfide bridge(s) in the extracellular region, and they are all cotranslationally N-glycosylated. Each of the two α-subunits carries at least part of an ACh binding site and can be labeled with α-bungarotoxin (αBgt), a potent competitive inhibitor of ACh.

3. The AChR is a channel-forming protein. The five subunits arrange in a circle around a fivefold axis of pseudosymmetry normal to the membrane plane. The order of the subunits, which is not definitely established, is probably $\alpha\gamma\alpha\beta\delta$ or $\alpha\beta\alpha\gamma\delta$; in any case, the two α-subunits are not vicinal. A cation-specific channel runs along the symmetry axis, lined by all five subunits. While the exact structure of the channel is not known, the bulk of the evidence indicates that it is lined by some of the hydrophobic segments, not by additional, hydrophilic transmembrane sequence segments (reviewed by Karlin, 1991, 1993; Changeux et al., 1992; Popot, 1993).

Biosynthesis of the AChR has been studied in a variety of systems, including primary cultures of myoblasts, transfected fibroblast lines, and *Xenopus* oocytes injected with mRNAs. The time course and efficiency of the various biosynthetic steps depend on the system used. Qualitatively, the main conclusions are the following.

1. *Subunit synthesis and folding.* Translation, posttranslational modifications, and initial folding of a subunit do not depend on the presence of the others. In the BC3H-1 muscle-like cell line, the α-subunit has been shown to undergo a conformational maturation in 15–30 min following synthesis (Merlie and Lindstrom, 1983). The mature α-subunit is monomeric and has acquired binding sites for αBgt and for conformation-dependent antibodies (in the latter case with somewhat lower affinities than mature AChR), but does not bind small cholinergic ligands like carbamylcholine or curare (reviewed by Blount and Merlie, 1991b; Conroy et al., 1990). The extracellular region of α contains one site for N-linked glycosylation and two disulfide bridges. Maturation depends on glycosylation and on the formation of one of the two bridges; nonglycosylated α-subunits are degraded rapidly ($\approx$20 min; Blount and Merlie, 1990). Immature but not mature subunits bind BiP (Blount and Merlie, 1991a). Since unassembled α-subunits, whether or not they have matured into the αBgt-binding form, are degraded with the same $t_{1/2}$ ($\approx$2 h), BiP has been suggested to prevent aggregation or to assist folding of immature subunits rather than to target them for degradation.

2. *Formation of heterodimers.* Assembly occurs in steps (see Blount et al., 1990; Saedi et al., 1991; Blount and Merlie, 1991b; Gu et al., 1991b; and references therein). The first step is the formation of $\alpha\gamma$- (or $\alpha\varepsilon$-) and $\alpha\delta$-heterodimers (and perhaps some $\alpha\gamma\alpha$-trimers). In the BC3H-1 cell line, this step requires 30–90 min (Merlie and Lindstrom, 1983). The $\alpha\delta$-dimer is much more stable than the isolated α-subunit ($>$13 h). Rather unexpectedly, immature α-sub-

units are competent for the formation of $\alpha\delta$-dimers. Dimerization does not prevent immature α-subunits from binding BiP and does not protect them against rapid degradation (see Blount and Merlie, 1990, 1991a, and references therein). Stable dimers exhibit high affinity for αBgt, for conformation-sensitive anti-α-antibodies, and for small cholinergic ligands, which means either that α has further matured into a more native-like form or that both subunits in the dimers contribute to forming the sites (or both). Interestingly, work with chimeric AChR subunits has shown that the luminal (extracellular) region of the ε is sufficient to ensure its association with α: while complex formation between the α- and β-subunits is very inefficient, a chimeric subunit carrying the extracellular sequences of ε and the transmembrane and cytosolic sequences of β assembles with α almost as well as ε itself (Yu and Hall, 1991; see also Gu et al., 1991a). More recent works have shown that the transmembrane region of the α-subunit can be replaced by those of the $GABA_A$ or glutamate receptors (Sumikawa, 1992) and that even truncated proteins comprised of the N-terminal extramembrane region of the α-, the γ-, or the δ-AChR subunits can compete for assembly with the full-length subunits (Verral and Hall, 1992).

3. *Formation of the pentamer.* The next step in assembly is probably the formation of $\alpha\gamma\alpha\delta$-tetramers (Saedi et al., 1991). The β-subunit, whose turnover, when expressed individually, is faster than that of the other subunits ($t_{1/2} \approx 12$ min; Claudio et al., 1989), is probably added last.[3] As with HA, only completed oligomers move from the ER to the Golgi, as judged from sugar modification (Smith et al., 1987; Blount et al., 1990; Ross et al., 1991). In the presence of tunicamycin, an inhibitor of N-linked glycosylation, the AChR can assemble, but it does not migrate to the plasma membrane (Sumikawa and Miledi, 1989).

4. *Regulation of assembly.* AChR expression is regulated both at the transcriptional level (which is beyond the scope of this review) and at later stages, including posttranslational one(s) (reviewed by Laufer and Changeux, 1989). It has been proposed that regulation of assembly (Carlin et al., 1986) and, more specifically, of the incorporation of the β-subunit (Claudio et al., 1989), determines the number of AChR pentamers that transit through the Golgi and reach the cell surface. Interestingly, efficiency of assembly depends on the level of cytosolic cAMP (Ross et al., 1991, and references therein). Since phosphorylation of the γ- and δ-subunits changes as they move along the biosynthetic pathway, it has been suggested that subunit phosphorylation regulates the assembly of the pentamer (see Ross et al., 1991; Green et al., 1991). This proposal is reminiscent of the way phosphorylation of IMPs of the photosynthetic chain determines their assembly with one or another complex (see later under Assembly of PSII Reaction Center).

---

3. **Note added in proof.** This sequence of events has recently been questioned by Green and Claudio (1993). These authors propose a very rapid formation of $\alpha\beta$, $\alpha\gamma$ and $\beta\gamma$ dimers, rapid trimerization of either of those into $\alpha\beta\gamma$ trimers by addition of the missing subunit, slow addition of δ, and final completion of the pentamer by very slow addition of the second α subunit. The last two steps would be dependent on slow intervening transconformations.

5. *About the formation of the channel.* Acquisition of the final structure of the transmembrane region of the AChR raises a particular problem. Because each of their purported transmembrane segments is overall hydrophobic (Table 3.1), insertion of the isolated subunits with native-like transmembrane regions would be energetically favorable. Successive formation of the $\alpha\gamma$-, $\alpha\delta$-, and $\alpha\gamma\alpha\delta$-intermediates by lateral association does not differ fundamentally from helix–helix packing within subunits. On the other hand, addition of β-subunit must be accompanied or followed by closure of the pentamer and the concomitant formation of a water-filled channel along its pseudosymmetry axis. In this process, a transmembrane region of each subunit becomes exposed to water to form the channel lining. Because the lining is rather hydrophobic, its exposure to water is expected to be energetically unfavorable. Rough estimates suggest that the free energy penalty for channel formation can be compensated easily by subunit–subunit interactions (see Popot and Engelman, 1990). Mechanistically, this last assembly step seems complex, and its activation energy is likely to be high.

In summary, it seems that despite important structural differences between HA and AChR, assembly steps are largely the same: independent synthesis of the subunits, maturation depending on glycosylation and on disulfide bond formation, oligomerization, and quality control before the completed protein exits from the ER. One difference is that, at variance with the AChR α-subunit and many other proteins (reviewed by Hurtley et al., 1989), normal immature HA0 apparently does not bind BiP. Another difference is that, while unglycosylated HA0 subunits rapidly yield aggregates in association with BiP, neither glycosylation of the AChR subunits nor the maturation of the α-subunit into an αBgt-binding form are prerequisites to AChR assembly, a surprising fact given the evidence that assembly further modulates the binding properties of the site. Finally, it should be mentioned that, while both unassembled AChR subunits and unassembled HA0 are retained in the ER, this is a common but not an absolutely general observation; export of unassembled subunits has been observed in some instances (reviewed by Hurtley and Helenius, 1989).

Regarding the extent of subunit transconformation following assembly, for which there is some evidence in AChR but not in HA, it should be noted that, particularly in multidomain proteins, various probes will report on different folding events. Because the AChR α-subunit binds a wide range of ligands, it has been possible to follow its conformational changes in greater detail than those of HA0. Lack of evidence in favor of a transconformation of HA0 upon trimerization does not prove that there is none. Indeed, as mentioned above, examination of the mature structure of HA does suggest that assembly is accompanied by a reorganization of the subunits. Current data bear only on the conformation of extramembrane regions. The extent of reorganization of the transmembrane region that has to be postulated for the AChR subunits depends on the nature of the transmembrane segments (see footnote 2, page 67) and is currently unknown. Nor is such information available for subunits of any other IMP. It seems reasonable to think, however, that the isolated L and N subunits of the reaction centers have the same transmembrane topology as the assembled subunits. The relative arrangement of the transmembrane helices within isolated subunits, however, is likely to differ from that in the mature ones, given the intimate association of these two subunits with each other and with prosthetic groups in the fully assembled complex.

Oligomerization in the Bacterial Plasma Membrane: the MalF/MalG Heterodimer

Somewhat paradoxically, given the sophistication of *E. coli* genetics, much less appears to be known about the process of IMP assembly in the bacterial plasma membrane than in the ER. A recent study, however, suggests that some of the same principles may apply. Namely, subunits are inserted independently one from the other, diffuse, and subsequently associate with one another.

As mentioned above, the MalF protein is part of a hetero-oligomeric ATP-driven transport system that also comprises another integral protein, MalG, and two copies of a cytosolic peripheral protein, MalK (Shuman, 1987; Davidson and Nikaido, 1991). Newly translated MalF expressed in spheroplasts is sensitive to externally applied proteases and chases progressively into a protease-resistant form. In the absence of either MalG or MalK, MalF remains protease sensitive even after a prolonged chase, suggesting that acquisition of resistance is linked to assembly. MalF and MalG are normally cotranslated from a single mRNA. Traxler and Beckwith (1992) have examined the protease resistance of MalF in a strain carrying an amber mutation in the *malG* gene and a tightly regulated amber suppressor. It was thus possible to express successively radiolabeled MalF, synthesized in the absence of MalG, followed by coexpression of unlabeled MalF and MalG. Examination of the susceptibility of labeled MalF to proteolysis showed that the MalG subunit synthesized in the second period was able to stabilize the MalF subunit synthesized during the first. These observations led Traxler and Beckwith (1992) to propose that MalF ordinarily inserts into the membrane independently from MalG and MalK. Following insertion, MalF and MalG would diffuse in the plane of the membrane and assemble, together with MalK, into a protease-resistant, functional transport complex.

Oligomerization in Organelles

Constraints on the Import of Integral Membrane Proteins into Organelles.
Mitochondria and chloroplasts import most of their soluble or peripheral proteins and only part of their integral proteins. Import is thought to be mainly posttranslational and involves (*1*) transient association of the proteins to be imported with cytosolic chaperones, (*2*) unfolding, (*3*) translocation, and (*4*) transient association with organelle chaperones (Pfanner and Neupert, 1990; Baker and Schatz, 1991; Wienhues and Neupert, 1992) (see later under Posttranslational Insertion and Translocation).

Even though the gene distribution between organelle and nucleus DNA varies according to the organism and organelle considered, many hydrophobic proteins are consistently encoded in the organelles (Borst, 1977; von Heijne, 1986b; Popot and de Vitry, 1990). The locus of synthesis is not simply determined by the average hydrophobicity of the protein, since the hydrophobicity distributions of imported and non-imported proteins overlap (Table 3.3, line 1). Similarly, although putative trans-

Table 3.3. Structural Properties of Integral Membrane Proteins from the Inner Membrane of Mitochondrion and from the Thylakoid Membrane as a Function of Gene Location

	Gene Location			
	Mitochondrial Proteins		Chloroplast Proteins	
	Nucleus	Mitochondrion	Nucleus	Chloroplast
Overall hydrophobicity of the whole mature sequence	-0.82 ± 0.85 (16)	$+0.45 \pm 0.41$ (13)	-0.59 ± 0.41 (6)	$+0.07 \pm 0.66$ (25)
Average hydrophobicity of transmembrane segments	$+1.78 \pm 0.41$ (38)	$+1.99 \pm 0.38$ (94)	$+1.45 \pm 0.39$ (14)	$+1.94 \pm 0.39$ (120)
Hydrophobicity of most hydrophobic segment	2.71	2.74	2.39	2.79
Number of proteins containing 1–3 or >3 hydrophobic transmembrane segments				
1–3	15	4	6	13
>3	1	9	0	12

Hydrophobicities (kcal/residue) were estimated using the GES scale as described in Table 1. Averages are given ± S.D. over the number of cases indicated in parentheses. The list of proteins and details of the analysis are given by Popot and de Vitry (1990).

membrane segments in imported proteins tend to be somewhat less hydrophobic than in nonimported proteins, the two distributions overlap largely (Popot and de Vitry, 1990; Heijne, 1986b) (see Table 3.3, line 2). At variance with what has been observed for the export of proteins toward bacterial outer membranes (see later under Constraints on the Structure of Outer Membrane Integral Proteins), there does not seem to be an upper limit beyond which the hydrophobicity of a given segment would make import impossible: the most hydrophobic segments in imported proteins are comparable to those present in locally synthesized proteins (line 3).

On the other hand, it is remarkable that, while the sequences of organelle-encoded proteins can contain numerous hydrophobic segments, imported proteins as a rule contain only one to three (Table 3.3, lines 4–5). The origin of this distribution is not certain. It has been suggested that hydrophobic segments appearing in the cytosol before the synthesis of the protein is completed (i.e., segments located too far from the C terminus), could cause mistargeting to the ER (von Heijne, 1986b). Alternatively, the presence of a large number of hydrophobic segments in a polypeptide could perturb import at several other steps, such as the achievement of a soluble conformation, its stabilization by association with chaperones, and protein unfolding or dissocation from chaperones (Popot and de Vitry, 1990). The striking abundancy in mitochondrial complexes of very small integral subunits encoded in the nucleus, many of them comprising a single putative transmembrane α-helix, may reflect at least in part such constraints on import. Import restrictions cannot be the only reason for the high frequency of these small subunits in organelles, however, since many of the one-helix subunits of photosynthetic complexes are coded by chloroplast genes (reviewed by Popot and de Vitry, 1990).

Some mitochondria, particularly in Protozoa, lack genes coding for integral proteins that are encoded in the mitochondrial genome of most other organisms. It is generally not known whether these proteins are at all present in these particular mitochondria and, if so, whether their structures present unusual characteristics resulting from the displacement of their site of synthesis from the mitochondrial matrix to the cytosol. A case in point is *Saccharomyces cerevisiae,* whose mitochondria lack genes coding for NADH-Q reductase. Reductases from other mitochondria contain subunits with up to 15 hydrophobic segments, the import of which would be atypical. This observation suggested that the yeast enzyme could have a simpler structure, such as is observed in some prokaryotes (Popot and de Vitry, 1990). Recently, the rotenone-insensitive internal (matrix-facing) NADH-Q reductase of mitochondria from *S. cervisiae* has indeed been reported to be of the latter type, comprising a single subunit with no strongly hydrophobic sequence segment (Marres et al., 1991).

In summary, integral complexes from the inner membrane of organelles characterize themselves by (*1*) the association of subunits synthesized locally with subunits imported from the cytosol; (*2*) the high frequency of very small integral subunits; and (*3*) a nonrandom distribution of subunits between imported and nonimported, polytopic subunits with many putative transmembrane α-helices being, as a rule, synthesized within the organelle.

Assembly of the PSII Reaction Center. As an example of organelle complex, we summarize below the current knowledge on the assembly of the PSII reaction center, an IMP complex from the thylakoid membrane of chloroplast. PSII RC is the green plant homologue of photosynthetic purple bacteria RC (see earlier under General Background). It effects the primary photochemistry of photosynthesis, generating a charge separation across the thylakoid membrane and splitting water with the concomitant evolution of oxygen. This multimolecular protein-pigment complex comprises four polytopic subunits, all of which are encoded in the chloroplast. Subunits D1 and D2 (five transmembrane α-helices each) are homologous to bacterial RC subunits L and M and, similarly, cooperate in binding the primary reactants (see Nanba and Satoh, 1987; Michel and Deisenhofer, 1988). Subunits P5 and P6 (six predicted transmembrane α-helices each) each bind about twenty chlorophylls and form the core antenna. PSII also comprises three peripheral subunits, OEE1/ OEE2/OEE3, imported from the cytosol and involved in oxygen evolution, and many small, one-helix integral subunits, most of which are encoded in the chloroplast (see de Vitry et al., 1991). The PSII RC is located in the stacked region of the thylakoid membranes, where it is associated with LHC (cf. earlier under Functions).

Several assembly steps (Fig. 3.3) have been detected by analyzing PSII mutants of *C. reinhardtii* (de Vitry et al., 1989; for reviews of random and site-directed PSII mutants, see Rochaix and Erickson, 1988; Nixon et al., 1994).

Step 1. The chloroplast-encoded PSII subunits are translated on ribosomes bound to unstacked regions of the thylakoids. Both synthesis of P6 and binding of chlorophyll by P5 and by P6, which occurs soon after or concomitantly with their synthesis, are independent of the presence of the other subunits. On the other hand, even in short (5 min) pulse-labeling experiments, mutants blocked in the synthesis of D1 accumulated less neosynthesized P5 than the wild type (WT), and mutants lacking D2 neosynthesized less D1 and P5 than WT. It is presently uncertain whether this

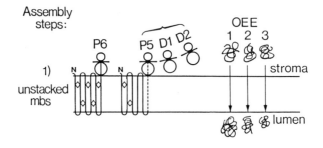

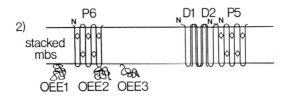

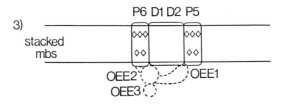

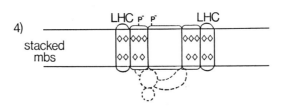

Fig. 3.3. Proposed steps in the assembly of photosystem II. Assembly steps are described in the text. Schematic polypeptide structures with predicted transmembrane α-helices and localization of the NH_2 terminus are given in schemes 1 and 2. A *bracket* indicates that synthesis of D1, D2, and P5 may be coupled. Some of the chlorophylls bound to the PSII core antenna (P5 and P6) and to the LHC are represented by *diamonds;* ligands bound to D1 and D2 are not represented. OEEs are not required for the assembly of the rest of PSII and are therefore drawn in *dashed lines.* (Adapted from de Vitry et al., 1989.)

coupling involves a rapid turnover of the unassembled subunits or a regulation at the translational level. Similar observations, interpreted as due to translational coupling, have been reported for the peripheral subunits α and β of chloroplast ATP synthase (Drapier et al., 1992).

Kim et al. (1991), using isolated barley chloroplasts, recently showed that the ribosomes paused at specific sites during the synthesis and cotranslational insertion of D1. The cause of pausing is unknown; longer retention of more hydrophobic segments within the ribosome tunnel and interaction of the nascent protein with a chaperone have been suggested. The authors speculated that such a pausing may facilitate cotranslational binding of liposoluble cofactors to newly formed transmembrane α-helices, a situation reminiscent of cotranslational glycosylation in the ER. As argued above, it is indeed to be expected that helices inserted into the membrane while translation proceeds would adopt a structure close to the one in the completed protein and could therefore provide specific binding sites for ligands. Organelle inner membranes are highly specialized and, as such, contain a restricted set of proteins and ligands at high concentration. This situation ought to facilitate cotranslational interactions of a nascent integral protein with its ligands or, possibly, with other proteins.

Step 2. The three subunits D1/D2/P5 form a heterotrimer and migrate (even in the absence of P6) to the stacked membrane regions, as does P6 alone. The incomplete complex remains sensitive to endogenous proteases until P6 is bound to form the PSII core complex. Cyanobacteria mutants lacking the *psbC* gene product (P6 equivalent) show light driven electron transfer from the secondary electron donor Z to the primary quinone electron acceptor Q_A, indicating that the core of the RC is functional (Rögner et al., 1991). The peripheral subunits OEE1–3 can accumulate in the thylakoid lumen in the absence of the main integral PSII subunits, although they bind only loosely to the membrane.

Step 3. The peripheral subunits associate to the core. OEE1 binds independently of the other two OEE subunits, while the presence of OEE2 is necessary to the binding of OEE3.

Step 4. The PSII complex and the LHC accumulate independently in thylakoid membranes. Phosphorylation of PSII subunits is correlated with the assembly of the PSII unit (PSII–LHC complex).

At a higher level of integration, part of the LHC can diffuse in the plane of the membrane and associate preferentially either with PSII, in the stacked regions, or with photosystem I (PSI), in the unstacked regions, as a function of the physiological state of the cell. This displacement is controlled by the extent of LHC phosphorylation (reviewed by Allen, 1992).

Synthesis and assembly of PSII are under the control of numerous nuclear genes acting at several levels. Nuclear control of transcript stability has been reported for genes *psbB* (P5; Jensen et al., 1986), *psbC* (P6; Sieburth et al., 1991), and *psbD* (D2; Kuchka et al., 1989). Nuclear control of translation has been reported for D2 (Kuchka et al. 1988) and P6 (Rochaix et al., 1989). In most species, processing of the C-terminus of D1 by a protease imported from the cytosol is required for stable assembly of the manganese cluster of the oxygen evolution site and proper binding of the OEE subunits (Marder et al., 1984; Diner et al., 1988). The functional significance of this processing step is not clear, since deletion of the C-terminal extension of D1 by genetic engineering does not appear to affect PSII assembly (Nixon et al.,

1992). At least one stromal protein factor is required to ensure insertion of LHC (which is imported for the cytosol) in the thylakoid membrane (Payan and Cline, 1991).

As already mentioned, the three peripheral subunits in PSII, OEE1-3, associate with the transmembrane region in a partially independent way. This is not generally true of peripheral organelle subcomplexes. In the case of mitochondrial NADH-Q dehydrogenase (complex I), an enzyme with very numerous peripheral and integral subunits, parallel assembly of the peripheral and the integral regions probably precedes association of the two subcomplexes (Tuschen et al., 1990). Similarly, the F_1 (peripheral) and F_0 (integral) regions of mitochondrial ATP synthase assemble independently from the presence of one another (see Senior, 1990).

Integral Proteins of Bacterial Outer Membranes

At variance with all other membranes that we have considered up till now, the outer membrane of gram-negative bacteria is not in contact with any biosynthetic compartment. Furthermore, the outer membrane is also the only membrane that, as far as we know, does not contain IMPs built up on the hydrophobic α-helix bundle scheme. Are these two peculiarities related, and in which way do they affect IMP folding and assembly?

Porin Folding and Assembly. As we have seen, it seems to be a fairly general principle that proteins built on the hydrophobic α-helix bundle scheme assemble after their insertion into the membrane. Porins, built on the β-barrel scheme, also singularize themselves in this respect, assembly being a prerequisite to insertion. The most extensive set of data relates to *E. coli* trimeric porins, i.e., the closely related OmpC, OmpF, and PhoE porins and the more distant maltoporin (LamB):

1. Porins are synthesized with a signal sequence that is cleaved upon export to the periplasm. The signal sequence in itself is sufficient to tag the protein for export. Signal sequences from outer membrane and periplasmic proteins are interchangeable and therefore do not determine the final location of the proteins (Tommassen et al., 1983; Jackson et al., 1985).
2. Specific insertion into the outer membrane does not seem to depend on an addressing sequence, but on the protein achieving a particular three-dimensional structure (for a review, see Nikaido and Reid, 1990).
3. OmpF porin secreted by spheroplasts (Sen & Nikaido, 1990) and signal sequence-less OmpF (Sen and Nikaido, 1991) or PhoE porins (de Cock et al., 1990) synthesized in vitro in the absence of membranes are found as soluble monomers. In the absence of added membranes, neither protein forms the SDS-resistant trimers characteristic of native porins. SDS-resistant trimers form, upon addition of either outer membrane fragments, lipopolysaccharide vesicles and/or detergent mixed micelles (de Cock et al., 1990; Sen and Nikaido, 1991).

These observations suggest that in vivo porins are secreted in a soluble, monomeric form into the periplasmic space and assemble into trimers only upon interaction with the outer membrane. Free mixing of monomers in the periplasmic space is consistent with the fact that, in vivo, coexpression of several porins results in the formation of heterologous trimers (Ichihara and Mizushima, 1979; Marchal and Hofnung, 1983; Gehring and Nikaido, 1989): as for HA in the ER and the MalF/MalG-heterodimer in *E. coli* plasma membrane, synthesis and assembly are not coupled, in the sense that proteins translated on different polysomes assemble randomly. Insertion into the outer membrane in vivo depends on the formation of trimers, as indicated, e.g., by mutagenesis studies on LamB (Boulain et al., 1986; see also Vos-Scheperkeuter and Witholt, 1984). At variance with coexpression, successive expression of two different porins does not lead to the formation of heterologous trimers (Ichihara and Mizushima, 1979), suggesting that formation of isolated, membrane-inserted monomers is energetically too costly for trimers to dissociate.

This sequence of events is consistent with the structure of porins. As argued before, insertion of isolated (or paired) β-strands is expected to be energetically very unfavorable, and a two-stage folding mechanism similar to that proposed for α-helical membrane proteins would be very unlikely. It is therefore logical that β-barrel formation should precede or accompany insertion. A requirement for trimerization would depend on the characteristics of the outer, lipid-exposed surfaces of the barrel. Two features of *Rhodob. capsulatus* porin argue in favor of trimerization preceding or accompanying insertion: (*1*) the rim of the barrel close to the symmetry axis of the trimer is not high enough to span the hydrophobic region of the membrane (see earlier under Secondary Structures and Transmembrane Topologies; Fig. 3.1*f*) and (*2*) the outer surface of the barrel in this region is rather polar (Schiltz et al., 1991). Exposure of this face of the barrel to lipids would make stable insertion of isolated monomers (or dissociation of an inserted trimer into monomers) problematical, in keeping with experimental data.

It has been reported that a fraction of monomeric PhoE synthesized in vitro acquires spontaneously, in the absence of added membranes, conformational epitopes characteristic of the mature protein (de Cock et al., 1990). To what extent the three-dimensional structure of these proteins resembles that of the native monomer is not clear. A monomer with a fully native-like fold would expose to its environment a largely hydrophobic outer surface. It is difficult to see how the protein could be driven to take up such a conformation unless by interaction with a hydrophobic surface, in which case a soluble, monomeric intermediate could hardly be expected to form. Further investigations are probably needed concerning the conformational state of porins while in the periplasmic space and their possible association with other proteins. In this respect, it is worth noting that Ried et al. (1990) have postulated the existence of a common periplasmic factor binding the precursors of several outer membrane proteins, a situation reminiscent of the role of chaperones in other cellular compartments. There is a precedent for the presence of a chaperone-like protein in the periplasm of *E. coli,* the PapD protein, which is required for assembly of the proteins that make up the pili (see Holmgren and Bränden, 1989; Hultgren et al., 1991; and references therein). It should be noted, however, that the periplasm does not contain the free ATP that is required to drive cycles of binding to and release from chaperones like GroE or mitochondrial hsp 70 (see later under Thermodynamic versus Kinetic Control of Folding and Assembly).

Constraints on the Structure of Outer Membrane Integral Proteins.
Sequences of outer membrane proteins (OMPs) are overall much less hydrophobic
than those of other IMPs (see, e.g., Nikaido and Reid, 1990). No OMP actually
contains long stretches of hydrophobic residues similar to those that form transmembrane segments in α-helical IMPs. This is shown in Figure 3.4, which compares the
hydrophobicity of the most hydrophobic segments found in OMPs from *E. coli* to
that of the most hydrophobic transmembrane segments found in (eukaryotic) plasma
membrane proteins. When hydrophobic segments are inserted into exported proteins
by genetic engineering, export is blocked (David and Model, 1985; MacIntyre et al.,
1988) (cf. Fig. 3.4). One possible reason why the structure of porins is built on the
β-barrel scheme, therefore, could well be the inability of the bacterium to export
toward its outer membrane the long hydrophobic stretches of residues that are needed
to build hydrophobic transmembrane α-helices (MacIntyre et al., 1988).

Conversely, one may ask why plasma membrane proteins apparently so seldom
make use of the β-barrel scheme. There is no obvious answer to this question, and it

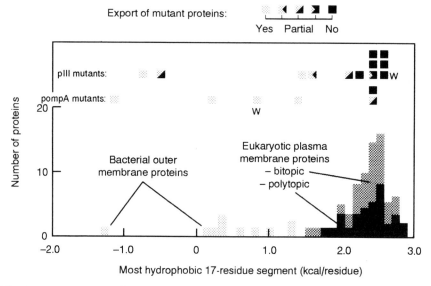

Fig. 3.4. A comparison of the highest peaks of local hydrophobicity in bacterial outer membrane proteins compared with plasma membrane proteins. Sequences were analyzed as
described in Table 3.1. Average hydrophobicity of the most hydrophobic 17 residue segment
in each sequence is expressed as ΔG° (kcal/residue) for transfer from lipids to water. Histograms describe the distributions of highest local hydrophobicities for bitopic *(dark gray)* and
polytopic *(black)* plasma membrane proteins from eukaryotes and for outer membrane proteins from *E. coli (light gray)*. (Data are from Tables 4 and 7 of Popot and de Vitry, 1990.)
In the *upper part* are indicated the highest local hydrophobicity and the extent of export of
two series of fusion proteins: *pIII*, the coat protein of phage pIII, the natural transmembrane
anchor of which had been deleted or substituted (*W* = natural anchor) (Davis and Model,
1985); and *pOmpA*, pro-OmpA containing hydrophobic inserts (*W* = most hydrophobic segment in wild-type OmpA) (MacIntyre et al., 1988). In both series, the hydrophobicity indicated is that of the most hydrophobic 17 residue segment encompassing (or encompassed by)
the insert. Extent of export is indicated by the *amount of light gray* in the symbol.

is not certain that the question is legitimate, inasmuch as our present knowledge of the structure of plasma membrane proteins is so patchy. Voltage-gated channels and, according to one model, chemically gated channels have been proposed to be structural hybrids between the α-helix bundle and the β-barrel schemes. Mitochondrial porin (VDAC) is inserted into the outer mitochondrial membrane posttranslationally, following its synthesis in the cytosol (reviewed by Hartl et al., 1989). Its sequence, like those of bacterial porins, does not contain extended hydrophobic stretches, and it is thought to be folded into a β-barrel (see, e.g., Blachly-Dyson et al., 1989; Mannella et al., 1992; De Pinto et al., 1992). Homologies between various families of porins, even those thought to be structurally very similar, can be extremely weak (cf. Jeanteur et al., 1991; Schiltz et al., 1991; and references therein). It is therefore possible that mitochondrial and bacterial porins share a common phylogenetic origin and that the β-sheet structure of mitochondrial porins (if confirmed) results from gene transfer rather than from convergent evolution (see Schiltz et al., 1991; Schirmer and Rosenbusch, 1991).

One factor that might favor the α-helix bundle scheme among IMPs from the plasma membrane and from membranes derived from it (during cell biogenesis or in the course of organelle evolution) is the existence of an elaborate machinery that facilitates co- or posttranslational insertion of hydrophobic α-helices (see later under Insertion, Folding, and Assembly as Assisted Processes). The existence of this machinery, together with the evolutionary potentialities offered by helix recombination (see earlier under α-Helix Autonomy and the Evolution of Integral Membrane Proteins), may have favored variations around the α-helix bundle theme over the development of β-barrel structures. Most membrane functions apparently can be carried out by α-helix bundles; the structure of gap junctions suggests that even aqueous channels as large as those of bacterial porins (but perhaps not of VDAC) can be built from α-helices (cf. Schwarzmann et al., 1981; and Unwin, 1989).

Voltage-Gated Cation Channels

Voltage-gated cation channels are presently the plasma membrane IMPs whose structures are the most likely to deviate from the pure hydrophobic α-helix bundle. These proteins form transmembrane channels specific for K^+, Na^+, or Ca^{2+}, the gating of which is regulated by the electric field across the plasma membrane or the sarcoplasmic reticulum membrane. As mentioned (see earlier under Gene Duplication and Fusion), K^+-channels of the *Shaker* family are thought to be homotetramers, while the monomeric Na^+ and Ca^{2+} channels feature four repeats, each one corresponding to one K^+-channel protomer (for reviews, see Stephenson, 1991; Stephan and Agnew, 1991).

Current topological models are based on hydrophobicity analysis, which suggests the existence of five hydrophobic transmembrane α-helices per module (K^+-channel monomer or Na^+ or Ca^{2+}-channel repeat), and on a combination of site-directed mutagenesis and electrophysiology, which suggests that the transmembrane region of each module also comprises two kinds of hydrophilic transmembrane segments: (*1*) a charged segment, containing one basic residue every turn in an otherwise hydrophobic helix; and (*2*) a hydrophilic loop, some 20 residues long, too short to form two conventional membrane-spanning helices. Electrophysiological data indicate that the charged helix is involved in voltage-controlled gating, albeit not in a straightforward manner (see Papazian et al., 1991, Liman et al., 1991, and references therein). They also demonstrate that the hydrophilic loop lines that part of the channel where most of the voltage drop occurs, i.e., most likely, the transmembrane region of the channel (Yellen et al., 1991; Hartmann et al., 1991; Yool and Schwarz, 1991). The assembled structure has been suggested to be an eight-strand β-barrel, each module contributing two strands, surrounded by 20 hydrophobic and 4 positively charged helices (Yool and Schwarz, 1991; Bogusz et al., 1992; Bogusz and Busath, 1992). A somewhat different, very detailed model of voltage-gated channel structure and activation has been developed by Guy and Conti [1990]. The model comprises a hollow cylinder made up of 16 hydrophobic helices, in the center of which lie shorter helices and, in the open conformation of the channels, a very short eight-strand β-barrel to which each module contributes two strands from nonadjacent sequence segments. Closure would involve transconformation of every other barrel strand to an α-helical structure, thereby dismantling the barrel and closing the pore. Some predictions of the model, however, are at odds with subsequent site-directed mutagenesis work [Liman et al., 1991; for further revision and discussion of the model, see the article by Durell and Guy (1992) and the discussion that accompanies it].)

If any of these models are correct, voltage-gated channels clearly depart from the hydrophobic α-helix bundle that is the expected outcome of two-stage folding. In no case could the charged helix insert independently. Nor is it to be expected that the loop thought to line the channel could remain exposed to lipids prior to subunit association, as the pore-lining residues in the acetylcholine receptor subunits may do (see earlier under Assembly of Hemagglutinin). Some sort of concerted conformational transition must be envisioned when subunits or repeats come together. As for the acetylcholine receptor, it would be of great interest to know whether the accessibility of proteolytic or antigenic sites located within the purported transmembrane hydrophilic segments changes upon assembly.

Insertion, Folding, and Assembly as Assisted Processes

Thermodynamic versus Kinetic Control of Folding and Assembly

Successful renaturation of proteins in vitro implies that their sequence contains all the information necessary for them to reach their native structure. In vivo, however, biosynthesis is assisted by numerous factors. In many cases, these factors can probably be considered as catalysts rather than antagonists of self-assembly. By facilitating certain reactions and blocking others, they speed up biosynthesis and increase its final yield.

For instance, folding and assembly of many soluble proteins are assisted by molecular chaperones (reviewed by Nilsson and Anderson, 1991; Ellis, 1991; Ellis and van der Vies, 1991; Zeils tra-Ralls et al., 1991; Gething and Sambrook, 1992). In bacteria, these chaperones are DnaK (associated factors DnaJ, GrpE) and GroEL (associated factor GroES). Eukaryotic hsp 70-class chaperones are homologous to DnaK. These chaperones are present in almost every subcellular compartment (nucleus, cytosol, lumen of the ER, matrix of the mitochondrion, stroma of the chloroplast). Eukaryotic chaperonins (cpn60 or hsp60) are homologous to GroEL; they include mitochondrial hsp60 and chloroplast Rubisco-binding protein (associated factor cpn10).

The mode of action of chaperones is not understood in detail. It seems that by virtue of their affinity for sequence segments rich in aliphatic residues (Flynn et al., 1991), which are normally buried in protein cores or at subunit–subunit interfaces, they are able to associate with folding or assembly intermediates and to prevent them from engaging into nonproductive pathways. Binding to GroE has been reported to stabilize the molten globule state of dihydrofolate reductase and of rhodanese (Martin et al., 1991). GroE is proposed to help folding of these proteins by cycles of binding and release of the molten globule, release being driven by ATP hydrolysis, until the protein reaches the native state and stops binding (see Creighton, 1991). Depending on exact conditions, folding may or may not be observed in the absence of chaperones. Renaturation of bacterial ribulose bisphosphate carboxylase-oxygenase (Rubisco), for instance, depends on GroE at 25°C, while at 15°C some active Rubisco can form slowly in its absence (see Ellis, 1991).

Other factors involved in IMP biosynthesis may also be considered to some extent as catalysts. For instance, in vitro translation experiments show that the red blood cell glucose carrier normally inserts cotranslationally into microsomes. Posttranslational insertion is possible, however, albeit with a lower efficiency (Mueckler and Lodish, 1986). *S. cerevisiae* cells survive disruption of the signal recognition particle (SRP; see below), because SRP-dependent targeting to the ER can be bypassed in vivo (Hann and Walter, 1991). Cotranslational targeting to the ER by SRP or binding of Rubisco to GroE affects the rate and yield of synthesis, but does not determine the final state of the protein (for a recent discussion, see Jaenicke, 1991).

As far as IMPs are concerned, the extent to which kinetic factors may contribute to determining the final structure is not established. We have already alluded (see earlier under Determinants of Transmembrane Topology) to the possible kinetic role of basic residues in favoring one transmembrane topology over another. It is obvious, to give another example, that targeting mechanisms will prevent newly synthesized proteins from inserting randomly into any cellular membrane, regardless that this would be thermodynamically favorable. It is beyond the scope of this chapter to review the very large field of factors that are or may be involved in the synthesis, targeting, insertion, and assembly of membrane proteins. We simply list below some of the best understood ones.

Cotranslational Insertion

Efficient integration into the ER of most eukaryotic membrane proteins depends on SRP, a component of the secretion machinery (reviewed by Hann and Walter, 1991). SRP first binds to the signal sequence of nascent proteins as it emerges from the ribosome and then to SRP receptors on the ER, directing association of the ribosome with the ER. A set of ER membrane proteins, whose identification is still in progress, catalyzes translocation or insertion of the nascent chain. As already mentioned, numerous ER-associated enzymes operate co- or posttranslationally in order to ensure cleavage of the signal sequence, glycosylation, proline imide bond isomerisation and disulfide bond shuffling. The lumen of the ER also contains BiP, a molecular chaperone of the hsp70 class, involved in assembly of both secreted and membrane proteins (see earlier under Oligomerization in the Endoplasmic Reticulum).

Posttranslational Insertion and Translocation

In eukaryotic and bacterial cells, factors have been identified that can associate with newly synthesized proteins in the cytosol and facilitate their posttranslational insertion or translocation. In bacteria, where insertion is considered to be mainly posttranslational, insertion of many (but not all) membrane proteins requires the *sec* gene products (reviewed in Wickner et al., 1991). SecB, a cytosolic chaperone, stabilizes precursor proteins. The SecB–protein complex binds to SecA, a peripheral membrane protein with ATPase activity. SecA interacts with two IMPs, SecY and SecE, which are involved in protein translocation. Both the presence of the signal sequence and association with chaperones contribute to maintaining proteins bound for the plasma membrane (or for organelles) in a state competent for translocation (reviewed in Wickner et al., 1991; Hartl et al., 1989).

Import into organelles is thought to be mainly posttranslational. Polypeptide precursors bind to outer membrane receptors and are translocated at contact sites between the outer and inner membranes of the mitochondrion or chloroplast envelope. Their addressing sequence is cleaved in the organelles, in one or two steps depending on their final destination (in the mitochondrion, matrix, inner membrane or intermembrane space; in the chloroplast, stroma, thylakoid membrane or thylakoid lumen; reviewed by Pugsley, 1989; Pfanner and Neupert, 1990; De Boer and Weisbeck, 1991). Translocation involves unfolding of the imported protein. As discussed (see earlier under Constraints on the Import of Integral Membrane Proteins into Organelles), and at variance with export to the bacterial outer membrane, the hydrophobicity of imported transmembrane segments can be very high, but there seems to be a restriction on the number of hydrophobic segments per polypeptide (cf. Table 3.3). Molecular chaperones of the hsp70 family and other proteins are involved in preventing aggregation or incorrect folding in the various cell compartments, in facilitating interactions of the targeting sequences with their receptors, and in presenting precursors in an import-competent form. In addition, binding of the polypeptide that is crossing the contact site to matrix or stroma hsp70 is proposed to provide the driving force for transport. Release from mitochondrial or plastid hsp70 requires hydrolysis of ATP. This step does not result in fully folded proteins, but is followed by interactions with other chaperones (cpn60) in the mitochondrial matrix or the plastid stroma, which play a role in folding and oligomerization: recent experiments indicate that the mitochondrial processing peptidase first binds to the mitochondrial hsp70, then to cpn60, and finally forms a complex with the processing enhancing protein (Manning-Krieg et al., 1991). It is presently not clear whether mitochondrial IMPs imported from the cytosol transit through a soluble state in the matrix before being inserted into the inner membrane.

Specific Factors

In addition to general purpose factors involved in the processing of many proteins, specific factors exist that will not be reviewed here. Some affect specific posttranslational modifications, for example, the protease mentioned earlier under Assembly of the PSII Reaction Center, which clips off the C terminus of the D1 protein of PSII and permits the formation of the oxygen evolving center. Other factors may resemble chaperones. A particularly interesting example is offered by the invariant chain of class II molecules of the major histocompatibility complex. The α- and β-subunits of class II molecules and the invariant chain all are bitopic proteins. The invariant chain (I) is not part of the final oligomer as expressed at the surface of antigen-presenting cells, but plays a key role in its biosynthesis. It associates in the ER with the newly synthesized α- and β-chains to form an $(\alpha\beta)_3I_3$ nonamer, which prevents the $\alpha\beta$-dimer from binding peptides resulting from the degradation of endogenous proteins and targets it to an endocytic compartment. Acidification causes dissociation of the invariant chain, binding of peptides originating from the degradation of endocytosed proteins, and targeting of the peptide-loaded $\alpha\beta$-dimer to the cell surface, where the peptides are offered for recognition by T cells (see Lotteau et al., 1990; Bakke and Dobberstein, 1990; Peters et al., 1991; Roche et al., 1991; and references therein). The invariant chain thus appears to modulate both the conformation and the traffic of the α- and β-chains (cf. Brodsky, 1990). Other examples of transiently associated integral subunits have been reviewed by Hurtley and Helenius (1989).

Conclusion

We have tried, in this chapter, to provide an overview of factors that contribute to determining the final structure of IMPs. The most salient conclusions are the following.

1. IMPs of known structures comply with a priori expectations based on energetic considerations: surfaces that are either buried into the protein or facing the lipids are overall hydrophobic, and the regular secondary structure of transmembrane segments permits most main chain hydrogen bonds to be formed. Two basic schemes allow these constraints to be met. (*a*) In most cases, the transmembrane region is comprised exclusively of α-helices, the surface of which is overall hydrophobic. Helices tend to present a relatively more polar face, turned toward the inside of the α-helix bundle, and a very hydrophobic face, facing outward. (*b*) In bacterial porins, on the other hand, a polypeptide that is overall hydrophilic folds into a wide water-filled β-barrel. On one side, the outer surface of the barrel is hydrophobic and faces lipids, while on the other side it is more polar and forms the interface with other subunits in the oligomer.

2. Hydrophobic transmembrane α-helices behave as autonomous folding domains. Information about the vectoriality of their insertion into the membrane is contained in the cytosolic loops. α-Helical transmembrane regions form by assembly of preformed transmembrane helices (two-stage folding). Integrity of the extramembrane loops connecting the helices is often dispensable: functional IMPs can be assembled from fragments containing one or a few transmembrane helices. Helix duplication, deletion, and shuffling probably have played a role in the evolution of α-helical IMPs.

3. In the best known cases, subunits with α-helical transmembrane regions insert independently from one another and subsequently diffuse in the plane of the bilayer before assembling into oligomers. Both transmembrane and extramembrane regions may contribute to the stability of the oligomer. Folding precedes assembly, but assembly is often accompanied by transconformation of the extramembrane regions and stabilization against proteolytic degradation. In most cases, subunit assembly probably does not affect the number and nature of transmembrane segments. However, the transmembrane topology proposed for cation-specific voltage-gated channels seems to imply the concerted insertion of hydrophilic transmembrane segments.

4. At variance with hydrophobic α-helices, isolated β-strands cannot form stable transmembrane entities. Indeed, β-barrel IMPs fold and oligomerize prior to or concomitantly with insertion into the membrane.

5. There are correlations between structure and cellular localization. Bacterial outer membranes probably contain only β-barrel IMPs. IMPs from the plasma membrane and from organelle inner membranes are mostly α-helical. Among those, organelle complexes are rich in very small integral subunits essentially comprised of a single transmembrane helix ("microassembly"). These differences reflect at least in part biosynthetic constraints on the nature or number of transmembrane segments.

6. While some IMPs have been refolded in vitro, folding and membrane insertion in the cell is usually catalyzed by chaperones and other factors. In the ER, posttranslational modifications, folding, and assembly generally must be completed before IMPs can move to the Golgi apparatus.

Because our knowledge of both structures and biosynthetic pathways is still fragmentary, these statements are bound to be in many respects too schematic. It seems clear, however, that a basic tenet of our argumentation, namely, the folding autonomy of transmembrane α-helices, is a relatively general and useful notion. Integral membrane proteins of the α-helix bundle persuasion are "collegial" structures, built up of prefolded elements. They are typical examples of the *architecture en étages* (construction by successive stages), which is characteristic of most biological structures (Jacob, 1970). In the simplest case, folding units (α-helices) combine to form a subunit, which itself associates with other subunits to form an oligomer, which itself may associate more or less strongly with other oligomers to form "supercomplexes" (Joliot et al., 1992) and/or large-scale organizations with more or less strictly determined geometries, such as the reaction center–antennae complexes or the gap junctions. Since polypeptide chain continuity is of secondary importance, individual α-helices may or may not be part of the same polypeptide, and subunits may remain distinct or become fused into larger chains. These variations are facilitated by the dispersion of signals defining the vectoriality of helix insertion throughout sequences. In this process, the definition of an oligomer may become somewhat blurred: there may exist a continuum of affinities between subunits such that observed associations will depend on investigation methods and/or on the functional state of the complex. While undoubtedly an oversimplification, the notion of transmembrane α-helices as independent building blocks should be of use when designing biochemical or genetic experiments, when considering possible schemes for the biosynthesis of membrane proteins, when building models of their structure, or when trying to understand their diversity and evolution.

Acknowledgments

We thank J. Beckwith, F. Boulay, I. Braakman, W. A. Cramer, E. Dassa, A. Devillers-Thiéry, M. Ehrmann, J.-L. Eiselé, D. M. Engelman, J.-L. Galzi, K. Gehring, A. Helenius, M. Hofnung, H. R. Kaback, W. Köster, J. P. Merlie, F. Pattus, W. Saurin, G.F.X. Schertler, G. E. Schulz, B. Traxler, and M. Yamaguchi, as well as many colleagues from the IBPC, for communication of unpublished information and/or comments on earlier drafts of this chapter. We are particularly grateful to S. Ketchner for her careful pruning of our English.

References

Akabas, N. H., Stauffer, D. A., Xu, M., and Karlin, A. (1992) Acetylcholine receptor channel probed in cysteine-substitution mutants. *Science* 258: 307.

Allen, J. F. (1992) Protein phosphorylation in regulation of photosynthesis. *Biochim. Biophys. Acta* 1098: 275.

Andersson, H., and von Heijne, G. (1991) A 30-residue-long "export initiation domain" adjacent to the signal sequence is critical for protein translocation across the inner membrane of *Escherichia coli. Proc. Natl. Acad. Sci. USA* 88: 9751.

Andersson, H., and von Heijne, G. (1993) *Sec*-dependent and *sec*-independent assembly of *E. Coli* inner membrane proteins. The topological rules depend on chain length. *EMBO J.* 12: 683.

Anfinsen, C. B., Harber, E., Sela, M., and White, F. H. (1961) The kinetics of formation of native ribonuclease during oxidation of the reduced polypeptide chain. *Proc. Natl. Acad. Sci. USA* 47: 1309.

Baker, K. P., and Schatz, G. (1991) Mitochondrial proteins essential for viability mediate protein import into yeast mitochondria. *Nature* 349: 205.

Bakke, O., and Dobberstein, B. (1990) MHC Class II–associated invariant chain contains a sorting signal for endosomal compartments. *Cell* 63: 707.

Baldwin, J. N. (1993) The probable arrangement of the helices in G protein-coupled receptors. *EMBO J.* 12: 1693.

Bibi, E., and Kaback, H. R. (1990) In vivo expression of the *lacY* gene in two segments leads to functional *lac* permease. *Proc. Natl. Acad. Sci. USA* 87: 4325.

Bibi, E., and Kaback, H. R. (1992) Functional complementation of internal deletion mutants in the lactose permease of *Escherichia coli. Proc. Natl. Acad. Sci. U.S.A.* 89: 1524.

Bibi, E., Verner, G., Chang, C.-Y., and Kaback, H. R. (1991) Organizaton and stability of a polytopic membrane protein: deletion analysis of the lactose permease of *Escherichia coli. Proc. Natl. Acad. Sci. USA* 88: 7271.

Bjorkman, P. J., Saper, M. A., Samraoui, B., Bennett, W. S., Strominger, J. L., and Wiley, D. C. (1987) Structure of the human class I histocompatibility antigen, HLA-A2. *Nature* 329: 506.

Blachly-Dyson, E., Peng, S. Z., Colombini, M., and Forte, M. (1989) Probing the structure of the mitochondrial channel, VDAC, by site-directed mutagenesis: a progress report. *J. Bioenerg. Biomembrane* 21: 471.

Blank, U., Ra, C., Miller, L., White, K., Metzger, H., and Kinet, J.-P. (1989) Complete structure and expression in transfected cells of high affinity IgE receptor. *Nature* 337: 187.

Blobel, G. (1980) Intracellular protein topogenesis. *Proc. Natl. Acad. Sci. USA* 77: 1496.

Blount, P., and Merlie, J. P. (1990) Mutational analysis of muscle nicotinic acetylcholine receptor subunit assembly. *J. Cell Biol.* 111: 2613.

Blount, P., and Merlie, J. P. (1991a) BiP associates with newly synthesized subunits of the mouse muscle nicotinic receptor. *J. Cell Biol.* 113: 1125.

Blount, P., and Merlie, J. P. (1991b) Biogenesis of the mouse muscle nicotinic acetylcholine receptor. *Curr. Top. Membrane Transport.* 39: 277.

Blount, P., Smith, McHardy, M., and Merlie, J. P. (1990) Assembly intermediates of the mouse muscle nicotinic acetylcholine receptor in stably transfected fibroblasts. *J. Cell Biol.* 111: 2601.

Bogusz, S., Boxer, A., and Basath, D. D. (1992) An SS1-SS2 β-barrel structure for the voltage-activated potassium channel. *Prot. Engin.* 5: 285.

Bogusz, S., and Busath, D. D. (1992) Is a β-barrel model of the K⁺ channel energetically feasible? *Biophys. J.* 62: 19.

Bormann, B.-J., and Engelman, D. M. (1992) Intramembrane helix–helix association in oligomerization and transmembrane signaling. *Annu. Rev. Biophys. Biomol. Struct.* 21: 223.

Bormann, B.-J., Knowles, W. J., and Marchesi, V. T. (1989) Synthetic polypeptides mimic the assembly of transmembrane glycoproteins. *J. Biol. Chem.* 264: 4033.

Borst, P. (1977) Structure and function of mitochondrial DNA. *Trends Biochem. Sci.* 2: 31.

Boulain, J. C., Charbit, A., and Hofnung, M. (1986) Mutagenesis by random linker insertion into the *lamB* gene of *Escherichia coli* K12. *Mol. Gen. Genet.* 205: 339.

Boulay, F., Doms, R. W., Webster, R. G., and Helenius, A. (1988) Posttranslational oligomerization and cooperative acid activation of mixed influenza hemagglutinin trimers. *J. Cell Biol.* 106: 629.

Boyd, D., and Beckwith, J. (1989) Positively charged amino acid residues can act as topogenic determinants in membrane proteins. *Proc. Natl. Acad. Sci. USA* 86: 9446.

Boyd, D., and Beckwith, J. (1990) The role of charged amino acids in the localization of secreted and membrane proteins. *Cell* 62: 1031.

Braakman, I., Helenius, J., and Helenius, H. (1992a) Role of ATP and disulphide bonds during protein folding in the endoplasmic reticulum. *Nature* 357: 260.

Braakman, I., Helenius, J., and Helenius, H. (1992b) Manipulating disulfide bond formation and protein folding in the endoplasmic reticulum. *EMBO J.* 11: 1717.

Braakman, I., Hoover-Litty, H., Wagner, K. R., and Helenius, A. (1991) Folding of influenza hemagglutinin in the endoplasmic reticulum. *J. Cell Biol.* 114: 401.

Brodsky, F. M. (1991) The invariant dating service. *Nature* 348: 581.

Broome-Smith, J. K., Tadayyon, M., and Zhang, Y. (1990) β-lactamase as a probe of membrane protein assembly and protein export. *Mol. Microbiol.* 4: 1637.

Büchel, D. E., Gronenborn, B., and Müller-Hill, B. (1980) Sequence of the lactose permease gene. *Nature* 283: 541.

Calamia, J., and Manoil, C. (1990) *lac* Permease of *Escherichia coli*: topology and sequence elements promoting membrane insertion. *Proc. Natl. Acad. Sci. USA* 87: 4937.

Cammarata, K. V., and Schmidt, G. W. (1992) In vitro reconstitution of a light-harvesting gene product: deletion mutagenesis and analysis of pigment binding. *Biochemistry* 31: 2779.

Capaldi, R. A. (1990) Structure and function of cytochrome *c* oxidase. *Annu. Rev. Biochem.* 59: 569.

Carlin, B. E., Lawrence, J. C., Lindstrom, J. M., and Merlie, J. P. (1986) Inhibition of acetylcholine receptor assembly by activity in primary cultures of embryonic rat muscle cells. *J. Biol. Chem.* 261: 5180.

Ceriotti, A., and Colman, A. (1990) Trimer formation determines the rate of influenza haemagglutinin transport in the early stages of secretion in *Xenopus* oocytes. *J. Cell Biol.* 111: 409.

Changeux, J.-P. (1990) Functional architecture and dynamics of the nicotinic acetylcholine receptor: an allosteric ligand-gated ion channel. In: *Fidia Research Foundation Neuroscience Award Lectures.* New York: Raven Press, vol. 4, p. 21.

Changeux, J.-P., Galzi, J.-L., Devillers-Thiéry, A., and Bertrand, D. (1992) The functional architecture of the acetylcholine nicotinic receptor explored by affinity labelling and site-directed mutagenesis. *Q. Rev. Biophys.* 25: 395.

Chepuri, V., Lemieux, L., Au, D.C.-T., and Gennis, R. B. (1990) The sequence of the *cyo* operon indicates substantial structural similarities between cytochrome *o* ubiquinol oxidase of *Escherichia coli* and the *aa₃*-type family of cytochrome *c* oxidases. *J. Biol. Chem.* 265: 11185.

Chothia, C., and Finkelstein, A. V. (1990) The classification and origins of protein folding patterns. *Annu. Rev. Biochem.* 59: 1007.

Claudio, T., Paulson, H. L., Green, W. N., Hartman, D., Ross, A. F., and Hayden, D. (1989) Fibroblasts transfected with *Torpedo* acetylcholine receptor β, γ, and δ subunit cDNAs express functional AChRs when infected with a retroviral α-recombinant. *J. Cell Biol.* 108: 2277.

Conroy, W. G., Saedi, M. S., and Lindstrom, J. (1990) TE671 cells express an abundance of a partially mature acetylcholine receptor alpha subunit which has characteristics of an assembly intermediate. *J. Biol. Chem.* 265: 21642.

Copeland, C. S., Doms, R. W., Bolzau, E. M., Webster, R. G., and Helenius, A. (1986) Assembly of influenza hemagglutinin trimers and its role in intracellular transport. *J. Cell Biol.* 103: 1179.

Cosson, P., Lankford, S. P., Bonifacio, J. S., and Klausner, R. D. (1991) Membrane protein association by potential intermembrane charge pairs. *Nature* 351: 414.

Costello, M. J., Escaig, J., Matsushita, K., Viitanen, P. V., Menick, D. R., and Kaback, H. R. (1987) Purified *lac* permease and cytochrome *o* oxidase are functional as monomers. *J. Biol. Chem.* 262: 17072.

Cramer, W. A., and Trebst, A. (1991) Membrane protein structure prediction: cytochrome *b*. *Trends Biochem. Sci.* 16: 207.

Cowan, S. W., Schirmer, T., Rummel, G., Steiert, M., Ghosh, R., Pauptit, R. A., Jansonius, J. N., and Rosenbusch, J. P. (1992) Crystal structures explain functional properties of two *E. coli* porins. *Nature* 358: 727.

Creighton, T. E. (1991) Unfolding protein folding. *Nature* 352: 17.

Curiale, M. S., and Levy, S. B. (1982) Two complementation groups mediate tetracycline resistance determined by *Tn*10. *J. Bacteriol.* 151: 209.

Dalbey, R. E. (1990) Positively charged residues are important determinants of membrane protein topology. *Trends Biochem. Sci.* 15: 253.

Dassa, E., and Hofnung, M. (1985) Homologie entre les protéines intégrales de membrane interne de systèmes de transport à protéine affine chez les entérobactéries. *Ann. Inst. Pasteur* 136A, 281.

Davidson, A. L., and Nikaido, H. (1991) Purification and characterization of the membrane-associated components of the maltose transport system from *Escherichia coli*. *J. Biol. Chem.* 266: 8946.

Davis, N. G., and Model, P. (1985) An artificial anchor domain: Hydrophobicity suffices to stop transfer. *Cell* 41: 607.

De Boer, A. D., and Weisbeek, P. J. (1991) Chloroplast protein topogenesis: import, sorting and assembly. *Biochim. Biophys. Acta* 1071: 221.

de Cock, H., Hendriks, R., de Vrije, T., and Tommassen, J. (1990) Assembly of an in vitro synthesized *Escherichia coli* outer membrane porin into its stable trimeric configuration. *J. Biol. Chem.* 265: 4646.

Deisenhofer, J., Epp, O., Miki, K., Huber, R., and Michel, H. (1985) Structure of the protein subunits in the photosynthetic reaction center of *Rhodopseudomonas viridis* at 3 Å resolution. *Nature* 318: 618.

Deisenhofer, J., and Michel, H. (1989) The photosynthetic reaction center from the purple bacterium *Rhodopseudomonas viridis*. *Science* 245: 1463.

De Pinto, V., and Palmieri, F. (1992) Transmembrane arrangement of mitochondrial porin or voltage-dependent anion channel (VDAC). *J. Bioeng. Biomemb.* 24: 21.

de Vitry, C., Diner, B. A., and Popot, J.-L. (1991) Photosystem II particles from *Chlamydomonas reinhardtii:* purification, molecular-weight, small subunit composition, and protein phosphorylation. *J. Biol. Chem.* 266: 16614.

de Vitry, C., Olive, J., Drapier, D., Recouvreur, M., and Wollman, F.-A. (1989) Posttranslational events leading to the assembly of photosystem II protein complex: a study using photosynthesis mutants from *Chlamydomonas reinhardtii*. *J. Cell Biol.* 109: 991.

Diner, B. A., Ries, D. F., Cohen, B. N., and Metz, J. G. (1988) COOH-terminal processing of polypeptide D1 of the photosystem II reaction center of *Scenedesmus obliquus* is necessary for the assembly of the oxygen-evolving complex. *J. Biol. Chem.* 263: 8972.

DiRienzo, J. M., Nakamura, K., and Inouye, M. (1978) The outer membrane proteins of gram-negative bacteria: biosynthesis, assembly, and functions. *Annu. Rev. Biochem.* 47: 481.

Doms, R. W., and Helenius, A. (1986) Quaternary structure of influenza virus hemagglutinin after acid treatment. *J. Virol.* 60: 833.

Drapier, D., Girard-Bascou, J., and Wollman, F.-A. (1992) Evidence for a nuclear control on the expression of the *atpA* and *atpB* chloroplast genes in *Chlamydomonas reinhardtii*. *Plant Cell* 4: 283.

Durrell, S. R., and Guy, H. R. (1992) Atomic scale structure and functional models of voltage-gated potassium channels. *Biophys. J.* 62: 238.

Ehrmann, M., and Beckwith, J. (1991) Proper insertion of a complex membrane protein in the absence of its amino-terminal export signal. *J. Biol. Chem.* 266: 16530.

Ehrmann, M., Boyd, D., and Beckwith, J. (1990) Genetic analysis of membrane protein topology by a sandwich gene fusion approach. *Proc. Natl. Acad. Sci. USA* 87: 7574.

Eiselé, J.-L., and Rosenbusch, J. P. (1990) In vitro folding and oligomerization of a membrane protein. *J. Biol. Chem.* 265: 10217.

Ellis, R. J. (1991) Chaperone function: cracking the second half of the genetic code. *Plant J.* 1: 9.

Ellis, R. J., and van der Vies, S. M. (1991) Molecular chaperones. *Annu. Rev. Biochem.* 60: 321.

Engelman, D. M., Adair, B. D., Hunt, J. F., Kahn, T. W., and Popot, J.-L. (1990) Bacteriorhodopsin folding in membranes: a two-stage process. *Curr. Top. Membrane Transport.* 36: 17.

Engelman, D. M., and Steitz, T. A. (1981) The spontaneous insertion of proteins into and across membranes: the helical hairpin hypothesis. *Cell* 23: 411.

Engelman, D. M., Steitz, T. A., and Goldman, A. (1986) Identifying nonpolar transbilayer helices in amino acid sequences of membrane proteins. *Annu. Rev. Biophys. Biophys. Chem.* 15: 321.

Finkelstein, A. V., and Ptitsyn, O. B. (1987) Why do globular proteins fit the limited set of folding patterns? *Prog. Biophys. Mol. Biol.* 50: 171.

Flynn, G. C., Pohl, J., Flocco, M. T., and Rothman, J. E. (1991) Peptide-binding specificity of the molecular chaperone BiP. *Nature* 353: 726.

Foster, D.L., Boublik, M., and Kaback, H. R. (1983) Structure of the *lac* carrier protein of *Escherichia coli. J. Biol. Chem.* 258: 31.

Froshauer, S., and Beckwith, J. (1984) The nucleotide sequence of the gene for *malF* protein, an inner membrane component of the maltose transport system of *Escherichia coli. J. Biol. Chem.* 259: 10896.

Froshauer, S., Green, G. N., Boyd, D., McGovern, K., and Beckwith, J. (1988) Genetic analysis of the membrane insertion and topology of MalF, a cytoplasmic membrane protein of *Escherichia coli. J. Mol. Biol.* 200: 501.

Fujii, J., Ueno, A., Kitano, K., Tanaka, S., Kadoma, M., and Tada, M. (1986) Complementary DNA-derived amino-acid sequence of canine cardiac phospholamban. *J. Clin. Invest.* 79: 301.

Garavito, R. M., and Picot, D. (1990) The art of crystallizing membrane proteins. In: *Methods: A Companion to Methods in Enzymology.* vol 1, p. 57, New York: Academic Press.

Garavito, R. M., and Rosenbusch, J. P. (1980) Three-dimensional crystals of an integral membrane protein: an initial x-ray analysis. *J. Cell Biol.* 86: 327.

Gavel, Y., Steppuhn, J., Herrmann, R., and von Heijne, G. (1991) The "positive-inside rule" applies to thylakoid membrane proteins. *FEBS Lett.* 282: 41.

Gehring, K. B., and Nikaido H. (1989) Existence and purification of porin heterotrimers of *Escherichia coli* K-12 OmpC, OmpF, and PhoE proteins. *J. Biol. Chem.* 264: 2810.

Gething, M.-J., McCammon, K., and Sambrook, J. (1986) Expression of wild-type and mutant forms of influenza hemagglutinin: the role of folding in intracellular transport. *Cell* 46: 939.

Gething, M.-J., and Sambrook, J. (1982) Construction of influenza hemagglutinin genes that code for intracellular and secreted forms of the protein. *Nature* 300: 598.

Gething, M.-J., and Sambrook, J. (1992) Protein folding in the cell. *Nature* 355: 33.

Ghélis, C., and Yon, J. (1982) *Protein Folding.* New York: Academic Press.

Green, N. M. (1991) The semiotics of charges. *Nature* 351: 349.

Green, W. N., and Claudio, T. (1993) Acetylcholine receptor assembly: subunit folding and oligomerization occur sequentially. *Cell* 74: 57.

Green, W. N., Ross, A. F., and Claudio, T. (1991) cAMP stimulation of acetylcholine receptor expression is mediated through posttranslational mechanisms. *Proc. Natl. Acad. Sci. USA* 88: 854.

Gu, Y., Camacho, P., Gardner, P., and Hall, Z. W. (1991a) Identification of two amino acid residues in the ε subunit that promote mammalian muscle acetylcholine receptor assembly in COS cells. *Neuron* 6: 879.

Gu, Y., Forsayet, J. R., Verrall, S., Yu, X. M., and Hall, Z. W. (1991b) Assembly of the mammalian muscle acetylcholine receptor in transfected COS cells. *J. Cell Biol.* 114: 799.

Guy, H. R., and Conti, F. (1990) Pursuing the structure and function of voltage-gated channels. *Trends Neurosci.* 13: 201.

Guy, H. R., and Hucho, F. (1987) The ion channel of the nicotinic acetylcholine receptor. *Trends Neurosci.* 10: 318.

Haley, J., and Bogorad, L. (1989) A 4-kDa maize chloroplast polypeptide associated with the cytochrome b_6-f complex: subunit 5, encoded by the chloroplast *petE* gene. *Proc. Natl. Acad. Sci. USA* 86: 1534.

Hann, B. C., and Walter, P. (1991) The signal recognition particle in *Saccharomyces cerevisiae. Cell* 67: 131.

Hargrave, P. A. (1991) Seven-helix receptors. *Curr. Biol.* 1: 575.

Hartl, F.-U., Pfanner, N., Nicholson, D. W., and Neupert, W. (1989) Mitochondrial protein import. *Biochim. Biophys. Acta* 988: 1.

Hartmann, E., Rapoport, T. A., and Lodish, H. F. (1989) Predicting the orientation of membrane-spanning proteins. *Proc. Natl. Acad. Sci. USA* 86: 5786.

Hartmann, H. A., Kirsch, G. E., Drewe, J. A., Tagliatella, M., Joho, R. H., and Brown, A. M. (1991) Exchange of conduction pathways between two related K^+ channels. *Science* 251: 942.

Heinemeyer, W., Alt, J., and Herrmann, R. G. (1984) Nucleotide sequence of the clustered genes for apocytochrome b_6 and subunit 4 of the cytochrome b/f complex in the spinach plastid chromosome. *Curr. Genet.* 8: 543.

Henderson, R., Baldwin, J. M., Ceska, T. A., Zemlin, F., Beckmann, E., and Downing, K. H. (1990) Model for the structure of bacteriorhodopsin based on high resolution electron cryo-microscopy. *J. Mol. Biol.* 213: 899.

Henderson, R., and Unwin, P.N.T. (1975) Three-dimensional model of purple membrane obtained by electron microscopy. *Nature* 257: 28.

Herrmann, R. G., Alt, J., Schiller, B., Widger, W. R., and Cramer, W. A. (1984) Nucleotide sequence of the gene for apocytochrome b-559 on the spinach plastid chromosome: implications for the structure of the membrane protein. *FEBS Lett.* 176: 239.

Heyn, M. P., Westerhausen, J., Wallat, I., and Seiff, F. (1988) High-sensitivity neutron diffraction of membranes: location of the Schiff base end of the chromophore in bacteriorhodopsin. *Proc. Natl. Acad. Sci. USA* 85: 2146.

Holmgren, A., and Bränden, C.-I. (1989) Crystal structure of chaperone protein PapD reveals an immunoglobulin fold. *Nature* 342: 248.

Huang, K.-S., Bayley, H., Liao, M.-J., London, E., and Khorana, H. G. (1981) Refolding of an integral membrane protein. Denaturation, renaturation, and reconstitution of intact bacteriorhodopsin and two proteolytic fragments. *J. Biol. Chem.* 256: 3802.

Hultgren, S. J., Normark, S., and Abraham, N. A. (1991) Chaperone-assisted assembly and molecular architecture of adhesive pili. *Annu. Rev. Microbiol.* 45: 383.

Hurtley, S. M., Bole, D. G., Hoover-Litty, H., Helenius, A., and Copeland, C. S. (1989) Interactions of misfolded influenza hemagglutinin with binding protein (BiP). *J. Cell Biol.* 108: 2117.

Hurtley, S. M., and Helenius, A. (1989) Protein oligomerization in the endoplasmic reticulum. *Annu. Rev. Cell Biol.* 5: 277.

Hyde, C. C., Ahmed, S. A., Padlan, E. A., Miles, E. W., and Davies, D. R. (1988) Three-dimensional structure of the tryptophan synthase $\alpha_2\beta_2$ multienzyme complex from *Salmonella typhimurium*. *J. Biol. Chem.* 263: 17857.

Ichihara, S., and Mizushima, S. (1979) Arrangement of proteins O-8 and O-9 in outer membrane of *Escherichia coli* K-12. *Eur. J. Biochem.* 100: 321.

Isacoff, E. Y., Jan, Y. N., and Jan, L. Y. (1991) Putative receptor for the cytoplasmic inactivation gate in the *Shaker* K^+ channel. *Nature* 353: 86.

Ishizuka, M., Machida, K., Shimada, S., Mogi, A., Tsuchiya, T., Ohmori, T., Souma, Y., Gonda, M., and Sone, N. (1990) Nucleotide sequence of the gene coding for four subunits of cytochrome c oxidase from the thermophilic bacterium PS3. *J. Biochem.* 108: 866.

Jackson, M. E., Pratt, J. M., Stoker, N. G., and Holland, I. B. (1985) An inner membrane protein N-terminal signal sequence is able to promote efficient localization of an outer membrane protein in *Escherichia coli. EMBO J.* 4: 2377.

Jacob, F. (1970) *La logique du vivant.* Paris: Gallimard.

Jacobs, R. E., and White, S. H. (1989) The nature of the hydrophobic binding of small peptides at the bilayer interface: implications for the insertion of transbilayer helices. *Biochemistry* 28: 3421.

Jaenicke, R. (1991) Protein folding: local structures, domains, subunits and assemblies. *Biochemistry* 30: 3147.

Jap, B. K., and Walian, P. J. (1990) Biophysics of the structure and function of porins. *Q. Rev. Biphys.* 23: 367.

Jeanteur, D., Lakey, J. H., and Pattus, F. (1991) The bacterial porin superfamily: sequence alignment and structure prediction. *Mol. Microbiol.* 5: 2153.

Jennings, M. L. (1989) Topography of membrane proteins. *Annu. Rev. Biochem.* 58: 999.

Jensen, K. H., Herrin, D. L., Plumley, F. G., and Schmidt, G. W. (1986) Biogenesis of photosystem II complexes: transcriptional, translational and posttranslational regulation. *J. Cell Biol.* 103: 701.

Joliot, P., Verméglio, A., and Joliot, A. (1992) Supramolecular membrane protein assemblies in photo-synthesis and respiration. *Biochim. Biophys. Acta* 141: 151.

Jubb, J. S., Worcester, D. L., Crespi, H. L., and Zaccaï, G. (1984) Retinal location in the purple membrane of *Halobacterium halobium:* a neutron diffraction study of membranes labelled in vivo with deuterated retinal. *EMBO J.* 3: 1455.

Kaback, H. R. (1992) In and out and up and down with the lactose permease of *Escherichia coli. Int Rev. Cytol.* 137A: 97.

Kahn, T. W. (1991) *The Contributions of Helix-Connectihg Loops and of Retinal to the Stability of Bacteriorhodopsin.* Ph.D. Thesis, Yale University.

Kahn, T. W., and Engelman, D. M. (1992) Bacteriorhodopsin can be refolded from two independently stable transmembrane helices and the complementary five-helix fragment. *Biochemistry* 31: 6144.

Kahn, T. W., Sturtevant, J. M., and Engelman, D. M. (1992) Thermodynamic measurements of the contributions of helix-connecting loops and of retinal to the stability of bacteriorhodopsin. *Biochemistry* 31: 8829.

Karlin, A. (1991) Explorations of the nicotinic acetylcholine receptor. *Harvey Lect.* 85: 71.

Karlin, A. (1993) Structure of nicotinic acetylcholine receptors. *Curr. Opinion Neurobiol.* 3: 299.

Khorana, H. G. (1992) Rhodopsin, photoreceptor of the rod cell. An emerging pattern for structure and function. *J. Biol. Chem.* 207: 1.

Khorana, H. G., Gerber, G. E., Herlihy, W. C., Gray, C. P., Anderegg, R. J., Nihel, K., and Biemann, K. (1979) Amino acid sequence of bacteriorhodopsin. *Proc. Natl. Acad. Sci. USA* 76: 5046.

Kim, J., Gamble Klein, P., and Mullet, J. E. (1991) Ribosomes pause at specific sites during synthesis of membrane-bound chloroplast reaction center protein D1. *J. Biol. Chem.* 266: 14931.

Kim, P. S., and Baldwin, R. L. (1990) Intermediates in the folding reactions of small proteins. *Annu. Rev. Biochem.* 59: 631.

Klausner, R. D. (1989) Architectural editing: determining the fate of newly synthesized membrane proteins. *New Biologist* 1: 3.

Klingenberg, M. (1990) Mechanism and evolution of the uncoupling protein of brown adipose tissue. *Trends Biochem. Sci.* 15: 108.

Kobilka, B. K., Kobilka, T. S., Daniel, K., Regan, J. W., Caron, M. G., and Lefkowitz, R. J. (1988) Chimeric α_2-β_2-adrenergic receptors: delineation of domains involved in effector coupling and ligand binding specificity. *Science* 240: 1310.

Köster, W. (1991) Iron(III) hydroxamate transport across the cytoplasmic membrane of *Escherichia coli. Biol. Metals* 4: 23.

Köster, W., and Braun, V. (1990) Iron(III) hydroxamate transport of *Escherichia coli:* Restoration of iron supply by coexpression of the N- and C-terminal halves of the cytoplasmic membrane protein FhuB cloned on separate plasmids. *Mol. Gen. Genet.* 223: 379.

Krauss, N., Hinrichs, W., Witt, I., Fromme, P., Pritzkow, W., Dauter, Z., Betzel, C., Wilson, K. S., Witt, H. T., and Saenger, W. (1993) Three-dimensional structure of system I of photosynthesis at 6 Å resolution. *Nature* 361: 326.

Kuchka, M. R., Goldschmidt-Clermont, M., van Dillewijn, J., and Rochaix, J.-D. (1989) Mutation at the *Chlamydomonas* nuclear *NAC2* locus specifically affects stability of the chloroplast *psbD* transcript encoding polypeptide D2 of PSII. *Cell* 58: 869.

Kuchka, M. R., Mayfield, S. P., and Rochaix, J.-D. (1988) Nuclear mutations specifically affect the synthesis and/or degradation of the chloroplast-encoded D2 polypeptide of photosystem II in *Chlamydomonas reinhardtii. EMBO J.* 7: 319.

Kühlbrandt, W. (1988) Three-dimensional cystallization of membrane proteins. *Q. Rev. Biophys.* 21: 429.

Kühlbrandt, W., and Wang, D. N. (1991) Three-dimensional structure of plant light-harvesting complex determined by electron cyrstallography. *Nature* 350: 130.

Kühlbrandt, W., Wang, D. N., and Fujiyoshi, Y. (1994) Atomic model of light-harvesting complex by electron crystallography. *Nature* 367: 614.

Laufer, R., and Changeux, J.-P. (1989) Activity-dependent regulation of gene expression in muscle and neuronal cells. *Mol. Neurobiol.* 3: 1.

Lemmon, M. A., Flanagan, J. M., Hunt, J. F., Adair, B. D., Bormann, B.-J., Dempsey, C. E., and Engelman, D. M. (1992a) Glycophorin A dimerization is driven by specific interactions between transmembrane α-helices. *J. Biol.Chem.* 267: 7683.

Lemmon, M. A., and Engelman, D. M. (1992) Helix-helix interactions inside lipid bilayers. *Curr. Opinion Struct. Biol.* 2: 511.

Lemmon, M. A., Flanagan, J. M., Treutlein, H. R., Zhang, J., and Engelman, D. M. (1992b) Sequence specificity in the dimerization of transmembrane α-helices. *Biochemistry* 31: 12719.

Lever, T. M., Palmer, T., Cunningham, I. J., Cotton, N.P.J., and Jackson, J. B. (1991) Purification and properties of the H^+-nicotinamide nucleotide transhydrogenase from *Rhodobacter capsulatus. Eur. J. Biochem.* 197: 247.

Li, J., Carroll, J., and Ellar, D. J. (1991) Crystal structure of insecticidal δ-endotoxin from *Bacillus thuringiensis* at 2.5 Å resolution. *Nature* 353: 815.

Li, J., and Tooth, P. (1987) Size and shape of the *Escherichia coli* lactose permease measured in filamentous arrays. *Biochemistry* 26: 4816.

Liao, M.-J., Huang, K.-S., and Khorana, H. G. (1984) Regeneration of native bacteriorhodopsin structure from fragments. *J. Biol. Chem.* 259: 4200.

Liao, M.-J., London, E., and Khorana, H. G. (1983) Regeneration of the native bacteriorhodopsin structure from two chymotryptic fragments. *J. Biol. Chem.* 258: 9949.

Liman, E. R., Hess, P., Weaver, F., and Koren, G. (1991) Voltage-sensing residues in the S4 region of a mammalian K^+ channel. *Nature* 353: 752.

Lotteau, V., Teyton, L., Peleraux, A., Nilsson, T., Karlsson, L., Schmid, S. L., Quaranta, V., and Peterson, P. A. (1991) Intracellular transport of class II MHC molecules directed by invariant chain. *Nature* 348: 600.

MacIntyre, S., Freudl, R., Eschbach, M.-L., and Henning, U. (1988) An artificial hydrophobic sequence functions as either an anchor or a signal sequence at only one of two positions within the *Escherichia coli* outer membrane protein OmpA. *J. Biol. Chem.* 263: 19053.

Mannella, C. A., Forte, M., and Colombini, M. (1992) Toward the molecular structure of the mitochondrial channel, VDAC. *J. Bioeng. Biomemb.* 24: 7.

Manning-Krieg, U. C., Scherer, P. E., and Schatz, G. (1991) Sequential action of mitochondrial chaperones in protein import into the matrix. *EMBO J.* 10: 3273.

Manoil, C. (1990) Analysis of protein localisation by use of gene fusions with complementary properties. *Proc. Natl. Acad. Sci. USA* 87: 4937.

Manoil, C., and Beckwith, J. (1986) A genetic approach to analyzing membrane protein topology. *Science* 233: 1403.

Manoil, C., Mekalanos, J. J., and Beckwith, J. (1990) Alkaline phosphatase fusions: sensors of subcellular location. *J. Bacteriol.* 172: 515.

Manolios, N., Bonifacino, J. S., and Klausner, R. D. (1990) Transmembrane helical intercations and the assembly of the T cell receptor complex. *Science* 249: 274.

Marchal, C., and Hofnung, M. (1983) Negative dominance in gene *lamB:* random assembly of secreted subunits issued from different polysomes. *EMBO J.* 2: 81.

Marder, J. B., Goloubinoff, P., and Edelman, M. (1984) Molecular architecture of the rapidly metabolized 32-kDa protein of photosystem II. *J. Biol. Chem.* 259: 3900.

Marres, C.A.M., de Vries, S., and Grivell, L. A. (1991) Isolation and inactivation of the nuclear gene encoding the rotenone-insensitive internal NADH: ubiquinone oxido-reductase of mitochondria from *Saccharomyces cerevisiae. Eur. J. Biochem.* 195: 857.

Martin, J., Langer, T., Boteva, R., Schramel, A., Horwich, A. L., and Hartl, F.-U. (1991) Chaperonin-mediated protein folding at the surface of groEL through a "molten globule"-like intermediate. *Nature* 352: 36.

McCrea, P. D., Engelman, D. M., and Popot, J.-L. (1988) Topography of integral membrane proteins: hydrophobicity analysis vs. immunolocalization. *Trends Biochem. Sci.* 13: 289.

McGovern, K., Ehrmann, M., and Beckwith, J. (1991) Decoding signals for membrane protein assembly using alkaline phosphatase fusions. *EMBO J.* 10: 2773.

Merlie, J. P., and Lindstrom, J. (1983) Assembly in vivo of mouse muscle acetylcholine receptor: identification of an α subunit species that may be an assembly intermediate. *Cell* 34: 747.

Michel, H. (ed.) (1991) *Crystallization of Membrane Proteins.* Boca Raton, FL: CRC Press.

Michel, H., and Deisenhofer, J. (1988) Relevance of the photosynthetic reaction center from purple bacteria to the structure of photosystem II. *Biochemistry* 27: 1.

Michel, H., and Deisenhofer, J. (1989) The photosynthetic reaction centre from the purple bacterium *Rhodopseudomonas viridis. EMBO J.* 8: 2149.

Michel, H., and Oesterhelt, D. (1980) Three-dimensional crystals of membrane proteins: bacteriorhodopsin. *Proc. Natl. Acad. Sci. USA* 77: 1283.

Milburn, M. V., Privé, G. G., Milligan, D. L., Scott, W. G., Yeh, J., Jancarik, J., Koshland, D. E. Jr., and Kim, S.-H. (1991) Three-dimensional structures of the ligand-binding domain of the bacterial aspartate receptor with and without a ligand. *Science* 254: 1342.

Mueckler, M., and Lodish, H. F. (1986) The human glucose transporter can insert posttranslationally into microsomes. *Cell* 44: 629.

Nanba, O., and Satoh, K. (1987) Isolation of a photosystem II reaction center consisting of D-1 and D-2 polypeptides and cytochrome b-559. *Proc. Natl. Acad. Sci. USA* 84: 109.

Nikaido, H., and Reid, J. (1990) Biogenesis of prokaryotic pores. *Experientia* 46: 174.

Nilsson, B., and Anderson, S. (1991) Proper and improper folding of proteins in the cellular environment. *Annu. Rev. Microbiol.* 45: 607.

Nitschke, W., and Rutherford, W. (1991): Photosynthetic reaction centers: variations on a common structural theme? *Trends Biochem. Sci.* 16: 241.

Nixon, P. J., Chisholm, D. A., and Diner, B. A. (1994): Isolation and functional analysis of random and site-directed mutants of photosystem II. In: *Plant Protein Engineering*. Cambridge: Cambridge University Press (in press).

Ovchinnikov, Y. A., Abdulaev, N. G., Feigina, M. Y., Kiselev, A., Lobanov, N. A. (1979) The structural basis of the functioning of the bacteriorhodopsin, an overview. *FEBS Lett.* 100: 219.

Pao, G. M., Wu, L.-F., Johnson, K. D., Höfte, H., Chrispeels, M. J., Sweet, G., Sandal, N. N., and Saier, Jr., M. H. (1991) Evolution of the MIP family of integral membrane transport proteins. *Mol. Microbiol.* 5: 33.

Papadopoulos, G., Dencher, N. A., Zaccaï, G., and Büldt, G. (1990) Water molecules and exchangeable hydrogen ions at the active center of bacteriorhodopsin localized by neutron diffraction. Elements of the proton pathway? *J. Mol. Biol.* 214: 15.

Papazian, D. M., Timpe, L. C., Jan, Y. N., and Jan, L. Y. (1991) Alteration of voltage-dependence of *Shaker* potassium channel by mutations in the S4 sequence. *Nature* 349: 305.

Parker, M. W., Pattus, F., Tucker, A. D., and Tsernoglou, D. (1989) Structure of the membrane-pore-forming fragment of colicin A. *Nature* 337: 93.

Patthy, L. (1991) Modular exchange principles in proteins. *Curr. Opin. Struct. Biol.* 1: 351.

Pattus, F. (1990) Membrane protein structure. *Curr. Opin. Cell Biol.* 2: 681.

Paulsen, H., Rümler, V., and Rüdiger, W. (1990) Reconstitution of chlorophyll *a,b*-containing complexes from LHCP overproduced in bacteria. *Planta* 181: 204.

Payan, L. A., and Cline, K. (1991) A stromal protein factor maintains the solubility and insertion competence of an imported thylakoid membrane protein. *J. Cell Biol.* 112: 603.

Persson, R., and Pettersson, R. F. (1991) Formation and intracellular transport of a heterodimeric viral spike protein complex. *J. Cell Biol.* 112: 257.

Peters, P. J., Neefjes, J. J., Oorschot, V., Ploegh, H. L., and Geuze, H. J. (1991) Segregation of MHC class II molecules from MHC class I molecules in the Golgi complex for transport to lysosomal compartments. *Nature* 349: 669.

Pfanner, N., and Neupert, W. (1990): The mitochondrial protein import apparatus. *Annu. Rev. Biochem.* 59: 331.

Picot, D., Loll, P. J., Garavito, R. M. (1994) The x-ray crystal structure of the membrane protein prostaglandin H_2 synthase-1. *Nature* 367: 243.

Pierre, Y., and Popot, J.-L. (1993) Identification of two 4 kDa miniproteins in the cytochrome $b_6 f$ complex from *Chlamydomonas reinhardtii*. *C. R. Acad Sci. (Paris) Ser. 3* (in press).

Popot, J.-L. (1993) Integral membrane protein structure: transmembrane α-helices as autonomous folding domains. *Curr. Opinion Struct. Biol.* 3: 532.

Popot, J.-L., and de Vitry, C. (1990) On the microassembly of integral membrane proteins. *Annu. Rev. Biophys. Biophys. Chem.* 19: 369.

Popot, J.-L., and Engelman, D. M. (1990) Membrane protein folding and oligomerization: the two-stage model. *Biochemistry* 29: 4031.

Popot, J.-L., Engelman, D. M., Gurel, O., and Zaccaï, G. (1989) Tertiary structure of bacteriorhodopsin: positions and orientations of helices A and B in the structural map determined by neutron diffraction. *J. Mol. Biol.* 210: 829.

Popot, J.-L., Gerchman, S.-E., and Engelman, D. M. (1987) Refolding of bacteriorhodopsin in lipid bilayers: a thermodynamically controlled two-stage process. *J. Mol. Biol.* 198: 655.

Popot, J.-L., Pham Dinh, D., and Dautigny, A. (1991) Major myelin proteolipid: the 4-α-helix topology. *J. Membrane Biol.* 120: 233.

Popot, J.-L., Trewhella, J., and Engelman, D. M. (1986) Reformation of crystalline purple membrane from purified bacteriorhodopsin fragments. *EMBO J.* 5: 3039.

Pugsley, A. P. (1989) *Protein Targeting*. San Diego: Academic Press.

Rees, D. C., Komiya, H., Yeates, T. O., Allen, J. P., and Feher, G. (1989) The bacterial photosynthetic reaction center as a model for membrane proteins. *Annu. Rev. Biochem.* 58: 607.

Reiss-Husson, F. (1992) In: *Crystallization of Protein and Nucleic Acids, a Practical Approach*, edited by R. Giegé and A. Ducruix. Oxford: IRL Press, ch. 8, p. 175.

Richardson, J. S. (1981) The anatomy and taxonomy of protein structure. *Adv. Protein Chem.* 34: 168.

Ried, G., MacIntyre, S., Mutschler, B., and Henning, U. (1990) Export of altered forms of an *Escherichia coli* K-12 outer membrane protein (OmpA) can inhibit synthesis of unrelated outer membrane proteins. *J. Mol. Biol.* 216: 39.

Rochaix, J.-D., and Erickson, J. (1988) Function and assembly of photosystem II: genetic and molecular analysis. *Trends Biochem. Sci.* 13: 56.

Rochaix, J.-D., Kuchka, K., Mayfield, S., Schirmer-Rahire, M., Girard-Bascou, J., and Bennoun, P. (1989) Nuclear and chloroplast mutations affect the synthesis or stability of the chloroplast *psbC* gene product in *Chlamydomonas reinhardtii*. *EMBO J.* 8: 1013.

Roche, P. A., Marks, M. S., and Cresswell, P. (1991) Formation of a nine-subunit complex by HLA class II glycoproteins and the invariant chain. *Nature* 354: 392.

Rögner, M., Chisholm, D. A., and Diner, B. A. (1991) Site-directed mutagenesis of the *psbC* gene of photosystem II: isolation and functional characteristics of CP43-less photosystem II core complexes. *Biochemistry* 30: 5387.

Rosenbusch, J. P. (1974) Characterization of the major envelope protein from *Escherichia coli*. Regular arrangement on the peptidoglycan and unusual dodecyl sulfate binding. *J. Biol. Chem.* 249: 8019.

Ross, A. F., Green, W. N., Hartman, D. S., and Claudio, T. (1991) Efficiency of acetylcholine receptor subunit assembly and its regulation by cAMP. *J. Cell Biol.* 113: 623.

Roth, M., Arnoux, B., Ducruix, A., and Reiss-Husson, F. (1991) Structure of the detergent phase and protein-detergent interactions in crystals of the wild-type (strain Y) *Rhodobacter sphaeroides* photochemical reaction center. *Biochemistry* 30: 9403.

Roth, M., Lewit-Bentley, A., Michel, H., Deisenhofer, J., Huber, R., and Oesterhelt, D. (1989) Detergent structure in crystals of bacterial photosynthetic reaction center. *Nature* 340: 659.

Rubin, R. A., and Levy, S. B. (1991) Tet protein domains interact productively to mediate tetracycline resistance when present on separate polypeptides. *J. Bacteriol.* 173: 4503.

Rubin, R. A., Levy, S. B., Heinrikson, R. L., and Kezdy, F. J. (1990) Gene duplication in the evolution of the two complementing domains of gram-negative bacterial tetracycline efflux proteins. *Gene* 87: 7.

Saedi, M. S., Conroy, W. G., and Lindstrom, J. (1991) Assembly of *Torpedo* acetylcholine receptors in *Xenopus* oocytes. *J. Cell Biol.* 112: 1007.

Samatey, F. A., Popot, J.-L., Etchebest, C., and Zaccaï, G. (1992) Rotational orientation of transmembrane α-helices in bacteriophodopsin studied by neutron diffraction. *Proceedings of the Vth International Conference on Retinal Proteins*, J.-L. Rigaud, ed. London: John Libbey, pp. 9–12.

Smatey, F. A., Zaccaï, G., Engelman, D. R., Etchebest, C., and Popot, J.-L. (1993) Rotational orientation of transmembrane α-helices in bacteriorhodopsin. A neutron diffraction study. *J. Mol. Biol.* (in press).

Saraste, M. (1990) Structural features of cytochrome oxidase. *Q. Rev. Biophys.* 23: 331.

Saraste, M., Metso, T., Nakari, T., Jalli, T., Lauraeus, M., and Van Der Oost, J. (1991) The *Bacillus subtilis* cytochrome *c* oxidase. *Eur. J. Biochem.* 195: 517.

Saurin, W., and Dassa, E. (1994) Sequence relationships between integral inner membrane proteins from binding protein-dependent transport systems. Evolution by recurrent gene duplications. *Protein Sci.* (in press).

Schertler, G.F.X., Villa, C., and Henderson, R. (1993) Projection structure of rhodopsin. *Nature* 362: 1770.

Schiltz, E., Kreusch, A., Nestel, U., and Schulz, G. E. (1991) Primary structure of porin from *Rhodobacter capsulatus. Eur. J. Biochem.* 199: 587.

Schirmer, T., and Rosenbusch, J. P. (1991) Prokaryotic and eukaryotic porins. *Curr. Opin. Struct. Biol.* 1: 539.

Schwarzmann, G., Wiegandt, H., Rose, B., Zimmerman, A., Ben-Haim, D., and Loewenstein, W. R. (1981) Diameter of the cell-to-cell junctional membrane channels as probed with neutral molecules. *Science* 213: 551.

Sen, K., and Nikaido, H. (1990) Trimerization of an in vitro synthesized OmpF porin of *Escherichia coli* outer membrane. *J. Biol. Chem.* 266: 11295.

Sen, K., and Nikaido, H. (1991) Lipopolysaccharide structure required for in vitro trimerization of *Escherichia coli* OmpF porin. *J. Bacteriol.* 173: 926.

Senior, A. E. (1990) The proton-translocating ATPase of *Escherichia coli. Annu. Rev. Biophys. Biophys. Chem.* 19: 7.

Shuman, H. A. (1987) The genetics of active transport in bacteria. *Annu. Rev. Genet.* 21: 155.

Sieburth, L. E., Berry-Lowe, S., and Schmidt, G. W. (1991) Chloroplast RNA stability in *Chlamydomonas:* rapid degradation of *psbB* and *psbC* transcripts in two nuclear mutants. *Plant Cell* 3: 175.

Sigrist, H., Wenger, R. H., Kislig, E., and Wüthrich, M. (1988) Refolding of bacteriorhodopsin. Protease V8 fragmentation and chromophore reconstitution from proteolytic V8 fragments. *Eur. J. Biochem.* 177: 125.

Singer, S. J. (1990) The structure and insertion of integral proteins in membranes. *Annu. Rev. Cell Biol.* 6: 247.

Singh, I., Doms, R. W., Wagner, K. R., and Helenius, A. (1990) Intracellular transport of soluble and membrane-bound glycoproteins: folding, assembly and secretion of anchor-free influenza hemagglutinin. *EMBO J.* 9: 631.

Smith, M. M., Lindstrom, J., and Merlie, J. P. (1987) Formation of the α-bungarotoxin binding site and assembly of the nicotinic acetylcholine receptor subunits occur in the endoplasmic reticulum. *J. Biol. Chem.* 262: 4367.

Stegmann, T., Doms, R. W., and Helenius, A. (1989) Protein-mediated membrane fusion. *Annu. Rev. Biophys. Biophys. Chem.* 18: 187.

Stephan, M., and Agnew, W. S. (1991) Voltage-sensitive Na^+ channels: motifs, modes and modulation. *Curr. Biol.* 3: 676.

Stephenson, F. A. (1991) Ion channels. *Curr. Biol.* 1: 569.

Sternberg, M.J.E., and Gullick, W. J. (1989) *Neu* receptor dimerization. *Nature* 339: 587.

Stühmer, W., Conti, F., Suzuki, H., Wand, X., Noda, M., Yahagi, N., Kubo, H., and Numa, S. (1989) Structural parts involved in activation and inactivation of the sodium ion channel. *Nature* 339: 597.

Sumikawa, K. (1992) Sequences on the N-terminus of ACh receptor subunits regulate their assembly. *J. Cell.Biochem.* 16E: 229.

Sumikawa, K., and Miledi, R. (1989) Assembly and *N*-glycosylation of all ACh receptor subunits are required for their efficient insertion into plasma membranes. *Mol. Brain Res.* 5: 183.

Sussman, J. L., Harel, M., Frolow, F., Oefner, C., Goldman, A., Toker, L., and Silman, I. (1991) Atomic structure of acetylcholinesterase from *Torpedo californica:* a prototypic acetylcholine-binding protein. *Science* 253: 872.

Tommassen, J., Van Tol, H., and Lugtenberg, B. (1983) The ultimate localization of an outer membrane protein of *Escherichia coli* K-12 is not determined by signal sequence. *EMBO J.* 2: 1275.

Traxler, B., and Beckwith, J. (1992) Steps in the assembly of a cytoplasmic protein—the malF component of the maltose transport complex. In: *Membrane Biogenesis and Protein Targeting,* edited by W. Neupert and R. Lill. (Series *New Comprehensive Biology*), pp. 49–61.

Traxler, B., Lee, C., Boyd, D., and Beckwith, J. (1992) The dynamics of assembly of a cytoplasmic membrane protein in *Escherichia coli. J. Biol. Chem.* 267: 5339.

Tuschen, G., Sackmann, U., Nehls, U., Haiker, H., Buse, G., and Weiss, H. (1990) Assembly of NADH: ubiquinone reductase (complex I) in *Neurospora* mitochondria. *J. Mol. Biol.* 213: 845.

Unwin, N. (1989) The structure of ion channels in membranes of excitable cells. *Neuron* 3: 665.

Unwin, N. (1993) Nicotinic acetylcholine receptor at 9 Å resolution. *J. Mol. Biol.* 229: 1101.

van der Goot, F. G., Gonzáles-Mañas, J. M., Lakey, J. H., and Pattus, F. (1991) A "molten-globule" membrane-insertion intermediate of the pore-forming domain of colicin A. *Nature* 354: 408.

Varghese, J. N., Laver, W. G., and Colman, P. M. (1983) Structure of the influenza virus glycoprotein antigen neuraminidase at 2.9 Å resolution. *Nature* 303: 35.

Verrall, S., and Hall, Z. W. (1992) The N-terminal domains of acetylcholine receptor subunits contain recognition signals for the initial steps of receptor assembly. *Cell* 68: 23.

von Heijne, G. (1986a) The distribution of positively charged residues in bacterial inner membrane proteins correlates with the trans-membrane topology. *EMBO J.* 5: 3021.

von Heijne, G. (1986b) Why mitochondria need a genome. *FEBS Lett.* 198: 1.

von Heijne, G. (1988) Transcending the impenetrable: how proteins come to terms with membranes. *Biochim. Biophys. Acta* 947: 307.

von Heijne, G. (1990) The signal peptide. *J. Membrane Biol.* 115: 195.

von Heijne, G., and Blomberg, C. (1979) Trans-membrane translocation of proteins. *Eur. J. Biochem.* 97: 175.

von Heijne, G., and Gavel, Y. (1988) Topogenic signals in integral membrane proteins. *Eur. J. Biochem.* 174: 671.

von Heijne, G., Wickner, W., and Dalbey, R. E. (1988) The cytoplasmic domain of *Escherichia coli* leader peptidase is a "translocation poison" sequence. *Proc. Natl. Acad. Sci. USA* 85: 3363.

Vos-Scheperkeuter, G. H., and Witholt, B. (1984) Assembly pathway of newly synthesized LamB protein an outer membrane protein of *Escherichia coli* K-12. *J. Mol. Biol.* 175: 511.

Weis, W., Brown, J. H., Cusack, S., Paulson, J. C., Skehel, J. J., and Wiley, D. C. (1988) Structure of the influenza virus haemagglutinin complexed with its receptor, sialic acid. *Nature* 333: 426.

Weiss, M. S., Kreusch, A., Schiltz, E., Nestel, U., Welte, W., Weckesser, J., and Schulz, G. E. (1991) The structure of porin from *Rhodobacter capsulatus* at 1.8 Å resolution. *FEBS Lett.* 280: 379.

Weiss, M. S., Wacker, T., Weckesser, J., Welte, W., and Schulz, G. E. (1990) The three-dimensional structure of porin from *Rhodobacter capsulatus* at 3 Å resolution. *FEBS lett.* 267: 379.

White, J. M. (1990) Viral and cellular membrane fusion proteins. *Annu. Rev. Physiol.* 52: 675.

White, S. H., and Jacobs, R. E. (1990) Observations concerning the topology and locations of helix ends of membrane proteins of known structure. *J. Membrane Biol.* 115: 145.

Wickner, W., Driessen, A.J.M., and Hartl, F.-U. (1991) The enzymology of protein translocation across the *Escherichia coli* plasma membrane. *Annu. Rev. Biochem.* 60: 101.

Widger, W. R., Cramer, W. A., Hermondson, M., and Herrmann, R. A. (1985) Evidence for a heterooligomeric structure of the chloroplast cytochrome *b*-599. *FEBS Lett.* 191: 186.

Wienhues, U., and Neupert, W. (1992) Protein translocation across mitochondrial membranes. *BioEssays* 14: 17.

Wiley, D. C., and Skehel, J. J. (1987) The structure and function of the hemagglutinin membrane glycoprotein of influenza virus. *Annu. Rev. Biochem.* 56: 365.

Wilson, I. A., Skehel, J. J., and Wiley, D. C. (1981) Structure of the haemagglutinin membrane glycoprotein of influenza virus at 3 Å resolution. *Nature* 289: 366.

Wistow, G. J., Pisano, M. M., and Chepelinsky, A. B. (1991) Tandem sequence repeats in transmembrane channel proteins. *Trends Biochem. Sci.* 16: 170.

Wrubel, W., Stochaj, U., Sonnewald, U., Theres, C., and Ehring, R. (1990) Reconstitution of an active lactose carrier in vivo by simultaneous synthesis of two complementary protein fragments. *J. Bacteriol.* 172: 5374.

Yamaguchi, M., and Hatefi, Y. (1991) Mitochondrial energy-linked nicotinamide nucleotide transhydrogenase. Membrane topography of the bovine enzyme. *J. Biol. Chem.* 266: 5728.

Yamaguchi, M., Hatefi, Y., Trach, K., and Hoch, J. A. (1988) The primary structure of the mitochondrial energy-linked nicotinamide nucleotide transhydrogenase deduced from the sequence of cDNA clones. *J. Biol. Chem.* 263: 2761.

Yamane, K., Akiyama, Y., Ito, K., and Mizushima, S. (1990) A positively charged region is a determinant of the orientation of cytoplasmic membrane proteins in *Escherichia coli*. *J. Biol. Chem.* 265: 21166.

Yellen, G., Jurman, M. E., Abramson, T., and MacKinnon, R. (1991) Mutations affecting internal TEA blockade identify the probable pore-forming region of a K^+ channel. *Science* 251: 939.

Yool, A. J., and Schwarz, T. L. (1991) Alteration of ionic selectivity of a K^+ channel by mutation of the H5 region. *Nature* 349: 700.

Yu, X.-M., and Hall, Z. W. (1991) Extracellular domains mediating ε subunit interactions of muscle acetylcholine receptor. *Nature* 352: 64.

Yun, C.-H., Van Doren, S. R., Crofts, A. R., and Gennis, R. B. (1991) The use of gene fusions to examine the membrane topology of the L-subunit of the photosynthetic reaction center and of the cytochrome *b* subunit of the *bc*1 complex from *Rhodobacter sphaeroides. J. Biol. Chem.* 266: 10967.

Zeilstra-Ralls, J., Fayet, O., and Georgopoulos, C. (1991) The universally conserved GroE (Hsp50) chaperonins. *Annu. Rev. Microbiol.* 45: 301.

Zuber, H. (1986) Primary structure and function of the light-harvesting polypeptides from cyanobacteria, red algae and purple photosynthetic bacteria. In: *Encyclopedia of Plant Physiology,* new series, vol. 19, *Photosynthesis III, Photosynthetic Membranes and Light Harvesting Centers.* A. Trebst and M. Avron, eds. Berlin: Springer, p. 238.

4

Hydropathy Plots and the Prediction of Membrane Protein Topology

STEPHEN H. WHITE

Plots of sliding-window averages of amino acid properties taken along amino acid sequences provide useful structural insights for both soluble (Rose, 1978; Rose and Roy, 1980; Kyte and Doolittle, 1982) and membrane (Argos et al., 1982; Kyte and Doolittle, 1982; Engelman et al., 1986) proteins. They have been especially important for membrane proteins, however, because the determination of three-dimensional structures is more problematic. The database of high-resolution crystallographic membrane protein structures contains only five examples of two types of proteins: two photosynthetic reaction centers (PSRC) from *Rhodopseudomonas viridis* (Deisenhofer et al., 1985) and *Rhodobacter sphaeroides* (Allen et al., 1987), a porin from *Rhodobacter capsulatus* (Weiss et al., 1991a), and two porins from *Escherichia coli* (Cowan et al., 1992). An excellent, but incomplete, structural model for bacteriorhodopsin (BR) from *Halobacterium halobium* has been determined by Henderson et al. (1990) using electron diffraction methods. More recently, an atomic model of plant light-harvesting complex, also determined by electron diffraction, has been reported by Kühlbrandt et al. (1994).

The small number of available structures makes it difficult to develop and test prediction algorithms for membrane proteins, although one should keep in mind that the prediction problem has not yet been solved for soluble proteins despite the hundreds of structures now available. But, the structure of membrane proteins may possibly be easier to predict because the fundamental thermodynamics of the problem are more constrained (at least for the membrane-embedded portions of the sequence). Overall, there is reason to be encouraged about the possibilities because the basic topology and identification of helices for BR predicted in 1980 by Engelman et al. proved to be remarkably accurate. This success also serves as a warning, however, in that the low-resolution structure of Henderson and Unwin (1975) had already revealed the seven transmembrane helices with little ambiguity. Furthermore, the optical properties of the retinal chromophore combined with the in situ two-dimensional crystallinity of the protein provided a large amount of spectroscopic and structural data not available for most other membrane proteins (reviewed recently by Lanyi, 1992; Oesterhelt et al., 1992; Rothschild, 1992; Zheng and Herzfeld, 1992).

For the great majority of membrane proteins, a hydropathy-plot analysis yields the first direct connection between sequence and structure. Hydropathy plots assume that transmembrane (TM) segments are comprised predominantly of hydrophobic residues (Segrest and Feldman, 1974) because of the low solubility of polar side chains in nonpolar environments such as lipid bilayers. Because the free-energy cost of transferring "open" hydrogen bonds (H-bonds) into nonpolar phases is excessive (Engelman and Steitz, 1981; Griko et al., 1988; Jacobs and White, 1989) for even the most hydrophobic side chains, the α-helix is an ideal TM segment because its H-bonds are satisfied internally. Although this issue was not generally appreciated at the time, the early proposal by Lenard and Singer (1966) that TM segments are α-helices was thermodynamically sound. The requirement for backbone hydrogen bonding is further emphasized by the observation that porins form β-barrels so that the TM β-strands are fully hydrogen bonded (Weiss et al., 1991a; Cowan et al., 1992).

The lengths of TM secondary-structure elements must be sufficient to span the hydrocarbon regions of fluid bilayers that are typically 30 Å thick (Levine and Wilkins, 1971; Wiener and White, 1992a). This establishes the minimum lengths of TM α-helices (1.5 Å rise per residue) and β-strands (3.3 Å rise per residue) as 20 and 9 amino acids, respectively, consistent with the observed lengths of 22 to 31 amino acids for PSRC TM helices (Deisenhofer et al., 1985; Allen et al., 1987) and 10 to 17 amino acids for the porin TM β-strands that contact with the bilayer (Weiss et al., 1991b). Assuming β-sheet TM structures of the porin type to be relatively uncommon, hydropathy plot analyses generally seek runs of 20 or more amino acids with a net hydrophobicity sufficient for thermodynamic stability as a helix in the bilayer. However, a major question, especially for very large proteins such as Na^+ channels (Lodish, 1988), is whether there are other more complex structural motifs not yet known that may allow for full backbone hydrogen bonding. The free energy of transfer of a 20 residue polyalanine α-helix from water into a lipid bilayer is about -42 kcal/mol, assuming that partitioning is determined solely by the hydrophobic effect (Engelman et al., 1986). This very favorable transfer will be reduced considerably if highly polar residues are also present, as is probably the case for most ion transporting proteins. If the transfer becomes marginal, then the cost of burying the backbone hydrogen-bonded pairs may be an issue, as discussed in detail by Roseman (1988). An experimental uncertainty of 0.5 kcal/mol per H-bond in the transfer free energy could cause a 10 kcal/mol uncertainty in the total helix transfer free energy.

Most hydropathy plot methods derive from studies of the partitioning of amino acids between water and bulk phases such as alkanes and alkanols because little direct information about the energetics of peptide–bilayer interactions was available during the period when the basic thermodynamic principles underlying the hydropathy plot were being enumerated. Furthermore, detailed structural images of fluid bilayers, which are crucial for understanding the interactions of proteins with bilayers, were not available. It is now clear that solute partitioning into bilayers is more complex than first expected and cannot be accurately described using bulk-phase partition coefficients (Huang and Charlton, 1972; Seelig and Ganz, 1991); Beschiaschvili and Seelig, 1992; Wimley and White, 1993; White and Wimley, 1994). I therefore begin with a brief overview of recent advances in our understanding of the structure of fluid bilayers and their interactions with peptides. I then discuss systematically the general principles of hydropathy plots and address the question of whether there is a perfect linear sliding-window method for the prediction of topology (the answer is *no*). Finally, I consider the practical problem of interpreting hydrophobicity analyses through comparisons of hydropathy plots of four membrane proteins of known topology, a detailed examination of the L subunit of the PSRC from *Rhodob. sphaeroides,* and an analysis of a potassium ion channel.

I emphasize throughout the chapter that the results of hydropathy-plot analyses should *never* be taken as the final word on topology subject only to fine tuning. The only proper use of hydropathy plots in their present form is for the construction of hypotheses for guiding experiments. No topological map should be considered satisfactory until it persistently survives direct experimental testing.

Fluid Bilayers: a Complex Solvent Phase for Proteins

Fluid-Bilayer Structure

Many different physical methods (Small, 1986; Marsh, 1990) have been used to characterize and understand lipid bilayers, but I discuss only the recent results of Wiener and White (1991a–c; 1992a; b) who used x-ray and neutron diffraction data to arrive at an accurate time-averaged image of the transbilayer distribution of the principal structural groups of dioleoylphosphocholine (DOPC) in fluid bilayers by means of a joint refinement method (Wiener and White, 1991b). An important feature of fluid bilayers is the high degree of thermal motion of the lipids. Because of the thermal disorder, it is not possible to locate single atoms by x-ray or neutron diffraction (Wiener and White, 1991a) unless they are specifically brominated (Wiener and White, 1991c) or deuterated (Wiener et al., 1991). It is possible, however, to locate chemically important structural groups (called *quasimolecular fragments*) such as the phosphates, cholines, and carbonyls. The structural image obtained consists of a series of gaussian probability distributions that represent the time-averaged projection of the fragments' positions onto an axis normal to the plane of the bilayer. The areas of the distributions are equal to the number of fragments represented so that the carbonyl distribution for one-half of a bilayer has an area of 2, the phosphate group an area of 1, and so forth. The positions and widths of these distributions can be determined with a precision of better than 0.5 Å so that, even though the exact position of a fragment at any instant of time is uncertain, the total range of motion and the most probable position are defined precisely.

The results of Wiener and White's structural analysis (1992b) are summarized in Figure 4.1*b, c.* Their measurements were made at low hydrations (5.4 waters/lipid); thus the thermal motion will be smaller than in the biologically more relevant condition of excess water. Nevertheless, the amount of thermal motion even at the low hydration used is impressive. The widths and overlaps of the distributions of the groups clearly show the extreme chemical heterogeneity of the bilayer. Particularly impressive is the fact that the double-bonds of the DOPC acyl chains explore almost the entire thickness of the hydrocarbon region. The physicochemical heterogeneity of the hydrocarbon core is revealed in Figure 4.1*c* by the distribution of the hexane dissolved in the bilayer determined by White et al. (1981) using neutron diffraction. The hexane is not uniformly distributed across the bilayer, consistent with the fact that the hydrocarbon core is not equivalent to a simple bulk alkyl phase (White, 1977, 1980; Simon et al., 1977).

Most cartoon images of bilayers focus on the hydrocarbon core and imply that the headgroups account for only a small amount of the total bilayer thickness. Such

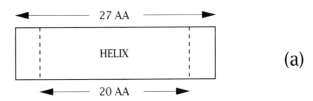

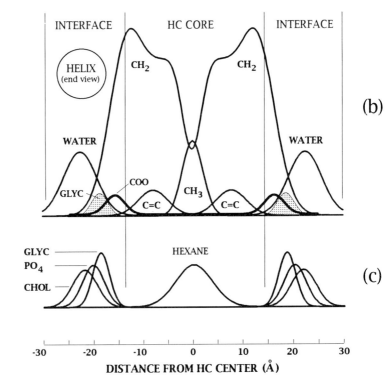

Fig. 4.1. Structure of a fluid bilayer (L_α phase). The "structure" consists of the projections onto the bilayer normal of the time-averaged transbilayer distributions of the principal structural groups of dioleoylphosphocholine (DOPC, 5.4 waters per lipid). The distributions represent probability density functions whose areas equal the number of components per lipid in the group. For example, the area under a water peak is 5.4, double-bond 2, glycerol 1, and so forth. The precisions of the positions and widths of the distributions are better than ± 0.5 Å. *a*: The dimensions of an α-helix with 27 amino acid acids, which is the typical length of a transmembrane helix. The expected minimum length required to span the hydrocarbon core of a bilayer is 20 amino acids (30 Å). *b*: The transbilayer distribution of DOPC structural groups and water except for the phosphocholines. Superimposed on the structure are *vertical lines* representing the approximate boundaries between the interfacial and hydrocarbon (HC) core regions. A *circle* representing an end-on helix has been placed in the interface to show that the interfacial region can comfortably accommodate an α-helix parallel to the bilayer. Note that the interface is a highly thermally disordered region containing both polar and nonpolar components. *c*: Distribution of the glycerol and phosphocholine components. All of the peaks have the same areas so that their widths indicate increasing thermal motion as one moves

images have led to the misconception of the bilayer as a thin hydrocarbon slab bounded by water. Figure 4.1*b*, however, shows that the hydrated headgroups, taken as the full widths of the water distributions, account for 50% of the total hydrated bilayer thickness. The headgroup region is thus of major importance to the problem of inserting and folding proteins in bilayer environments. To place these results in the context of transmembrane helices in bilayers, the approximate physical dimensions of helices are indicated in Figure 4.1*a, b*. The minimum 20 amino acid helix length and the average helix length of 27 amino acids observed in the PSRC are shown in Figure 4.1*a*. The 20 amino acid marker corresponds closely the hydrocarbon core thickness, while the amino acids beyond 20 are contained well within the interface region consisting of the phosphocholines and water. This comparison emphasizes that the amino acids of TM helices are in a highly nonuniform chemical environment; the amino acids near the center of the helix are in an environment different from those near the ends. Models of helix–bilayer interactions based on bulk-phase partition coefficients are, at best, gross estimates of reality. Another important structural comparison is that of the diameter of a helix relative to the hydrated headgroup distribution shown in Figure 4.1*b*; a helix placed in the bilayer interface parallel to the bilayer plane is easily accommodated. Importantly, a parallel helix in this region is in a highly heterogeneous region and can easily contact water, hydrocarbon, and phosphocholines.

Peptide–Bilayer Interactions

Given the structure and complexity of the bilayer interface, it is not surprising that interactions there strongly affect peptide conformations and can induce secondary structure (Kaiser and Kezdy, 1983, 1984; Sargent and Schwyzer, 1986; Wattenbarger et al., 1990). Jacobs and White (1986, 1987, 1989) have used a homologous series of hydrophobic tripeptides to examine the thermodynamic and structural consequences of interactions with fluid bilayers. Structural studies using neutron diffraction methods clearly show that the tripeptides are located in the interface and cause significant changes in bilayer structure. This emphasizes an important difference between bilayers and bulk phases: the solvent properties of the bilayer are strongly affected by the solute. Unlike partitioning into bulk nonpolar phases that is determined almost exclusively by the hydrophobic effect, bilayer partitioning involves additional thermodynamic contributions related to the thermodynamic response of the bilayer to the partitioning process (Wimley and White, 1993; White and Wimley, 1994). Estimating the free energy of transfer of peptides into bulk phases is simple because the contribution of the hydrophobic effect is easily calculated from the accessible surface area of the solute (Nozaki and Tanford, 1971; Reynolds et al., 1974;

---

outward toward the water region. The distribution of hexane dissolved in the bilayer is also shown in order to illustrate that the HC is not uniformly available to dissolved nonpolar molecules. GLYC, glycerol; CHOL, choline; COO, carbonyl; PO_4, phosphate; $C{=}C$, double bonded carbon; CH_2, methylene; and CH_3, methyl. The distributions of the structural groups of DOPC are based on Wiener and White (1992a) and the distribution of hexane dissolved in the bilayer upon White et al. (1981).

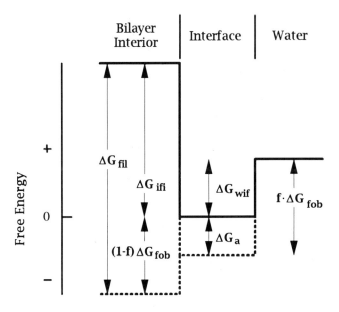

(a) Available hydrophobic free energy:

$$\Delta G_{fob} = C_s \cdot A_a$$

(b) Transfer from water to interface:

$$\Delta G_{wif} = f \cdot \Delta G_{fob} + \Delta G_a$$

(c) Transfer from interface to interior (extended chain):

$$\Delta G_{ifi} = (1\text{-}f) \cdot \Delta G_{fob} + \Delta G_{fil}$$

$$\Delta G_{fil} = \underset{\text{main chain} \rfloor}{\Delta G_{mc}} + \underset{\lfloor \text{side chain}}{\Delta G_{sc}}$$

(d) Free energy change with helix formation:

$$\Delta G_{hlx} = \Delta G_{ifi} - \Delta G_{mcH} - h \cdot \Delta G_{sc}$$

$$IFH(h) \equiv - \Delta G_{hlx}(h)$$

Fig. 4.2. Thermodynamic basis for describing the interaction of peptides with lipid bilayers based on the work of Jacobs and White (1989). The interface is a highly favorable region for the partitioning of all amino acids because both polar and nonpolar interactions can be satisfied simultaneously (see Fig. 4.1 and text).

Sharp et al., 1991). Although transfer of free energies into bilayers can sometimes be estimated in this way, great discrepancies are the rule rather than the exception and have led to the concept of the "nonclassic" hydrophobic effect in bilayers (Huang and Charlton, 1972; Seelig and Ganz, 1991; Beschiaschvili and Seelig, 1992). No general rules for estimating the bilayer contributions to partitioning have yet emerged.

Jacobs and White's thermodynamic studies of the interactions of hydrophobic tri-peptides with fluid bilayers (1989) have revealed the importance of the bilayer inter-face in peptide–bilayer interactions and have provided a general thermodynamic for-malism that has proved useful in simulations of protein insertion into bilayers (Milik and Skolnick, 1992, 1993). Although the formalism presently ignores specific con-tributions of bilayer thermodynamic changes to peptide partitioning, it does focus attention on the importance of hydrogen-bonding groups and the bilayer interface in peptide partitioning as summarized in Figure 4.2. The main driving force for par-titioning is taken to be the hydrophobic effect that provides a maximum free energy of partitioning of $\Delta G_{fob} = C_s A_a$, where C_s is the solvation parameter and A_a the acces-sible surface area of the peptide (Fig. 4.2a). If the value of C_s is -25 cal/mol·Å^2, as frequently assumed (Reynolds et al., 1974), then Jacobs and White's measure-ments (1989) indicate that a fraction $f \approx 0.5$ of the available hydrophobic effect free energy is consumed upon binding to the interface even though peptides do not pen-etrate deeply into the bilayer hydrocarbon interior. Opposing this favorable free energy of binding is an unfavorable free energy change ΔG_a associated with the reduction of entropy caused by partitioning into the interface (Fig. 4.2b). It should be emphasized, however, that the proper value of the C_s to use under these circum-stances is uncertain because of questions about what partition coefficient units should be used (Sharp et al., 1991; Wimley and White, 1992, 1993; White and Wimley, 1994). In any case, the analysis and results emphasize that the bilayer is a hetero-geneous phase and that important thermodynamic processes occur at the interface without the penetration of peptides into the hydrocarbon core to a significant extent. The major reason that the interface is a favorable region is that solutes with mixed nonpolar and polar character can simultaneously satisfy hydrophobic and hydro-philic interactions (see Fig. 4.1b).

The fraction $(1 - f)$ of hydrophobic free energy not consumed upon binding to the interface is available for partitioning the peptide between the interface and the hydrocarbon core (Fig. 4.2c). However, the favorable hydrophilic interactions between bilayer headgroups and water and the peptide's main chain and side chain polar groups must be disrupted for the peptide to move into the center of the bilayer (Fig. 4.2c). The disruption of these hydrophilic interactions is, for the most part, energetically very unfavorable unless compensating polar interactions can be estab-lished within the bilayer hydrocarbon core through peptide–peptide or peptide–lipid interactions. Of particular importance for TM hydrophobic segments are the main chain hydrogen bonds that are easily satisfied when the TM segment forms an α-helix. The favorable free energy of membrane insertion ΔG_{hlx} that accompanies the formation of a helix can be estimated by the addition of two terms to the generally unfavorable free energy of transfer ΔG_{ifi} from the bilayer interface to the bilayer inte-rior (Fig. 4.2d). One of the terms, $-\Delta G_{mcH}$, accounts for the favorable free energy of main chain hydrogen bonding, and the other, $-h\Delta G_{SC}$, accounts for possible favorable interactions within the bilayer of the side chain hydrogen-bonding groups.

The satisfaction of side chain hydrogen bonds depends on the number of hydrogen-bonding groups of the side chain and the availability of hydrogen-bonding partners. The factor h, which can have values between 0 and 1, was introduced to allow the energetic contribution of side chains to be examined under various assumptions about side chain H-bond formation. This general approach allows one to define an interfacial hydrophobicity index, $IFH(h) = -\Delta G_{hlx}$, as in Figure 4.2d, that is useful for searching protein sequences for TM helices (Jacobs and White, 1989; White and Jacobs, 1990b).

The Hydropathy Plot: a Sliding-Window Recognizer

Hydropathy plot analysis was first introduced by Rose (1978) as a means of identifying chain turns in soluble proteins, but it was the paper of Kyte and Doolittle (1982) that brought it into widespread use. There is now a bulk of literature on hydropathy analysis that is too large and diverse to review here, but the general principles are the same for all of the methods and are illustrated in Figure 4.3. In the simplest case, one performs a moving average or sum of amino acid hydrophobicity values along a sequence that yields plots of hydrophobicity versus window position (see Fig. 4.6, below). The average hydrophobicity at a sequence position extends over a "window" of length W amino acids and is most commonly an unweighted average. Computer programs of varying sophistication can be written to produce hydropathy plots, but the simplest approach is to use a microcomputer spreadsheet program (Vickery, 1987). The values of hydrophobicity are generally derived from measured or estimated values for the free energy of transfer of the natural amino acids from a nonpolar phase to water (Kyte and Doolittle, 1982; Engelman and Steitz, 1981) so that positive peaks identify possible TM helices. Because other amino acid properties such as secondary structure preference or charge can also be examined by this approach, I will use the more generic terminology of *sliding-window recognizer* (SWR), which includes the hydropathy plot as a particular case. A more accurate term for a SWR is *linear convolutional recognizer* (LCR) (Edelman and White, 1989) because, mathematically, one is convoluting a window function (w) with a sequence of weights H_m ($m = 1, 2, \ldots, N$). The resulting function (e.g., hydropathy plot) is a decision function D_m that is interpreted against a decision threshold T that might, for example, represent the global average of the H_m; regions of the sequence with $D_m > 0$ are candidates for the structural feature sought (e.g., TM helix). This mathematical approach emphasizes that the essential elements of an SWR are (*1*) a numerical scale of weights for the amino acid property, (*2*) a threshold or reference level, and (*3*) a window or weighting function used for the moving average. Consideration of these three elements allows one to distinguish, compare, and evaluate the various hydropathy plot schemes that have been devised during the past fifteen years.

Hydropathy Scales

Scales are generally derived from experimental measurements of the partitioning of amino acids between polar and nonpolar phases (Nozaki and Tanford, 1971; Fauch-

Sliding Window Recognizer (SWR)

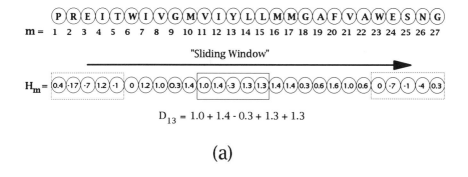

$$D_{13} = 1.0 + 1.4 - 0.3 + 1.3 + 1.3$$

(a)

Decision Function:

$$D_m = \sum_n H_{(m-n)} w_n - T$$

mathematical value of AA ⌐ ⌐ threshold level

└ window function centered at m

Favorable decision when $D_m > 0$

(b)

Window Functions:

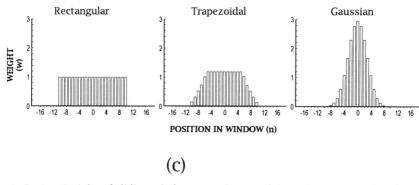

(c)

Fig. 4.3. Basic principles of sliding window recognizers. *a*: Schematic representation of an SWR applied to an amino acid sequence. *b*: Mathematical representation of an SWR showing that the SWR plot (decision function, D_m) consists of the convolution of a window function, w_n, with a sequence of amino acid weights H_m. Each type of amino acid $i = 1, 2, \ldots, 20$ is assigned a weight H_i so that the H_i constitute a scale or index of physical or statistical properties. The constant T is the threshold level for a favorable decision. *c*: Three different window functions. The rectangular function weights all amino acids equally but a function that emphasizes the center of the window, such as a trapezoid or gaussian, is probably better (see text).

105

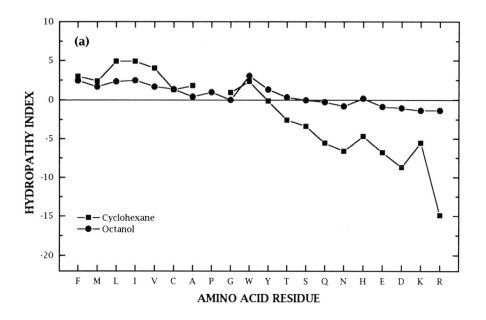

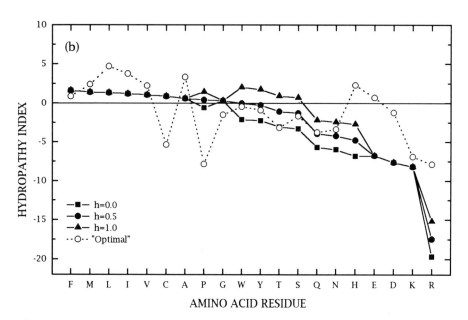

Fig. 4.4. Several different hydropathy scales. *a*: Hydropathy indices derived from the partitioning of amino acid model compounds between water and cyclohexane or octanol (Radzicka and Wolfenden, 1988). The amino acids along the abscissa have been rank ordered according to the IFH(0.5) scale in *b*. The hydropathy index is the free energy of transfer from the organic phase to water. Note that the octanol values have about the same relative order as the cyclohexane values. The absolute values of the free energies for the polar compounds are much smaller than for cyclohexane because of the hydrogen-bonding capability of octanol. *b*: Com-

ere and Pliska, 1983; Radzicka and Wolfenden, 1988), physicochemical estimates based on partitioning studies and other considerations (von Heijne, 1981; Kyte and Doolittle, 1982; Engelman et al., 1986; Jacobs and White, 1989), statistical considerations of proteins of known structure (Michel et al., 1986; Cornette et al., 1987; Edelman and White, 1989; Degli Esposti et al., 1989), or from combined statistical and physical considerations (Rao and Argos, 1986). Degli Esposti et al. (1990) have reported a systematic comparison of a large number of scales that reveals, not surprisingly, a high correlation between them. Because of the small number of membrane proteins of known structure, the accuracy of statistical scales is uncertain, and one cannot generally be encouraged about the possibilities considering that our ability to predict the secondary structure of soluble proteins has never exceeded 65% accuracy despite the large number of protein structures available (Rooman and Wodak, 1988; Qian and Sejnowski, 1988; Garnier, 1990). As for soluble proteins, the best long-term solution for predicting membrane protein structure is to understand the physical principles of folding, which focuses attention on scales derived from partitioning studies.

As discussed earlier, the fluid bilayer is a highly heterogeneous and anisotropic surface phase that *cannot* be accurately represented as a bulk phase. Nevertheless, the bilayer is predominantly hydrophobic, and one therefore expects bulk nonpolar phases to provide at least an estimate of the *relative* bilayer solubilities of amino acid side chains even though the absolute values may be unreliable. This is illustrated in Figure 4.4a for scales derived from the partitioning of amino acid derivatives from water into cyclohexane and octanol (Radzicka and Wolfenden, 1988). The rank orders of the hydropathy values of the amino acids are very similar despite large differences in absolute values that arise from the fact that the free energies of transfer from octanol to water are much smaller than from cyclohexane because of the polar hydroxyl group of octanol. The relative ordering is more important in terms of the mathematics of SWRs, because scales with the same rank ordering of amino acids can always be rescaled to an arbitrary absolute scale. The absolute values are not important if one wishes only to establish the locations of the most hydrophobic segments of a sequence. Indeed, a simple binary scale with hydrophobes assigned a value of 1 and hydrophiles a value of 0 is perfectly adequate for that purpose (White and Jacobs, 1990a). Absolute values become critically important, however, when one wishes to interpret hydropathy plots thermodynamically.

The number of different hydrophobicity scales is extraordinarily large. Cornette et al. (1987) examined thirty-eight scales in the context of amphiphilic helix predic-

---

parison of the IFH(h) hydropathy indices of Jacobs and White (1989) that take into account different assumptions about the satisfaction of side chain hydrogen bonding in membranes by means of the parameter h that is 0 if there are no H-bonds and 1 if there is a maximum number. The "optimal" scale is that of Edelman and White (1989) based on linear optimization of the amino acid weights and windows in an SWR that uses the known PSRC structures as reference standards. Note that some values are drastically different from thermodynamic expectations. This is probably because (*1*) polar residues are located near helix ends but are counted as being part of transmembrane helices and (*2*) specific structural and physiological requirements cannot be accounted for by hydropathy alone.

tion, and Degli Esposti et al. (1990) looked at eighteen scales in terms of TM helix prediction. An important conclusion of the later study was that the prediction accuracy of a scale appeared to depend on the class of membrane protein examined. However, prediction accuracy also depends on the choice of decision threshold and window function (Edelman and White, 1989). Overall, the physicochemical GES (read "guess") scale of Engelman et al. (1986) is probably the most reasonable general purpose scale if one wishes to ignore the heterogeneous nature of the bilayer by treating it as a very thin bulk phase. The scale is a derived one in that a wide variety of data from many sources have been combined with rational assumptions about polar side chain interactions in folded membrane proteins. Its principal value is that it is an absolute scale constructed to answer the question of whether the transfer of a putative TM helix into a bilayer is energetically favorable. Engelman et al. (1986) also recognized that pairs of amino acids of opposite charge located at i and $i + 3$ positions on a helix could neutralize one another. Their implementation of hydropathy plots took this possibility into account by assigning a less polar hydrophobicity value to such pairs.

The analysis of peptide–bilayer interactions of Jacobs and White (1989) and the resulting interfacial hydrophobicity scales, described earlier, help to clarify the origin of some of the differences between various hydrophobicity scales because one of the crucial issues in the development of scales is the status of hydrogen-bonding groups of the side chains. Thus, most scales will place phenylalanine and leucine at the extreme nonpolar end and lysine and arginine at the extreme polar end. The differences between the scales usually are found in the relative positions of the amino acids of mixed polarity such as proline, tryptophan, and threonine for which assumptions about their hydrogen bonding play a critical role in scale placement (Engelman et al., 1986). To illustrate this point, the interfacial hydrophobicity scales of Jacobs and White (1989) created with $h = 0, 0.5$, and 1.0 are compared in Figure 4.4b. A comparison of these scales with the cyclohexane- and octanol-based scales (Fig. 4.4a) reminds us again of the importance of hydrogen bond considerations; the solubility of polar side chains is much higher in octanol because of favorable hydrogen bonding. A particular advantage of Jacob and White's formalism (1989) is that one can compare the free energy of transfer of TM segments into the bilayer interior taking either the water or the interface as the reference phase. The comparison, as will be described below, reveals that interfacial interactions can account for a significant fraction of the favorable free energy of transfer from water to the bilayer interior. Thus, binding to the bilayer interface can be quite favorable for many amino acid residues, whereas transfer from interface to interior can be quite unfavorable. The assumption that the bilayer is a uniform nonpolar slab with diminutive interfaces can lead to overly optimistic estimates of the probability of finding a TM segment within the hydrocarbon interior.

Decision Threshold

The selection of a region in a hydropathy plot as the location of a TM helix depends on the decision threshold. By tradition, the data are plotted so that positive peaks indicate potential TM helices. This is equivalent for thermodynamic scales to plotting the free energy transfer from the bilayer to the aqueous phase. Thermodynamics-based hydropathy plots (Engelman et al., 1986; Jacobs and White, 1989) must, of course, use the zero free energy level as the decision threshold. A single point above zero means that, in principle, the net free energy of transfer of the sequence segment included in the window favors the nonpolar phase. If one is only interested in finding the most hydrophobic domains in a sequence, then the mean hydrophobicity of the sequence is an appropriate choice and has the advantage that one can distinguish to some extent soluble from membrane proteins using the mean values (Kyte and Doo-little, 1982). Statistics-based plots derived from Chou and Fasman (1974) analyses of amino acid preferences logically use 1 as a decision threshold (Degli Esposti et al., 1989). In the optimization-based statistical analysis of Edelman and White (1989), the decision threshold was absorbed into the determination of optimal weights so that $T = 0$.

How much of a particular peak must be above the threshold level for the peak to be considered a TM segment? An ideal SWR should have $D_m > 0$ over the length of the TM segment, but this is not easy to accomplish in practice because of the close coupling between the scale, decision threshold, and window function used in the SWR. The shapes of the peaks of D_m must depend strongly, for example, on the window function. Furthermore, one must decide the structural meaning of $D_m > 0$, since TM helices tend to be longer than the hydrocarbon thickness of the bilayer and to have polar ends. The ideal SWR would identify the full length the TM helix and the subregion corresponding to the hydrocarbon thickness. Most hydropathy plot methods are not that ambitious; they tend to identify the most hydrophobic peaks and to assume that a peak's maximum is near the center of a TM helix that is nineteen to twenty-one amino acids long. White and Jacobs (1990b) and Edelman and White (1989) have considered the problem of determining the full length of TM helices.

Window Function

The most common window function is a simple rectangular one (Fig. 4.3c) in which all amino acids are equally weighted. The width of the window is frequently chosen as nineteen or twenty-one amino acids, corresponding roughly to the expected min-imum length of a transmembrane helix, but windows of five to eleven amino acids are also used (White and Jacobs, 1990b; Kyte and Doolittle, 1982), depending on how much "detail" is desired. An odd number is usually chosen for the width for reasons of symmetry. Because TM segments tend to have polar residues at their ends, a window function that assigns higher weights to the central part of the window is a reasonable refinement (Fig. 4.3c) of the hydropathy plot method that is consistent with the structure of the bilayer (Fig. 4.1) and statistical analyses (Edelman and White, 1989; Edelman, 1993). The simplest of these is a trapezoidal window that has been used by White and Jacobs (1990b) and by von Heijne (1992). Rao and Argos (1986) have recommended multiple cycles of smoothing, i.e., sliding-window averages of sliding-window averages using rectangular windows. As pointed out by White and Jacobs (1990b), multiple-cycle refinements are equivalent to a single slid-ing-window average using a window obtained by multiple convolutions of the win-dow function. The result of an infinite number of convolutions of a rectangular func-tion is gaussian (Blass and Halsey, 1981) so that the use of a gaussian window shape (Fig. 4.3c) is equivalent to using a large number of refinement cycles.

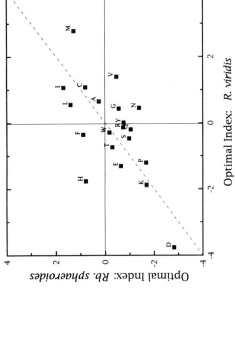

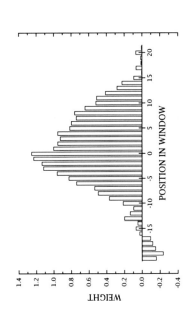

Optimal Index: *R. viridis*

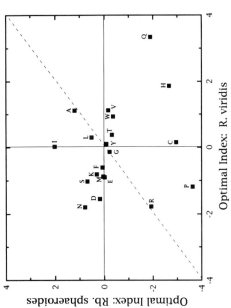

LINEAR OPTIMIZATION

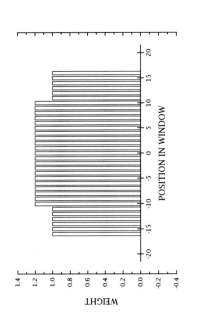

QUADRATIC OPTIMIZATION

Is There a "Perfect" Hydropathy Plot Method?

The large number of hydrophobicity scales described in the literature is the result of the search for a highly reliable, if not perfect, SWR that accurately predicts all of the TM helices. Our failure thus far to find such an SWR could mean that we have not yet found the right combination of hydrophobicity scale and window function or because the physical determinants of membrane protein structure are too complex to be revealed by any simple SWR. Recognizing that simple SWRs, i.e., those that depend on a single set of amino acid weights and the linear convolution of a window function with the sequence of weights, are all mathematically equivalent, Edelman and White (1989) sought the ideal weights and window function through a linear optimization procedure. If a perfect simple SWR exists, they reasoned that the perfect window function and set of weights could be found by mathematical optimization procedures using a single membrane protein of known structure. There were two high-resolution photosynthetic reaction center PSRC structures available from closely related species of purple bacteria, *Rhodop. viridis* (Deisenhofer et al., 1985) and *Rhodob. sphaeroides* (Allen et al., 1987). The optimization procedure applied to these two examples should result in the same weights and window function if the perfect simple SWR exists. Although the linear optimization procedure turned out to be too computationally intense to allow weights and windows to be optimized simultaneously, it was possible to optimize window shape within the rectangular and trapezoidal families. The results are summarized in two left-hand panels of Figure 4.5. The best window, a "stepped" rectangular window function, weighted the center of the window more than the ends, consistent with the existence of polar residues on helix ends. The central part of the window corresponded to a length of twenty-one amino acids, consistent with the expectation of transmembrane helices with lengths of 30 Å. However, the two hydrophobicity scales obtained by optimizing against the two PSRC structures were only marginally correlated despite the close similarities of the structures! This result indicates immediately that there is not a perfect hydrophobicity scale probably because multiple factors determine protein conformation.

A better correlation of the *Rhodop. viridis* and *Rhodob. sphaeroides* amino acid weights has subsequently been achieved by Edelman (1993), who used a quadratic optimization scheme as shown in the right-hand panels of Figure 4.5. The major advantage of this scheme is that simultaneous optimization of both the window func-

---

Fig. 4.5 *(opposite).* Comparisons of optimal hydropathy scales and window shapes derived from linear optimization (Edelman and White, 1989) and quadratic optimization (Edelman, 1993) of SWRs. The question of the existence of a "perfect" scale can be addressed by comparing scales derived from optimization using PSRC structures from two different species of purple bacteria (see text). If there were a perfect scale, the points would fall on the *dashed lines;* they do not and therefore the existence of a perfect scale seems unlikely. Linear optimization is computationally more intense so only a limited number of classes of window functions could be examined such as the stepped window shown. Quadratic optimization, however, permits simultaneous optimization of both the scale and the window functions. The quadratic scheme suggests that window functions that weight the center of the window more heavily than the ends are preferred. This is consistent with the observation that small, nonpolar solutes prefer the center of the hydrocarbon core of bilayers (see Fig. 4.1).

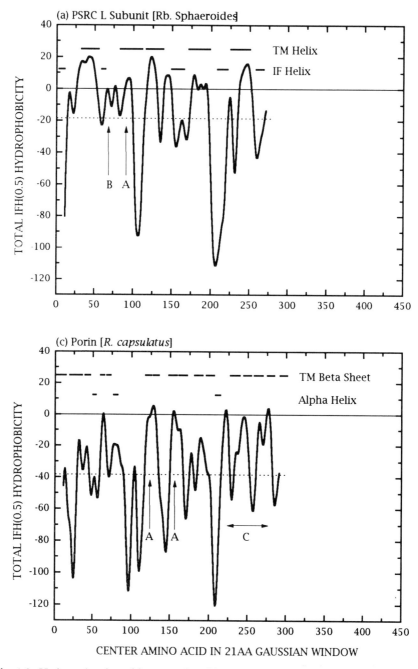

Fig. 4.6. Hydropathy plots of four proteins of known structure or topology. All plots use the same scale, window function, and abscissa length to facilitate comparisons and interpretations of similar features in different plots (see text). Locations of known structural features are indicated by the *heavy horizontal lines*. Comparisons such as these allow an investigator to gain experience with the interpretation of hydropathy plots using particular scales and window

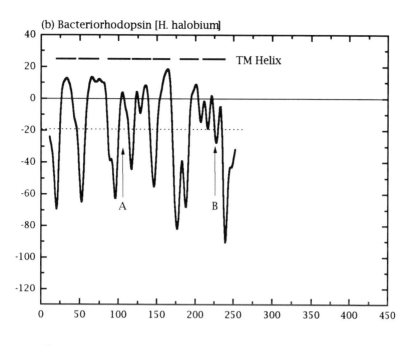

(b) Bacteriorhodopsin [H. halobium]

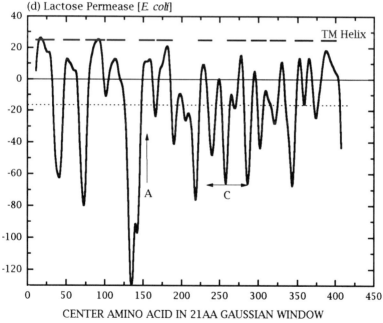

(d) Lactose Permease [E. coli]

CENTER AMINO ACID IN 21AA GAUSSIAN WINDOW

functions. Here the IFH(0.5) scale (1989) and a gaussian window have been used. Degli Esposti et al. (1990) have observed that different classes of membrane proteins seem to require different scales. (The known secondary structures of the various proteins are from Allen et al., 1987 [PSRC], Engelman et al., 1980 [BR], Weiss et al., 1991b [porin], and Calamia and Manoil, 1990 [lac permease].

tion and weights can be achieved. The resulting window function has, grossly, a triangular shape that weights the central amino acids very heavily. It is interesting that the window is somewhat asymmetric and has negative values on the N-terminal side. Despite the improvements in the agreement of the two scales, it is clear that no "perfect" scale emerges from the optimization approach.

The major conclusion that follows from attempts to find the perfect scale is that a reliably accurate simple SWR for TM helices probably does not exist. This indicates that the best approach for predicting TM helices is to examine more than just hydrophobicity. Thus, the general approach of Argos et al. (1982) of using multiple physical parameters is probably the best one.[1] White and Jacobs (1990b) found it useful to consider both hydrophobicity and reverse-turn potential as a minimum set of parameters. Recently, von Heijne (1992) has made considerable progress by taking into account the transmembrane distribution of charged residues (see von Heijne, Chapter 2).

Learning about SWR Analysis

The main goal of SWR analysis of membrane proteins is to identify accurately the TM segments of the sequence. Because there is no perfect combination of scale and window that achieves this, the practical goal is to develop a set of *possible* topologies to guide experiments. The beginner is advised to gain as much experience as possible with SWR analysis by examining membrane proteins of known structure (all four of them!) and/or topology using a variety of physical scales and window functions in order to gain experience with the uncertainties of TM helix prediction. The best way to begin is by comparing SWR plots using a single hydrophobicity scale and window shape as has been done in Figure 4.6 for four proteins of known topology (PSRC L subunit, bacteriorhodopsin [BR], porin, and lactose permease). The IFH(0.5) scale and a twenty-one amino acid gaussian window have been used, and the lengths of the x and y axes for all of the plots are the same so that the relative widths and heights of the peaks can be compared. The difficulty of deciding which peaks are TM segments is revealed by comparing peaks of similar appearance in different proteins. The peaks marked A in the four plots in Figure 4.6 are all rather modest but nevertheless correspond to true TM segments. Note, however, that for porin (Fig. 4.6c) the A peaks are TM β-strands rather than helices. The B regions of the PSRC L subunit and BR have a very similar appearance, but only in BR do they indicate a TM helix. Similarly, the C region of porin arising from four or five β-strands is very similar to the comparison region in the lactose permease plot that arises from two TM helices.

The lactose permease plot (Fig. 4.6d) is remarkably complex. It is not surprising that early analyses predicted variously eight to fourteen TM segments (Beyreuther et al., 1982; Overath and Wright, 1983; Juretic and Williams, 1991; Vogel et al., 1985) prior to the correct identification of twelve segments by means of gene fusions (Calamia and Manoil, 1990). Empirically, it appears to be easier to predict helical TM segments when the number of helices per unit length is relatively small, as in the case of the PSRC L and M subunits, with about two helices per hundred residues compared with lactose permease and BR, with about three per hundred residues. The connecting loops between helices in the latter cases are very short so that the distinction between TM and non-TM segments is blurred. The presence of physiologically important charged groups within the membrane as for BR and, probably, lactose permease can cause true TM segments to appear to be too polar, as in region *B* of BR (Fig. 4.6*b*), and therefore overlooked in hydropathy analyses.

The second important step in learning to use SWRs is to examine a wide variety of physical properties rather than relying on hydrophobicity alone. This approach is demonstrated in Figure 4.7 for the PSRC L subunit of *Rhodob. sphaeroides* whose structure is known to high resolution (Allen et al., 1987). The known elements of secondary structure for the subunit are indicated in Figure 4.7 by heavy horizontal lines labeled *TM* for transmembrane helices and *IF* for interfacial helices. The latter are helices located at the membrane surface that run generally parallel to the membrane plane. This arrangement of TM helices connected by IF helices may be a general structural motif of membrane proteins (Shon et al., 1991; Nambudripad et al., 1991).

Figure 4.7*a* shows three hydrophobicity plots using the IFH(*h*) hydrophobicity scale, with *h* = 0, 0.5, and 1.0, which indicate, respectively, the consequences of having 0, 50, and 100% of the side-chain hydrogen bonds satisfied (White and Jacobs, 1990b). The importance of side chain hydrogen-bonding assumptions in hydropho-

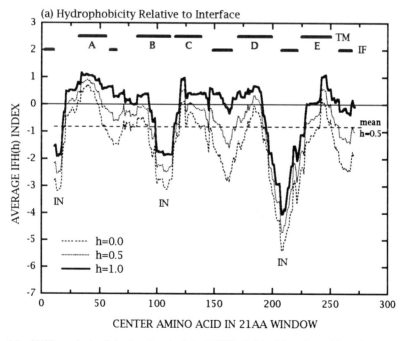

Fig. 4.7. SWR analysis of the L subunit of the PSRC of *Rhodob. sphaeroides.* The secondary structure, indicated by *heavy horizontal lines,* consists of five transmembrane (*TM*) helices and five connecting-link helices that lie in and parallel to the membrane interface (*IF*) (Allen et al., 1987). *a*: Hydropathy plots using the IFH(*h*) scale with three different values of *h*. Notice that the non-TM segments that must cross the membrane during assembly are much more sensitive to *h* than are those that do not. (*continued overleaf*)

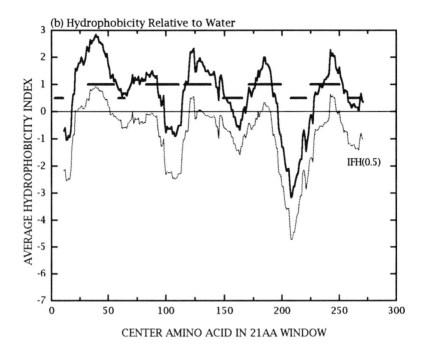

(b) Hydrophobicity Relative to Water

AVERAGE HYDROPHOBICITY INDEX

CENTER AMINO ACID IN 21AA WINDOW

IFH(0.5)

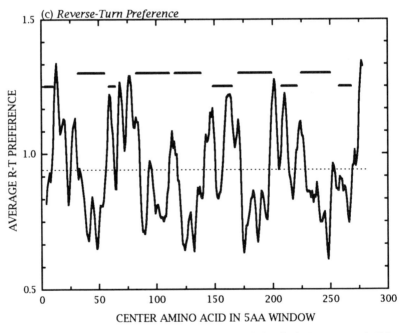

(c) *Reverse-Turn Preference*

AVERAGE R-T PREFERENCE

CENTER AMINO ACID IN 5AA WINDOW

Fig. 4.7 (continued) *b*: Comparison of plots using scales defined relative to water (solid curve) and the interface *(dashed curve)*. The difference between the plots measures how much of the hydrophobic free energy available for driving insertion can be consumed through interfacial partitioning prior to insertion into the hydrocarbon core of the bilayer (see text). *c*: A narrow-window SWR analysis (White and Jacobs, 1990b) of reverse-turn (R-T) propensity using the R-T preferences determined by Levitt (1978). Notice that the ends of the helices correspond strongly to maxima in R-T preference.

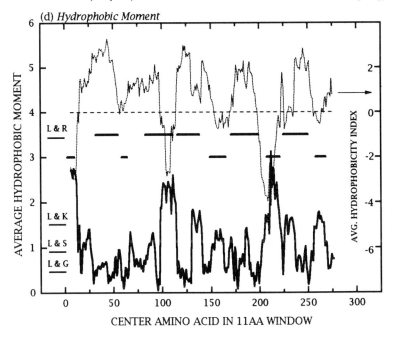

Fig. 4.7 (continued) *d*: An SWR analysis using hydrophobic moments (Eisenberg et al., 1984) that identify segments that could form amphiphilic helices. The hydrophobic moment SWR *(solid line)* and hydrophobicity *(dashed line; right-hand scale)* use the IFH(h)-based scale defined relative to water. The horizontal lines marked with *L & R, L & K, L & S,* and *L & G* correspond to the hydrophobic moments of amphiphilic helices formed from leucine and arginine, lysine, serine, or glycine. Notice that the peaks tend to correspond to *IF* helices but that the ends of some *TM* helices are also very amphiphilic. Especially note that the hydrophobic moment of the *IF* helix between *TM* segments D and E is exceptionally strong and corresponds to the most polar region of the protein (cf. appearance of the S4 segment in Fig. 4.8).

bicity scales is clearly revealed. The hydrophobicities of the extracellular TM helix connecting links have the greatest sensitivity to the value of h, which helps to visualize the topology of the proteins. This sensitivity suggests that transient side chain hydrogen bonds may be important for insertion and folding (White and Jacobs, 1990b). The IFH(h) scales use the bilayer interface as the reference phase so that positive values indicate favorable free energies of transfer from the interface to the bilayer interior. The consequences of using the water phase as the reference is illustrated in Figure 4.7*b* by the heavy solid curve. The difference between the solid and dashed curves illustrates how much of the free energy of transfer can be consumed during the transfer to the interface and emphasizes the difficulty of treating the bilayer as a bulk phase. Figure 4.7*a* and 4.7*b* fairly clearly indicate that there are five strong hydrophobicity peaks corresponding roughly to the five TM helices. Helix B is interesting because its C-terminal end is very polar, causing the major width of its hydrophobicity peak (Fig. 4.7*b*) to be a poor marker of the true helix length. One might be tempted, in the absence of a structure, to assign the TM helix to a region closer to the N terminus. Similar misassignments could occur for helices A, C, and E as well.

The ambiguities in the selection of the precise location of a helix within a hydrophobicity maximum illustrate the importance of using physical properties other than hydrophobicity to identify and locate TM helix positions. As for soluble proteins, the secondary structure of membrane proteins tends to be bounded by amino acids with a high propensity for reverse turn formation (Rose, 1978; Presta and Rose, 1988; Rose and Wetlaufer, 1977; Richardson and Richardson, 1988). The usefulness of reverse-turn propensity (Levitt, 1978) in SWR analysis is illustrated in Figure 4.7c, where a narrow five amino acid sliding window has been used (White and Jacobs, 1990b) because reverse turns generally occur within segments of that length. It should be noted that all of the helices, including the IF helices, are neatly bounded by reverse-turn maxima. Jacobs and White (1990b) found that a reverse-turn peak occurred 1 $\pm$ 1.9 residues before the N termini of TM helices and 3 $\pm$ 1.5 residues after the C termini.

If it is correct that TM helices connected by IF helices is a common structural motif of membrane proteins, the identification of possible IF helices must be an important goal of SWR analysis. The hydrophobic moment concept introduced by Eisenberg and his colleagues (1984) is useful for this purpose, assuming that the IF helices are amphiphilic. The basic idea of a hydrophobic-moment analysis is that amphiphilic helices will have a 3.6 residue periodicity in the polar–apolar character of their amino acids that can be detected by Fourier transformation of the hydrophobicity function. Eisenberg et al. (1989) found that the secondary structure elements of proteins could be classified into broad categories based on the magnitudes of their average hydrophobicity and hydrophobic moments so that lytic (surface-preferring) peptide sequences could be distinguished from TM helices and from amphiphilic helices of globular proteins. TM helices tend to have high hydrophobicity and low hydrophobic moments, whereas surface-preferring peptides tend to be less hydrophobic while having high hydrophobic moments.

Although computationally more intense than a regular hydrophobicity plot, one can easily perform sliding-window hydrophobic-moment plots as illustrated in Figure 4.7d, where an eleven amino acid window has been used in order to be consistent with the analysis of Eisenberg et al. (1989). The solid curve (left-hand axis) is the sliding-window hydrophobic moment plot and the dashed curve the hydrophobicity (right-hand axis) relative to the aqueous phase. Indicated at the left of the plots are the values of hydrophobic moment expected for amphiphilic helices composed of leucine and a series of more polar amino acids ranging from glycine to arginine. A comparison of the two curves shows that the TM helices and the IF helices adhere to the expectations of the analysis of Eisenberg et al. (1989). The hydrophobic moment of the IF helix connecting link between helices D and E of the PSRC L and M subunits is impressively high. But, as is invariably the case in SWR analyses, there are ambiguities. For example, the C termini of helices B and C have very high hydrophobic moments but are not parts of IF helices.

The ambiguities that arise in the analysis of membrane protein sequences are illustrated by the SWR analysis of the rat RCK1 potassium channel (Stuhmer et al., 1989) shown in Figure 4.8. The top frame shows a hydropathy plot using a twenty-one amino acid gaussian window and the bottom frame the hydrophobic-moment plot using a rectangular eleven amino acid window. The narrow horizontal lines labeled S1 through S6 indicate the locations of the generally accepted, but putative,

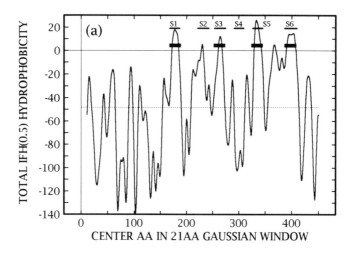

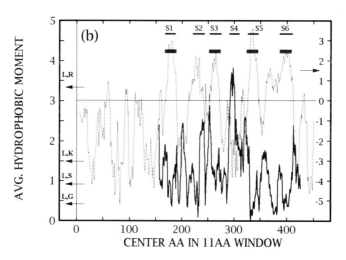

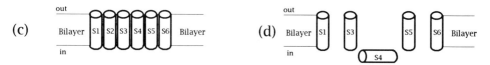

Fig. 4.8. SWR analysis of the RCK1 potassium channel protein (Stuhmer et al., 1989) that illustrates the ambiguities that can result in different topologies. *a*: A hydropathy plot using a gaussian window (cf. with Fig. 4.6). The *thin horizontal lines* labeled *S1–S6* indicate putative transmembrane segments (Stuhmer et al., 1989) illustrated in *c*, while the *thick horizontal lines* indicate an alternate four transmembrane segment model illustrated in *d*. *b*: Hydrophobic moment plot of the RCK1 sequence showing that the S4 segment could also be an interface helix (see Fig. 4.7). If that is true and S4 lies on the inside of the membrane, then a four transmembrane segment model is more likely. Note, however, that both S2 and S3 have high hydrophobicities and low hydrophobic moments, a combination that suggests they could both be transmembrane segments (Eisenberg, 1984). The various ambiguities can only be resolved through experiment.

TM helices. The broad horizontal lines indicate the most likely TM helices based on the IFH(0.5) scale and on a twenty-one amino acid gaussian window. The now famous S4 helix, which is often assumed to line the channel in a tetrameric assembly of RCK1 monomers, seems an unlikely candidate for a TM structure based on the lack of a major peak in hydrophobicity. In addition, S4 has an extraordinarily high hydrophobic moment. Using the L subunit as a reference standard, one could conclude that S4 is a surface helix rather than a TM helix. The rationale for choosing S4 as a TM is the perceived need to have a channel with a very polar lining, but that may not be a good assumption (Popot and Engelman, 1990). If S4 is not a TM helix, then the generally accepted topology of the potassium channel protein could be in error. For example, if S4 is an IF helix, its most likely location would be intracellular. Because both the N- and C-terminal domains of the sequence are very polar, they must both be intracellular. Four TM helices rather than six would be a more reasonable topology under these conditions, which would mean that S2 is a connecting link rather than a TM segment. It could be structurally similar to the segment represented by the minor peak between S5 and S6, which seems to be some kind of hairpin structure (Guy and Conti, 1990; Yellen et al., 1991; Hartmann et al., 1991; Yool and Schwarz, 1991) lining the pore of the channel.

   The important conclusion from the analysis of the potassium channel is that one can conceive of several alternative topologies that depend on the details of the SWR analysis, experience derived from a small repertoire of membrane proteins, assumptions about specific structural requirements for physiological function, and incomplete knowledge of peptide–bilayer interactions. The identification of the regions of a sequence of high hydrophobicity is straightforward, but the correct identification of true TM segments is not. As for soluble proteins, the ultimate key to structure prediction is a detailed understanding of the physicochemical rules for folding and how these rules are encoded in the sequence. An additional problem for membrane proteins is that their sequences must also carry information related to targeting and insertion (see Chapter 2). Until these problems are solved, the wise course of action is to adopt a skeptical attitude about conclusions derived solely from SWR analyses and to recognize that there is no substitute for experiments.

Acknowledgements

This research was supported by grants from the National Institutes of Health (GM-46823) and the National Science Foundation (DMB-880743).

References

Allen, J. P., Yeates, T. O., Komiya, H., and Rees, D. C. (1987) Structure of the reaction center from *Rhodobacter sphaeroides* R-26: the protein subunits. *Proc. Natl. Acad. Sci. USA* 84: 6162–6166.
Argos, P., Rao, J.K.M., and Hargrave, P. A. (1982) Structural prediction of membrane-bound proteins. *Eur. J. Biochem.* 128: 565–575.
Beschiaschvili, G., and Seelig, J. (1992) Peptide binding to lipid bilayers—nonclassical hydrophobic effect and membrane-induced pk shifts. *Biochemistry* 31: 10044–10053.
Beyreuther, K., Muller-Hill, B., Overath, P., and Wright, J. K. (1982) Lactose permease and the molecular biology of transport. *Hoppe-Seylers Z. Physiol. Chem.* 363: 1409–1414.

Blass, W. E., and Halsey, G. W. (1981) *Deconvolution of Absorption Spectra.* New York: Academic Press.

Calamia, J., and Manoil, C. (1990) *lac* Permease of *Escherichia coli:* Topology and sequence elements promoting membrane insertion. *Proc. Natl. Acad. Sci. USA* 87: 4937–4941.

Chou, P. Y., and Fasman, G. D. (1974) Conformational parameters for amino acids in helical, beta-sheet, and random coil regions calculated from proteins. *Biochemistry* 13: 211–222.

Cornette, J. L., Cease, K. B., Margalit, H., Spouge, J. L., Berzofsky, J. A. and DeLisi, C. (1987) Hydrophobicity scales and computational techniques for detecting amphipathic structures in protein. *J. Mol. Biol.* 195: 659–679.

Cowan, S. W., Schirmer, T., Rummel, G., Steiert, M., Ghosh, R., Pauptit, R. A., Jansonius, J. N., and Rosenbusch, J. P. (1992) Crystal structures explain functional properties of two *E. coli* porins. *Nature* 358: 727–733.

Crofts, A. R. (1992) pSAAM for Windows®. A program for protein sequence analysis and modeling. Programs run under Windows® 3.x. Copyright 1992–1994 by University of Illinois.

Degli Esposti, M., Ghelli, A., Luchetti, R., Crimi, M., and Lenaz, G. (1989) New approaches to the prediction of the folding of membrane proteins with redox function. *Italian J. Biochem.* 38: 1–22.

Degli Esposti, M., Crimi, M., and Venturoli, G. (1990). A critical evaluation of the hydropathy profile of membrane proteins. *Eur. J. Biochem.* 190: 207–219.

Deisenhofer, J., Epp, O., Miki, K., Huber, R., and Michel, H. (1985) Structure of the protein subunits in the photosynthetic reaction centre of *Rhodopseudomonas viridis* at 3 Å resolution. *Nature* 318: 618–624.

Edelman, J. (1993) Quadratic minimization of predictors for protein secondary structure: Application for transmembrane alpha helices. *J. Mol. Biol.* 232: 165–191.

Edelman, J., and White, S. H. (1989) Linear optimization of predictors for secondary structure—application to transbilayer segments of membrane proteins. *J. Mol. Biol.* 210: 195–209.

Eisenberg, D. (1984) Three-dimensional structure of membrane and surface proteins. *Annu. Rev. Biochem.* 53: 595–623.

Eisenberg, D., Weiss, R. M., and Terwilliger, T. C. (1984) The hydrophobic moment detects periodicity in protein hydrophobicity. *Proc. Natl. Acad. Sci. USA* 81: 140–144.

Eisenberg, D., Wesson, M., and Wilcox, W. (1989) Hydrophobic moments as tools for analyzing protein sequences and structures. In: *Prediction of Protein Structure and the Principles of Protein Conformation,* edited by G. D. Fasman. New York: Plenum, pp. 635–646.

Engelman, D. M., Henderson, R., McLachlan, A. D., and Wallace, B. A. (1980) Path of the polypeptide in bacteriorhodopsin. *Proc. Natl. Acad. Sci. USA* 77: 2023–2027.

Engelman, D. M., Steitz, T. A., and Goldman, A. (1986) Identifying nonpolar transbilayer helices in amino acid sequences of membrane proteins. *Annu. Rev. Biophys. Biophys. Chem.* 15: 321–353.

Engelman, D. M., and Steitz, T. A. (1981) The spontaneous insertion of proteins into and across membranes: the helical hairpin hypothesis. *Cell* 23: 411–422.

Fauchere, J.-L., and Pliska, V. (1983) Hydrophobic parameters of pi amino-acid side chains from the partitioning of *N*-acetyl-amino-acid amides. *Eur. J. Med. Chem. Chim. Ther.* 18: 369–375.

Garnier, J. (1990) Protein structure prediction. *Biochimie* 72: 513–524.

Guy, H. R., and Conti, F. (1990) Pursuing the structure and function of voltage-gated channels. *Trends Neurosci.* 13: 201–206.

Hartmann, H. A., Kirsch, G. E., Drewe, J. A., Taglialatela, M., Joho, R. H., and Brown, A. M. (1991) Exchange of conduction pathways between 2 related K$^+$ channels. *Science* 251: 942–944.

Henderson, R., Baldwin, J. M., Ceska, T. A., Zemlin, F., Beckmann, E., and Downing, K. H. (1990) Model for the structure of bacteriorhodopsin based on high-resolution electron cryo-microscopy. *J. Mol. Biol.* 213: 899–929.

Henderson, R., and Unwin, P.N.T. (1975) Three-dimensional model of purple membrane obtained by electron microscopy. *Nature* 257: 28–32.

Huang, C.-H., and Charlton, J. P. (1972) Interactions of phosphatidylcholine vesicles with 2-*p*-toluidinylnaphthalene-6-sulfonate. *Biochemistry* 11: 735–740.

Jacobs, R. E., and White, S. H. (1986) Mixtures of a series of homologous hydrophobic peptides with lipid bilayers: a simple model system for examining the protein-lipid interface. *Biochemistry* 25: 2605–2611.

Jacobs, R. E., and White, S. H. (1987) Lipid bilayer perturbations induced by simple hydrophobic peptides. *Biochemistry* 26: 6127–6134.

Jacobs, R. E., and White, S. H. (1989) The nature of the hydrophobic binding of small peptides at the bilayer interface: implications for the insertion of transbilayer helices. *Biochemistry* 28: 3421–3437.

Kaiser, E. T., and Kezdy, F. J. (1983) Secondary structures of proteins and peptides in amphiphilic environments (a review). *Proc. Natl. Acad. Sci. USA* 80: 1137–1143.

Kaiser, E. T., and Kezdy, F. J. (1984) Amphiphilic secondary structure: design of peptide hormones. *Science* 223: 249–255.

Kühlbrandt, W., Wang, D. N., and Fujiyoshi, Y. (1994) Atomic model of plant light-harvesting complex by electron crystallography. *Nature* 367: 614–621.

Kyte, J., and Doolittle, R. F. (1982) A simple method for displaying the hydropathic character of a protein. *J. Mol. Biol.* 157: 105–132.

Lanyi, J. K. (1992) Proton transfer and energy coupling in the bacteriorhodopsin photocycle. *J. Bioenerg. Biomembranes* 24: 169–179.

Lenard, J., and Singer, S. J. (1966) Protein conformation in cell membrane preparations as studied by optical rotatory dispersion and circular dichroism. *Proc. Natl. Acad. Sci. USA* 56: 1828–1835.

Levine, Y. K., and Wilkins, M.H.F. (1971) Structure of oriented lipid bilayers. *Nature New Biol.* 230: 69–72.

Levitt, M. (1978) Conformational preferences of amino acids in globular proteins. *Biochemistry* 17: 4277–4285.

Lodish, H. F. (1988) Multi-spanning membrane proteins: how accurate are the models? *Trends Biochem. Sci.* 13: 332–338.

Marsh, D. (1990) *CRC Handbook of Lipid Bilayers*. Boca Raton, FL: CRC Press.

Michel, H., Weyer, K. A., Gruenberg, H., Dunger, I., Oesterhelt, D., and Lottspeich, F. (1986) The "light" and "medium" subunits of the photosynthetic reaction centre from *Rhodopseudomonas viridis*: isolation of the genes, nucleotide and amino acid sequence. *EMBO J.* 5: 1149–1158.

Milik, M., and Skolnick, J. (1992) Spontaneous insertion of polypeptide chains into membranes—a monte-carlo model. *Proc. Natl. Acad. Sci. USA* 89: 9391–9395.

Milik, M., and Skolnick, J. (1993) Insertion of peptide chains into lipid membranes—an off-lattice monte-carlo dynamics model. *Protein Struct. Funct. Genet.* 15: 10–25.

Nambudripad, R., Stark, W., Opella, S. J., and Makowski, L. (1991) Membrane-mediated assembly of filamentous bacteriophage-Pf1 coat protein. *Science* 252: 1305–1308.

Nozaki, Y., and Tanford, C. (1971) The solubility of amino acids and two glycine peptides in aqueous ethanol and dioxane solutions. Establishment of a hydrophobicity scale. *J. Biol. Chem.* 246: 2211–2217.

Oesterhelt, D., Tittor, J., and Bamberg, E. (1992) A unifying concept for ion translocation by retinal proteins. *J. Bioenerg. Biomembranes* 24: 181–191.

Overath, P., and Wright, J. K. (1983) Lactose permease: a carrier on the move. *Trends Biochem. Sci.* 8: 404–408.

Popot, J.-L., and Engelman, D. M. (1990) Membrane protein folding and oligomerization—the 2-stage model. *Biochemistry* 29: 4031–4037.

Presta, L. G., and Rose, G. D. (1988) Helix signals in proteins. *Science* 240: 1632–1641.

Qian, N., and Sejnowski, T. J. (1988) Predicting the secondary structure of globular proteins using neural network models. *J. Mol. Biol.* 202: 865–884.

Radzicka, A., and Wolfenden, R. (1988) Comparing the polarities of the amino acids: side-chain distribution coefficients between the vapor phase, cyclohexane, 1-octanol, and neutral aqueous solution. *Biochemistry* 27: 1664–1670.

Rao, J.K.M., and Argos, P. (1986) A conformational preference parameter to predict helices in integral membrane proteins. *Biochem. Biophys. Acta* 869: 197–214.

Reynolds, J. A., Gilbert, D. B., and Tanford, C. (1974) Empirical correlation between hydrophobic free energy and aqueous cavity surface area. *Proc. Natl. Acad. Sci. USA* 71: 2925–2927.

Richardson, J. S., and Richardson, D. C. (1988) Amino acid preferences for specific locations at the ends of α-helices. *Science* 240: 1648–1652.

Rooman, M. J., and Wodak, S. J. (1988) Identification of predictive sequence motifs limited by protein structure data base size. *Nature* 335: 45–50.

Rose, G. D. (1978) Prediction of chain turns in globular proteins on a hydrophobic basis. *Nature* 272: 586–590.

Rose, G. D., and Roy, S. (1980) Hydrophobic basis of packing in globular proteins. *Proc. Natl. Acad. Sci. USA* 77: 4643–4647.

Rose, G. D., and Wetlaufer, D. B. (1977) The number of turns in globular proteins. *Nature* 268: 769–770.

Roseman, M. A. (1988) Hydrophobicity of the peptide C = O . . . H–N hydrogen-bonded group. *J. Mol. Biol.* 201: 621–625.

Rothschild, K. J. (1992) FTIR difference spectroscopy of bacteriorhodopsin: toward a molecular model. *J. Bioenerg. Biomembranes* 24: 147–167.

Sargent, D. F., and Schwyzer, R. (1986) Membrane lipid phase as catalyst for peptide–receptor interactions. *Proc. Natl. Acad. Sci. USA* 83: 5774–5778.

Seelig, J., and Ganz, P. (1991) Nonclassical hydrophobic effect in membrane binding equilibria. *Biochemistry* 30: 9354–9359.

Segrest, J. P., and Feldman, R. J. (1974) Membrane proteins: amino acid sequence and membrane penetration. *J. Mol. Biol.* 87: 853–858.

Sharp, K. A., Nicholls, A., Friedman, R., and Honig, B. (1991) Extracting hydrophobic free energies from experimental data—relationship to protein folding and theoretical models. *Biochemistry* 30: 9686–9697.

Shon, K. J., Kim, Y. G., Colnago, L. A., and Opella, S. J. (1991) NMR studies of the structure and dynamics of membrane-bound bacteriophage-Pf1 coat protein. *Science* 252: 1303–1304.

Simon, S. A., Lis, L. J., MacDonald, R. C., and Kauffman, J. W. (1977) The noneffect of a large linear hydrocarbon, squalene, on the phosphatidylcholine packing structure. *Biophys. J.* 19: 83–90.

Small, D. M. (1986) *The Physical Chemistry of Lipids*, New York: Plenum.

Stuhmer, W., Ruppersberg, J. P., Schroter, K. H., Sakmann, B., Stocker, M., Giese, K. P., Perschke, A., Baumann, A., and Pongs, O. (1989) Molecular basis of functional diversity of voltage-gated potassium channels in mammalian brain. *EMBO J.* 8: 3235–3244.

Vickery, L. E. (1987) Interactive analysis of protein structure using a microcomputer spreadsheet. *Trends Biochem. Sci.* 12: 37–39.

Vogel, H., Wright, J. K., and Jahnig, F. (1985) The structure of the lactose permease derived from Raman spectroscopy and prediction methods. *EMBO J.* 4: 3625–3631.

von Heijne, G. (1981) On the hydrophobic nature of signal sequences. *Eur. J. Biochem.* 116: 419–422.

von Heijne, G. (1992) Membrane protein structure prediction—hydrophobicity analysis and the positive-inside rule. *J. Mol. Biol.* 225: 487–494.

Wattenbarger, M. R., Chan, H. S., Evans, D. F., Bloomfield, V. A., and Dill, K. A. (1990) Surface-induced enhancement of internal structure in polymers and proteins. *J. Chem. Phys.* 93: 8343–8351.

Weiss, M. A., Abele, U., Weckesser, J., Welte, W., Schiltz, E., and Schulz, G. E. (1991a) Molecular architecture and electrostatic properties of a bacterial porin. *Science* 254: 1627–1630.

Weiss, M. S., Kreusch, A., Schiltz, E., Nestel, U., Welte, W., Weckesser, J., and Schulz, G. E. (1991b) The structure of porin from *Rhodobacter capsulatus* at 1.8 Å resolution. *FEBS Lett.* 280: 379–382.

White, S. H. (1977) Studies of the physical chemistry of planar bilayer membranes using high precision measurements of specific capacitance. *Ann. N. Y. Acad. Sci.* 303: 243–265.

White, S. H. (1980) How electric fields modify alkane solubility in lipid bilayers. *Science* 207: 1075–1077.

White, S. H., King, G. I., and Cain, J. E. (1981) Location of hexane in lipid bilayers determined by neutron diffraction. *Nature* 290: 161–163.

White, S. H., and Jacobs, R. E. (1990a) Statistical distribution of hydrophobic residues along the length of protein chains—implications for protein folding and evolution. *Biophys. J.* 57: 911–921.

White, S. H., and Jacobs, R. E. (1990b) Observations concerning topology and locations of helix ends of membrane proteins of known structure. *J. Membrane Biol.* 115: 145–158.

White, S. H., and Wimley, W. C. (1994) Peptides in bilayers: Structural and thermodynamic basis for partitioning and folding. *Curr. Opinion. Struct. Biol.* 4: 79–86.

Wiener, M. C., King, G. I., and White, S. H. (1991) The structure of a fluid dioleoyl phosphatidylcholine bilayer determined by joint refinement of x-ray and neutron diffraction data. I. Scaling of neutron data and the distribution of double-bonds and water. *Biophys. J.* 60: 568–576.

Wiener, M. C., and White, S. H. (1991a) Fluid bilayer structure determination by the combined use of x-ray and neutron diffraction. I. Fluid bilayer models and the limits of resolution. *Biophys. J.* 59: 162–173.

Wiener, M. C., and White, S. H. (1991b) Fluid bilayer structure determination by the combined use of x-ray and neutron diffraction II. "Composition-Space" Refinement Method. *Biophys. J.* 59: 174–185.

Wiener, M. C., and White, S. H. (1991c) The transbilayer distribution of bromine in fluid bilayers containing a specifically brominated analog of dioleoylphosphatidylcholine. *Biochemistry* 30: 6997–7008.

Wiener, M. C., and White, S. H. (1992a) Structure of a fluid dioleoylphosphatidylcholine bilayer determined by joint refinement of x-ray and neutron diffraction data. II. Distribution and packing of terminal methyl groups. *Biophys. J.* 61: 428–433.

Wiener, M. C., and White, S. H. (1992b) Structure of a fluid dioleoylphosphatidylcholine bilayer determined by joint refinement of x-ray and neutron diffraction data. III. Complete structure. *Biophys. J.* 61: 434–447.

Wimley, W. C., and White, S. H. (1992) Partitioning of tryptophan side-chain analogs between water and cyclohexane. *Biochemistry* 31: 12813–12818.

Wimley, W. C., and White, S. H. (1993) Membrane partitioning: distinguishing bilayer effects from the hydrophobic effect. *Biochemistry* 32: 6307–6312.

Yellen, G., Jurman, M. E., Abramson, T., and Mackinnon, R. (1991) Mutations affecting internal TEA blockade identify the probable pore-forming region of a K^+ channel. *Science* 251: 939–942.

Yool, A. J., and Schwarz, T. L. (1991) Alteration of ionic selectivity of a K^+ channel by mutation of the H5 region. *Nature* 349: 700–704.

Zheng, L., and Herzfeld, J. (1992) NMR studies of retinal proteins. *J. Bioenerg. Biomembranes* 24: 139–146.

Notes

1. The software package pSAAM (Protein Sequence Analysis and Modeling) written by A. R. Crofts (1992) that runs under Microsoft Windows® is excellent in this regard in that it allows the user to choose from a large number of hydrophobicity and propensity scales, window functions, smoothing, etc. It is available for a modest fee from the Biotechnology Center, University of Illinois, 105 Observatory, 901 S. Mathews, Urbana, IL 61801 or free by anonymous ftp over the Internet. Initiate a ftp connection to nemo.life.uiuc.edu and log on as "anonymous" using your email address as the password then change directory path to /pub/psaam.

II. Biochemical and Molecular
Biological Approaches: Protein Topology

After the sequencing has been done and the hydropathy analysis performed, the most important next step is to determine the correct topology of the membrane protein. I cannot emphasize enough the importance of this step because, obviously, an incorrect topology will cause the wrong questions to be asked. There is a strong tendency for researchers who are not primarily motivated by protein structure to want to believe what they believe about their hydropathy plots and to get on with the "interesting" experiments. Avoid the temptation if possible! For many biological systems, of course, the determination of topology may not be straightforward. In those cases one should at least keep an open mind and think carefully about the limitations of hydropathy plot analyses. Often one can learn a good deal about topology in the process of studying function, as in the case of the ion channels.

How can the topology be tested? The earliest methods, with are still frequently used, included antibodies, enzymatic digestion or labeling, and chemical labeling. David Cafiso reviews these methods in the first chapter of this section and then describes a novel and highly reliable method that uses proteolysis and mass spectrometry. Dana Boyd describes gene fusion methods that provide virtually definitive answers for proteins expressed in *Esherichia coli*. This method has been a boon not only to protein structure–function studies but also to membrane protein targeting and insertion studies. He also discusses the use of glycosylation sites as a topology-determination tool and considers the use of gene fusions in eukaryotic systems. The final chapter in this section, by Mario Amzel and his colleagues, may be taken as a case study of how hydropathy and topological analyses can be combined to arrive at reasonable models for membrane proteins; in this case, the F_1F_0ATPase complex. Dr. Amzel's perspective on the problem is particularly useful because his point of view is that of the structural biologist. Although Dr. Cafisio's chapter is concerned with general issues of topology determination, he uses the acetylcholine receptor as his primary example and thus provides an additional case study.

A final word of caution is in order and especially so for large membrane proteins such as the sodium channel. We generally make the facile assumption that membrane proteins must be largely α-helical in their transbilayer domains. While this may be true for most membrane proteins we do not yet have enough direct structural information to be sure. There is a thermodynamic necessity for internal hydrogen bonding for transbilayer segments that make direct contact with the lipid bilayer's hydrocarbon core, but for large proteins one can imagine a bilayer–protein interface region comprised of α-helices, for example, that surrounds a complex domain with other folding motifs (Lodish, 1988). There will surely be surprises as the structures of more membrane proteins are determined. This has certainly been true for globular proteins, although it does not happen as often these days as it did earlier. An interesting case in point is the recent discovery of a β-helix motif in the globular plant protein pectate lyase C (Yoder et al., 1993) that has its hydrogen bonds satisfied internally and can thus be considered a candidate for a transmembrane motif. A β-helix motif of quite a different type has been observed for the channel-forming peptide gramicidin (see Chapter 14 by Andrew Woolley and Bonnie Wallace).

References

Lodish, H. F. (1988) Multi-spanning membrane proteins: how accurate are the models? *Trends Biochem. Sci.* 13: 332–338.

Yoder, M. D., Keen, N. T., and Jurnak, F. (1993) New domain motif: the structure of pectate lyase C, a secreted plant virulence factor. *Science* 260: 1503–1507.

5

Experimental Determination of the Topography of Membrane Proteins: Lessons from the Nicotinic Acetylcholine Receptor, a Multisubunit Polytopic Protein

DAVID S. CAFISO

The sequencing and cloning of a large number of membrane proteins has stimulated both experimental and theoretical approaches to determine membrane protein structure. One of the most fundamental structural questions about a membrane protein is the transmembrane arrangement of its sequence (the term *topography* will be used here). Determining the cytoplasmic and extracellular domains is often a major step in formulating reliable and detailed models for membrane protein structures, models that can then be tested with specific chemical and spectroscopic techniques. Theoretical approaches have been motivated by the view that an understanding of the forces working during the biogenesis of membrane proteins can yield a likely topography based on the protein's sequence. By estimating the free-energy of transfer of amino acid side chains from the aqueous to the membrane phase, a reasonable first guess as to the likely topography of membrane protein can be made (see White, Chapter 4). In addition to hydrophobicity, electrostatic forces appear to play a major role; for example, clusters of positively charged residues appear to be responsible for localizing sequences to the cytoplasmic surface (see, for example, Hartman et al., 1989; Dalbey, 1990; Nilsson and von Heijne, 1990). This could result from the interactions of positive charges with negative membrane surface potentials or with the internal membrane dipole potential (for a more detailed discussion of these effects, see Cafiso, 1991; Kim et al., 1991; Mosior and McLaughlin, 1992; von Heijne, Chapter 2). A better understanding of the steps involved in the biogenesis of membrane proteins and the forces involved in protein–membrane interactions should improve the reliability of predictions for membrane protein topography. Clearly, experimental procedures to determine the topography of membrane proteins will play an important role in defining the forces and mechanisms that function during the synthesis and assembly of membrane proteins.

In this chapter, several chemical and immunological approaches that are routinely used to determine the transmembrane topography of membrane proteins will be described. In addition, a number of the difficulties that can be encountered with these methods will be discussed. The nicotinic acetylcholine receptor provides an excellent example for many of the experimental considerations that arise in the determination of membrane protein topography, and this chapter will focus on experimental work on this system. The use of mass spectrometry to examine membrane proteins will also be discussed. This methodology has improved dramatically in terms of mass range and sensitivity and provides a powerful new methodology to sequence proteins and identify sites of chemical derivatization. Techniques that utilize a genetic approach have also been developed, but will not be discussed in this chapter (see, for example, Charbit et al., 1991; Boyd et al., 1987). These promising methods are discussed elsewhere in this volume (see Boyd).

The Nicotinic Acetylcholine Receptor: an Example of a Complex Polytopic Membrane Protein

Determining the transmembrane folding or "topography" of a membrane protein is often the first step in determining its structure. While this is in principle a simple question that can be easily addressed, in some membrane protein systems it has been very difficult to answer. The nicotinic acetylcholine receptor (AChR) provides a good example of some of the problems that can arise in the investigation of membrane protein topography. The AChR is a large (290 kDa) multisubunit protein that functions as a receptor ion channel in the postsynaptic membrane. In size and complexity it is typical of ion channels and other membrane proteins found in the nervous system. The subunit make-up of the AChR is $\alpha_2\beta\gamma\delta$, and there is homology among the four subunits. Based on a hydropathy analysis of the amino acid sequences, each subunit has four hydrophobic stretches labeled MI to MIV that have been proposed to be membrane-spanning α-helices (Noda et al., 1983). The signal sequence for the AChR is cleaved, implying that the N terminus is extracellular (ie., synaptic) (Sabatini, 1982; Anderson et al., 1982). Several assumptions are inherent in most of the models for its transmembrane topography. First, because of its homology, each subunit is assumed to display the same transmembrane topography. Another assumption, based on thermodynamic arguments and the finding that hydrophobic membrane-associated helices appear to be highly stable structures, is that transmembrane protein segments are likely to be α-helical (for a discussion, see Popot and Engleman, 1990). With these assumptions and initial data, the first model that was proposed (see Fig. 5.1a) has each subunit of the receptor peptide spanning the membrane four times with both the C terminus and N terminus lying in the synaptic space (Noda et al., 1983).

In a portion of the sequence between MIII and MIV, the frequency of charged amino acids allows the formation of a strongly amphipathic helix. This led to the proposal that an additional helix, MA, made up the ion conductive pathway and was structured across the membrane (Guy, 1984; Finer-Moore and Stroud, 1984). Evidence for this folding model, which is shown in Figure 5.1b, was subsequently obtained from monoclonal antibody binding data that indicated that the C terminus had a cytoplasmic location (Lindstrom et al., 1984; Ratnam and Lindstrom, 1984;

Young et al., 1985). However, at least one report using antibodies directed at the α-subunit indicated that the C terminus was extracellular (Barkas et al., 1984). Further work using antibodies provided evidence for a cytoplasmic localization of epitopes on the N-terminal side of the hydrophobic MI segment. This led to a proposed model involving seven transmembrane passes of the receptor peptide (Criadio et al., 1984a,b). This model was subsequently refined by work with immunochemical approaches that provided evidence for a cytoplasmic location of M4, MA, and the C terminus (Ratnam et al., 1986). This "immunochemical" model is shown in Figure 5.1c. Because the glycosylated residue at α141 is only 11 residues away from a sequence that was determined to be cytoplasmic, the transmembrane segment MVI, shown in Figure 5.1c, is nonhelical.

A large amount of work has been carried out on the receptor since these original models were proposed, and several features of the AChR topography are now generally agreed on. The portion of the receptor sequence that includes MI, MII, and MIII appears to be buried and is not readily accessible to proteases or antibodies. The amphipathic helix (MA) is not directly involved in forming the ion channel. This is not surprising, given that amphipathic helices do not need to be highly charged to form functional channels (Lear et al., 1988; Popot and Engelman, 1990). The helix MII (rather than MA) appears to participate in the channel structure and likely has the orientation shown in Figure 5.1 (Imoto et al., 1988).

Surprisingly, a large number of features of the receptor topography remain unresolved. While immunochemical work places the C terminus on the cytoplasmic surface, direct chemical approaches place this portion of the sequence on the synaptic surface (Dunn et al., 1986; McCrea et al., 1987; DiPaola et al., 1989). The model shown in Figure 5.1a is the only one consistent with this orientation for the C terminus. Proteolysis data from sealed lipid vesicles containing intact oriented AChR are also consistent with a synaptic location of the C terminus and provide evidence for a synaptic location of the domain between MIII and MIV (Moore et al., 1989). This arrangement is not predicted by any of the folding models. Although the immunolocalization model has not received strong support, more recent work (which appears to be carefully executed) provides strong evidence for the existence of the two cytoplasmic crossings shown in Figure 5.1c. Low-resolution images of the AChR obtained by electron microscopy also provide some insight into the likely folding models (Toyoshima and Unwin, 1988). These images indicate that a relatively small fraction of the receptor mass is in the cytoplasmic domain, with about 50% of the receptor in the synaptic domain. Considering peptide mass alone (ignoring carbohydrate), the model shown in Figure 5.1c places too high a proportion of the protein in the cytoplasm.

The evolution of the folding models and current controversy regarding the AChR demonstrate that a determination of membrane protein topography can be a nontrivial problem. The reasons for the striking discrepancies seen in much of the experimental work on the AChR are not known. As with many experiments on large labile biological molecules, it is likely that some of the discrepancy is due to differences in preparation and the instability of the protein. It is also likely that the interpretation of some of the data has been based on reasonable but erroneous assumptions. Some of these assumptions, along with the strengths and problems associated with certain approaches, are discussed below. Our understanding of the application of many tech-

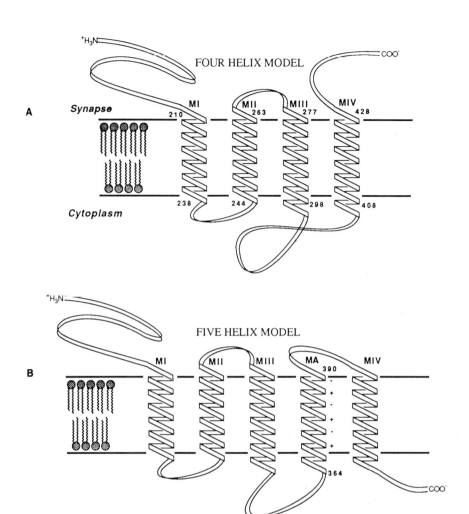

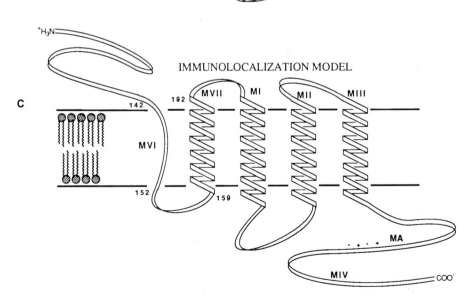

niques such as antibody binding has improved dramatically, and many of the potential problems that can be encountered with methodologies used to examine membrane protein topography are now better understood.

General Approaches to Determine Topography

The problem of membrane protein topography can be approached with a wide range of techniques, which may be no fewer in number than the number of membrane protein systems that have been studied. In general there are two types of probes that are used to determine membrane protein topography: chemical probes based on covalent derivatization and proteins or probes based on molecular recognition. Sites of post-translational modification, such as sites for carbohydrate attachment, provide information on topography since these sites are normally extracellular. In addition, the processing of signal sequences, as indicated above for the AChR, provides evidence for the extracellular or cytoplasmic location of the protein N terminus.

Antibodies

Both polyclonal and monoclonal antibodies are widely used as tools to determine the transmembrane disposition of segments in membrane proteins. Antibodies can be produced that recognize epitopes on membrane-bound proteins using several methods. These include immunization with synthetic fragments corresponding to specified segments of the membrane protein and immunization with the intact protein or fragments of the intact protein. Antibody binding allows a determination of the transmembrane disposition of the epitope, provided that the epitope to which the antibody binds has been correctly determined (or mapped).

Several techniques have been employed to map epitopes. For example, antibodies that were generated to sodium dodecyl sulfate (SDS) denatured subunits of the nicotinic acetylcholine receptor (nAChR) were mapped to specific epitopes by examining their binding to proteolytic fragments of the receptor and synthetic receptor peptides (Pedersen et al., 1990). Information on the transmembrane disposition of these epitopes was then obtained by localizing the antibody binding to either the cytoplasmic or extracellular surface. For the LamB protein of *E. coli,* epitopes were mapped by immunoblotting against specific LamB mutants (Molla et al., 1989).

A number of approaches can be used to detect the binding of antibodies and to assign the epitopes to a specific surface. If the antibody binding is strong enough, it can be coupled to colloidal gold and its transmembrane disposition determined using

---

Fig. 5.1 *(opposite)*. Several of the models that have been proposed for the transmembrane topography of the nicotinic acetylcholine receptor, AChR. *A*: The "four helix" model, which was based primarily on a hydropathy analysis of the receptor sequence. *B*: The "five helix" model, which includes an additional charged amphipathic transmembrane helix (*MA*). In this model, *MA* is thought to form part of the ion-conductive path. The C terminus also has a cytoplasmic location. *C*: A model based on immunolocalization studies using antibodies. The C terminus is cytoplasmic in this model, and two additional transmembrane segments are included on the amino side of MI.

thin section or freeze-etch electron microscopy (see, for example, Young et al., 1985; Bridgman et al., 1987). Immunofluorescence of fluorescein-conjugated antibodies (Pedersen et al., 1990), precipitation with immobilized protein A (Young et al., 1985), and the enzyme-linked immunosorbent assay (ELISA) are examples of a few of the methods that have been used to assess antibody binding. A comparison of the antibody binding in intact right-side-out membrane preparations to samples of which the cytoplasmic surface of the membrane protein is exposed is often employed to determine the sidedness of epitopes. Exposure of the cytoplasmic epitopes has been achieved by a wide range of approaches, including the addition of a mild detergent (Cradio et al., 1985a), alkaline treatment of the membrane (Cradio et al., 1985b), or complete solubilization of the membrane protein (Young et al., 1985). In the case of thylakoid membranes an elegant approach was taken by examining antibody binding to inside-out and right-side-out populations of the membrane preparation. These two populations of vesicles were separated by phase partitioning in a two-phase polymer system composed of dextran and polyethylene glycol (Tae et al., 1988). This approach eliminates some of the problems that may arise from the addition of detergents or other permeabilizing agents (see below).

Epitope Specificity. High-affinity antibodies provide a potentially powerful methodology for the determination of membrane protein topography. However, a critical step in the prudent application of this methodology is an analysis of the epitope specificity. For example, it has been demonstrated that antibodies directed at peptides will not necessarily have specificity for the immunizing peptide (Maelicke et al., 1989). Antipeptide antibodies can exhibit dramatic cross-reactivities; for example, when antisera are produced to a synthetic portion of the α-subunit of the acetylcholine receptor (α387–392), antibodies are found that bind to two unrelated epitopes preferentially to the epitope that contained the immunizing sequence (Maelicke et al., 1989). Even if the antibody shows preferential specificity for the intended epitope, it can show affinity for additional epitopes that have sequences with no homology to the immunizing peptide. This cross-reactivity can be a particular problem with procedures that require high concentrations of antibody such as electron microscopy (see McCrea et al., 1987).

From a chemical point of view, the antibody cross-reactivity that is found is not surprising. Antibodies recognize three-dimensional determinants, not linear sequences. A large number of three-dimensional conformations are likely to be accessible to synthetic peptides, or proteolytic fragments of membrane proteins, and it is difficult to ensure that a unique determinant resembling the desired structure in the native protein has been used in the immunization. In view of this consideration, it is perhaps more surprising that binding to the intended epitope can often be obtained.

To improve the chances of obtaining an antibody that will recognize the appropriate sequence, it has been suggested that peptides of only five to seven residues be used in the immunization (Maelicke et al., 1989). This represents a minimal size necessary to evoke an immune response and appears to maximize the possibility that the antibody recognizes the linear sequence. Unfortunately, antibodies to these shorter peptides often have lowered affinity and may not permit studies using electron microscopy. This lowered affinity is not surprising given that antibody-binding sites may contact two to three times this number of residues (Amit et al., 1986). A series of criteria for the immunolocalization of sites on proteins has been discussed (see Pedersen et al., 1990). These criteria include ensuring the purity of the antibody, establishing that the antibody binds to a short linear sequence present in the native and denatured protein, the use of immunoelectron microscopy in combination with direct binding measurements, and defining the epitope to which the antibody binds by linear mapping.

Detergents, Reconstitution, and Membrane Permeabilization. The absence of antibody binding to intact native membranes, but a subsequent binding upon the addition of agents to "permeabilize" membranes is often taken as evidence for a cytoplasmic localization of epitopes. Binding to reconstituted membranes (which have a population of inside-out protein) as well as binding to detergent-solubilized membrane proteins has also been used as evidence for a cytoplasmic localization of epitopes (Pedersen et al., 1990). While these are appropriate experiments to test for a cytoplasmic disposition of epitopes, there are several potential problems that must be controlled for before the results can be unambiguously interpreted.

The structure and activity of many membrane proteins are sensitive to the lipid environment and to the presence of detergents (for examples of the effects of membrane physical chemistry on protein function, see Gennis, 1989). In the case of the AChR, the stability of the protein during reconstitution requires the presence of lipid (Lindstrom et al., 1980; Heidmann et al., 1980), and increasing the level of detergent even in the presence of lipid can result in irreversible inactivation of this membrane protein (Jones et al., 1988). The structure of the protein also appears to be sensitive to the lipid composition; for example, the content of sterol and negative phospholipid was found to alter the secondary structure of reconstituted AChR as determined by infrared spectroscopy (Fong and McNamee, 1987). As a result, the addition of detergents to expose cytoplasmic determinants may also expose epitopes that are not cytoplasmic simply as a result of structural changes in the protein. This possibility should be considered when antibody binding data are interpreted or when any other technique that employs recognition at sites on a protein is employed.

Membrane proteins can exist at a high density in native membranes, and this close packing may prevent the association of large molecules such as antibodies (or enzymes) to epitopes on the membrane exterior. The addition of detergent or reconstitution can lower the density of membrane protein so that extracellular epitopes that were previously inaccessible now bind antibodies. Indeed, the AChR is much more rapidly proteolyzed in reconstituted membranes with a high lipid to protein ratio than in native membranes (Moore, 1989). As far as can be determined, the reconstituted AChR is correctly oriented and fully functional in reconstituted membranes (McCrea et al., 1987).

It should be noted that a number of the concerns mentioned here are not only important for the interpretation of antibody accessibility, but are also a concern for other approaches involving molecular recognition (e.g., proteolysis) or chemical derivatization.

Enzymatic Approaches

Proteolytic enzymes have been widely utilized to address questions of regarding membrane protein topography. In principle these enzymes are similar to antibodies except that they are less specific and may act on a large number of sites on a membrane protein. For small membrane proteins, proteolysis can provide a relatively simple test for topography. For example, trypsin cleavage has been used to determine the orientation of the leader peptidase protein in *Escherichia coli* (an aqueous loop in this protein contains a single proteolytic site; Nilsson and von Heijne, 1990). For larger proteins, proteolysis is likely to yield a large number of fragments some of which are small and difficult to identify. A number of approaches can be taken to identify proteolytic fragments of these proteins. A newer and particularly promising approach to examine proteolytic fragments of proteins involves the use of mass spectrometry (discussed below). For example, mass spectrometry was used to identify over 50 peptide fragments from reconstituted membranes containing right-side-out AChR (Moore et al., 1989) These fragments ranged in molecular weight from about 600 to over 3,500 and could be identified in impure mixtures of peptides.

As is the case for other large molecules such as antibodies, the use of proteolytic enzymes requires that membranes remain impermeable to these enzymes. Proteolytic enzymes have been observed to alter the morphology of membranes containing the AChR (Klymkowsky et al., 1980), and it is important to determine that the action of the enzyme does not itself alter membrane permeability (perhaps by generating peptides that are lytic). The protease may also alter the folding of the protein; for example, there is some evidence from the tryptic treatment of bacteriorhodopsin and cytochrome b_6 that proteolysis can destabilize membrane-bound segments of proteins (see, for example, Dumont et al., 1985; Szczepaniank and Cramer, 1990).

Proteolysis of the protein from both the extracellular and cytoplasmic surfaces can be useful to determine whether the protein is transmembrane and what the orientation of epitopes is (see, for example, Strader and Raftery, 1980; Tae et al., 1988). This can be accomplished in a number of ways, for example, by trapping enzymes on the cytoplasmic side or performing proteolysis using right-side-out and inside-out vesicle systems. Care should be taken when trapping proteolytic enzymes such as trypsin within vesicles; for example, when a freeze-thaw procedure was used to trap trypsin on the interior of membrane vesicles, trypsin remained active even at 4° C (Moore, 1989). As a result, limited proteolysis of the external domains of membrane proteins occurred before the external trypsin could be removed or inactivated by inhibitor. For the AChR, inside versus outside proteolysis produced different fragments as determined on gels; however, these results were reproduced by proteolytic treatment for short versus long times from the external surface only.

A number of enzymatic procedures can be used to label membrane proteins in a surface-specific manner, and these have proven to be important tools for determining topography. Lactoperoxidase-catalyzed iodination is one of the more popular enzymatic systems that has been employed for this purpose. In the presence of H_2O_2, lactoperoxidase catalyzes the iodination of the side groups of tyrosines. However, the presence of excess H_2O_2 is reported to result in the labeling of phospholipids and the aggregation of membrane proteins (Fung and Hubbell, 1978). A milder procedure using glucose oxidase and glucose to produce the peroxide (Hubbard and Cohn, 1972) was found to overcome this problem. Iodination using lactoperoxidase was used to examine the topography of the AChR (see, for example, Hartig and Raftery, 1977; St. John et al., 1982). Treatments that make the AChR membrane permeable have little effect on the level of iodination of the AChR, which provides evidence that a relatively small fraction of the receptor protein is on the cytoplasmic surface.

Chemical Reagents

Chemical reagents that act on specific sites or residues are widely used to provide information on topography. For example, lysine and cysteine residues provide convenient nucleophiles for chemical derivatization by aqueous nonpermeant reagents. Modification of lysines with pyridoxal phosphate followed by reduction of the Schiff's base linkages with sodium borohydride is a procedure that was used to investigate the transmembrane disposition of lysine residues in the AChR (Dwyer, 1988, 1991). In these experiments, binding and quantitation of the derivatized peptides was simplified by the use of immunoabsorption. An interesting approach was recently taken to label internally exposed lysines of the AChR in a vesicle system (Perez-Ramirez and Martinez-Carrion, 1989). In these experiments, pyridoxine phosphate was trapped into vesicles along with pyridoxine phosphate oxidase. At 37° C, enzymatic oxidation of pyridoxine phosphate produced pyridoxal phosphate, which then reacted with the cytoplasmic lysines. Cytochrome c was added externally to scavenge any pyridoxal phosphate that might have leaked.

The use of chemical reagents to define membrane protein topography can exploit very specific features of the membrane protein. The nAChR can exist as a dimer that is disulfide linked through a cystine that is the penultimate residue on the δ-subunit. This feature of the AChR was used to localize the C terminus by examining the rate of reduction of the disulfide. Reduction of the AChR dimer by glutathione or mercaptoethanesulfonic acid, reagents that were shown to be impermeable, occurred much more rapidly for right-side-out receptor than for inside out receptor, indicating that the C terminus was on the extracellular (synaptic) surface (see McCrea et al., 1987; DiPaola et al., 1989).

Residues such as lysine are believed to reside primarily on the surfaces of proteins facing aqueous phases (Chothia, 1976). To label hydrophobic residues, which presumably lie at the lipid protein interface in membrane proteins, several methods have been employed. Some of these reagents include pyrenesulfonyl azide, adamantanediazirine, iodonaphthyl azide, and trifluoromethyliodophenyldiazirine (TID). Labeling with reagents such as TID has been used to determine those regions of a membrane protein that are in contact with the membrane hydrocarbon. For example, TID labeling of the AChR provides evidence that the peptide containing MIV (see Fig. 6.1) is in contact with the hydrocarbon; however, the N-terminal third of the protein does not incorporate the label, which was taken as evidence that the AChR has no transmembrane segments on the amino side of MI (White and Cohen, 1988). It is not clear with these experiments how strongly the lack of labeling can be taken as evidence against the existence of a transmembrane segment. Indeed, a later study by this laboratory concluded that the receptor does have additional transmembrane segments in the N-terminal region (based on antibody binding) and that the lack of labeling by TID was likely due to the lack of exposure of the protein to the hydrocarbon (Pedersen et al., 1990). In the case of bacteriorhodopsin, where most of the protein is in the membrane, TID was used to examine the exposure of the protein to the hydrocarbon. Photolabeling of bacteriorhodopsin with TID and an analysis of the labeling pattern shows that the label incorporated at an interval of residues that would be expected if one surface of an α-helix were exposed to the label. These data were used as evidence supporting a specific orientation of helix C in the protein with respect to the membrane hydrocarbon (Brunner et al., 1985).

A final concern that might be raised concerning TID is the extent to which it can label portions of membrane proteins that are outside the membrane. For example, unlike bacteriorhodopsin, most of the mass of the AChR is not in the membrane, and TID could label a hydrophobic (interior) portion of the protein in the aqueous phase. This does not appear to be the case for the AChR, where TID partitions strongly to the membrane and labeling apparently occurs primarily through the lipid domain (White and Cohen, 1988).

Another approach that has been taken to label the lipid-exposed domains of membrane proteins involves the use of labels incorporated into lipid analogs. For example, an analysis of the lipid in contact with the AChR was carried out with phospholipids derivatized in either the acyl chain or headgroup with the photoreactive arylazido group (see, for example, Giraudat et al., 1985; Blanton and Wang, 1990). Chain labels placed at different positions relative to the headgroup were also used to infer the position of a reactive cysteine in the AChR membrane (Giraudat et al., 1985). While interesting differences in labeling are seen between labels placed at different positions on the alkyl chain, interpreting the labeling patterns can be difficult. Labels attached to an alkyl chain can exhibit a wide spatial distribution due to the high mobility and low order of the alkyl chain segments (see, for example, Ellena et al., 1988).

Mass Spectrometry

Mass spectrometry is currently growing in importance as a technique to analyze the structure of large biological molecules. Because this is not widely thought of as a tool for determining protein topography and because of its growing potential for studying complex membrane proteins, its use and some of the basic principles behind its application will be discussed here.

Mass spectrometry has been used to sequence proteins and to determine sites of posttranslational modification such as glycosylation and phosphorylation (see, for example, Hunt et al., 1991). It is also a technique that has been used to examine the topography of membrane proteins. For example, the sites of glycosylation of the AChR (as well as the structures of the oligosaccharides) were determined using mass spectrometry and provided evidence for the typography of the receptor (Poulter et al., 1988, 1989). Mass spectrometry was also used to identify rapidly over 50 peptides produced by external trypsin and/or *Staphylococcus aureus* V8 protease treatment of the AChR reconstituted in predominantly right-side-out sealed lipid vesicles (Moore et al., 1989). Because the vesicles remain sealed during proteolysis and internally trapped water-soluble proteins were not cleaved by proteases, these data provided evidence for the extracellular location of the released peptides.

Sequencing by Mass Spectrometry

The rapid analysis of large numbers of fragment peptides by mass spectrometry is possible, because this technique can utilize relatively impure mixtures of peptides.

A

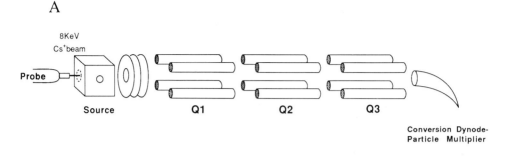

B

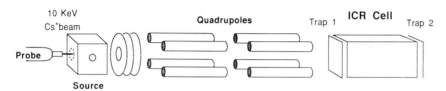

Fig. 5.2. *A*: Schematic diagram of a triple quadrupole mass spectrometer used for protein sequencing. Peptide ions are produced by bombarding the sample in an acidic thioglycerol matrix with 6–10 keV Cs^+ ions. With *Q1* and *Q2* set to act as ion-focusing devices, *Q3* is used as a mass filter to identify primary ions corresponding to the peptides in solution. In the sequencing mode, *Q2* is filled with about 5 mtorr of argon, and a peptide ion that is passed to *Q2* undergoes a collisionally activated decomposition. *Q3* is then utilized to analyze the fragment masses (see Hunt et al., 1986). *B*: Schematic of a tandem quadrupole mass spectrometer. In the tandem quadrupole machine, peptides are sent to an ion cyclotron resonance cell (ICR). An rf pulse on the ICR produces coherent orbits of the peptide ions, which then dephase. Fourier transformation of the signal produces a mass spectrum (see Hunt et al., 1987).

The analysis by mass spectrometry of proteolytic fragments of a protein can be carried out on samples containing mixtures of ten to fifteen peptides (Hunt et al., 1986). With the development of new ionization procedures (see below) the ability of mass spectrometry to handle complex mixtures will improve. Shown in Figure 5.2 are diagrams for two mass spectrometers that have been used to sequence and make mass determinations on proteins. The triple quadrupole mass spectrometer shown in Figure 5.2*a* can be run in one of two modes. With the first two quadrupoles (Q_1 and Q_2) acting as ion-focusing devices, Q_3 is used as a mass filter to provide a spectrum of the $(M + H)^+$ ions corresponding to the molecular weights of peptides in the sample. In a second or sequencing mode, one of these peptides is selected by mass and passed to Q_2 where it collides with argon atoms at low pressure and fragments at the amide linkages. The fragments are then analyzed by Q_3 to provide the sequence (see below). The diagram shown in Figure 5.2*b* depicts a tandem quadrupole Fourier-transform spectrometer that was constructed using a 7-T superconducting magnet (Hunt et al., 1987). In this instrument, peptide ions are passed to an ion cyclotron resonance (ICR) cell in which an rf pulse accelerates the ions and forces them to orbit coherently at their characteristic frequencies. Fourier transformation of the induced rf signal produces a mass spectrum. In this machine, peptide ions can also undergo collision-activated decomposition or laser-induced photodissociation to provide sequence information (see Hunt et al., 1987).

The collisionally activated decomposition of the gas phase peptide ions occurs as depicted in Figure 5.3. In the gas phase, the charged peptide can be protonated at one of the amide linkages (the proton affinities of the amide linkage and amines in the gas phase are similar). When the oligopeptide undergoes collisions with argon atoms, the peptide gains vibrational energy that can result in fragmentation at the protonated amide bond. The fragmentation occurs via two major pathways and results in the production of ions that contain either the original N terminus (type B) or the original C terminus (type Y"). Because each molecule fragments more or less randomly at one of the amide linkages, the resulting collision-activated decomposition spectrum yields masses that correspond to the sequence of the peptide. A typical collision-activated decomposition spectrum showing the assigned peptide sequence as well as the masses of the corresponding B and Y" type ions is shown in Figure 5.4.

Many of the experimental limitations with mass spectrometry have been associated with the ionization techniques. For example, until the development of secondary

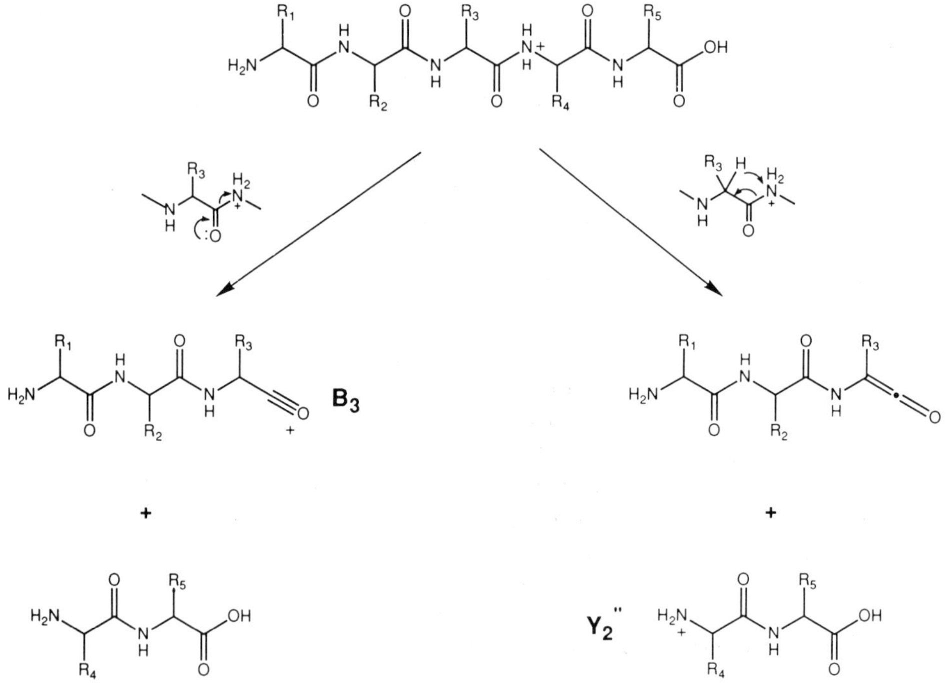

Fig. 5.3. A diagram showing the major fragmentation pathways for peptide ions that undergo collision-activated decomposition. To a first approximation, the peptide can be protonated randomly at any amide linkage, and low energy collisions with argon atoms produce a single break resulting in either a B-type ion (containing the original amino terminus) or a Y"-type ion (containing the original C terminus). The distribution between Y"- and B-type ions can be affected by the composition of the peptide (see Hunt et al., 1986, for a more detailed discussion of this process).

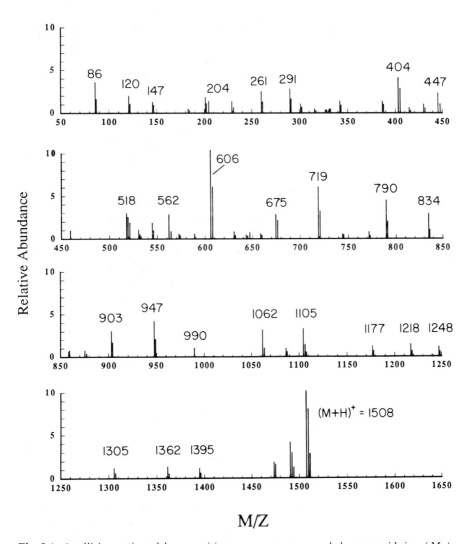

Fig. 5.4. A collision-activated decomposition mass spectrum recorded on a peptide ion, $(M + H)^+$, of m/z = 1,508. The amino acid sequence determined from this spectrum is IFADDIDISDISGK. The Y''- and B-type ions that are produced from this sequence are also shown. This peptide is a tryptic fragment from the α-subunit of the acetylcholine receptor from *T. californica*, α341–354.

ion (SIMS) and fast atom bombardment (FAB) ionization procedures, mass spectrometry was limited to relatively low mass ranges and relatively large sample requirements. The more recently employed SIMS and FAB approaches increase the mass range, but suffer from other experimental difficulties. For example, the sensitivity of detection of a given peptide, particularly in complex mixtures, can vary greatly using SIMS or FAB ionization procedures. When the kinetics of tryptic proteolysis of the AChR was examined, ion currents were often seen to decrease for peptides that were increasing in concentration (Moore, 1989). This "suppression" of an ion current is thought to occur in more complex mixtures as a result of the selective partitioning of more hydrophobic peptides to the interface of the glycerol or thioglycerol matrix used in SIMS (see Naylor et al., 1986). However, the potential of mass spectrometry as a technique to examine biological macromolecules has dramatically improved in recent years, primarily because of the development of new ionization methods that allow large, fragile molecules to be placed nondestructively into the vacuum of the mass spectrometer. Two of these techniques, electrospray ionization (see Fenn et al., 1989; Smith et al., 1990) and matrix-assisted laser desorption (see Beavis and Chait, 1990; Bornsen et al., 1991), now permit accurate mass measurements on proteins in excess of 100 kDa at the femtomole to picomole level. With these developments, techniques utilizing mass spectrometry provide a new, powerful approach to examine protein structure and covalent modification. The application of this methodology to examine membrane protein topography is also attractive, since the results of proteolysis or chemical derivatization can be identified rapidly and accurately by this methodology. This methodology should provide an important complement to more traditional biochemical and immunological approaches to examine membrane protein topography.

Summary and Conclusions

The determination of topography can employ a wide range of techniques and is an extremely important step in defining the structure of a membrane protein. Approaches using antibodies are attractive and powerful because numerous specific epitopes can be targeted; however, the specificity of the antibody to the intended epitope must be ensured. Procedures such as proteolysis also recognize specific sites, but are less specific than antibodies. In addition, a number of chemical approaches can be employed depending on the chemistry of the membrane protein in question. With all these approaches, it is imperative that the membrane system under investigation be rigorously defined. New procedures to detect and characterize proteins using mass spectrometry have developed in recent years, and this should provide an important tool for examining membrane protein topography when combined with other chemical and enzymatic approaches.

Acknowledgments

I thank Drs. Donald Hunt and Jeffrey Shabanowitz for helpful discussions on the use of mass spectrometry for protein analysis and sequence determination. Portions of the research described in this work were supported by grant BNS-8908692 from the National Science Foundation.

References

Amit, A. G., Mariuzza, R. A., Phillips, S.E.V., and Poljak, R. J. (1986) Three-dimensional structure of an antigen-antibody complex at 2.8 Å resolution. *Science* 233: 747–753.

Anderson, D. J., Walter, P., and Blobel, G. (1982) Signal recognition protein is required for the integration of acetylcholine receptor δ subunit, a transmembrane glycoprotein, into the endoplasmic reticulum membrane. *J. Cell Biol.* 93: 501–506.

Barkas, T., Juillerat, M., Kistler, J., Schwendimann, B., and Moody, J. (1984) Antibodies to synthetic peptides as probes of acetylcholine receptor structure. *Eur. J. Biochem.* 143: 309–314.

Beavis, R. C., and Chait, B. T. (1990) Rapid, sensitive analysis of protein mixtures by mass spectrometry. *Proc. Natl. Acad. Sci. USA* 87: 6873–6877.

Blanton, M. P., and Wang, H. P. (1990) Photoaffinity labeling of the *Torpedo californica* nicotinic acetylcholine receptor with an aryl azide derivative of phosphatidylserine. *Biochemistry* 29: 1186–1194.

Bornsen, K. O., Schar, M., Gassmann, E., and Steiner, V. (1991) Analytical applications of matrix-assisted laser desorption and ionization mass spectrometry. *Biol. Mass Spec.* 20: 471–478.

Boyd, D., Manoil, C., and Beckwith, J. (1987) Determinants of membrane protein topology. *Proc. Natl. Acad. Sci. USA* 84: 8525–8529.

Bridgman, P. C., Carr, C., Pedersen, S. E., and Cohen, J. B. (1987) Visualization of the cytoplasmic surface of *Torpedo* postsynaptic membranes by freeze-etch and immunoelectron microscopy. *J. Cell. Biol.* 105: 1829–1846.

Brunner, J., Franzusoff, A. J., Lusher, B., Zuglaiani, C., and Semenza, G. (1985) Membrane protein topology: amino acid residues in a putative transmembrane α-helix of bacteriorhodopsin labeled with the hydrophobic carbene-generating reagent 3-(trifluoromethyl)-3-(m-[^{125}I]iodophenyl) diazirine. *Biochemistry* 24: 5422–5430.

Cafiso, D. S. (1991) Lipid bilayers: membrane–protein electrostatic interactions. *Curr. Opin. Struct. Biol.* 1: 185–190.

Charbit, A., Ronco, J., Michel, A., Werts, C., and Hofnung, M. (1991) Permissive sites and topology of an outer membrane protein with a reporter epitope. *J. Bacteriol.* 173: 262–275.

Chothia, C. (1976) The nature of the accessible and buried surfaces in proteins. *J. Mol. Biol.* 105: 1–14.

Criado, M., Hochschwender, S., Sarin, V., Fox, L. J., and Lindstrom, J. (1985a) Evidence for unpredicted transmembrane domains in acetylcholine receptor subunits. *Proc. Natl. Acad. Sci. USA* 82: 2004–2008.

Criado, M., Sarin, V., Fox, L. J., and Lindstrom, J. (1985b) Structural localization of the sequence α235–242 of the nicotinic acetylcholine receptor. *Biochem. Biophys. Res. Commun.* 128: 864–871.

Dalbey, R. E. (1990) Positively charged residues are important determinants of membrane protein topology. *Trends Biochem. Sci.* 15: 253–257.

DiPaola, M., Czajkowski, C., and Karlin, A. (1989) The sidedness of the COOH terminus of the acetylcholine receptor δ subunit. *J. Biol. Chem.* 264: 15457–15463.

Dumont, M. E., Trewhella, J., Engelman, D. M., and Richards, F. M. (1985) Stability of transmembrane regions in bacteriorhodopsin studied by progressive proteolysis. *J. Membrane Biol.* 88: 233–247.

Dunn, S. M., Conti-Tronconi, B. M., and Raftery, M. A. (1986) Acetylcholine receptor dimers are stabilized by extracellular disulfide bonding. *Biochem. Biophys. Res. Commun.* 139: 830–837.

Dwyer, B. P. (1988) Evidence for the extramembranous location of the putative amphipathic helix of acetylcholine receptor. *Biochemistry* 27: 5586–5592.

Dwyer, B. P. (1991) Topological dispositions of lysine α380 and lysine γ486 in the acetylcholine receptor from *Torpedo californica*. *Biochemistry* 30: 4105–4112.

Ellena, J. F., Archer, S. J., Dominey, R. N., Hill, B. D., and Cafiso, D. S. (1988) Localizing the nitroxide group of fatty acid and voltage-sensitive spin-labels in phospholipid bilayers. *Biochim. Biophys. Acta* 940: 63–70.

Fenn, J. B., Mann, M., Meng, C. K., Wong, S. R., and Whitehouse, C. M. (1989) Electrospray ionization for mass spectrometry of large biomolecules. *Science* 246: 64–71.

Finer-Moore, J., and Stroud, R. M. (1984) Amphipathic analysis and possible formation of the ion-channel in an acetylcholine receptor. *Proc. Natl. Acad. Sci. USA* 81: 155–159.

Fong, T. M., and McNamee, M. G. (1987) Stabilization of acetylcholine receptor secondary structure by cholesterol and negatively charged phospholipids in membranes. *Biochemistry* 26: 3871–3880.

Fung, B. K.-K., and Hubbell, W. L. (1978) Organization of rhodopsin in membranes. 2. Transmembrane organization of bovine rhodopsin: evidence from proteolysis and lactoperoxidase-catalyzed iodination of native and reconstituted membranes. *Biochemistry* 17: 4403–4410.

Gennis, R. B. (1989) *Biomembranes: Molecular Structure and Function.* New York: Springer-Verlag.

Giraudat, J., Montecucco, C., Bisson, R., and Changeux, J.-P. (1985) Transmembrane topology of acetylcholine receptor subunits probed with photoreactive phospholipids. *Biochemistry* 24: 3121–3127.

Guy, H. R. (1984) A structural model of the acetylcholine receptor channel based on partition energy and helix pacing calculations. *Biophys. J.* 45: 249–261.

Hartig, P. R., and Raftery, M. A. (1977) Lactoperoxidase catalyzed membrane surface labeling of the acetylcholine receptor from *Torpedo californica. Biochem. Biophys. Res. Commun.* 78: 16–22.

Hartman, E., Rapoport, T. A., Lodish, H. F. (1989) Predicting the orientation of eukaryotic membrane-spanning proteins. *Proc. Natl. Acad. Sci. USA* 86: 5786–5790.

Heidmann, T., Sobel, A., Popot, J.-L., and Changeux, J.-P. (1980) Reconstitution of a functional acetylcholine receptor. Conservation of the conformational and allosteric transitions and recovery of the permeability response: role of lipids. *Eur. J. Biochem.* 110: 35–55.

Hubbard, A. L., and Cohn, Z. A. (1972) The enzymatic iodination of the red cell membrane. *J. Cell Biol.* 55: 390–405.

Hunt, D. F., Alexander, J. E., McCormick, A. L., Martino, P. A., Michel, H., Shabanowitz, J., and Sherman, N. (1991) Mass spectrometric methods for protein and peptide sequence analysis. In: *Techniques in Protein Chemistry II,* edited by J. J. Villafranca. New York: Academic Press, p. 441–454.

Hunt, D. F., Shabanowitz, J., Yates, J. R., Zhu, N.-Z., Russell, D.-H., and Castro, M. E. (1987) Tandem quadrupole Fourier-transform mass spectrometry of oligopeptides and small proteins. *Proc. Natl. Acad. Sci. USA* 84: 620–623.

Hunt, D. F., Yates, J. R., Shabanowitz, J., Winston, S., and Hauer, C. R. (1986) Protein sequencing by tandem mass spectrometry. *Proc. Natl. Acad. Sci. USA* 83: 6233–6237.

Imoto, K., Busch, C., Sakmann, B., Mishina, M., Konno, T., Nakai, J., Bujo, H., Mori, Y., Fukuda, K., and Numa, S. (1988) Rings of negatively charged amino acids determine the acetylcholine receptor channel conductance. *Nature* 335: 645–648.

Jones, O. T., Eubanks, J. H., Earnest, J. P., and McNamee, M. G. (1988) A minimum number of lipids are required to support the functional properties of the nicotinic acetylcholine receptor. *Biochemistry* 27: 3733–3742.

Kim, J., Mosior, M., Chung, L. A., Wu, H., and McLaughlin, S. (1991) Binding of peptides with basic residues to membranes containing acidic phospholipids. *Biophys. J.* 60: 135–148.

Klymkowsky, M. W., Heuser, J. E., Stroud, R. M. (1980) Protease effects on the structure of acetylcholine receptor membranes from *Torpedo californica. J. Cell Biol.* 85: 473–496.

Lear, J. D., Wasserman, Z. R., DeGrado, W. F. (1988) Synthetic amphiphilic peptide models for protein ion channels. *Science* 240: 1177–1181.

Lindstrom, J., Anholt, R., Einarson, B., Engel, A., Osame, M., and Montal, M. (1980) Purification of acetylcholine receptors, reconstitution into lipid vesicles, and study of agonist-induced cation channel regulation. *J. Biol. Chem.* 255: 8340–8350.

Lindstrom, J., Criado, M., Hochschwender, S., Fox, J. L., and Sarin, V. (1984) Immunochemical tests of acetylcholine receptor subunit models. *Nature* 311: 573–575.

Maelicke, A., Plumer-Wilk, R., Fels, G., Spencer, S. R., Engelhard, M., Veltel, D., and Conti-Tronconi, B. M. (1989) Epitope mapping employing antibodies raised against short synthetic peptides: a study of the nicotinic acetylcholine receptor. *Biochemistry* 28: 1396–1405.

McCrea, P. D., Popot, J.-L., and Engelman, D. M. (1987) Transmembrane topography of the nicotinic acetylcholine receptor δ subunit. *EMBO J.* 6: 3619–3626.

Molla, A., Charbit, A., Le Guern, A., Ryter, A., and Hofnung, M. (1989) Antibodies against synthetic peptides and the topology of LamB, an outer membrane protein from *Escherichia coli* K12. *Biochemistry* 28: 8234–8241.

Moore, C. R. (1989) *Transmembrane Topography of the Nicotinic Acetylcholine Receptor From* Torpedo *Determined From Proteolytically Sensitive Sites of the Reconstituted Protein.* Ph.D. Thesis, Charlottesville: University of Virginia.

Moore, C. R., Yates, J. R., Griffin, P. R., Shabanowitz, J., Martino, P. A., Hunt, D. R., and Cafiso, D.

S. (1989) Proteolytic fragments of the nicotinic acetylcholine receptor identified by mass spectrometry: implications for receptor topography. *Biochemistry* 28: 9184–9191.

Mosior, M., and McLaughlin, S. (1992) Binding of basic peptides to acidic lipid in membranes: effects of inserting alanine(s) between the basic residues. *Biochemistry* 31: 1767–1773.

Naylor, S., Findeis, A. F., Gibson, B. W., and Williams, D. H. (1986) An approach toward the complete FAB analyis of enzymatic digests of peptides and proteins. *J. Am. Chem. Soc.* 108: 6359–6363.

Nilsson, I., and von Heijne, G. (1990) Fine-tuning the topology of a polytopic membrane protein: role of positively and negatively charged amino acids. *Cell* 62: 1135–1141.

Noda, M., Takahashi, H., Tanabe, T., Toyosato, M., Kikyotani, S., Furutani, Y., Hirose, T., Takashima, H., Inayama, S., Miyata, T., and Numa, S. (1983) Structural homology of *Torpedo californica* acetylcholine receptor subunits. *Nature* 302: 528–532.

Pedersen, S. E., Bridgman, P. C., Sharp, S. D., and Cohen, J. B. (1990) Identification of a cytoplasmic region of the *Torpedo* nicotinic acetylcholine receptor α-subunit by epitope mapping. *J. Biol. Chem.* 265: 569–581.

Perez-Ramirez, B., and Martinez-Carrion, M. (1989) Pyridoxal phosphate as a probe of the cytoplasmic domains of transmembrane proteins: application to the nicotinic acetylcholine receptor. *Biochemistry* 28: 5034–5040.

Popot, J.-L., and Engleman, D. M. (1990) Membrane protein folding and oligomerization: the two-stage model. *Biochemistry* 29: 4031–4037.

Poulter, L., Earnest, J. P., Stroud, R. M., and Burlingame, A. L. (1988) Cesium ion liquid secondary ion mass spectrometry of membrane-bound glycoproteins: structural and topological considerations of acetylcholine receptor from *Torpedo californica*. *Biomed. Environ. Mass Spec.* 16: 25–30.

Poulter, L., Earnest, J. P., Stroud, R. M., and Burlingame, A. L. (1989) Structure, oligosaccharide structures, and posttranslationally modified sites of the nicotinic acetylcholine receptor. *Proc. Natl. Acad. Sci. USA* 86: 6645–6649.

Ratnam, M., and Lindstrom, J. (1984) Structural features of the nicotinic acetylcholine receptor revealed by antibodies to synthetic peptides *Biochem. Biophys. Res. Commun.* 122: 1225–1233.

Ratnam, M., Nguyen, D. L., River, J., Sargent, P. B., and Lindstrom, J. (1986) Transmembrane topography of nicotinic acetylcholine receptor: immunochemical tests contradict theoretical predictions based on hydrophobicity profiles. *Biochemistry* 25: 2633–2643.

Sabatini, D. D., Kreibich, G., Morimoto, T., and Adesnik, M. (1982) Mechanisms for the incorporation of proteins in membranes and organelles. *J. Cell Biol.* 92: 1–22.

Smith, R. D., Loo, J. A., Edmonds, C. G., Barinaga, C. J., and Udseth, H. R. (1990) New developments in biochemical mass spectrometry: electrospray ionization. *Anal. Chem.* 62: 882–899.

Strader, C. D., and Raftery, M. A. (1980) Topographic studies of *Torpedo* acetylcholine receptor subunits as a transmembrane complex. *Proc. Natl. Acad. Sci. USA* 77: 5807–5811.

St. John, P. A., Froehner, S. C., Goodenough, D. A., and Cohen, J. A. (1982) Nicotinic postsynaptic membranes from *Torpedo:* sidedness, permeability to macromolecules, and topography of major polypeptides. *J. Cell Biol.* 92: 333–342.

Szczepaniak, A., and Cramer, W. A. (1990) Thylakoid membrane protein topography. Location of the termini of the chloroplast cytochrome b6 on the stromal side of the membrane. *J. Biol. Chem.* 265: 17720–17726.

Tae, G.-S., Black, M. T., Cramer, W. A., Vallon, O., and Bogorad, L. (1988) Thylakoid membrane protein topography: transmembrane orientation of the chloroplast cytochrome *b*-559 *pbsE* gene product. *Biochemistry* 27: 9075–9080.

Toyoshima, C., and Unwin, N. (1988) Ion channel of acetylcholine receptor reconstructed from images of postsynaptic membranes. *Nature* 336: 247–250.

White, B. H., and Cohen, J. B. (1988) Photolabeling of membrane-bound *Torpedo* nicotinic acetylcholine receptor with the hydrophobic probe 3-trifluoromethyl-3-(m-[^{125}I]iodophenyl)diazirine. *Biochemistry* 27: 8741–8751.

Young, E. F., Ralston, E., Blake, J., Ramachandran, J., Hall, Z. W., Stroud, R. M. (1985) Topological mapping of acetylcholine receptor: evidence for a model with five transmembrane segments and a cytoplasmic COOH-terminal peptide. *Proc. Natl. Acad. Sci. USA* 82: 626–630.

6

Use of Gene Fusions to Determine
Membrane Protein Topology

DANA BOYD

The topological model of an integral membrane protein specifies which parts of the protein lie on which side of the membrane and which parts are embedded within it. The topological model can be considered a set of constraints on the possible three-dimensional structures for the protein. As such, a simple topological model contains a great deal of information about the structure of the protein, since it greatly limits the number of possible three-dimensional structures. Predicting topological structures and testing these predictions is therefore of great interest.

A preliminary topological model for a membrane protein, prokaryotic or eukaryotic, can be generated readily by hydropathy analysis of its primary amino acid sequence (Degli Esposti et al., 1990; Fasman and Gilbert, 1990; see also White, Chapter 4). Although none of the various methods for carrying out this kind of analysis appears to be perfect, and different methods occasionally produce different models, useful, testable topological models are readily generated. The orientation of membrane proteins is determined at least in part by the distribution of basic residues in short hydrophilic domains (Boyd and Beckwith, 1990; von Heijne and Manoil, 1990; see also von Heijne, Chapter 2). Analysis of the distribution of charged residues in short hydrophilic domains is therefore useful for predicting the orientation of membrane proteins.

In the last few years, several gene fusion methods for studying membrane protein topology have been developed. With these methods, a DNA fragment coding for a reporter molecule is joined to the gene for the membrane protein. The hybrid protein produced from such a construct consists of an N-terminal part from the membrane protein and a C-terminal reporter moiety. The reporter moiety behaves as if it were part of the membrane protein and is localized in the same way as the part of the membrane protein to which it is joined. The topology of the membrane protein is then inferred from study of localization of the reporter moiety in a set of fusion proteins. Such an approach provides information about the orientation of the membrane protein that cannot be predicted by hydropathy analysis.

This chapter deals with the methods available for carrying out such gene fusion studies, how these methods work, what constitutes an adequate study of topology using these methods, and what the limitations of these methods are. Finally, it addresses what may be inferred about the determination of membrane protein topology by the success of gene fusion methods and what is understood about how they work. The intent is to provide an introduction to the technology for potential users and, more importantly, to provide a framework for the general reader to assess critically current and future gene fusion topology studies.

The most widely used of these gene fusion methods is the alkaline phosphatase fusion method (Manoil and Beckwith, 1986), which can be applied in a large number of different bacterial species (Manoil et al., 1990). Although I focus on this most widely used and best studied method, many of the salient features of the alkaline phosphatase fusion method must be features of any such reporter gene fusion method. Therefore, while some of what follows is specific to this system, much of it can be considered general. Moreover, the approach may not be limited to the study of bacterial proteins. The bacterial inner membrane is in many ways equivalent to the eukaryotic cytoplasmic membrane. Since bacteria have no endoplasmic reticulum, membrane proteins must insert directly into the inner membrane. While very little is known about the process of insertion, it is clear from sequence comparisons that the signals within membrane proteins that determine topology must be similar in eukaryotes and prokaryotes (von Heijne, 1986; von Heijne and Gavel, 1988). Some eukaryotic membrane proteins have been functionally expressed in bacteria (Marullo et al., 1988; Sarkar et al., 1988). In addition, all reporter gene fusions have much in common. (See Table 6.1 for examples of gene fusion studies of membrane protein topology.)

The alkaline phosphatase fusion approach is based on two findings. The first is that export signals from other proteins can replace the signal sequence of alkaline phosphatase and direct its export out of the cytoplasm (Hoffman and Wright, 1985; Manoil and Beckwith, 1985). The second is that alkaline phosphatase is not enzymatically active if it is not exported (Boyd et al., 1987a; Derman and Beckwith, 1991; Michaelis et al., 1986). The idea is illustrated in Figure 6.1. When alkaline phosphatase, lacking its own signal sequence, is fused to a membrane protein at site 1, which is normally exported across the membrane, the alkaline phosphatase moiety of the fusion protein is also exported across the membrane and becomes enzymatically active. However, when alkaline phosphatase is fused at site 2, which is normally retained in the cytoplasm, it is also retained in the cytoplasm where it remains enzymatically inactive. Alkaline phosphatase can be considered a neutral reporter moiety in the sense that it can be efficiently localized to either side of the membrane in appropriate constructs. Note that in fusions of this type the C-terminal part of the membrane protein is deleted and replaced by the reporter moiety. Such fusions may therefore be called *C-terminal deletion fusions*. A set of such fusions to a polytopic membrane protein should consist of alternating groups of active and inactive fusions corresponding to cytoplasmic and extracytoplasmic regions of the membrane protein. Such a simple picture does not always materialize, however (see below). This method has been successfully applied to a number of integral membrane proteins whose topology is either fully or partially confirmed by other methods (Calamia and Manoil, 1990; Chun and Parkinson, 1988; Manoil and Beckwith, 1986; San Millan et al., 1989; Yun et al., 1991).

Table 6.1. A Representative Sample of Membrane Proteins Studied by Gene Fusion Methods

Reporter Membrane Protein	References
Acid phosphatase	
Yeast arginine permease	Ahmad and Bussey (1988)
Yeast uracil permease	Silve et al. (1991)
Alkaline phosphatase	
E. coli Sec Y protein	Akiyama and Ito (1987)
E. coli H(+)-ATPase a subunit	Bjrbaek et al. (1990)
E. coli MalF protein	Boyd et al. (1987b)
E. coli MalG protein	Boyd et al. (1993)
E. coli lactose permease	Calamia and Manoil (1990)
E. coli FtsQ protein	Carson et al. (1991)
E. coli cytochrome *o* terminal oxidase complex	Chepuri and Gennis (1990)
E. coli MotB protein	Chun and Parkinson (1988)
E. coli SecD and SecF proteins	Gardel et al. (1990)
E. coli colicin A immunity protein	Geli et al. (1989)
E. coli sn-glycerol-3-phosphate permease	Gött and Boos (1988)
E. coli IucD protein	de Herrero et al. (1988)
Bacteriophage fl gene I protein	Horabin and Webster (1988)
E. coli HisQ and HisM proteins	Kerppola and Ferro-Luzzi Ames (1992)
E. coli F1F0-ATP synthase α subunit	Lewis et al. (1990)
E. coli Uhp protein	Lloyd and Kadner (1990)
Vibrio cholerae ToxR protein	Miller et al. (1987)
Respiratory syncytial virus membrane fusion protein	Martin-Gallardo et al. (1989)
E. coli prolipoprotein signal peptidase	Muñoa et al. (1991)
E. coli TonB protein	Roof et al. (1991)
E. coli leader peptidase	San Millan et al. (1989)
E. coli SecE protein	Schatz et al. (1989)
E. coli colicin E1 immunity protein	Song and Cramer (1991)
E. coli mannitol permease	Sugiyama et al. (1991)
E. coli serine chemoreceptor	Manoil and Beckwith (1986), Gebert et al. (1988)
Bacillus subtilis cytochrome *c*-550	von Wachenfeldt and Hederstedt (1990)
E. coli CpxA protein	Weber and Silverman (1988)
Agrobacterium tumefaciens VirA protein	Winans et al. (1989), Melchers et al. (1989)
Rhodobacter sphaeroides bc1 cyt b subunit	Yun et al. (1991)
Rhodobacter sphaeroides PSRC L subunit	Yun et al. (1991)
β-Galactosidase	
E. coli MalF protein	Froshauer et al. (1988)
E. coli cytochrome *d* terminal oxidase	Georgiou et al. (1988)
E. coli sn-glycerol-3-phosphate permease	Gött and Boos (1988)

Table 6.1.—*Continued*

Reporter Membrane Protein	References
E. coli IucD protein	de Herrero et al. (1988)
E. coli serine chemoreceptor	Manoil, (1991), Gebert et al. (1988)
E. coli olicin E1 immunity protein	Song and Cramer (1991)
β-Lactamase	
E. coli penicillin binding protein 3	Bowler and Spratt (1989)
Yeast Ste2 protein	Cartwright and Tipper (1991)
E. coli penicillin binding protein 1B	Edelman et al. (1987)
E. coli EnvZ protein	Forst et al. (1987)
Salmonella typhimurium TonB protein	Hannavy et al. (1990)
E. coli HlyB protein	Wang et al. (1991)
Sheep NaK ATPase β subunit	Zhang and Broome-Smith (1990)
Yeast Ste2 protein	Cartwright and Tipper (1991)
Galactokinase	
Yeast arginine permease	Green et al. (1989)
Glycosylation site insertion	
Mouse muscle nicotinic acetylcholine receptor	Chavez and Hall (1991)
Histidinol reductase	
Yeast HMG CoA reductase	Sengstag et al. (1990)
α-Globin with glycosylation site	
Hepatitis B surface antigen	Eble et al. (1987)

Construction of Fusions

Alkaline phosphatase fusions may be generated by a variety of methods. The transposon vector Tn*phoA* (Manoil and Beckwith, 1985) has been used to obtain many membrane protein–alkaline phosphatase fusions. Tn*phoA* is a derivative of the transposon Tn5 in which the gene for alkaline phosphatase, missing its signal sequence, is inserted at one end. When Tn*phoA* transposes in the correct orientation and reading frame into an expressed gene, a fusion protein is synthesized. The fusion protein has phosphatase activity only if the target gene has an export signal that can replace the signal sequence. This method has the advantage that fusions into a target as large as an average gene cloned on a plasmid are easily obtained. At the beginning of a topology study this may be the method of choice to obtain a few active fusions quickly. However, many genes have favored sites for Tn*phoA* transposition, and fusions in only one of the six possible reading frames are informative. Since some out of frame fusions have low, but significant, levels of alkaline phosphatase activity (presumably due to translational restarting), finding cytoplasmic fusions by such a random method can be difficult.

To complete a topology study of a complex membrane protein, it is usually necessary to have fusions in specific regions. Fusions to a small target, such as a short

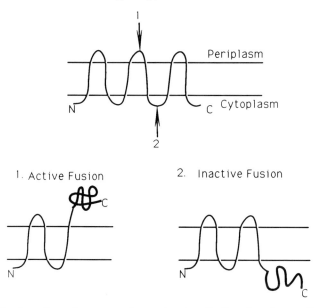

Fig. 6.1. Indication of membrane protein topology by alkaline phosphatase. When the gene for the mature part of alkaline phosphatase is joined to the gene for an expressed membrane protein, a fusion protein is generated. The alkaline phosphatase moiety is represented by the thicker line at the C terminus. The alkaline phosphatase moiety behaves as if it were part of the membrane protein (Manoil and Beckwith, 1986). It is exported out of the cytoplasm to the periplasm if it is joined to a part of the membrane protein that is exported, site *1*. It is retained in the cytoplasm if it is attached to a part of the membrane protein that is cytoplasmic, site *2*. Fusion alkaline phosphatase is active if it is exported, as in *1*, but inactive if retained in the cytoplasm, as in *2*. Such a simple picture is not always obtained when the fusion disrupts a topogenic signal. Note that in fusion proteins of this type the alkaline phosphatase moiety replaces the C terminus of the membrane protein.

hydrophilic loop between a pair of putative membrane-spanning stretches, can be much more difficult (or perhaps impossible) to obtain by transposition. An oligo-nucleotide-directed deletion mutagenesis method has been used to construct fusions precisely at preselected sites (Boyd et al., 1987b). With this method a downstream fusion to the same gene (or to a subsequent gene on the same plasmid) is used as a parent in construction of the desired fusion. Polymerase chain reaction methods can also be used to construct exact fusions (Boyd et al., 1993). Unlike the oligonucleotide-directed deletion method, this method is not limited to making fusions that are shorter than existing fusions. The target membrane protein gene and the phosphatase gene need not be on the same DNA molecule.

An advantage of these methods is that the fusions produced have sequences iden-tical to those that would be obtained by Tn*phoA* transpositions to the same sites. Thus such fusions can be safely compared with those obtained by transposition as well as to one another. Several vectors with one or more restriction sites usable for generating alkaline phosphatase fusions have been constructed (Gutierrez and Devedjian, 1989; Hoffman and Wright, 1985; Zozulia et al., 1990). An in vitro dele-tion method employing an exonuclease and restriction sites for constructing a nested set of random alkaline phosphatase fusions has recently been described (Sugiyama et al., 1991). An issue in the use of restriction sites to generate fusions is that the amino acid sequence at the fusion joint is dictated by the restriction site and the vector used. Sequence variation at the fusion joint is a possible source of activity variation in a set of fusions and should be avoided. The Tn*phoA* method discussed above gives fusions with one of four different residues at the fusion joint, depending on the base pair at which it is fused. It does not seem to matter which one of these four is present, but the neutrality of other single residues or short sequences at the fusion joint has not been assessed.

Choice of Sites for Fusion

If the objective of a gene fusion topology study is to suggest or provide experimental evidence for a topological model, a minimal requirement for a complete topological analysis is one fusion in each extramembrane domain. In a typical study, hydropathy analysis of the amino acid sequence (determined from DNA sequence) has suggested one or more topological models, and the goals are to determine orientation and to provide experimental support for one model. It is therefore important to consider all possible topologies and to construct fusions that will discriminate between them, to the extent that this is possible.

In choosing the sites for construction of fusions, it is important to consider what the reporter molecule responds to. Our current understanding of how the gene fusion method works (see below) is that the reporter moiety in each fusion protein responds either to an export signal or, after the first export signal, to a cytoplasmic localization signal (Blobel, 1980). Cytoplasmic domains contain information that contributes to determination of their own localization (Boyd and Beckwith, 1989; Boyd et al., 1987b; McGovern et al., 1991; Nilsson and von Heijne, 1990; San Millan et al., 1989). For this reason, a fusion near the N terminus of a cytoplasmic domain, which deletes most or all of the domain, may not be as useful as fusions at the C terminus of the same domain. This point is illustrated by data taken from the published study of the *Escherichia coli* MalF protein (Fig. 6.2) (Boyd et al., 1987b). MalF is an integral inner membrane protein involved in maltose transport. The topological model shown is derived from hydropathy analysis of its sequence (Froshauer and Beckwith, 1984) The alkaline phosphatase activity data shown are generally consistent with the model, but there are significant exceptions. In support of the model, fusions to exported (periplasmic) domains of the MalF protein have uniformly high activities, and fusions to the C termini of cytoplasmic domains (fusions A, D, M, P, and R) have at least tenfold lower activities. However, fusions at the C termini of incoming transmembrane stretches (C, K, L, and O) have 5- to 20-fold higher activity than the corresponding fusions at the C termini of the same cytoplasmic domain. In the C, K, L, and O fusions the short hydrophilic cytoplasmic loops are deleted. Since the pattern of increased activity was similar in all three cytoplasmic loops and the short hydrophilic sequences (there are 12 residues between the L and M fusions joints, for example) were unlikely to be transmembrane stretches, it could be concluded that the hydrophilic segments contain information that contributes to the cytoplasmic localization of the later fusion. A similar pattern has been observed with the *E. coli.* lactose

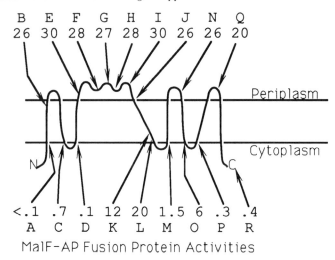

Fig. 6.2. The topology of the *E. coli* MalF protein. The name and activities of alkaline phosphatase fusions to the MalF protein are shown together with *arrows* pointing to the positions of the fusion joints in the topological model. The alkaline phosphatase activity is that measured in a strain expressing a single copy of the fusion gene on the chromosome. All fusion proteins are synthesized at similar rates (except for the A fusion protein; see text). (Adapted from Boyd et al., 1987b.)

permease protein Lac Y (Calamia and Manoil, 1990), *E. coli.* leader peptidase (San Millan et al., 1989), and also with the HlyB protein, where a different reporter moiety was used (Wang et al., 1991).

In the case of MalF, this phenomenon has been investigated extensively. Proteolysis and fractionation experiments have shown that the activity of the K, L, and M, and O fusions can be attributed to export of a fraction of the fusion alkaline phosphatase and not to activation of alkaline phosphatase in the cytoplasm (Traxler et al., 1993). Since native alkaline phosphatase, i.e., that which gives rise to the enzymatic activity, is resistant to proteolysis, treatment of spheroplasts (bacterial cells with the outer membrane removed) with proteases results in the release of the alkaline phosphatase moiety owing to cleavage at or near the fusion joint. With the K, L, M, and O fusions, the activity can be quantitatively released from the surface by proteolysis. Pulse-chase experiments showed that the amount of released protease resistant fragment corresponds to the amount expected if the fusion protein consisted of a fully active periplasmic fraction and an inactive cytoplasmic fraction. The released fragment corresponds to two-thirds of what is synthesized in the case of L and to one-tenth of what is synthesized in the case of M. Thus the M fusion alkaline phosphatase is retained more efficiently in the cytoplasm. In this case it has been shown that basic residues within the short hydrophilic loop between the sites of the L and M fusions are responsible for its effect on localization (Boyd and Beckwith, 1989). This suggests that these basic residues play a role in determining the cytoplasmic localization of this loop in the native MalF protein too.

It is not known why a fraction of the fusion alkaline phosphatase in fusions such as K, L, and O is exported. Since interpretation of data from such fusions can lead to incorrect topological assessments, construction of fusions at the N termini of hydrophilic stretches should be avoided. Conversely, added significance should be given to fusions at the C termini of hydrophilic regions in assessment of a set of fusion data.

In short, a set of fusions consisting of one fusion at the C terminus of each hydrophilic domain may be sufficient for determination of topology. Of course, such an approach is not entirely objective in that it is assumed that all transmembrane segments can be identified by hydropathy analysis. In the case of the LacY protein, for example, hydropathy analysis does not suggest a unique structure (Calamia and Manoil, 1990). The alkaline phosphatase fusion approach was used to distinguish between two possible topologies for LacY. In the region where the two models differed, fusions were constructed at several sites that would maximize discrimination between the models.

Of course, hydropathy analysis will not identify all transmembrane stretches if there exist membrane-spanning segments that are actually hydrophilic. These are often present in models of channel proteins. The potassium channel is postulated to contain such segments (Miller, 1991). Electrophysiological evidence indicates that some residues within a hydrophilic region that is primarily on one side of the membrane are exposed to the other side. A pair of short hydrophilic membrane-spanning stretches is proposed to account for this. Since such membrane-spanning stretches would not be identified by hydropathy analysis, they would be would be missed if the strategy of constructing fusions only at the C-terminal ends of hydrophilic domains were followed. For this reason some studies have included construction of fusions approximately every thirty residues within hydrophilic regions. Although such a course would seem especially prudent, it is unlikely that a large deletion fusion reporter like alkaline phosphatase is suited to detecting such specialized transmembrane segments. Their origin and stability would presumably depend on protein–protein interactions that would be disrupted in the fusion protein.

Characterization of Fusions

Once a set of fusions has been constructed and the site of the fusion joints determined or confirmed by DNA sequence analysis, it must be decided which fusions have high and which have low activity. Often this can be determined just by observation of the color of the colonies on indicator plates (Manoil, 1991). Colonies expressing high levels of alkaline phosphatase activity are dark blue when grown on solid media containing the indicator dye 5-bromo-4-chloro-3-indolylphosphate (XP). Colonies with little or no alkaline phosphatase activity are pale blue or white. Accurate measurement of alkaline phosphatase activity requires an enzyme assay (Manoil, 1991). Whereas properly localized cytoplasmic domain fusions have 10% or less of the activity of exported domain fusions, exported domain fusions have a specific activity that is similar to native alkaline phosphatase. Observation or measurement of activity levels alone is, however, insufficient to indicate topology. The level of expression and the stability of the fusion proteins must also be considered.

If the members of a set of fusion proteins are synthesized at different levels, differences in activity levels may reflect different amounts of protein rather than different localization. The MalF fusion proteins of Figure 6.2 are all synthesized at similar levels (except for the completely inactive A fusion, which is made at a fivefold higher level than the others), but this is not always the case. Therefore, an estimate of the level of synthesis is an essential part of a topology study. This is illustrated in Figure 6.3 by the analysis of the *E. coli* leader peptidase (San Millan et al., 1989). As a study of a protein of known topology, this should serve as a model for studies of proteins of unknown topology. Within the single, large periplasmic domain of this protein the measured levels of alkaline phosphatase activity varied by a factor of 40-fold. The large differences in activity levels, however, did not reflect the topology but were the consequence of widely differing levels of synthesis. Some of the fusions to this protein were synthesized at much lower rates than others. Only when the activity of each of these proteins was compared with its rate of synthesis was a consistent picture of the topology generated. This "relative activity," the amount of phosphatase activity relative to the rate of synthesis of the fusion protein, comprises the essential data for determining topology.

Synthesis level is best assessed by measurement of the rate of synthesis of the fusion protein relative to that of other proteins by pulse labeling and immunoprecipitation followed by electrophoresis and quantitative autoradiography. Western blot analysis is generally inappropriate for this purpose, since cytoplasmic phosphatase is usually unstable (Boyd et al., 1987b; Calamia and Manoil, 1990; San Millan et al., 1989). Consequently, the steady-state levels of fusion proteins measured by Western blot analysis often represent the active fractions only. Of course if only the active fraction is considered, all fusions, whether cytoplasmic (and fractionally exported) or extracytoplasmic (and fully exported), would be calculated to have the same specific activity as deduced from Western blot analysis, and no information would be gained. This point has not been universally appreciated.

A hypothetical case of a membrane protein with a single membrane-spanning stretch can serve as an example. A fusion preceding the membrane-spanning stretch

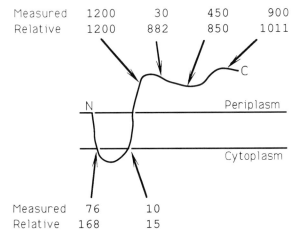

Fig. 6.3. The topology of the *E. coli* leader peptidase. As in Figure 6.2, the *arrows* point to the positions of the fusion joints in the topological model of the protein. The activity was measured in a strain expressing the fusion gene on a low copy plasmid. Relative activity gives the measured activity normalized to expression level as measured by pulse labeling, immunoprecipitation, and SDS-PAGE. (Data are from San Millan et al., 1989.)

would be expected to have very low activity as it would have no export signal. A fusion following the first membrane-spanning stretch would be expected to have higher activity either because it is efficiently exported as are fusions to external domains or because it would be inefficiently, but detectably, exported as are most fusions to cytoplasmic domains. In both cases the second fusion would be expected to have higher activity than the first. Discrimination between the two possible topologies, in this case, would depend on determination of the relative activity (activity normalized to the rate of synthesis) and comparison to alkaline phosphatase or another active fusion protein!

How Does the Alkaline Phosphatase Fusion Method Work?

It is now clear from the studies with characterized proteins (Calamia and Manoil, 1990; Chun and Parkinson, 1988; Manoil and Beckwith, 1986; San Millan et. al., 1989; Yun et. al., 1991) that the alkaline phosphatase fusion method does, when applied properly, indicate membrane protein topology correctly. At this point it may be instructive to ask how it does this. The alkaline phosphatase fusion method has been analyzed sufficiently that a few questions can be answered.

Alkaline phosphatese indicates topology because it is inactive in the cytoplasm and becomes active only after it crosses the membrane into the periplasm. A likely reason for this is that its two intrachain disulfide bonds are essential for its activity. When disulfide bond formation was prevented by the change of a cysteine to another residue, the mutant enzymes had little or no activity (DuBose and Hartl, 1990). Further evidence for this comes from a mutant strain deficient in a protein that enhances the rate of disulfide bond formation in the periplasm. In this strain, nascent exported phosphatase remains in a protease-sensitive (presumably unfolded and inactive) state (Bardwell et al., 1991). Under these conditions the majority of it is broken down in vivo. Recently it has been shown that the disulfide bonds of alkaline phosphatase do not form if it is retained in the cytoplasm but do form immediately when the nascent protein enters the periplasm (Derman and Beckwith, 1991). It has been suggested that the dependence on disulfide bond formation for activation may prevent inappropriate, and possibly deleterious, activation of unexported alkaline phosphatase in the cytoplasm (Derman and Beckwith, 1991).

A recently published study of the kinetics of export of fusion alkaline phosphatases examines another aspect of the mechanism by which alkaline phosphatase indicates topology. The results suggest that the rate of export of the phosphatase moiety may be correlated with the level of activity measured (Traxler et al., 1992). It has been noted above that the level of activity is proportional to the fraction of the amount synthesized that becomes protease resistant. The rate of appearance of the protease-resistant alkaline phosphatase moiety was estimated from pulse chase experiments with MalF fusion proteins. The resistant moiety appeared quickly in the case of the active periplasmic J and N fusions in Figure 6.2. The 10% of the M fusion protein alkaline phosphatase moiety that became protease resistant, however, appeared very slowly. The K and L fusions, which are intermediate in activity, show an intermediate rate of appearance of the protease-resistant form intermediate. The periplasmic Q fusion protein may be preceded by a poor export signal like the atypical one in the

LacY protein described below. There is a charged residue in the hydrophobic stretch preceding the fusion joint. It has lower activity, similar to the L fusion, and its resistant alkaline phosphatase moiety appears slowly like that of the L fusion. Since cytoplasmic fusion proteins are usually unstable, a simple kinetic competition between export and degradation may determine the amount of fusion alkaline phosphatase that is finally exported.

Sandwich Fusions

The fusion proteins thus far discussed are C-terminal deletion fusions in which the C-terminal part of the membrane protein is replaced by the reporter moiety. It may seem somewhat surprising that such a method could work at all, since the structure of the membrane protein is so severely perturbed. Such an approach to structure determination would not work at all with soluble proteins where protein–protein interactions involved in folding and stability would be eliminated by the deletion of the parts of the protein following the fusion joint. However, in exceptional cases where fusions were made between domains, the native-like structure of the N-terminal domains might be obtained. Therefore, the usefulness of C-terminal deletion fusions in the study of membrane protein topology may mean that each transmembrane stretch, together with its flanking hydrophilic regions, functions as an independent domain interacting with the membrane or the insertion machinery during membrane insertion (Boyd et al., 1990; Singer, 1990). In fact, it has been shown that five of the six transmembrane stretches that precede periplasmic domains in the LacY protein are capable of independently exporting alkaline phosphatase when expressed with their flanking hydrophilic domains as truncated fusion proteins (Calamia and Manoil, 1993). The other transmembrane stretch functions poorly as an export signal both in the context of the entire N-terminal part of the LacY protein and when expressed independently. An arginine residue in this transmembrane stretch has been shown to be responsible for this poor capability as an export signal in both contexts.

A fusion method to examine the possibility that C-terminal signals may contribute to the topological determination of N-terminal parts of the protein has been described (Ehrmann et al., 1990). In this sandwich fusion approach the alkaline phosphatase reporter moiety is inserted into the membrane protein so as to interrupt it rather than to truncate it. Thus there are fusion joints at both N and C termini of alkaline phosphatase, as shown in Figure 6.4. Sandwich fusions corresponding to a subset of the MalF fusions of Figure 6.2 have been constructed. Exported domain sandwich fusions are approximately as active as the corresponding deletion fusions when corrected for their slightly lower rate of synthesis. Sandwich fusions corresponding to the anomalous high-activity K and L deletion fusions, which are cytoplasmic in the model, have very low activities, as do other cytoplasmic domain fusions. Thus, the sandwich fusion method gives a more accurate picture of topology in this case. It has not yet been tried in the context of a poor export signal such as that described above for the LacY protein.

Sandwich fusions can be difficult to work with. Those in the MalF protein inhibit cell growth when expressed at high levels. Such effects can be eliminated by use of a

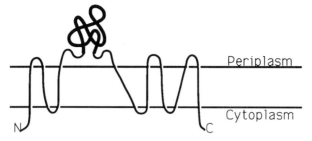

Fig. 6.4. Sandwich fusion. In sandwich fusion, the gene for alkaline phosphatase, lacking its signal sequence, is inserted into the gene for the membrane protein (Ehrmann et al., 1990). The resulting fusion protein consists of the entire sequence of the membrane protein with the mature sequence of alkaline phosphatase, indicated by the *thicker line,* inserted into it.

regulatable promoter and a low copy plasmid vector or insertion into the chromosome (Boyd and Beckwith, 1989; Boyd et al., 1987b). Instability has also been a problem with some sandwich fusions.

β-Lactamase Fusions

Another reporter protein that has been extensively used is the TEM β-lactamase (Broome-Smith and Spratt, 1986; Broome-Smith et al., 1990). Unlike alkaline phosphatase, β-lactamase folds into an active form both when retained in the cytoplasm and when exported. It confers high-level resistance to β-lactam antibiotics, however, only when it is exported. Thus a set of β-lactamase fusion proteins indicates membrane protein topology similarly to a set of alkaline phosphatase fusions. External domains are identified as having fusions that form colonies on plates containing a β-lactam antibiotic, ampicillin. Methods for random generation of fusions, including a transposon, have been described (Broome-Smith et al., 1990). Several studies of bacterial membrane proteins (Bowler and Spratt, 1989; Edelman et al., 1987; Wang et al., 1991) and one of a eukaryotic membrane protein expressed in *E. coli* have been reported (Zhang and Broome-Smith, 1990).

This system appears in many ways to be very similar to the alkaline phosphatase method discussed above. However, no direct comparison of the two methods has been reported yet. The principal difference is that the phenotype that indicates localization is scorable only by lethal selection. Fully exported fusions are identified as having a high minimal inhibitory concentration of antibiotic when plated at low cell density. In frame, cytoplasmic fusions can be identified by plating at high cell density. Under these conditions, lysis of a fraction of the cell population liberates enough of the cytoplasmic β-lactamase to permit growth of surviving cells. Out of frame fusions, since they have lower levels of cytoplasmic enzyme, are even less resistant. This may provide better discrimination between in frame and out of frame fusions than the alkaline phosphatase method, as has been claimed (Broome-Smith and Spratt, 1986; Broome-Smith et al., 1990), but it is not clear why this should be true. As with alkaline phosphatase fusions, out of frame fusions have been isolated, some cytoplasmic fusions have anomalous, high resistance, and some fusion proteins may be lethal when expressed at high levels (Edelman et al., 1987). Without direct comparison of the two approaches by construction of pairs of fusions to the same protein, it is not clear which approach would minimize these problems.

Since β-lactamase folds into an active form in the cytoplasm and folding, in general, interferes with export, it is possible that the amount of β-lactamase fusion protein exported depends on the relative rates of export and cytoplasmic folding. This suggestion is based on the ideas about kinetic competition between the rates of fusion alkaline phosphatase export and cytoplasmic degradation outlined above. In this case, cytoplasmic folding should prevent further export of fusion β-lactamase.

β-Galactosidase Fusions

Other proteins have also been used as reporter moieties in topology studies. Fusions to β-galactosidase have properties that are in some ways complementary to alkaline phosphatase and β-lactamase fusions. It has long been known that fusion of β-galactosidase to proteins whose export is directed by signal sequences results in fusion proteins with little or no β-galactosidase activity (Silhavy and Beckwith, 1985). Fusions to exported domains of membrane proteins are also inactive while fusions to cytoplasmic domains are active (Froshauer et al., 1988; Georgiou et al., 1988; Manoil, 1990).

Interestingly, the reason for inactivity in the case of fusions to membrane proteins may be different from that responsible for inactivity of secreted proteins. In both cases, folding of β-galactosidase in the cytoplasm may prevent its export (Lee et al., 1989). In the case of fusions to secreted proteins there appears to be an inactive complex formed between the fusion protein and the secretion machinery. The evidence for this is genetic (Schatz and Beckwith, 1990). It suggests that both the function of the secretion apparatus and the folding of β-galactosidase into its active state are blocked in the inactive complex.

Host mutants selected for increased β-galactosidase activity of a membrane protein fusion on the other hand are found in a gene that codes for a protein that is responsible for formation of disulfide bonds in the *E. coli* periplasm (Bardwell et al., 1991). A reasonable hypothesis for the inactivity of the fusions in the wild-type background

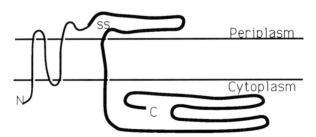

Fig. 6.5. Hypothetical structure of the MalF-β-galactosidase 102 fusion protein. The *thicker line* represents the inactive β-galactosidase moiety. *SS* represents a putative disulfide bond formed in the periplasm of a wild-type strain between cysteine residues present in the early part of the β-galactosidase moiety. (From Bardwell et al., 1991.)

is therefore that export of the N terminus of the fusion β-galactosidase by the membrane protein export signal is followed by oxidation of cysteine residues present in that part of the protein. This is illustrated in Figure 6.5. This would prevent folding of an active cytoplasmic β-galactosidase moiety. With the rate of disulfide bond formation greatly diminished in the mutant strain, it has been suggested, the active fusion protein could fold in the cytoplasm. The striking difference in these two similar phenomena may point to a fundamental difference between the mechanism of protein secretion and membrane protein insertion in bacteria.

Many methods for construction of β-galactosidase fusions exist (Krebs and Reznikoff, 1988; Silhavy and Beckwith, 1985). Noteworthy are in vivo methods for converting alkaline phosphatase fusions to β-galactosidase fusions (Manoil, 1990; Wilmes-Riesenberg and Wanner, 1992).

Eukaryotic Membrane Proteins Expressed in Prokaryotes

The methods discussed above depend on prokaryotic systems and have been applied mainly to prokaryotic membrane proteins. As mentioned above, the apparent similarity between eukaryotic and prokaryotic membrane protein sequences suggests that the same principles govern determination of topology in both cases (von Heijne, 1986; von Heijne and Gavel, 1988). Eukaryotic proteins that can be functionally expressed in bacteria (Marullo et al., 1988; Sarkar et al., 1988) can be studied using gene fusions in the prokaryotic system. A study of the β-subunit of sheep-kidney Na$^+$,K$^+$-ATPase has been reported (Zhang and Broome-Smith, 1990). Information about the topology of a eukaryotic protein in bacteria is most reliable if it can be shown that the protein is expressed in a functional state and that most of it, not just a small fraction, is in that state. However, this approach carries the caveat that the rules for determination of topology in prokaryotes and eukaryotes may not really be identical (Boyd and Beckwith, 1990; Hartmann et al., 1989).

Gene Fusions in Eukaryotic Systems

In eukaryotes glycosylation often permits the identification of exported domains of membrane proteins. Since the enzymes involved in N-linked glycosylation are located in the lumen of the endoplasmic reticulum (Hirschberg and Snider, 1987), only exported domains can be glycosylated. However, not all exported domains have glycosylation sites, and not all potential sites are glycosylated. It is often easy to correlate topology and glycosylation patterns for simple proteins like glycophorin (Tomita et al., 1978) or VSV G protein (Rothman and Lodish, 1977), but with complex proteins the study of natural glycosylation sites provides only a small piece of the information necessary to determine a topology. Band 3 protien (Kopito et al., 1985) and the human glucose transporter (Mueckler et al., 1986) provide examples of complex proteins wherein a single glycosylated domain provides information about orientation. However, this single piece of information cannot be used to deduce a detailed topology.

Glycosylation sites have been utilized in topology studies by inserting glycosylation sites into membrane proteins (Chavez and Hall, 1991), by making fusions to a gly-cosylatable reporter protein, acid phosphatase (Ahmad and Bussey, 1988; Silve et al., 1991), and by inserting a glycosylation site into a C-terminal reporter gene (Eble et al., 1987). Both in vivo and in vitro techniques for studying glycosylated proteins are available (Wessels et al., 1991). Highly glycosylated proteins have greatly reduced electrophoretic mobility. Glycosylation can be demonstrated by blocking it in vivo with the antibiotic globomycin or in vitro by removal of N-linked glycosyl residues by hydrolysis with endo-β-N-acetylglucosaminidase H (endo H). The results can then be analyzed by electrophoresis and immunological identification of the protein.

In yeast, histidinol dehydrogenase has been used as a reporter molecule in a topology study of the 3-hydroxy-3-methylglutaryl-coenzyme A reductases (Sengstag et al., 1990). Yeast strains unable to synthesize histidine, expressing histidinol dehydrogenase in the cytoplasm and carrying a mutation that allows efficient uptake of histidinol, can grow on media containing histidinol. When the histidinol dehydrogenase is exported out of the cytoplasm either by an N-terminal signal sequence (Deshaies and Schekman, 1987) or by an export signal in a membrane protein (Sengstag et al., 1990), histidinol cannot be used to satisfy the histidine requirement and there is no growth on histidinol media. The exported reporter moiety is glycosylated in the endoplasmic reticulum, and this may prevent it from becoming active, but it is not definitively known why the cells cannot utilize histidinol.

Also, in yeast, the topology of arginine permease has been studied by measuring the translocation of a fused galactokinase moiety across the membrane of the endoplasmic reticulum in vitro (Green et al., 1989).

Conclusions

It is now clear that gene fusion methods, when properly applied, can yield valuable information about membrane protein topology. The methods have in common that neutral reporter moieties will respond to signals within membrane proteins to be localized to either side of the membrane. Since the topologies determined by these methods are generally accurate, it is likely that the same signals determine the topology of the membrane proteins themselves. Since large portions of the membrane protein can be deleted and topology is still indicated correctly, it can be concluded that each signal acts locally and independently of the others. Studies using a variety of approaches (von Heijne, 1986, 1989; von Heijne and Gavel, 1988), including the use of gene fusions (Boyd and Beckwith, 1989), indicate that a signal is comprised of a hydrophobic stretch together with its flanking hydrophilic regions. Basic residues within short hydrophilic regions are determinants of cytoplasmic localization and can determine the orientation of transmembrane stretches. Other classes of cytoplasmic localization signals may exist. Since folding interferes with export, a small, and therefore quickly synthesized, rapidly folding domain should act similarly to orient transmembrane stretches.

A study of alkaline phosphatase fusions has revealed a direct correlation between the rate of fusion alkaline phosphatase export and the total amount that is exported (Traxler et al., 1992). If this is generally the case, then the signals that reporter moieties respond to may function primarily by determining the rate of reporter moiety export. This suggests that, in native membrane proteins, the signals, that determine topology may function by modulating the local rate of export of the polypeptide chain (Boyd et al., 1990). Such a mechanism would of course be sufficient to determine a membrane protein's topology. In this view the topology of membrane proteins may be determined by the local kinetics of the insertion process rather than the overall thermodynamics.

Acknowledgments

I am grateful to Colin Manoil, Giovanna Ferro-Luzzi Ames, and Barry Wanner for providing information prior to publication. I thank Alan Derman and Jon Beckwith for criticism of this manuscript and the National Science Foundation for support.

References

Ahmad, M., and Bussey, H. (1988) Topology of membrane insertion in vitro and plasma membrane assembly in vivo of the yeast arginine permease. *Mol. Microbiol.* 2: 627–635.

Akiyama, Y., and Ito, K. (1987) Topology analysis of the SecY protein, an integral membrane protein involved in protein export in *Escherichia coli. EMBO J.* 6: 3465–3470.

Bardwell, J.C.A., McGovern, K., and Beckwith, J. (1991) Identification of a protein required for disulfide bond formation in vivo. *Cell* 67: 581–589.

Bjrbaek, C., Föersom, V., and Michelsen, O. (1990) The transmembrane topology of the a [corrected] subunit from the ATPase in *Escherichia coli* analyzed by PhoA protein fusions. *FEBS Lett.* 260: 31–34.

Blobel, G. (1980) Intracellular protein topogenesis. *Proc. Natl. Acad. Sci. USA* 77: 1496–1500.

Bowler, L. D., and Spratt, B. G. (1989) Membrane topology of penicillin-binding protein 3 of *Escherichia coli. Mol. Microbiol.* 3: 1277–1286.

Boyd, D., and Beckwith, J. (1989) Positively charged amino acid residues can act as topogenic determinants in membrane proteins. *Proc. Natl. Acad. Sci. USA* 86: 9446–9450.

Boyd, D., and Beckwith, J. (1990) The role of charged amino acids in the localization of secreted and membrane proteins. *Cell* 62: 1031–1033.

Boyd, D., Guan, C.-D., Willard, S., Wright, W., Strauch, K., and Beckwith, J. (1987a) Enzymatic activity of alkaline phosphatase precursor depends on its cellular location. In: *Phosphate Metabolism and Cellular Regulation in Microorganisms*, edited by A. Torriani-Gorini et al. Washington, D. C: American Society for Microbiology, p. 89–93.

Boyd, D., Manoil, C., and Beckwith, J. (1987b) Determinants of membrane protein topology. *Proc. Natl. Acad. Sci. USA* 84: 8525–8529.

Boyd, D., Manoil, C., Froshauer, S., San Millan, J.-L. Green, N., McGovern, K., Lee, C., Beckwith, J. (1990) Use of gene fusions to study membrane protein topology. In: *Protein Folding: Deciphering the Second Half of The Genetic Code*, edited by L. M. Gierasch and J. King. Washington, D.C.: American Association for the Advancement of Science, p. 314–322.

Boyd, D., Traxler, B., and Beckwith, J. (1993) Analysis of the topology of a membrane protein by using the minimum number of alkaline phosphatase fusions. *J. Bacteriol.* 175: 553–556.

Broome-Smith, J. K., and Spratt, B. G. (1986) A vector for the constructton of translational fusions to TEM beta-lactamase and the analysis of protein export signals and membrane protein topology. *Gene* 49: 341–349.

Broome-Smith, J. K., Tadayyon, M., and Y. Zhang (1990) Beta-lactamase as a probe of membrane protein assembly and protein export. *Mol. Microbiol.* 4: 1637–1644.

Calamia, J., and Manoil, C. (1990) *lac* Permease of *Escherichia coli*: topology and sequence elements promoting membrane insertion. *Proc. Natl. Acad. Sci. USA* 87: 4937–4941.

Calamia, J., and Manoil, C. (1993) Membrane protein insertion: function of individual spanning segments as export signals. *Science* (in press).

Carson, M. J., Barondess, J., and Beckwith, J. (1991) The FtsQ protein of *Escherichia coli:* membrane topology, abundance, and cell division phenotypes due to overproduction and insertion mutations. *J. Bacteriol.* 173: 2187–2195.

Cartwright, C. P., and Tipper, D. J. (1991) In vivo topological analysis of Ste2, a yeast plasma membrane protein, by using beta-lactamase gene fusions. *Mol. Cell. Biol.* 11: 2620–2628.

Chavez, R. A., and Hall, Z. A. (1991) The transmembrane topology of the amino terminus of the alpha subunit of the nicotinic acetylcholine receptor. *J. Biol. Chem.* 266: 15532–15538.

Chepuri, V., and Gennis, R. B. (1990) The use of gene fusions to determine the topology of all of the subunits of the cytochrome *o* terminal oxidase complex of *Escherichia coli. J. Biol. Chem.* 265: 12978–12986.

Chun, S. Y., and Parkinson, J. S. (1988) Bacterial motility: membrane topology of the *Escherichia coli* MotB protein. *Science* 239: 276–278.

Degli Esposti, M., Crimi, M., and Venturoli, G. (1990) A critical evaluation of the hydropathy profile of membrane proteins. *Eur. J. Biochem.* 190: 207–219.

de Herrero, M.L.V., and Neilands, J. B. (1988) Nucleotide sequence of the *iucD* gene of the pColV-K30 aerobactin operon and topology of its product studied with *phoA* and *lacZ* gene fusions. *J. Bacteriol.* 170: 56–64.

Derman, A., and Beckwith, J. (1991) *Escherichia coli* alkaline phosphatase fails to acquire disulfide bonds when retained in the cytoplasm. *J. Bacteriol* 173: 7719–7722.

Deshaies, R. J., and Schekman, R. (1987) A yeast mutant defective at an early stage in import of secretory protein precursors into the endoplasmic reticulum. *J. Cell. Biol.* 105: 633–645.

DuBose, R. F., and Hartl, D. L. (1990) The molecular evolution of bacterial alkaline phosphatase: correlating variation among enteric bacteria to experimental manipulations of the protein. *Mol. Biol. Evol.* 7: 547–577.

Eble, B. E., MacRae, D. R., Lingappa, V. R., and Ganem, D. (1987) Multiple topogenic sequences determine the transmembrane orientation of the hepatitis B surface antigen. *Mol. Cell. Biol.* 7: 3591–3601.

Edelman, A., Bowler, L., Jk, B.-S. and Spratt, B. G. (1987) Use of a beta-lactamase fusion vector to investigate the organization of penicillin-biding protein 1B in the cytoplasmic membrane of *Escherichia coli. Mol. Microbiol.* 1: 101–106.

Ehrmann, M., Boyd, D., and Beckwith, J. (1990) Genetic analysis of membrane protein topology by a sandwich gene fusion approach. *Proc. Natl. Acad. Sci. USA* 87: 7574–7578.

Fasman, G. D., and Gilbert, W. A. (1990) The prediction of transmembrane protein sequences and their conformation: an evaluation. *TIBS* 15: 89–92.

Forst, S., Comeau, D., Norioka, S., and Inouye, M. (1987) Localization and membrane topology of EnvZ, a protein involved in osmoregulation of OmpF and OmpC in *Escherichia coli. J. Biol. Chem.* 262: 16433–16438.

Froshauer, S., and Beckwith, J. (1984) The nucleotide sequence of the gene for MalF protein, an inner membrane component of the maltose transport system of *Escherichia coli. J. Biol. Chem.* 259: 10896–10934.

Froshauer, S., Green, G. N., Boyd, D., McGovern K., and Beckwith, J. (1988) Genetic analysis of the membrane insertion and topology of MalF, a cytoplasmic membrane protein of *Escherichia coli. J. Mol. Biol.* 20: 501–511.

Gardel, C., Johnson, K., Jacq, A., and Beckwith, J. (1990) The secD locus of *E. coli* codes for two membrane proteins required for protein export. *EMBO J.* 9: 3209–3216.

Gebert, J. F., Overhoff, B., Manson, M. D., and Boos, W. (1988) The Tsr chemosensory transducer of *Escherichia coli* assembles into the cytoplasmic membrane via a SecA-dependent process. *J. Biol. Chem.* 263: 16652–16660.

Geli, V., Baty, D., Pattus, F., and Lazdunski, C. (1989) Topology and function of the integral membrane protein conferring immunity to colicin A. *Mol. Microbiol.* 3: 679–687.

Georgiou, C. D., Dueweke, T. J., and Gennis, R. B. (1988) Beta-galactosidase gene fusions as probes for the cytoplasmic regions of subunits I and II of the membrane-bound cytochrome d terminal oxidase from *Escherichia coli. J. Biol. Chem.* 263: 13130–13137.

Gött, P., and Boos, W. (1988) The transmembrane topology of the sn-glycerol-3-phosphate permease of *Escherichia coli* analysed by phoA and lacZ protein fusions. *Mol. Microbiol.* 2: 655–663.

Green, G. N., Hansen, W., and Walter, P. (1989) The use of gene-fusions to determine membrane protein topology in Saccharomyces cerevisiae. *J. Cell Sci.* Suppl. 11: 109–113.

Use of Gene Fusions to Determine Membrane Protein Topology   **161**

Gutierrez, C., and Devedjian, J. C. (1989) A plasmid facilitating in vitro construction of *phoA* gene fusions in *Escherichia coli*. *Nucleic Acids Res.* 17: 3999.

Hannavy, K., Barr, G. C., Dorman, C. J., Adamson, J., Mazengera, L. R., Gallagher, M. P., Evans, J. S., Levine, B. A., Trayer, I. P., and Higgins, C. F. (1990) TonB protein in *Salmonella typhimurium*. A model for signal transduction between membranes. *J. Mol. Biol.* 216: 897–910.

Hartmann, E., Rapoport, T. A., and Lodish, H. F. (1989) Predicting the orientation of eukaryotic membrane-spanning proteins. *Proc. Natl. Acad. Sci. USA* 86: 5786–5790.

Hirschberg, C. B., and Snider, M. (1987) Topography of glycosylation in the rough endoplasmic reticulum and golgi apparatus. *Annu. Rev. Biochem.* 56: 63–87.

Hoffman, C. S., and Wright, A. (1985) Fusions of secreted proteins to alkaline phosphatase: an approach for studying protein secretion. *Proc. Natl. Acad. Sci. USA* 82: 5107–5111.

Horabin, J. I., and Webster, R. E. (1988) An amino acid sequence which directs membrane insertion causes loss of membrane potential. *J. Biol. Chem.* 263: 11575–11583.

Kerppola, R. E., and Ferro-Luzzi Ames, G. (1992) Topology of the hydrophobic membrane-bound components of the histidine periplasmic permease. Comparison with other members of the family. *J. Biol. Chem.* 267: 2329–2336.

Kopito, R. R., and Lodish, H. F. (1985) Primary structure and transmembrane orientation of the murine anion exchange protein. *Nature* 316: 234–238.

Krebs, M., and Reznikoff, W. S. (1988) Use of a Tn5 derivative that creates lacZ translation fusions to obtain a transposition mutant. Gene 63: 277–285.

Lee, C., Li, P., Inouye, H., and Beckwith, J. (1989) Genetic studies on the inability of beta-galactosidase to be translocated across the *E. coli* cytoplasmic membrane. *J. Bacteriol.* 171: 4609–4616.

Lewis, M. J., Chang, J. A., and Simoni, R. D. (1990) A topological analysis of subunit alpha from *Escherichia coli* F1F0-ATP synthase predicts eight transmembrane segments. *J. Biol. Chem.* 265: 10541–10550.

Lloyd, A. D., and Kadner, R. J. (1990) Topology of the *Escherichia coli* uhpT sugar-phosphate transporter analyzed by using Tn*phoA* fusions. *J. Bacteriol.* 172: 1688–1693.

Manoil, C. (1990) Analysis of protein localizaton by use of gene fusions with complementary properties. *J. Bacteriol.* 172: 1035–1042.

Manoil, C. (1991) Analysis of membrane protein topology using alkaline phosphatase and beta-galactosidase gene fusions. *Methods Cell Biol.* 34: 61–75.

Manoil, C., and Beckwith, J. (1985) TnphoA: a transposon probe for protein export signals. *Proc. Natl. Acad. Sci. USA* 82: 8129–8133.

Manoil, C., and Beckwith, J. (1986) A genetic approach to analyzing membrane protein topology. *Science* 233: 1403–1408.

Manoil, C., Mekalanos, J. J., and Beckwith, J. (1990) Alkaline phosphatase fusions: sensors of subcellular location. *J. Bacteriol.* 172: 515–518.

Martin-Gallardo, A., Deich, R. A., Fien, K. A., Metcalf, B. J., Anilionis, A., and Paradiso, P. R. (1989) Alkaline phosphatase fusions to the respiratory syncytial virus F protein as an approach to analyze its membrane topology. *DNA* 8: 659–667.

Marullo, S., Delavier, K. C., Eshdat, Y., Strosberg, A. D., and Emorine, L. (1988) Human beta 2-adrenergic receptors expressed in *Escherichia coli* membranes retain their pharmacological properties. *Proc. Natl. Acad. Sci. USA* 85: 7551–7555.

McGovern, K., Ehrmann, M., and Beckwith, J. (1991) Decoding signals for membrane protein assembly using alkaline phosphatase fusions. *EMBO J.* 10: 2773–2782.

Melchers, L. S., Regensburg, T. T., Bourret, R. B., Sedee, N. J., Schilperoort, R. A., and Hooykaas, P. J. (1989) Membrane topology and functional analysis of the sensory protein VirA of *Agrobacterium tumefaciens*. *EMBO J.* 8: 1919–1925.

Michaelis, S., Hunt, J., and Beckwith, J. (1986) Effects of signal sequence mutations on the kinetics of alkaline phosphatase export to the periplasm in *Escherichia coli*. *J. Bacteriol.* 167: 160–167.

Miller, C. (1991) 1990: annus mirabilis of potassium channels. *Science* 252: 1092–1096.

Miller, V. L., Taylor, R. K., and Mekalanos, J. J. (1987) Cholera toxin transcriptional activator toxR is a transmembrane DNA binding protein. *Cell* 48: 271–279.

Mueckler, M., Caruso, C., Baldwin, S. A., Panico, M., Blench, I., Morris, H.R., Allard, W. J., Lienhard, G. E., and Lodish H. F. (1986) Sequence and structure of a human glucose transporter. *Science* 229: 941–945.

Muñoa, F. J., Miller, K. W., Beers, R., Graham, M., and Wu, H. C. (1991) Membrane topology of

Escherichia coli prolipoprotein signal peptidase (signal peptidase II). *J. Biol. Chem.* 266: 17667–17672.

Nilsson, I., and von Heijne, G. (1990) Fine-tuning the topology of a polytopic membrane protein: role of positively and negatively charged amino acids. *Cell* 62: 1135–1141.

Roof, S. K., Allard, J. D., Bertrand, K. P., and Postle, K. (1991) Analysis of *Escherichia coli* TonB membrane topology by use of PhoA fusions. *J. Bacteriol.* 173: 5554–5557.

Rothman, J. E., and Lodish, H. F. (1977) Synchronized transmembrane insertion and glycosylation of a nascent membrane protein. *Nature* 269: 775–780.

San Millan, J. L., Boyd, D., Dalbey, R., Wickner, W., and Beckwith, J. (1989) Use of phoA fusions to study the topology of the *Escherichia coli* inner membrane protein leader peptidase. *J. Bacteriol.* 171: 5536–5541.

Sarkar, H. K., Thorens, B., Lodish, H. F., and Kaback, H. R. (1988) Expression of the human erythrocyte glucose transporter in *Escherichia coli. Proc. Natl. Acad. Sci. USA* 85: 5463–5467.

Schatz, P. J., and Beckwith, J. (1990) Genetic analysis of protein export in *Escherichia coli. Annu. Rev. Genet.* 24: 215–248.

Schatz, P. J., Riggs, P. D., Jacq, A., Fath, M. J., and Beckwith, J. (1989) The secE gene encodes an integral membrane protein required for protein export in *E. coli. Genes Dev.* 3: 1035–1044.

Sengstag, C., Stirling, C., Schekman, R., and Rine, J. (1990) Genetic and biochemical evaluation of eucaryotic membrane protein topology: multiple transmembrane domains of *Saccharomyces cerevisiae* 3-hydroxy-3-methylglutaryl coenzyme A reductase. *Mol. Cell. Biol.* 10: 672–680.

Silhavy, T. J., and Beckwith, J. (1985) Use of lac fusions for the study of biological problems. *Microbiol. Rev.* 49: 398–418.

Silve, S., Volland, C., Garnier, C., Jund, R., Chevallier, M. R., and Haguenauer, T. R. (1991) Membrane insertion of uracil permease, a polytopic yeast plasma membrane protein. *Mol. Cell. Biol.* 11: 1114–1124.

Singer, S. J. (1990) The structure and insertion of integral proteins in membranes. *Annu. Rev. Cell Biol.* 6: 247–296.

Song, H. Y., and Cramer, W. A. (1991) Membrane topography of ColE1 gene products: the immunity protein. *J. Bacteriol.* 173: 2935–2943.

Sugiyama, J. E., Mahmoodian, S., and Jacobson, G. (1991) Membrane topology analysis of *Escherichia coli* mannitol permease by using a nested-deletion method to create mtlA–phoA fusions. *Proc. Natl. Acad. Sci. USA* 88: 9603–9607.

Tomita, M., Furthmayr, H., and Marchesi, V. T. (1978) Primary structure of human erythrocyte glycophorin A. Isolation and characterization of peptides and complete amino acid sequence. *Biochemistry* 17: 4756–4770.

Traxler, B., Lee, C., Boyd, D., and Beckwith, J. (1992) The dynamics of assembly of a cytoplasmic membrane protein in *Escherichia coli. J. Biol. Chem.* 267: 5339–5345.

von Heijne, G. (1986) The distribution of positively charged residues in bacterial inner membrane proteins correlates with the trans-membrane topology. *EMBO J.* 5: 3021–3027.

von Heijne, G. (1989) Control of topology and mode of assembly of a polytopic membrane protein by positively charged residues. *Nature* 341: 456–458.

von Heijne, G., and Gavel, Y. (1988) Topogenic signals in integral membrane proteins. *Eur. J. Biochem.* 174: 671–678.

von Heijne, G., and Manoil, C. (1990) Membrane proteins: from sequence to structure. *Protein Eng.* 4: 109–112.

von Wachenfeldt, C., and Hederstedt, L. (1990) *Bacillus subtilis* 13-kilodalton cytochrome *c*-550 encoded by cccA consists of a membrane-anchor and a heme domain. *J. Biol. Chem.* 265: 13939–13948.

Wang, R., Seror, S. J., Blight, M., Pratt, J. M., Broome-Smith, J. K., and Holland, I. B. (1991) Analysis of the membrane organization of an *Escherichia coli* protein translocator, HlyB, a member of a large family of prokaryote and eukaryote surface transport proteins. *J. Mol. Biol.* 217: 441–454.

Weber, R. F., and Silverman, P. M. (1988) The cpx proteins of *Escherichia coli* K12. Structure of the cpxA polypeptide as an inner membrane component. *J. Mol. Biol.* 203: 467–478.

Wessels, H. P., Beltzer, J. P., and Spiess, M. (1991) Analysis of protein topology in the endoplasmic reticulum. *Methods Cell Biol.* 34: 287–302.

Wilmes-Riesenberg, M. R., and Wanner, B. L. (1992) TnphoA and TnphoA prime elements for making and switching fusions to study transcription, translation and cell surface localization. *J. Bacteriol.* 174: 4558–4575.

Winans, S. C., Kerstetter, R. A., Ward, J. E., and Nester, E. W. (1989) A protein required for transcriptional regulation of *Agrobacterium virulence* genes spans the cytoplasmic membrane. *J. Bacteriol.* 171: 1616–1622.

Yun, C. H., Van, D. S., Crofts, A. R., and Gennis, R. B. (1991) The use of gene fusions to examine the membrane topology of the L-subunit of the photosynthetic reaction center and of the cytochrome b subunit of the bc1 complex from *Rhodobacter sphaeroides. J. Biol. Chem.* 266: 10967–10973.

Zhang, Y. B., and Broome-Smith, J. K. (1990) Correct insertion of a simple eukaryotic plasma-membrane protein into the cytoplasmic membrane of *Escherichia coli. Gene* 96: 51–57.

Zozulia, S. A., Obukhova, T. A., Shirokova, E. P., and Babalov, P. R. (1990) Plasmid expression vectors with elements of the *E. coli* alkaline phosphatase gene [Rus]. *Bioorg. Khim.* 16: 1339–1347.

7

Structure of F_0F_1ATPases Determined by Direct and Indirect Methods

L. MARIO AMZEL, MARIO A. BIANCHET, and PETER L. PEDERSEN

ATP synthesis—the phosphorylation of ADP by inorganic phosphate (P_i) in mitochondria, chloroplast, and bacteria—is a very important and complex biochemical pathway. The reaction involves the utilization of the proton electrochemical gradient, produced by either the oxidation of substrates or the utilization of light quanta, for the generation of ATP levels up to 10^8 times the concentration expected from the hydrolytic equilibrium $(ATP + H_2O = ADP + P_i)$. The reaction in which the dissipation of the H^+ gradient is coupled to the phosphorylation of ADP is carried out by a large, complex enzyme system: the ATP synthase. The membranes of bacteria, chloroplasts, and mitochondria contain ATP synthases that utilize H^+ gradients generated across their membranes for the formation of as much as 98% of the ATP required by living organisms. All the ATP synthases are composed of two main sectors: the integral membrane portion F_0 and the membrane associated portion F_1 (see reviews by Futai and Kanazawa, 1983; Futai et al., 1989; Senior, 1990; Kagawa, 1984). Both F_0 and F_1 are multisubunit proteins. (At least thirteen subunits have been identified in mammalian ATP synthases (Hatefi, 1985; Godinot & Di Pietro, 1986; Walker et al., 1987), while only eight subunits exist in bacteria (Filligame, 1981; Schneider and Altendorf, 1987). It has been demonstrated that F_0 forms a transmembrane H^+ channel that directs H^+ ions to the F_1 sector where their translocation is coupled to the synthesis of ATP. The F_1 sector contains all the catalytic and noncatalytic nucleotide-binding sites. ATP synthases have been the subject of extensive structural studies that utilized direct and indirect methods aimed at providing three-dimensional structural information about the enzyme. The most relevant and recent studies will be discussed in this chapter; no attempt is made to make this a comprehensive review of all the ATP synthase literature.

Structure of the F_0 Sector

The F_0 sector of the ATP synthase is an integral membrane multisubunit protein. The number of different subunits in the complex depends on the organism and varies from three different subunits in *Escherichia coli* to eight or more different subunits in bovine heart mitochondria (Walker et al., 1985). The sequences of all three sub-units have been determined in *E. coli* (Walker et al., 1984) as well as in several other bacteria. The three F$_0$ subunits of *E. coli*—**a**, **b**, and **c**—have 271, 156, and 79 amino acids, respectively. There is one copy of a, two copies of b, and ten or more (Filligame, 1981) copies of c in one complex. No direct three-dimensional structural information is available for any of these subunits, but they were the subject of extensive modeling studies (structure predictions).

Although secondary structure predictions are in general unreliable, they are used in conjunction with hydropathy plots (Kyte and Doolittle, 1982) to model the trans-membrane portion of membrane proteins. Possible models are based on the presence of stretches of about twenty-five hydrophobic amino acids in the sequences that would fold into 40 Å long membrane-spanning α-helices. From the hydropathy curves presented in Figures 7.1*a*, 7.2*a* and 7.3*a*, it is possible to postulate the models for the three *E. coli* F$_0$ subunits shown in Figures 7.1*b*, 7.2*b*, and 7.3*b*.

The a subunit (also called protein 6) probably contains six to eight transmembrane segments and small external domains connecting these segments. Recently, Lewis et al. (1990) reported a very elegant study of the topology of the *E. coli* a subunit using gene fusion with alkaline phosphatase. After engineering fusion proteins linking dif-ferent N-terminal fragments of the a subunit with alkaline phosphatase the bacteria are tested for periplasmic alkaline phosphatase activity. The presence of the activity is taken as an indication that the place of the insertion corresponds to a periplasmic portion of the intact **a** subunit. Surprisingly, these experiments suggest that the **a** subunit contains eight transmembrane spans, several of them shorter than what is necessary to span the membrane as an α-helix. These segments probably traverse the membrane in extended, nonhelical conformations and are thought to contain residues that are important for the function of the subunit. Both the N and the Carboxy ter-mini were found to be in the periplasmic space, and a large globular domain was identified in the cytoplasmic side of the membrane.

The **b** subunit shows an extremely strong helical prediction in a region where the sequence is very hydrophilic, suggesting that this subunit has long extramembrane helices. The two termini (amino acids 1 to 25 and 127 to 156) are mostly hydrophobic (see Fig. 7.2*a*), leading to the suggestion that the subunit has one (the N end) or both termini inserted into the membranes and two long, antiparallel helices (residues 25 to 80 and 85 to 120 or 140) protruding out of the membrane with a turn at residues 80 to 85. (There is some suggestion that the terminal portions that are inserted in the membrane are also helical.) This overall architecture is in agreement with other experimental evidence that suggests that the b subunit may work as a column or shaft that inserts in both the membrane and the F$_1$ sector and provides one of the main attachments for the F$_1$ sector.

The **c** subunit has been sequenced from a very large number of sources (Hoppe and Sebald, 1984). In all cases the protein has about 75 amino acids (79 in *E. coli*) with the same hydropathy distribution (see Fig. 7.3*a*): residues 1 to 7 are amphi-pathic, residues 8 to 36 are hydrophobic, residues 37 to 47 are amphipathic, and res-idues 48 to the end are hydrophobic. This leads to the suggestion that the peptide forms two transmembrane helices (residues 8 to 36 and 48 to the end) with an exposed loop between residues 37 and 47 (see Fig. 7.3*b*). Asp[61] (in *E. coli*) has been identified (Walker et al., 1985) as the residue that when it is labeled by N,N′-dicy-

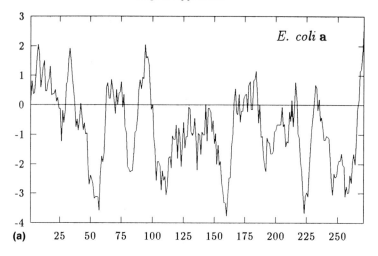

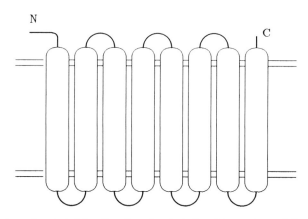

Fig. 7.1. *a*: Hydropathy plot of the *E. coli* a subunit. *b*: Possible topology of *E. coli* a subunit. The first five transmembrane segments are probably α-helical while the last three—if present—are probably more extended.

lohexylcarbodiimide (DCCD) inhibits the translocation of protons through the F_0 sector (Sebald et al., Wachter, 1980). This and other evidence suggests that the 10 to 12 copies of the **c** subunit form the transmembrane channel for the translocation of protons. Despite early reports to the contrary (Schindler and Nelson, 1982), it appears that the **a** subunit is also necessary for proton translocation activity. Mutations in the **a** subunit of *E. coli* strongly affect proton translocation as well as attachment of F_1 to the membrane (Eya et al., 1988; Cain and Simoni, 1989).

Structure of the F_1 Sector

Sequence and Modeling

The F_1 sector of the ATP synthase—the soluble portion of the enzyme—is an oligomeric protein of five different subunits (α, β, γ, δ, and ϵ) with a stoichiometry of

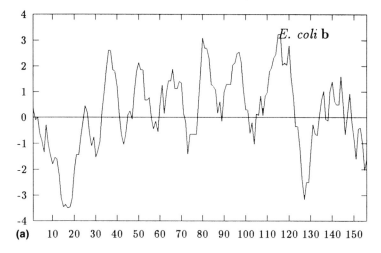

(a)

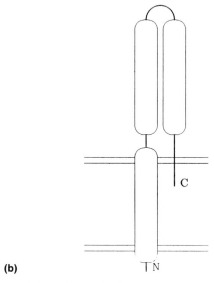

(b)

Fig. 7.2. *a*: Hydropathy plot the *E. coli* b subunit. *b*: Possible topology of the *E. coli* b subunit. Some of the proposed models do not have the C terminus in the membrane.

$\alpha_3\beta_3\gamma\delta\epsilon$. A sixth subunit, called δ', is present in the mitochondria of dycotiledonean plants (see Table 7.1). A very comprehensive review from our laboratory summarizes the most important findings (Ysern et al., 1988). The amino acid sequences of the subunits of F_1 are now known in many species—a result of the efforts of several laboratories. The total number of residues in each subunit, depending on the species, is α, 509–513; β, 459–480; γ, 272–286; δ, 177–190; and ϵ, 132–146 (molecular weights are presented in Table 7.1).

Sequence comparisons between different species have shown that the α- and β-subunits are well conserved in all species, while the minor subunits show a lesser degree of homology. The fraction of identical residues between different species

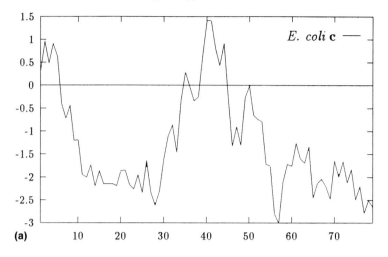

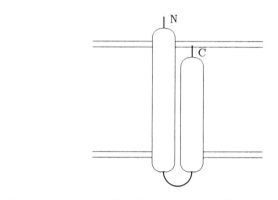

Fig. 7.3. *a*: Hydropathy plot the *E. coli* c subunit. *b*: Possible topology of *E. coli* c subunit.

found for the α-subunit is greater than 60%; for the β-subunit the homology is even higher (Walker et al., 1990). Alignment of the α- with β-subunit shows sequence similarities throughout the polypeptide chains, suggesting that the two major sub-units are evolutionarily related and share the same polypeptide fold. In addition, local homologies with proteins of different activities have been found for several regions of the α- and the β-subunits. For β, the first homology region A (Walker et al., 1982), known as the "glycine-rich loop" (Fry et al., 1986) of sequence GXXXXGK($-$)(T/S), where X is any residue, is centered around amino acid 175 (spinach sequence numbering) and the second homology region B—sequence (R/K)X($-$)XGXXXLZZZ(X)$_{0-2}$D, where Z is a nonpolar residue—around amino acid 264. Among the proteins with homologies in these two regions there are several with known three-dimensional structure; of those, adenylate kinase (AK) has been used extensively to model the nucleotide-binding site of the β-subunit (Duncan et al., 1986; Taylor and Green, 1989). Although it is very likely that both β and α have a nucleotide-binding (or catalytic) site that contains the "glycine-rich loop" the more

Table 7.1. Subunit Molecular Mass (kDa) of F_1 ATPase Subunits from Several Sources

Source	Subunit						References
	α	β	γ	δ	δ'	ϵ	
Mammalian Mitochondrial							
Bovine	53	50	33	17		7.5	Walker et al. (1984)
Rat	55	50	33	15.1		5.7	Lee et al. (1990; Garboczi et al. (1988)
Bacterial							
E. coli	57.2	52.5	31.5	20.5		14.5	Spitsberg et al. (1985)
Thermophilic PS3	54.6	51.1	31.7	20.0		14	Kagawa (1984), Yoshida et al. (1975), Ohta et al. (1988)
Plant Mitochondrial F_1							
Sweet potato	52.5	51.5	35.5	27.0	23	12	Iwasaki and Asahi (1983)
Pea	57	55	36.5	26.5	22.5	8	Horak and Packer (1985)
Faba bean	52	51	34	23.8		22.9	βouty et al. (1983)
Maize	58	55	35	22		12	Spitsberg et al. (1985)
Chloroplast CF_1							
Maize	60	56	40	22.5		15.5	Spitsberg et al. (1985)

detailed models proposed for the complete nucleotide-binding domain of β are probably largely inadequate.

In the most detailed study (Duncan et al., 1986), a proposal was made for the detailed fold of residues 141 to 321 of the β-subunit of the *E. coli* enzyme based on the three-dimensional structure of AK. Since the total extent of the two regions that show certain degrees of homology between AK and β is no more than 40 residues, the authors rely mainly on secondary structure predictions to align the rest of the β-sequence with the AK structure. Simple tests such as using their secondary structure prediction algorithm on AK to see if they could correctly predict the fold of the known parent structure were not performed. The authors used the proposed model for designing and interpreting mutagenesis experiments (Parsonage et al., 1987, 1988). These mutagenesis studies provided excellent new information, but at the same time highlighted the inadequacies of the structural model. Mutagenesis experiments designed and interpreted with an experimentally determined structure should be extremely informative.

Labeling with Affinity and Photoaffinity Substrate Analogs. The identification of labeled subunits after reaction of F_1 ATPases with radioactive affinity or photoaffinity analogs of ATP and ADP substrates have shown the presence of six nucleotide-binding sites on the α- and β-subunits of mitochondrial and bacterial enzymes (Cross and Nalin, 1982; Wise et al., 1983; Xue et al., 1987; Girault et al., 1988). As there are three copies of the two major subunits in the holoenzyme, it might be inferred that these sites are equally distributed between these subunits. The facts agree with the existence of adenine nucleotide–binding sites in isolated α- and β-

subunits from bacterial F_1 ATPases (Otha et al., 1980; Dunn and Futai, 1980; Rao et al., 1988). Three of the sites behave as catalytic sites (Cross and Nalin, 1982; Wise et al., 1983), showing strong positive catalytic cooperativity (Kalayar et al., 1977; Gresser et al., 1982); they appear to be entirely on the β-subunit. The functional role of the other three sites is poorly understood and thus are called *noncatalytic*. These sites appear to be present at the interfaces of α- and β-subunits (Bullough and Allison, 1986; Lunardi et al., 1987; Bullough et al., 1988; Verbug and Allison, 1990).

   Many studies, especially those of the laboratory of Allison, have used labels to identify residues that participate in catalytic and noncatalytic nucleotide-binding sites. In the F_1 of bovine heart mitochondria, Tyr^{311}, Tyr^{345}, Tyr^{368}, and His^{427} of the β-subunit have been labeled with covalent inhibitors of the enzyme. In the α subunit, Tyr^{244} has been identified in the same way. Mutagenesis experiments have been used in *E. coli* to identify important residues on the F_1 sector. Residues Tyr^{297} and Tyr^{331} (corresponding to Tyr^{311} and Tyr^{345}, respectively, of beef heart mitochondria) were found to be in contact in nucleotides bound at the catalytic site of the enzyme.

Reconstitution Experiments. The isolated subunits of the F_1 ATPase do not have detectable enzymatic activity, but the enzyme can be reconstituted from mixtures of either native or denatured individual subunits. The reconstitution of different parts of the enzyme ($\alpha_3\beta_3\gamma$, $\alpha_3\beta_3\delta$, $\alpha_3\beta_3$, and so forth) was used to analyze the interrelation between the subunits and their spatial relationship in the complex. Reconstitution experiments were carried out with native subunits in *E. coli* (Futai, 1977; Dunn, and Futai, 1980) and with both native and denatured subunits in thermophilic bacterium PS3(TF) (Yoshida et al., 1977). Early reconstitution experiments for 31 possible subunit mixtures were performed by Kagawa et al. (1979). Successful reconstitution, judged by functional and structural considerations, were found for the complex $\alpha + \beta + \gamma$ in *E. coli* (Futai, 1977) and PS3(TF$_1$) (Yoshida et al., 1977) and similar results for the $\alpha_3\beta_3\delta$ oligomer in the PS3 (TF$_1$) (Yoshida et al., 1977). Recently Miwa and Yoshida (1989) reconstituted the $\alpha_3\beta_3$ oligomer and found that it has about 20% of ATPase activity of TF$_1$ and about 50% the rate of $\alpha_3\beta_3\gamma$ complex and that its enzymatic properties are similar to those of native TF$_1$. No active $\alpha_3\beta_3$ has been confirmed in any other system.

Minor Subunits. The structure and function of three minor subunits of the F_1 sector are much less understood than those of the α- and β-subunits. At the present time there is considerable experimental effort being devoted toward elucidating the role of small subunits in the F_0F_1 ATPase. Comparison of the amino acid sequences of the minor subunits of the F_1 ATPases from several sources shows that only the α-, β-, and γ-subunits of mammalian and higher plant mitochondria have a direct counterpart in bacteria and chloroplasts. In addition to the α- and β-subunits, the γ-subunits from different sources show several regions of significant sequence conservation (Walker et al., 1985). Important homology also exists between the δ-subunits of the mitochondrial F_1 and ϵ-subunits of bacteria and chloroplasts, but the mammalian ϵ-subunit does not have a counterpart in the other sources (Table 7.2).

   Mabuchi et al. (1981) found similar hydropathy profiles for the δ-subunit from different sources, and secondary structure predictions suggest that the δ-subunit is a polypeptide with a high a helical content (Sternweis and Smith, 1977). Recently

Table 7.2. Correspondence of Minor Subunits between F_1
ATPases from Several Sources

Bacteria	Plant		Mammalian Mitochondrial F_1
	CF_1	Mitochondrial F_1	
γ	γ	γ	γ
δ	δ	δ	OSCP*
ϵ	ϵ	$\delta'\dagger$	δ
		ϵ	ϵ

*OSCP is part of the F_0 portion in the F_1F_0-ATPase.
†In dicotyledonous plants
From Kimura et al. (1989).

Lunardi et al. 1989) probed the accessibility of the δ-subunit in F_1 and the F_0F_1 complex using monoclonal antibodies. Circular dichroism (CD) measurements (Sterweis and Smith, 1977; Miwa and Yoshida, 1989) are also consistent with a 60% helical content. Small-angle x-ray diffraction of the δ-subunit of chloroplast F_1 (Schmidt and Paradies, 1977) were interpreted as corresponding to a 25×90 Å ellipsoid. Based on all this information it is proposed that the δ-subunit forms a 50 residue long helical stretch (75 Å length). The δ-subunits of the bacterial F_1, chloroplast CF_1, and plant mitochondrial F_1 are homologous to the oligomycin-sensitivity-conferring protein (OSCP) of the eukaryotic mitochondrial F_0F_1 complex (Table 7.2). Recently Morikami et al. 1992) found strong similarities between the amino acid sequences of the δ-subunit of plant mitochondria and the δ-subunit of animal mitochondria (Table 7.2).

Crystallographic Studies on F_1. Single crystals of the F_1 sector have been described in three systems: rat liver mitochondria (Amzel and Pedersen, 1978), beef heart mitochondria (Walker et al., 1990), and thermophilic bacterium PF3 (Shirakihara et al., 1991); of those, a structure determination using x-ray diffraction methods has been reported for the rat liver enzyme. Using data to 3.6 Å resolution, a molecular model of F_1 was presented (Bianchet et al., 1991) that describes the most salient features of the enzyme's quaternary structure. In the crystal, the rat liver enzyme sits on a crystallographic threefold axis (parallel to the c axis of the hexagonal cell) that relates the three copies of each major subunit. Both the α- and the β-subunits have similar ellipsoidal shapes and sizes—α of dimensions $48 \times 48 \times 50$ Å (Fig. 7.4) and β of $40 \times 48 \times 50$ Å. The major axis of the β-subunit is almost parallel to the threefold axis, while that of the α is tilted by about 30°. Starting at the plane defined by three twofold axes ($z = 0$, "bottom"), one finds density corresponding to the three α-subunits; they are elongated in the plane in such a way that they interact with each other at the threefold axis. They continue in a very similar arrangement for a total of about 50 Å measured along the z direction. The β-subunits start at about 10–15 Å from the $z = 0$ plane with their major axes running parallel to the z direction, and the center of the subunits approximately 30 Å from the threefold axis. In this arrangement the β-subunits interact strongly with the α-subunits, but little or not at all with each other. Since the α-subunits are tilted, the relative

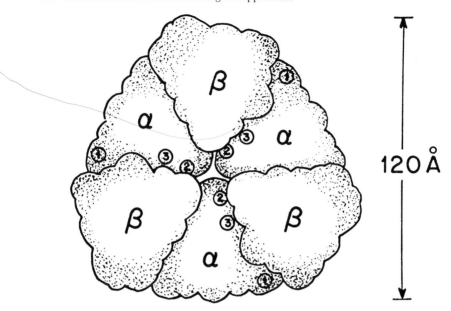

120 Å

Fig. 7.4. Schematic representation of F_1 ATPase. The important features of the quaternary structure (Bianchet et al., 1991) are schematically represented, as are the arrangements of αs and βs and the positions of three mercury heavy atoms. The heavy atom (*1*) is on the Cys^{201} spatially close to the "glycine-rich loop" and the interface between α- and β-subunits. (From Bianchet et al., 1991.)

arrangement of the α- and the β-subunits varies from plane to plane, but on average can be described as having the center of the α-subunits at 40 degrees to 50 degrees from the center of the β-subunits. At the "top" of the molecule, about 75 Å from the "bottom," only the β-subunits are present, leaving the region surrounding the three-fold axis devoid of density.

Electron Microscopy. The structure of F_1 obtained with x-ray diffraction methods can be used to interpret the results of the electron microscopic studies reported in the past. As expected, the six stain-excluding regions observed in the micrographs correspond to the three α- and the three β-subunits. Not discernible from the micrographs is the fact that the α- and β-subunits are not oriented the same way with respect to the threefold axis of symmetry. Studies that used sixfold averaging not only averaged α- with β-subunits but also averaged the two subunits in different orientations; the resulting images incorrectly overemphasized the apparent hexagonal arrangement of subunits. Similar errors probably affected studies that used averaging of multiple particles: in aligning different individual images it is extremely difficult (if not impossible, at the resolution of the images) to discriminate between the correct alignment and one with α-subunits aligned with β-subunits and β-subunits with αs.

Many of these difficulties were overcome in studies with immunolabeling. From the pioneering work of Lünsdorf et al. (1984) to the very definitive work of Gogol et al. (1989b), these studies correctly concluded that in F_1 three copies of each of the major subunits were related by a 120° rotation. Also, using F_1 ATPase of *E. coli* decorated with Fab' fragments of monoclonal antibodies prepared against the β-subunit, Capaldi and coworkers produce evidence that a central mass is asymmetrically arranged with respect to the β-subunits. Similar observations without identification of the subunit involved have been done in mitochondria (Boekema et al., 1986) and chloroplast (Boekema et al., 1988).

Another recent study (Gogol et al., 1989a) used tilted images of negatively stained bidimensional crystals and cryoelectron microscopy of unstained specimens to produce a three-dimensional model of F_1. This model, although correct in many of its features, has α- and β-subunits that are 90 Å long ellipsoids of 30 Å diameter. These ellipsoids run the whole length of the F_1 in an approximate hexagonal arrangement. In projection, this model is very similar to the x-ray structure. However, in the x-ray structure the α- and the β-subunits are wider and shorter and are offset by about 15 Å in the direction parallel to the threefold axis. This offset can explain the triangular appearance of the top and the bottom of the model of Gogol et al. (1989b). The authors used the symmetry of the diffraction intensities along the z^* direction about the $z^* = 0$ point to suggest that the symmetry of the molecule was higher than C3, namely, C6 (Schoenflies symbols). Considering the limited tilt used, their data are equally compatible with the molecule having symmetry D3 (32 in crystallographic symbols). The excessive elongation of the subunits probably is due to the limited tilts utilized, which reduce the resolution in the vertical direction. This distortion also contributes to making the object appear more hexagonal. The images from cryoelectron microscopy were mostly of the pseudohexagonal projection (top view); only a few images were identified as side views, but these images can also be explained as distorted or incomplete top views.

Functional Implications of the X-Ray Model. Comparison of the amino acid sequences of the α- and the β-subunits shows weak but significant homology. It shows, in addition, similarities with other ATP-utilizing enzymes, including the two regions of AK thought to be involved in nucleotide binding. Many of the previous proposals for the quaternary structure of the F_1 emphasized a hexagonal arrangement of subunits. The implied C6 symmetry is such that equivalent regions of α- and β-subunits can only be spatially close in the center of the molecule. For example, a catalytic site made by the nucleotide-binding domains of the α- and the β-subunits could only exist close to the threefold axis. In the x-ray model, the F_1 is formed by the threefold repetition of one α/β pair. The relation between the α- and β-subunits in each pair is such that equivalent regions of the two subunits (e.g., the nucleotide-binding sites of α and β) can be close to each other in structure. One of the cysteine residues we identified (Cys[201] rat sequence numbering) is close, both spatially and in sequence, to the loop that is thought to be involved in binding the ATP phosphate. That particular cysteine is on the surface of the α-subunit and is close to the interface with β-subunits. Titration of this cysteine with mercurials could be responsible for the effects of the mercurials on the catalytic activity of the enzyme (Catterall and Pedersen, 1974).

Mechanism of the Enzyme. One of the most interesting aspects of ATP synthesis is the ability of F_1 to synthesize enzyme-bound ATP from ADP and P_i (the equilibrium constant for the enzyme-bound reaction $ADP + P_i = ATP + H_2O$ is approximately 1.0). This observation has led to proposals in which H^+ ions from the H^+ gradient bring about the release of enzyme-bound ATP; both direct and indirect effects of the H^+ ions have been proposed. Most of the proposals invoke a complex pattern of nucleotide binding and release involving conformational changes in the enzyme: the binding change mechanism. According to this mechanism, the ATP-binding catalytic sites on each of the three β-subunits exhibit different affinities for nucleotide depending on whether only one or more of the sites is occupied; when F_1 binds only 1 mol of ATP(Mg) such that only one catalytic β-site is occupied per 1 mol of enzyme (unisite conditions), that 1 mol of ATP(Mg) is very strongly bound ($K_d \simeq 10^{-12}$ M) (Grubmeyer et al., 1982). This bound ATP undergoes a reversible hydrolysis at that site, with a Keq $\simeq 1$, but products are not readily released. To exhibit high steady-state ATPase activity ($K_{cat} \simeq 600$ sec^{-1}), additional ATP(Mg) must promote product release by filling at least one other catalytic site (multisite conditions).

The complex kinetics of cooperation between the catalytic sites of F_1 suggests that the enzyme has at least two equivalent catalytic (exchangeable) sites that are assumed to function alternately. Thus, the binding change mechanism is characterized as an "alternating site-binding change" process. Whether two or three catalytic sites on the β-subunits actually operate in an alternating sequence during steady-state ATP hydrolysis and synthesis is a subject of some controversy. However, changes in the affinity for nucleotides at these β-sites depending on whether one or more of them is filled seems to be a very consistent observation. These mechanisms have explicit structural implications that need to be evaluated as soon as atomic structural information becomes available. As a result of this scrutiny, some proposals will be discarded while others will be modified, leading to a new round of mechanistic experimental studies.

Acknowledgments

This work was supported by National Institutes of Health grants GM 25432 and CA 10951.

References

Amzel L. M., and Pedersen P. L. (1978) Adenosine triphosphate from rat liver mitochondria. Crystallization and x-ray diffraction studies of F_1-component of enzyme. *J Biol. Chem.* 253(7): 2067–2069.

Bianchet M., Ysern X., Hullihen J., Pedersen P. L., and Amzel L. M. (1991) Mitochondrial ATP synthase: Quaternary structure of F_1 moiety at 3.6 Å determined by x-ray diffraction analysis. *J. Biol. Chem.* 266: 21197–21201.

Boekema E. J., Berden J. A., and Gräber P. (1988) Structure of ATPsynthase from chloroplasts studied by electron microscopy and image processing. *Biochim. Biophys. Acta* 933: 365–373.

Boekema E. J., Berden J. A., and Van Heel G. M. (198) Structure of mitochondrial F_1-ATPase studied by electron microscopy and image processing. *Biochim. Biophys. Acta* 851: 353–360.

Bouty M., Briquet M., and Goffeau A. (1983) The α subunit of plant mitochondrial F_1-ATPase is translated in mitochondria. *J. Biol. Chem.* 258: 8524–8526.

Bullough D. A., and Allison W. S. (1986) Three copies of β subunit must be modified to achieve complete inactivation of bovine mitochondrial F_1-ATPase by 5′-p-fluorsulfonylbenzoyladenosine. *J. Biol. Chem.* 261(13): 5722–5730, 1986.

Bullough D. A., Brown E. L., Saario J. D., and Allison W. S. (1988) On the location and function of the noncatalytic sites on the bovine heart mitochondrial F_1ATPase. *J. Biol. Chem.* 263(28): 14053–14060.

Cain B. D. and Simoni R. D. (1989) Proton translocation by A the F_1F_0ATPase of *Escherichia coli*. Mutagenic analysis of the **a** subunit. *J. Biol. Chem.* 264(6): 3292–3300.

Catterall W. A., and Pedersen P. L. (1974) Structural and catalytic properties of mitochondrial adenosine triphosphatase. *Biochem Soc. Spec. Publ.* 4: 63–88.

Cross R. L., and Nalin C. M. (1982) Adenosine nucleotide binding sites of beef heart F_1ATPase, evidence for three exchageable sites that are distinct from three noncatalytic sites. *J. Biol. Chem.* 257: 2874–2881.

Duncan T. M., Parsonage D., and Senior A. E. (1986) Structure of the nucleotide-binding domain in the β-subunit of *Escherichia coli* F_1-ATPase. *FEBS Lett.* 208: 1–6.

Dunn S. D., and Futai M. (1980) Reconstitution of functional coupling factor from isolated subunits of *Escherichia coli* F_1-ATPase. *J. Biol. Chem.* 255: 113–118.

Eya S., Noumi T., Maeda M., and Futai M. (1988) Intrinsic membrane sector (F_0) of H^+ ATPase (F_1F_0) from *Escherichia coli*. *J. Biol. Chem.* 263(21): 10056–10062.

Filligame R. H. (1981) Biochemistry and genetics of bacterial H^+-translocating ATPases. *Curr. Top. Bioenerg.* 11: 35–106.

Fry D. C., Kuby S. A., and Mildvan A. S. (1986) ATP binding site of adenylate kinase: Mechanistic implications of its homology with ras encoded p21, F_1-ATPase, and other nucleotide binding proteins. *Proc. Natl. Acad. Sci. USA* 83: 907–911.

Futai M. (1977) Reconstitution of ATPase activity from isolated α, β, and γ subunits of the coupling factor F_1 of *Escherichia coli*. *Biochem. Biophys. Res. Commun.* 79: 1231–1237.

Futai M., and Kanazawa H. (1983) Structure and function of proton-translocating adenosine triphosphatase (F_0F_1): Biochemical and molecular biological approaches. *Microbiol. Rev.* 47: 285–312.

Futai M., Noumi T., and Maeda M. (1989) ATP synthase (H^+-ATPase): Results by combined biochemical and molecular biological approaches. *Annu. Rev. Biochem.* 58: 111–136.

Garboczi D. N., Fox A. H., Gerring S. L., Thomas P. J., and Pedersen P. L. (1988) β Subunit of rat liver mitochondrial ATP synthase. *Biochemistry* 27: 553–560.

Girault G., Berger G., Galmiche J. M., and Andre F. (1988) Characterizations of six nucleotide-binding sites of chloroplast coupling factor and one site on its purified β subunit. *J. Biol. Chem.* 263: 14690–14695.

Godinot C., and Di Pietro A. (1986) Structure and function of the ATPase-ATPsynthase complex of mitochondria as compared to chloroplast and bacteria. *Biochimie* 68: 367–374.

Gogol E. P., Aggeler R., Sagermann M., and Capaldi R. A. (1989) Cryoelectron microscopy of *Escherichia coli* F_1 adenosinetriphosphatase decorated with monoclonal antibodies to individual subunits of the complex. *Biochemistry* 28: 4717–4724.

Gogol E. P., Lücken T. B., and Capaldi R. A. (1989) Molecular architecture of *Escherichia coli* F_1 adenosinetriphosphatase. *Biochemistry* 28: 4709–4716.

Gresser M. J., Myer J., and Boyer P. D. (1982) Catalytic site cooperativity of beef heart mitochondrial F_1 adenosine triphosphatase. *J. Biol. Chem.* 257(20): 12030–12038.

Hatefi Y. (1985) The mitochondrial electron transport and oxidative phosphorylation system. *Annu. Rev. Biochem.* 54: 1015–1069.

Hoppe J., and Sebald W. (1984) The proton conducting F_0-part in bacterial ATPsynthases. *Biochim. Biophys. Acta* 768: 1–27.

Horak A., and Packer M. (1985) Coupling factor activity of the purified pea mitochondrial F_1-ATPase. *Biochim. Biophys. Acta* 810: 310–318.

Iwasaki Y., and Asahi T. (1983) Purification and characterization of soluble form of mitochondrial adenosinetriphosphate from sweet potato. *Arch. Biochem. Biophys.* 227: 164–173.

Kagawa Y. (1984) *New Comprehensive Biochemistry,* volume 9 of *Bionergetics,* pages 149–186. Elsevier, Amsterdam, first edition.

Kagawa Y., Sone N., Hirata, H., and Okamoto H. (1979) Structure and function of H^+-ATPase. *J. Bioenerg. Biomembr.* 11: 39–78.

Kalayar C., Rosing J., and Boyer P. D. (1977) An alternative site sequence for oxidative phosphorylation suggested by measurement of substrate binding patterns and exchange reaction inhibitions. *J. Biol. Chem.* 252: 2486–2491.

Kimura T., Nakamura K., Hattori H., Nelson N., and Asahi T. (1989) Correspondence of minor Subunits of plant mitocondrial F_1-ATPase to F_1F_0-ATPase subunits of other organisms. *J. Biol. Chem.* 264: 3183–3186.

Kyte J., and Doolite R. F. (1982) A simple method for displaying the hydropathic character of a protein. *J. Mol. Biol.* 157: 105–132.

Lee J. H., Garboczi D. N., Thomas P. J., and Pedersen P. L. (1990) Mitochondrial ATP synthase. *J. Biol. Chem.* 265: 4664–4669.

Lewis M. J., Chang J. A., and Simoni R. D. (1990) A topological analysis of subunit a from *Escherichia coli* F_1F_0 ATP synthase predicts eight transmembrane segments. *J. Biol. Chem.* 27(18): 10541–10550.

Lunardi J., Dupuis A., Frobert Y., Grassi J., and Vignais P. V. (1989) Exploration of delta-subunit interactions in beef heart mitochondrial f1-ATPase by monoclonal antibodies. *FEBS Lett.* 245: 223–228.

Lunardi J., Garin J., Issartel J. P., and Vignais P. V. (1987) Mapping of nucleotide-depleted mitochondrial F_1-ATPase with 2-azido-[α-^{32}P]adenosine diphosphatase. *J. Biol. Chem.* 262(31): 15172–15181.

Lünsdorf H., Ehrig K., Friedl P., and Schairer H. U. (1984) Use of monoclonal antibodies in immunoelectron microscopy for determination of subunit stoichiometry in oligomeric enzymes. *J. Mol. Biol.* 173: 131–136.

Mabuchi K., Kanazawa H., Kayano T., and Futai M. (1981) Nucleotide sequence of the gene coding for the δ subunit of proton-translocating ATPase of *Escherichia coli. Biochem. Biophys. Res. Commun.* 102: 172–179.

Miwa K., and Yoshida M. (1989) The $\alpha_3\beta_3$ complex, the catalytic core of F_1-ATPase. *Proc. Natl. Acad. Sci. USA* 86(17): 6484–6487.

Morikami A., Aiso K., Asahi T., and Nakamura K. (1992) The delta'-subunit of higher plant 6-subunit mitochondrial f1-ATPase is homologous to the delta-subunit of animal mitochondrial F_1-ATPase. *J. Biol. Chem.* 267: 72–76.

Otha S., Tsuboi M., Oshima T., Yoshida M., and Kagawa Y. (1980) Nucleotide binding to isolated α and β subunits of proton translocating adenosinetriphosphate studied with circular dichroism. *J. Biochem. (Tokyo)* 87: 1609–1617.

Ohta S., Yohda M., Ishizuka M., Hirata H., Hammamoto T., Otawara-Hammamoto Y., Matsuda K., and Kagawa Y. (1988) Site-directed mutagenesis of stable adenosine triphosphate synthase. *Biochim. Biophys. Acta* 933: 141–155.

Parsonage D., Al-Shawi M. K., and Senior A. E. (1988) Directed mutation of strongly conserved lysine 155 in the catalytic nucleotide-binding domain of β-subunit of F_1-ATPase from *Escherichia coli. J. Biol. Chem.* 263(10): 4740–4744.

Penefsky H. S., and Grubmeyer C. (1984) *H^+-ATPase (ATP Synthase): Structure, Function, Biogenesis of the F_0F_1 Complex of Coupling Membranes*, ICSU Press, Adriatica Editrice, Bari Italy, pp. 195–204.

Rao R., Al-Shawi M. K., and Senior A. E. (1988) Trinitrophenyl-ATP and ADP bind to a single nucleotide site on isolated β-subunit of *Escherichia coli* F_1-ATPase. *J. Biol. Chem.* 263: 5569–5573.

Schindler H., and Nelson N. (1982) Proteolipid of adenosinetriphosphate from yeast mitochondria. Forms proton-selective channels in planar lipid bilayers. *Biochemistry* 21: 5787–5794.

Schmidt V. D., and Paradies H. (1977) The structure of the δ-subunit from chloroplast coupling factor (CF$_1$) in solution. *Biochem. Biophys. Res. Commun.* 78: 1043–1052.

Schneider E., and Altendorf K. (1987) Bacterial adenosine 5'-triphosphatase synthase (F_1F_0): Purification and reconstitution of F_0 complexes and biochemical and functional characterization of their subunits. *Microbiol. Rev.* 51: 477–497.

Sebald W., Machleidt W., and Wachter E. (1980) N,N'-Dicyclohexylcarbodiimide binds specifically to a single glutamyl residue of proteolipid subunit of mitochondrial adenosinetriphosphatase from *Neurospora crassa* and *Saccharomyces cerevisiae. Proc. Natl. Acad. Sci. USA* 77: 785–789.

Senior A. E. (1990) The proton-translocating ATPase of *Escherichia coli. Annu. Rev. Biophys. Chem.* 19: 7–41.

Shirakihara Y., Yohda M., Kagawa Y., Yokoyama K., and Yoshida M. (1991) Purification by dye-ligand chromatography and a crystallization study of the F_1-ATPase and its major subunits, β and α, from a thermophilic bacterium, PS3. *J. Biochem.* 109(3): 466–471.

Spitsberg V. L., Pfeiffer N. E., Partridge B., Wylie D. E., and Schuster S. M. (1985) Isolation and antigenic characterization of corn mitochondrial F_1-ATPase. *Plant Physiol. (Bethesda)* 77: 339–345.

Sterweis P. C., and Smith J. B. (1977) Characterization of the purified membrane attachment (δ) subunit of proton translocating adenosine triphosphatase from *Escherichia coli*. *Biochemistry* 16: 4020–4025.

Taylor W. R., and Green N. M. (1989) The predicted secondary structure of nucleotide-binding sites of six cation-transporting ATPases lead to a probable tertiary fold. *FEBS Lett.* 179: 241–248.

Verbug J. G., and Allison W. S. (1990) Tyrosine α244 is derivatized when the bovine heart mitochondrial F_1-ATPase is inactivated with 5′-p-fluorosulfonylbenzoylethenoadenosine. *J. Biol. Chem.* 265: 8065–8074.

Walker J. E., Fearnley I. M., Gay N. J., Gibson B. W., Northop F. D., Powell S. J., Runswick M. J., Saraste M., and Tybulewicz V.L.J. (1985) Primary structure and subunit stoichiometry of F_1ATPase from bovine mitochondria. *J. Mol. Biol.* 184: 677–701.

Walker J. E., Fearnley I. M., Lutter R., Todd R. J., and Runswick M. J. (1990) Structural aspects of proton pumping ATPases. *Phil. Trans. R. Soc. Lond.* B326: 367–378.

Walker J. E., Runswick M. J., and Poulter L. (1987) ATP synthase from bovine mitochondria. *J. Mol. Biol.* 197: 89–100.

Walker J. E., Saraste M., and Gay N. J. (1984) The unc operon: Nucleotide sequence, regulation and structure of ATP synthase. *Biochim. Biophys. Acta* 768: 164–200.

Walker J. E., Saraste M., Runswick J. J., and Gay N. J. (1982) Distantly related sequences in the α- and β-subunits of ATP synthase, myosin, kinases and other ATP-requiring enzymes and the common nucleotide binding fold. *EMBO J.* 1(8): 945–981.

Wise J. G., Duncan T. M., Cox L. R., and Senior A. E. (1983). Properties of F_1-ATPases from the uncD412 mutant of *Escherichia coli*. *Biochem. J.* 215: 343–350.

Yoshida M., Okamoto H., Hirata H., and Kagawa Y. (1977) Reconstitution of adenosine triphosphatase of thermophilic bacterium from purified individual subunits. *Proc. Natl. Acad. Sci. USA* 74: 963–940.

Yoshida M., Sone N., Hirata J., and Kagawa Y. (1975) A highly stable adenosine triphosphatase from a thermophilic bacterium. *J. Biol. Chem.*, 250: 7910–7916.

Ysern X., Amzel L. M., and Pedersen P. L. (1988) ATP synthases: structure of the F_1 moeity and its relationship to function and mechanism. *J. Bioener. Biomembr.* 20: 423–450.

Xue Z., Zhou J. M., Melese T., Cross R. L., and Boyer P. D. (1987) Chloroplast F_1-ATPase has more than three nucleotide binding sites, and 2-azido-ADP or 2-azido-ATP at both catalytic and noncatalytic sites labels the β-subunit. *Biochemistry* 26: 3749–3753.

III. Direct Structural Approaches

The great difficulties involved in producing three-dimensional crystals of membrane proteins precludes the use of standard crystallography as a routine direct structural approach. We must therefore rely on other methods to gain direct structural information. Although most of them are highly specialized and quite beyond the technical capabilities of the average laboratory, it is important to know what is possible. The most widely available methods for obtaining useful information on the secondary structures of proteins are circular dichroism (CD) and infrared (IR) spectroscopy but, as Robert Williams points out in his thorough discussion of these methods, membrane proteins present special problems. Nevertheless, CD and IR spectroscopy are extremely important tools that can give accurate and invaluable information.

The first direct three-dimensional structure of a membrane protein was obtained by high-resolution electron crystallography of bacteriorhodopsin (BR) that naturally forms two-dimensional crystals. The collection and analysis of such data is a long and demanding process but eventually can yield excellent models at moderately high resolution as for BR (Henderson et al., 1990). Membrane proteins exist naturally in the quasi-two-dimensional lipid bilayer, and it follows that they are more likely to form two-dimensional crystals than three-dimensional ones. Efforts are now being devoted to forming such crystals from proteins that do not form them naturally. Henderson and his colleagues (see Schertler et al., 1993) have recently succeeded in obtaining so-called projection maps of rhodopsin in this way. Werner Kühlbrandt, who has focused his research on the structure of the light harvesting complex, describes this important approach in his chapter.

Magnetic resonance methods are proving to be extremely useful structural tools for membrane proteins. The chapter by Wayne Hubbell and Christian Altenbach describes what they call site-directed spin labeling that takes good advantage of the fact that one can replace virtually any amino acid in a membrane protein by cysteine through site-directed mutagenesis. Nitroxide spin labels can then be attached at these sites to obtain information by electron paramagnetic resonance. One of the most important developments in structural biology has been the use of multidimensional nuclear magnetic resonance (NMR) to determine the solution structure of small proteins. This approach can also be used for small membrane proteins by the use of uniform isotopic labeling and solid-state NMR methods. This method is described in the chapter by Stanley Opella, who has used it very successfully in studies of the Pf1 viral coat protein.

The three-dimensional crystallization of the photosynthetic reaction center (PSRC) required the use of detergents that produced an arrangement of the reaction centers in the unit cell that was quite unlike their native two-dimensional arrangement (see Chapter 1 by Douglas Rees and his colleagues). A question that naturally arose was whether the structure derived from the three-dimensional crystals was the same as in the native membrane. A major effort was subsequently devoted to dealing with this issue. What was generally overlooked was the fact that the issue had been settled by Kent Blasie and his colleagues several years before the PSRC structure had been determined to high resolution (Pachence et al., 1979). The basic approach of Blasie and his group was to form oriented arrays of the PSRC in lipid multilayers from which they could determine the profile of the PSRC projected onto an axis normal to the bilayer. Those profiles, it turned out, were in excellent agreement with those calculated from the atomic-resolution structure of the PSRC. This general approach, described by Dr. Blasie in his chapter, has been refined to the extent that it is now possible to obtain useful diffraction data from oriented protein monolayers.

References

Henderson, R., Baldwin, J. M., Ceska, T. A., Zemlin, F., Beckmann, E., and Downing, K. H. (1990) Model for the structure of bacteriorhodopsin based on high-resolution electron cryo-microscopy. *J. Mol. Biol.* 213: 899–929.

Pachence, J. M., Dutton, P. L., and Blasie, J. K. (1979) Structural studies on reconstituted reaction center–phosphatidylcholine membranes. *Biochim. Biophys. Acta* 548: 348–373.

Schertler, G.F.X., Villa, C., and Henderson, R. (1993) Projection structure of rhodopsin. *Nature* 362: 770–772.

8

Experimental Determination of Membrane Protein Secondary Structure Using Vibrational and CD Spectroscopies

ROBERT W. WILLIAMS

Experimentalists interested in obtaining spectroscopic measurements of membrane protein secondary structure must keep in mind one general critical issue: the measurements must be reliable and specific enough to help distinguish between competing models of structure or function. An example of how this issue plays itself out can be seen in a series of papers beginning with that of Jap et al. (1983), in which it was proposed that some of the images in the in-plane electron diffraction map of bacteriorhodopsin may be due to transmembrane β-sheets instead of helices. This proposal was supported by circular dichroism (CD) and infrared (IR) measurements of secondary structures. The calculated helix content was only about 50%, and β-sheet content was about 20%. The investigators carefully corrected for differential light scattering in their CD measurements, but (according to subsequent studies) did not correct for absorption flattening effects. IR spectra were clearly not consistent with the hypothesis that the protein was 80% helix. The amide I maximum was at about 1,686 cm^{-1}, while an 80% helical protein should have an amide I maximum at about 1,652 cm^{-1}. Other CD results by Wallace and Mao (1984) that corrected for the absorption flattening effects did not support the β-sheet hypothesis. Their calculated helix content was about 80%. However, this calculation included a normalization of the results to correct for what was assumed to be an inaccurate determination of protein concentration. The data upon which it was based was actually similar to those obtained by Jap et al. (1983). Glaeser and Jap (1985) subsequently made a convincing argument that the normalization procedure was not valid. Nevertheless, in the face of recent evidence, Glaeser et al. (1991) subsequently acknowledged that all of the transmembrane segments are clearly helical and that their β-sheet hypothesis was wrong.

This scenario presents a challenge to investigators who perform or develop methods to make measurements of membrane protein secondary structure with CD and vibrational spectroscopy. CD and IR spectra of bacteriorhodopsin have not changed in the past 10 years. By conventional empirical interpretations, they still indicate substantially less helix content than is now known to exist. Glaeser et al. (1991) suggest that this situation indicates something unusual about the structure of the helices in bacteriorhodopsin that cannot currently be detected by other methods. Computational studies by Krimm and Dwivedi (1982) have long indicated that this may be the case and that the unusual amide I spectrum may be due to α_{II}-helices. Glaeser et al. (1991) also observed that what appears to be a failure of two different techniques is actually an invitation to refine our understanding—of both CD and Fourier-transform IR (FTIR) spectroscopy and of why they have yielded anomalous results. Unless such a refinement can be accomplished, it will be difficult to place much confidence in spectroscopic measurements of membrane protein secondary structure content in the future. Preliminary studies have shown that the anomalous amide I frequency of purple membrane may be due to transition dipole coupling (Hunt et al., 1993).

A variety of new empirical methods for protein secondary structure determination using FTIR spectroscopy have become available recently. Many of these methods remain untried in measurements of membrane protein secondary structure, and they may have sources of artifacts arising from the presence of membranes that are not as well understood as those present in CD measurements. It appears unlikely that any of these new methods will give the desired results in measurements of bacteriorhodopsin, however. These problems need to be studied.

Three spectroscopic methods are currently used to measure membrane protein secondary structure (and the conformation of prosthetic groups); they are FTIR, Raman, and CD. This chapter presents discussions of some of the developments in these fields and of the relative strengths and weaknesses of these methods when they are applied to membrane proteins. Suggestions are made that may lead to improvements in the information that may be obtained from vibrational spectroscopy.

Comprehensive reviews of some of these methods are given elsewhere. FTIR methods applied to membrane protein structure and, more specifically, to measurements of the dynamics of prosthetic groups have been discussed recently in the excellent review by Braiman and Rothschild (1988). Consequently, most of those techniques are not discussed here. Another outstanding review of FTIR methods, by Surewicz and Mantsch (1988), also treats membrane protein structure and focuses on resolution enhancement techniques. Methods for CD estimation of globular protein structure are summarized by Yang et al. (1986).

The use of these methods in studies of membrane proteins differs from their application to soluble proteins where they must overcome problems arising from the presence of lipids. Lipids with carbon–carbon double bonds have vibrational frequencies that interfere strongly with measurements of the protein amide I region of the spectrum, where the secondary structure information is to be found in FTIR and Raman measurements. The intense spectrum of water in FTIR spectra is shifted by the presence of lipids, making the results of corrections for the spectrum of water ambiguous. Lipids tend to increase the background fluorescence and decrease the signal-to-noise ratio in Raman measurements. Liposomes cause light scattering artifacts in CD measurements, decrease confidence in determinations of protein concentration, and make the collection of data below 200 to 190 nm practically impossible with many of the available instruments. Under some circumstances the presence of lipid membranes becomes an advantage; such is the case with attenuated total reflection FTIR measurements. To a significant extent the interpretation of the spectra of membrane proteins and peptides is the same as it is for soluble proteins, and, in the interests of clarity, some of the discussion here related to vibrational spectra will emphasize results from water-soluble peptides.

Vibrational Spectroscopy

Vibrational spectroscopy may be used to obtain information about secondary structure through a combination of empirical, theoretical, and computational methods. Empirical methods (described later under Fourier-Transform Infrared Spectroscopy and under Raman Spectroscopy) give relatively accurate estimates of percentages of helix, β-sheet, reverse turn, and unfolded structure present in globular proteins. However, as with CD methods, these measurements, which quantitate only the average secondary structure content, have a limited usefulness. New techniques are being developed that will allow the measurement of conformational information about specific amino acid residues. These techniques are readily applicable to membrane-bound peptides and can be extended to proteins. The application of these techniques will require the combined use of both empirical methods and normal mode calculations with theoretically derived force fields.

Computational methods for predicting the vibrational spectra of proteins have been advanced in significant ways in the past few years. They are now approaching a stage at which they can be truely useful to the biophysicist interested in measuring peptide and protein structures. Normal mode calculations and their applications in vibrational spectroscopy to measure protein structure have been reviewed by Krimm and Bandekar (1986). Another review by Fogarasi and Pulay (1985) describes the scaled quantum mechanical force field (SQMFF) methodology that is currently the state of the art in methods for obtaining accurate vibrational force fields. A particularly important development has made it possible to transform SQMFFs into parameters for molecular mechanics potential functions (Palmö et al., 1991). This will allow more accurate molecular mechanics simulations of protein structure and dynamics to be tested using vibrational spectroscopy.

Secondary structure information about membrane-bound peptides and proteins is obtained primarily from the amide I mode, which is composed of the amide $C=O$ stretching mixed with some in-plane N–H bending and some amide C–N stretching vibrations. An illustration of the amide I modes of two forms of L-Ala-L-Ala are shown in Figure 8.1. The two structures on the left represent the right-hand helix conformation in terms of ψ–ϕ space, while the structure on the right is in the β-sheet region of ψ–ϕ space. The calculated amide I frequencies shown in Figure 8.1 agree reasonably well with the measured frequencies shown in Figures 8.2 and 8.3. The difference between the frequencies of these two forms is due primarily to the charge difference. Differences observed between the spectra of helical and β-sheet peptides, on the other hand, are due almost entirely to transition dipole coupling, which is accounted for in *ab initio* calculations and which can also be calculated independently for very large proteins (Krimm and Bandekar, 1986; Torii and Tasumi, 1992). This information from the combined experimental and computational results can be used to distinguish between amino acids in a polypeptide that are in the helix or β-sheet regions of ψ space. Significantly, the amide I frequencies for individual peptide groups in a relatively large peptide can be measured using the isotope effect in conjunction with difference spectroscopy. This approach is described below.

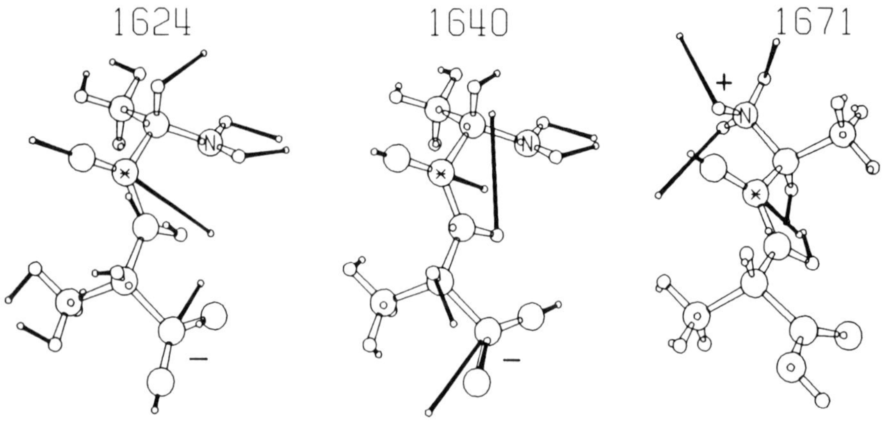

Fig. 8.1. Ortep drawings of normal modes and calculated frequencies for the amide I vibrations of L-Ala-L-Ala in helical and extended conformations. Atomic displacements shown here *(solid dark lines)* have been emphasized by multiplying them by a factor of five. These structures were obtained using the gaussian 90 system of programs (Frisch et al., 1989) from full ab initio SCF energy minimizations using the 4-31G basis set. Frequencies and scaled quantum mechanical force fields were calculated as described by Williams et al. (1991), using a single scale factor of 81.06%. In the positively charged extended molecule (ψ, ϕ = 155.8, −166.1) on the right, a hydrogen atom on the amine terminus interacts with the amide carbonyl oxygen. In the negatively charged helical molecule (ψ,ϕ = −14.9,−163.3), *middle and left*, a weak interaction may be formed between the amine terminus nitrogen atom and the amide hydrogen. A helical structure cannot be obtained when the amine terminus is positively charged. An extended structure can be obtained when the amine terminus is neutral, but the calculated amide I frequency is still at 1,670 or 1,680 cm^{-1}. The calculated frequency for the COOH group C=O stretch (mode not shown) is 1,730 cm^{-1}. Calculated frequencies shown here closely match the experimentally observed spectra shown in Figures 8.2 and 8.3.

Other modes are less likely to be useful in studies of membrane proteins, particularly for obtaining information about the conformation of specific amino acids. The amide II mode, composed of amide C–N stretching, N–H bending, and a proportion of C=O stretching vibrations, is useful in IR measurements. However, this band does not show the strong relationship between frequency and conformation that can be useful for obtaining information from difference spectra. The amide III mode is a complex mixture of in-plane N–H bending and C–H bending. It can be used to give information about the dihedral angle ϕ in limited cases (Weaver and Williams, 1990; Williams et al., 1990). However, the amide III mode overlaps with C–H bending vibrations of lipid acyl chains, which tend to vary slightly in frequency among samples. This variation shows up in difference spectra and interferes with interpretations of shifts in the amide III mode.

Stable Isotope Substitution

Information about the conformation of a specific amino acid in a polypeptide can be obtained through synthesis of the polypeptide with an amino acid incorporating ^{13}C at the position of the main chain carbonyl carbon atom. This method has not been tried on relatively large polypeptides or proteins. However, there currently does not

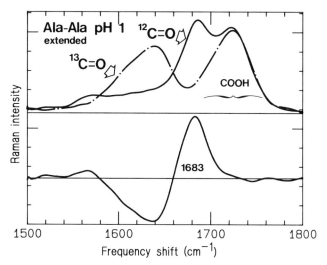

Fig. 8.2. Raman spectra of stable isotopomers of L-Ala-L-Ala in solution at pH 1. ^{13}C in the amide carbonyl carbon shifts the amide I frequency down by 49 cm^{-1}. *Top: solid line,* Ala-Ala with ^{12}C at the amide carbonyl carbon (indicated by the asterisks in Fig. 8.1); *line with dot,* Ala-Ala with ^{13}C at the amide carbonyl carbon. *Bottom:* difference spectrum showing that vibrations not coupled to the amide C=O stretch, such as the carboxylic acid C=O stretch, are canceled. A similar shift occurs at pH 7, from 1,677 to 1,624 cm^{-1}. This isotope effect can be used to identify the conformation of a single amino acid in a relatively large peptide.

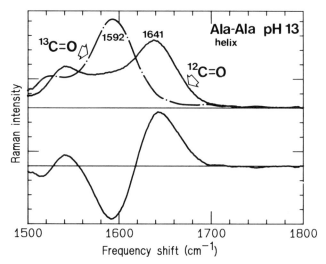

Fig. 8.3. Raman spectra of stable isotopomers of L-Ala-L-Ala in solution at pH 13. ^{13}C in the amide carbonyl carbon shifts the amide I frequency down by about 45 cm^{-1}. *Top: solid line,* Ala-Ala with ^{12}C in the amide carbonyl group; *line with dot,* Ala-Ala with ^{13}C in the amide carbonyl group. *Bottom:* difference spectrum. The amide I band in this spectrum of the ^{12}C isotopomer is broader than it is in spectra of the extended molecule (pH below 10), indicating that this form possibly has more structural heterogeneity. A Raman spectrum of Ala-Ala at a pH near 10, at the midpoint of the titration of the amine group, shows two amide I bands, one at each of the frequencies shown here and in Figure 8.2, with intensities that indicate the structural equilibrium.

1659   1688

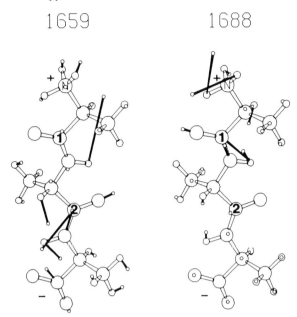

Fig. 8.4. Ortep drawings of normal modes and calculated frequencies for the amide I vibrations of L-Ala-L-Ala-L-Ala in the extended conformation, showing that scaled quantum mechanical force field calculations yield accurate predictions of the spectra of small peptides. Atomic displacements *(solid dark lines)* have been emphasized by multiplying them by a factor of five. This structure was obtained from a gaussian 90 (Frisch et al., 1989) ab initio SCF energy minimization using the 4-31G basis set. Frequencies and the scaled quantum mechanical force field were calculated as described by Williams et al. (1991), using a single scale factor of 81.06%. Calculated frequencies shown here closely match the experimentally observed spectra given in Figure 8.5. Using a differentially scaled force field optimized for peptides in solution, two amide I modes appear at 1,657 and 1,687 cm^{-1} corresponding to the second and first amide groups, respectively (Williams and Lowrey, unpublished data).

appear to be any experimental or computational obstacles for its application to studies of peptide–lipid interactions in which hydrophobic or amphiphilic peptides can be chemically synthesized. The best position for ^{13}C substitution is shown in Figure 8.1 as the atom marked with an asterisk. Figures 8.2 and 8.3 show Raman spectra of the L-Ala-L-Ala peptide with ^{12}C and ^{13}C in this position. This substitution shifts the amide I band downward by more than 40 cm^{-1} so that difference spectra of the [12]C- and ^{13}C-substituted isotopomers (also shown in the figures) clearly indicate the frequency of each band. By measuring a number of isotopomers of a peptide, each one having a different ^{13}C-labeled amino acid replacement, the amide I frequency of each amide group can be determined.

With this isotope substitution approach, assignments of β-sheet and α-helical structures can be made to many specific amino acid residues based solely on empirically determined rules for the amide I frequencies of these structures. Empirical methods for measuring protein secondary structure (described below) show that α-helical structures have an amide frequency at (or near) 1,649 cm^{-1} and that β-sheet

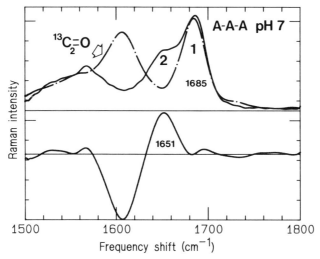

Fig. 8.5. Raman spectra of two stable isotopomers of L-Ala-L-Ala-L-Ala in solution at pH 7. *Top: solid line,* Ala-Ala with ^{12}C in both amide carbonyl groups; *line with dot,* Ala-Ala with ^{13}C in the *number 2* amide carbonyl group. *Bottom:* difference spectrum. The ^{12}C-labeled isotopomer has two amide I bands, one at 1,651 and one at 1,685 cm^{-1}. ^{13}C in the *number 2* amide carbonyl carbon shifts one of the amide I frequencies for that group down by about 47 cm^{-1}. The amide I frequency for the *number 1* amide group is shifted down by about 2 cm^{-1} by the isotope effect. These spectra are accurately predicted by the scaled quantum mechanical force field calculations. This figure illustrates that the amide I spectrum of a single ^{13}C-labeled amide group in a peptide can be identified and that the difference spectrum can be used, in conjunction with normal mode calculations, to obtain information about the conformation of that single peptide group.

structures show at least two amide I frequencies: a strong Raman band and a weak IR band at 1,670 cm^{-1} and a strong IR band at (or near) 1,630 cm^{-1}.

However, for nonrepeating structures such as reverse turns, the ends of helices and β-sheets, and the ends of the peptide as a whole, where the transition dipole coupling and amide I frequencies of adjacent peptide groups vary, empirical rules cannot be applied with confidence. This can be seen in Figures 8.4 and 8.5, where, although both peptide groups in the polypeptide L-Ala-L-Ala-L-Ala are in the extended conformation, the computational and experimental amide I frequencies for these two peptide groups are quite different (the transition dipole coupling interactions are negligible in this case). Under these circumstances, normal mode calculations using a force field obtained through the SQMFF method, combined with independent calculations of the transition dipole coupling, can be used to predict accurately the splitting of amide I vibrations for hypothetical structures.

Figure 8.4 shows an example of results from normal mode calculations; here are two predicted amide I normal modes, and the corresponding calculated frequencies, for the extended structure of Ala-Ala-Ala. Both the structure and its force field were computed using *ab initio* methods combined with the SQMFF methodology with a single scale factor (Williams et al., 1990). (The splitting predicted by the *ab initio* calculation was not changed by scaling.) Although the two amide groups in extended

Ala-Ala-Ala have similar conformations, the predicted amide I frequencies differ significantly.

Figure 8.5 shows the experimentally measured amide I spectra of ^{12}C and ^{13}C isotopomers of Ala-Ala-Ala. Difference spectra are also shown. The replacement of the number 2 amide group carbonyl carbon with ^{13}C identifies the amide I frequency for this group at 1,651 cm^{-1}, in good agreement with the calculated frequency. Several other local-energy-minimized conformations of Ala-Ala-Ala do not yield calculated splittings of the amide I frequencies that match the experimentally measured frequencies this well (R. Williams and A. Lowrey, unpublished data). While empirical rules would fail to yield a correct conformational interpretation of the amide I spectrum of Ala-Ala-Ala, normal mode calculations with a scaled quantum mechanical force field clearly eliminate several possibilities and put forward a probable preferred structure for Ala-Ala-Ala in water. This approach can easily be extended to membrane-bound peptides.

An assumption built into all empirical methods of secondary structure estimation using vibrational spectra is that the amide I band of a protein is a linear combination of the amide I bands of each amide group in the protein. Figure 8.5 shows that this assumption is not strictly valid and indicates to some extent the degree to which normalization of the amide I band employed in empirical methods is an approximation.

Figure 8.6 shows Raman spectra of magainin F and of magainin F-(Ala^{18}-1-^{13}C) associated with dipalmitoylphosphatidylcholine (DPPC) in a mole ratio of 12 lipid to 1 peptide. Magainin F associates with DPPC in a dramatic way, irreversibly turning turbid suspensions of liposomes quite clear when heated to the liquid crystalline phase transition of the lipid. The difference spectrum shows a sharp peak at 1,651 cm^{-1}. This can be interpreted empirically and with some confidence as indicating that Ala^{18} is in an α-helix. However, the band at 1,630 cm^{-1} cannot be interpreted empirically with the same confidence. Sharp amide I bands observed in difference spectra using other ^{13}C-labeled amino acids are observed at 1,660 cm^{-1} (data not shown). Midway between the frequencies expected for α-helical and β-sheet conformations, these bands are also difficult to interpret empirically. Frequencies from other nearby specific amide groups, FTIR spectra, which may not show all of the same frequencies, and normal mode calculations with an SQMFF are required to provide a full understanding. While normal mode calculations on large peptides may not be able to sort out all of the frequencies and all of the assignments, they can probably give specific information about the amide I frequencies and the conformations that give rise to them when combined with experimental frequencies from each amino acid.

Stable isotope substitution can be accomplished by automated chemical synthesis for short peptides such as melittin and magainin, but this approach can also be used for membrane proteins that cannot be chemically synthesized. In this strategy, two proteins could be synthesized in vivo. In one of these proteins, the specific residue to be probed would be replaced by site-directed mutagenesis by an alternative amino acid that does not (or is not expected to) alter significantly the conformation of neighboring residues. Let us say that a valine is replaced by an isoleucine. This mutated protein would then be produced under conditions in which all of the isoleucines are labeled with ^{13}C at the amide carbonyl carbon atom. The second protein would contain the native sequence; it would not incorporate the replacement of valine by an

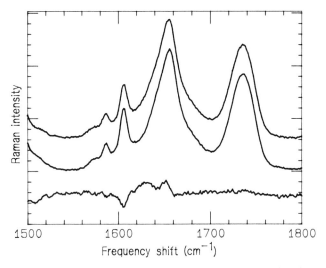

Fig. 8.6. Raman spectra of magainin F *(top)* and magainin F-(Ala[18]-1-^{13}C) (GIGKFLHS-AKKFAKAFV*A*EIMNS–NH$_2$) *(middle)*, both associated with DPPC in a mole ratio of 12 lipid to 1 peptide, and the difference *(bottom)*. The broad band at 1,735 cm^{-1} is the lipid ester C=O stretching mode. Relatively narrow peaks are observed in the difference at 1,651 (15 cm^{-1} wide) and 1,605 cm^{-1}. A broader positive peak is observed at 1,630 (20 cm^{-1} wide), which appears to increase in intensity as the mole ratio of lipid to peptide is increased from zero up to 12 (not shown). The positive peaks in this difference spectrum are the amide I bands of the A[18]–E[19] amide group. The negative band is the amide I band of the corresponding A[18]-1-^{13}C–E[19] amide group. The frequency shift between the positive and negative bands is typically 45 cm^{-1}. The width of these bands, at about 15 cm^{-1}, is typical of short crystalline peptides and indicates that there is a homogeneous population of conformations present. The width of the amide I bands for the two and three amino acid peptides shown in Figures 8.2, 8.3, and 8.5, at 30 to 50 cm^{-1}, indicates that there is a heterogeneous population of conformations and gives some measure of what the conformational distribution is. Total data collection time for each spectrum was 5 h, using 100 mW of sharply focused 514.5 nm light.

isoleucine, but it would also be synthesized under conditions that uniformly incorporates ^{13}C-labeled isoleucine. The difference spectrum between these two proteins would reveal information about the conformation of the valine in the native structure, since these two proteins, from the spectroscopic point of view, differ by a single ^{13}C-labeled amino acid substitution. By uniformly replacing all valines with ^{13}C-labeled valine, the conformation of the replacement isoleucine could also be probed.

The most problematic limitation in applications of this approach to proteins (appart from the labor requirements) may be the extent to which the alternative amino acid used in the site-directed mutagenesis alters the conformations of neighboring residues. These alterations themselves introduce features into difference spectra that may complicate interpretations of the differences due to isotope replacement. We have found that many single amino acid residue changes in site-directed mutants of staphylococcal nuclease yield Raman difference spectra characteristic of small changes in the conformations of one or two residues (R. Williams, A. Wen, and D. Shortle, unpublished results). However, difference spectra between mutant and wild-type proteins that do not have stable isotope substitutions should, in principle, identify those features that are due to conformational changes. This should help to discriminate differences due to conformational changes from those due to the isotope effect.

This approach applied to relatively large proteins would have a number of other technical limitations. For a protein with 200 residues, the amide I band of a single residue will represent only 0.5% of the area under the amide I spectrum. Consequently, the signal to noise ratio of the spectra must be very high. More importantly, the stability of the frequency calibration of the instrument must be excellent. FTIR instrumentation is automatically held in calibration by the interferometer and should easily provide the required stability. Raman instrumentation does not have this stability. However, it may be possible to avoid temporal drift in the frequency calibration of a Raman instrument by constructing a sample-holding apparatus that measures two samples simultaneously. Charge coupled device detectors (CCD) are readily suited to this kind of experiment.

Computationally, predictions of vibrational frequencies will be limited only by the maximum size of a protein that can be accommodated with molecular mechanics methods. Force fields calculated using the SQMFF methodology can be transformed into parameters for molecular mechanics wave functions that yield accurate vibrational frequencies (Palmö et al., 1991). (Molecular mechanics calculations have not, in the past, yielded useful predictions of vibrational frequencies.) So, limitations on the size of the problem available to ab initio methods will not effect calculations of frequencies for proteins using these force fields.

Both IR and Raman spectroscopy can give different and complementary information about the amide I spectrum. For example, the amide I spectrum of β-sheet secondary structure shows an intense Raman band at 1,670 cm^{-1} and an FTIR band at (or near) 1,630 cm^{-1}. Normal mode calculations can give an accurate prediction of the relative intensity of the FTIR bands. The combined information from both methods is necessary to resolve ambiguities in conformational interpretations of spectra.

Fourier-Transform Infrared Spectroscopy

There has been a recent surge of interest in using FTIR for secondary structure measurements of proteins. Six new methods have appeared since the start of 1990 (Dong et al., 1990; Goormaghtigh et al., 1990; Dousseau and Pézolet, 1990; Kalnin et al., 1990; Lee et al., 1990; Sarver and Krueger, 1991). Methods that use FTIR to obtain estimates of secondary structure fall into two main categories, those that use deconvolution or resolution enhancement techniques and those that use linear least-squares fits to spectra of proteins with known structures. The last four of the methods cited above are in the latter category, and these are currently (in this author's opinion) the methods of choice for FTIR secondary structure content determinations.

The best least-squares methods follow the general strategy described by Provencher and Glöckner (1981) or Hennessey and Johnson (1981), whereby spectra of proteins with known structures are fitted to the spectrum of the unknown protein. The solution to this least-squares problem is then transformed into fractions of secondary structure. Several different least-squares algorithms have been described.

Those that are least vulnerable to numerical instability are probably those that use singular value decomposition (Lawson and Hanson, 1974), also refered to as *factor analysis*. Singular value decomposition gives rise to a set of "eigenspectra" (involving eigenvectors of spectra of the knowns) that contain all of the significant information present in the specctra of the knowns. These eigenspectra are fit to the spectrum of the unknown (Hennessey and Johnson, 1981). As with CD methods, details regarding the differences between the various approaches involving computational algorithms are probably not as important as the differences that exist between sets of reference proteins and artifacts that may arise due to the presence of membranes.

Sources of Error

The primary sources of error in FTIR measurements of membrane proteins and peptides have probably not become fully appreciated, since FTIR methods have only recently been applied to membrane proteins. Some of them probably contribute only a small error to the analysis. However, unlike the case for CD in which much effort has been devoted to understanding the artifacts caused by membranes, systematic studies of some of the possible errors inherent in FTIR of membrane proteins have not been carried out. This should be the focus of some of the work to be done in the next few years. Possible sources of artifacts are (*1*) incorrect assignment of secondary structures to frequencies in resolution enhancement techniques; (*2*) incomplete deuterium exchange (in methods that require D_2O as solvent); (*3*) inadequate correction for the spectrum of membrane-bound water; (*4*) interference from amino acid side chains, end groups, and lipids; and (*5*) the choice of reference proteins.

Resolution Enhancement Techniques

The technique known as *resolution enhancement* or *fourier self-deconvolution* was introduced by Susi and Byler (1983) and was developed into a useful tool (Susi and Byler, 1986, 1987, 1988; Surewicz and Mantsch, 1988). Two new methods have adopted this approach for secondary structure analysis of IR spectra (Goormaghtigh et al., 1990; Dong et al., 1990). This approach uses a mathematical transformation of the spectrum to cause narrowing of overlapping bands detected in the original spectrum in order to make the resolution appear to be better than it is. The resulting bands are fit, using least-squares methods, with gaussian and/or lorentzian bandshapes at theoretically and empirically derived frequencies or are otherwise analyzed for secondary structure information according to their integrated area and frequency.

Errors will result if the experimentally measured frequencies and their associated secondary structure type are not correctly matched. Several examples of conflicting assignments can be found in the literature. For example, amide I frequencies observed and calculated by Krimm and Bandekar (1986) show that intense bands due to β-turns can occur at three frequencies assigned by Susi and Byler (1986) to unordered ($1,645 \pm 4$ cm^{-1}), helix ($1,653 \pm 4$ cm^{-1}), and extended chain ($1,675 \pm 5$ cm^{-1}) structures. Dong et al. (1990) make the following different assignments to virtually the same frequencies: β-sheet ($1,642 \pm 1$ cm^{-1}), unordered ($1,650 \pm 1$ cm^{-1}), and turn ($1,672 \pm 1$ cm^{-1}).

Fourier self-deconvolution is also subject to the introduction of artifacts arising from a loss of intensity information, reduction in the signal to noise ratio, distortions of spectral band shapes, and the use of subjective judgements in choosing deconvolution parameters (Surewicz and Mantsch, 1988). Use of the integrated intensities of resolution-enhanced bands is subject not only to errors arising from the loss of intensity information but also to differences that may systematically occur in the amide I intensities of bands due to different structure types. Moreover, resolution enhancement appears to be unnecessary to obtain accurate estimates of protein secondary structure, since the least-squares methods described above achieve a reasonable accuracy without using resolution enhancement methods.

Resolution enhancement methods continue to be used (Wu and Lentz, 1991) because for a limited number of proteins they appear to give an agreement with x-ray results that is better than that reported for the complete set of reference proteins in least-squares methods. Byler and Susi (1986) report excellent results for 11 proteins, for which standard deviations from x-ray–derived estimates (Levitt and Greer, 1977) for helix and β-sheet (or extended structure) are 2.3% and 4.3%, respectively. (The 4.3% value includes corrected values for the x-ray percent β-sheet for carbonic anhydrase and concanavalin A.) However, as more proteins are added to these statistics the agreement becomes worse. When only hemoglobin and myoglobin are added to the list, the standard deviations for helix and β-sheet become 4.9% and 9.8%, respectively. β-Sheet is not reliably measured in predominantly helical proteins. Moreover, the errors for helix content in helical proteins are about 10%, indicating that this approach is not useful for helical membrane proteins.

Nevertheless, these techniques do increase the extent to which overlapping bands can be visualized, and they do provide information about the average positions of bands due to different secondary structure types. In this respect they can be an important aid in accurately assigning frequencies to crowded vibrational modes, a step in the development of a force field, and in understanding, through visualization, the amide I spectrum of proteins. As vibrational force fields continue to be developed and refined, particularly with the aid of the SQMFF methodology (Fogarasi and Pulay, 1985), and if the errors for predominantly helical proteins can be corrected, Fourier self-deconvolution methods may find new applications.

Methods That Require Deuterium Exchange

Early attempts to devise a method for quantitating secondary structure using IR spectroscopy required that D_2O be used as the solvent (Grosse et al., 1972; Chirgadze et al., 1973; Chirgadze and Brazhnikov, 1974; Eckert et al., 1977; Byler and Susi, 1986). In this way, the very strong HOH bending absorption band between 1,600 and 1,680 cm^{-1} was avoided, allowing an analysis of the amide I' vibrations. Although this approach was partly successful, it required that all of the amide hydrogens in a protein should be completely exchanged with deuterium. This could not be guaranteed in every case for relatively large proteins. These methods may still be useful for measuring the conformation of smaller peptides in their interactions with membranes, where complete exchange can be ensured. Artifacts due to the unsubtracted spectrum of membrane-bound water could be avoided in this way. However, Dousseau and Pézolet (1990) have observed that their least-squares method is less accurate when it is applied to proteins in D_2O. Hydrogen–deuterium exchange is still used, nevertheless, to give information about membrane protein structure (Earnest et al., 1990).

Membrane-Bound Water

The spectrum of water bound to membranes is different from that of bulk water. This difference may be observed by subtracting the spectrum of bulk water from the spectrum of a lipid dispersion. This may present an obstacle to FTIR measurements of membrane protein secondary structure, particularly when the concentration of protein in the membrane is relatively low. The intense IR bending vibrations of H_2O overlap with the amide I region of the spectrum. Current methods for analyzing FTIR spectra of soluble proteins are successful at subtracting the spectrum of bulk water from this region. However, these methods have not been successfully applied to lipid dispersions (Dousseau and Pézolet, 1990). A possible solution to this problem is to subtract the spectrum of an aqueous lipid dispersion from the spectrum of the membrane-bound protein so that spectra of both bulk and bound water are eliminated. However, some assurances should be made that the lipid surface area in the blank is close enough to that in the sample so that the correction is adequate. The sample may also be dried to a point where it is hydrated by only the ambient humidity.

Interference from Amino Acid Side Chains, End Groups, and Lipids

Some amino acid side chains, and the peptide end groups, contribute significantly to the IR spectrum in the region of the amide I and II bands, interfering with the analysis of bands in this region for secondary structure information. This does not appear to be a serious problem for globular proteins in which the average distribution of side chains in each is about the same. However, membrane proteins, and peptides in general, may have a distribution of side chains that is different enough to cause artifacts. For example, the ionized side chains of aspartic and glutamic acids have a strong COO antisymmetrical stretching band at 1,560 cm^{-1}, and the ionized amine group of lysine has significant bands at 1,522 and 1,637 cm^{-1}, corresponding to the symmetrical and antisymmetrical bending modes of the NH_3^{+1} group. Venyaminov and Kalnin (1990a,b) have developed a procedure for subtracting the contributions from side chains and observe a marked improvement in the estimates of protein secondary structure when this procedure is used (Kalnin et al., 1990). This method appears to involve some subjective judgement, but shows the best agreement with secondary structure contents derived from x-ray coordinates (using the Levitt and Greer [1977] H-bond criteria) among the methods for analyzing IR spectra.

Lipid molecules also have vibrations that interfere in the amide I region. These vibrations include carbon–carbon double bonds, the ester $C=O$ stretch, the amine groups of phosphatidylethanolamine and phosphatidylserine, and the carboxylate group of phosphatidylserine. Most of these groups can be avoided in the selection of lipid, but this approach requires reconstitution. The ester $C=O$ stretch appears mostly above 1,700 cm^{-1}, but significant overlap with the amide I band can occur at high lipid to protein ratios. Subtraction of the spectrum of protein-free liposomes may not correct for this band, since it shifts in the presence of proteins. Subtraction of the ester $C=O$ stretch may be approximated by fitting the spectrum with gaussian or lorentzian functions.

Choice of Reference Proteins

The choice of reference proteins should ideally include representatives of the type and amount of secondary, and perhaps tertiary, structures contained in the unknown. The importance of this requirement is illustrated by the controversy surrounding the anomalous results obtained using both FTIR and CD of bacteriorhodopsin. If some of the helices in bacteriorhodopsin contain a significant amount of α_{II}-helix, as suggested by Krimm and Dwivedi (1982), a reference protein containing this structure is required. However, it may not be desirable to include this reference in the analysis of proteins with no α_{II}-helix, and it may not be possible to obtain a priori knowledge about which reference proteins to use.

Attenuated Total Reflection

Attenuated total reflection (reviewed by Braiman and Rothschild, 1988) can be used to determine secondary structure content, orientation of secondary structures, and the lipid to protein ratio (Goormaghtigh et al., 1990). While the secondary structure content estimates from this approach have a standard deviation of 8.6%, too high to be useful, the information about orientation (also reviewed by Braiman and Rothschild, 1988) is of interest.

Examples of the Use of FTIR Spectra for Membrane Protein Structure

Some examples of the use of FTIR in studies of membrane protein structure include the following. Measurements of secondary structure have been performed on porin (Kleffel et al., 1985), and measurements of the orientation of β-sheets have been performed in porin (Nabedryk et al., 1988), the photosystem II reaction center (He et al., 1991), myelin basic protein (Surewicz et al., 1987), gastric H^+,K^+-ATPase (Mitchell et al., 1988), acetylcholine receptor (Fong and McNamee, 1987), uncoupling protein from mitochondria (Rial et al., 1990), apolipoproteins in human HDL_3 particles (Herzyk et al., 1988), and a membrane-bound channel-forming peptide of colicin E1 (Rath et al., 1991). Orientation of secondary structure in bacteriorhodopsin has been studied recently by Draheim et al. (1991). Studies of the proton-pumping mechanism in bacteriorhodopsin have been performed by Braiman et al. (1988a,b). Han et al. (1991) have studied the structure of the formyl group on heme A.

Raman Spectroscopy

Raman spectroscopy is a measurement of the intensity of light scattered by the sample at frequencies shifted from the incident light frequency. A laser beam enters the sample cell (usually a small melting point capillary tube), and the scattered light is focused into a spectrometer. The incident laser light can be ultraviolet, blue, green, red, or infrared. Most of the light that is scattered by the sample is the same color as the incident light (Rayliegh scattering), but a very small fraction of that light is shifted in frequency. The spectrometer measures frequencies of the scattered light. The arithmetic difference between the incident laser frequency and the scattered light frequency is a vibrational frequency of the chemical group that gave rise to the scattered light. One of the best general introductions to Raman spectroscopy is still the review by Yu (1977).

A variety of methods for measuring protein secondary structure using Raman have been developed (Lippert et al., 1976; Pézolet et al., 1976; Williams et al., 1980a,b; Williams and Dunker, 1981; Williams, 1983, 1986; Thomas and Agard, 1984; Berjot et al., 1987; Bussian and Sander, 1989). The method used most frequently in measurements of membrane proteins (Williams, 1983, 1986) employs least-squares techniques, described above for FTIR methods. The standard deviations for this method are 4%, 3%, and 2% for helix, β-strand, and reverse-turn structures, respectively, using the singular value decomposition approach. Constrained least-squares yields estimated errors that are 1% higher. However, as with FTIR and CD results, the presence of membranes probably yields errors that are higher. The most recent method (Bussian and Sander, 1989) uses the reference data from Williams (1986), but simplifies the computational analysis.

Sources of Error

The primary sources of error in Raman measurements of membrane proteins are likely to be (*1*) poor signal to noise ratio due to background fluorescence; (*2*) overlapping bands due to side chains and lipids; (*3*) inadequate subtraction of the spectrum of water; (*4*) frequency shifts due to errors in spectrometer calibration; and (*5*), as with FTIR methods, the choice of reference spectra.

Fluorescence

The most serious obstacle to the collection of Raman spectra of membrane proteins is the background fluorescence that is excited from extremely small amounts of chromophoric impurities by the extraordinarily intense monochromatic laser light. The presence of lipids makes this problem worse because fluorescent impurities that partition into the hydrophobic lipid bilayer are no longer subject to quenching from low-lying electronic states to the high-frequency vibrational states of water, and native membranes frequently bring many fluorescent "impurities" with them. The fluorescence background can typically be 10 to 30 times as intense as the spectrum of the membrane, in measurements that are successful, and higher levels frequently make measurements of membranes impossible. Colored membrane proteins such as bacteriorhodopsin that absorb the incident laser radiation, typically green light at 514.5 nm, cannot be studied with conventional Raman instruments. For colorless samples, it is difficult to obtain a noise-free spectrum of a membrane protein in a reasonable amount of time. Data collection may require as much as 24 hours of laser time for a single spectrum. This makes it difficult and expensive to collect large numbers of spectra—as a function of the concentration of one of the components, for example.

There are some measures that can reduce the fluorescence problem to levels that make measurements possible. Charcoal can be added to the sample at various stages during purification and preparation to bind hydrophobic impurities. This step can dramatically reduce fluorescence in some samples, but care must be taken that the charcoal does not adversely change the sample composition, and particles of charcoal must not be in the laser beam path. Impurities may be photobleached by long exposures to the laser light, and this is almost always necessary to some extent, but care must be taken that the sample is not overheated by the beam. This may be achieved by starting at low power levels with an unfocused beam. Other strategies may include preparing and storing samples under nitrogen and using very pure lipids in reconstitution experiments. However, more effective alternatives have become available. CCD detectors, used in conjunction with laser frequencies above 700 nm, may provide a solution to the fluorescence problem and may allow Raman secondary structure measurements of chromophoric proteins such as bacteriorhodopsin. Fourier-transform Raman instruments also provide a solution to the fluorescence problem.

Charge-Coupled Device Detectors

The CCD facilitates avoidance of the fluorescence that can be a serious problem in visible Raman measurements of membranes. CCDs have as much as three times the quantum efficiency of photomultiplier tubes and intensified diode arrays (IDAs), and the sensitivity extends further into the red, going as far as 1,000 nm. This allows the detector to be used effectively with red laser illumination of the sample. Consequently, using laser illumination at wavelengths near or longer than 750 nm, interference from fluorescence can be virtually eliminated. A number of lasers can be used to provide light at these frequencies. The krypton ion laser with a line at 752 nm appears to be a good choice. Titanium-sapphire lasers are tunable and allow adjustments to avoid fluorescence between 700 and 1,000 nm. A description of the CCD detector and examples of its usefulness in Raman measurements of fluorescent samples can be found in the article by Pemberton et al. (1990).

CCDs have several advantages over IDAs. CCDs have a dynamic range that is about 40 times that of IDAs. IDAs also suffer from a higher level of background noise than CCDs. The dark current from cooled IDA detectors is generally more than 100,000 times as high as it is from liquid-nitrogen-cooled CCDs. CCDs also have a substantially larger surface area than do diode array detectors due to their larger vertical dimension (10.25 vs. 2.5 mm). This allows the CCD to collect four to five times as much light as the diode array. Alternatively, it can allow simultaneous collection of data from two samples, providing a means of obtaining shift-free difference spectra. The high sensitivity of the CCD allows Raman measurements of solutes at concentrations as low as 0.002% by weight (2×10^{-5} g/ml) with only 15 min of integration time using only 25 mw of 620 nm He–Ne radiation (Pemberton et al., 1990).

Studies of membrane protein secondary structure using CCD detection have not appeared yet. Unforseen problems may appear as instruments of this type become more prevalent. However, it is more likely that these instruments will make an important contribution to vibrational measurements of membrane proteins.

Fourier-Transform Raman Spectroscopy

FT-Raman instruments consist essentially of a YAG laser emitting 1,064 nm light and an FTIR instrument to measure light scattered from the sample. The 1,064 nm excitation produces virtually no fluorescence, so that even with an extremely weak signal (the light scattering intensity at this wavelength suffers from the $1/\lambda^4$ dependence) it is possible to obtain Raman spectra of colored samples. Studies of membrane protein secondary structure using FT-Raman measurements have not appeared, however. This is probably at least partly due to the relative newness of this technique and to the relative paucity of instruments. There are some technical difficulties associated with aqueous samples and temperature control, but until more experimental results are reported it will be difficult to predict how well this technique will overcome the difficulties associated with dispersive Raman experiments.

Overlapping Bands from Side Chains and Lipids

Raman amide I spectra are subject to interference from side chains and lipid bands as are FTIR measurements (see earlier under Fourier-Transform Infrared Spectroscopy). Corrections for the amide groups of asparagine and glutamine have not improved secondary structure estimates of the water-soluble reference proteins (Williams, 1986), but they may be necessary for membrane proteins and peptides. An example of corrections for bands from lipid acyl chains is given by Williams et al. (1986).

Corrections for the Spectrum of Water

Raman spectra of membrane proteins probably suffer less from the subtraction of the spectrum of water than do FTIR spectra. The intensity of IR absorption bands is proportional to dipole moment strength, whereas Raman band intensity is proportional to the molecular polarizability. Carbon–carbon bonds that have a low dipole moment and a high polarizability show stretching frequency bands that are weak in the IR spectrum and strong in the Raman spectrum. Water, on the other hand, has a high dipole moment and consequently shows very strong absorption bands in the IR, but relatively weak Raman scattering. Consequently, artifacts from subtraction of the spectrum of water from the Raman spectrum of a membrane protein are likely to be substantially smaller than they are in FTIR spectra. The presence of lipids can also lower the accuracy of subtractions of the spectrum of water from both Raman and FTIR spectra. This can occur because the lipid ester $C=O$ stretch, from about $1{,}700 \text{ cm}^{-1}$ to about $1{,}770 \text{ cm}^{-1}$, interferes with the region of the spectrum that can be used to gauge the intensity of the H–O–H bending spectrum of water. As with FTIR spectra, the subtraction of the spectrum of a liposome blank may lessen these artifacts, but the ester $C=O$ stretch may be shifted significantly by the presence of membrane-bound proteins.

Frequency Shifts due to Errors in Calibration

Dispersive Raman instruments are subject to drift in their wave number calibration due to small shifts in the mechanical tolerances and temperature fluctuations. Spectra of the same sample collected on subsequent days may differ by a fraction of a wave number (cm^{-1}). This makes the use of difference spectra to detect small structural changes and isotope effect shifts difficult. Over time these shifts can amount to several wave numbers in some instruments. As observed earlier (Williams, 1986), a 1 cm^{-1}

shift from the calibration setting at which the reference spectra were collected will produce a 3% shift in the relative content of β-strand and helix. The use of a CCD detector may reduce or solve the problem related to difference spectra. A daily log of the spectrometer shift, relative to a known mercury vapor line such as 546.074 nm, will solve the calibration problem. Investigators who use the database measured in this laboratory (Williams, 1986; Bussian and Sander, 1989) should keep in mind that these reference spectra are shifted 1.7 Δcm^{-1} higher than they would be if the spectrometer were perfectly adjusted. This means that spectra of unknowns should be shifted upward by 1.7 Δcm^{-1} prior to the least-squares procedure.

Examples of the Use of Raman Spectra for Membrane Protein Structure

Raman measurements have been made on a variety of membrane proteins and peptides. For example, protein secondary structure measurements have been made of lipid–fd coat protein complexes (Dunker et al., 1982), the acetylcholine receptor (Yager et al., 1984), lactose permease (Vogel et al., 1985), the calcium pump protein in sarcoplasmic reticulum (Williams et al., 1986), outer membrane proteins of *E. coli* (Vogel and Jähnig, 1986a), melittin in membranes (Vogel and Jähnig, 1986b), substance P in liposomes (Williams and Weaver, 1990), and the antimicrobial frog peptides magainin and PGLa (Williams et al., 1990).

Circular Dichroism Spectroscopy

There are several methods currently in use to quantitate secondary structure using CD spectroscopy (Bolotina et al., 1980, 1981; Brahms and Brahms, 1980; Chang et al., 1978; Hennessey and Johnson, 1981; Provencher and Glöckner, 1981; Compton and Johnson, 1986; Manavalan and Johnson, 1987). Investigators interested in performing these calculations should read the article by Yang et al. (1986) (with which software is included). The calculations for membrane proteins are the same as those for soluble proteins, except where wavelength limits are a factor and where corrections for absorption flattening may be performed. Those methods that use the general approach described by Provencher and Glöckner (1981), in which spectra of proteins with known structure are fitted to the spectrum of the unknown protein via a singular value decomposition (Lawson and Hanson, 1974) of those spectra into "eigenspectra" (Hennessey and Johnson, 1981), and the results are then transformed into fractions of secondary structure, are generally acknowledged to be the best. Other details regarding the differences between these methods, involving computational algorithms, are probably not important relative to the artifacts that enter the equation due to the presence of membranes.

Sources of Error

The primary sources of error in CD measurements of membrane proteins and peptides are (*1*) inaccurate determinations of protein concentration (or choice of reference spectra), (*2*) circular differential absorption flattening (CDAF), (*3*) circular differential scattering (CDS), (*4*) lack of data below 200 nm, and (*5*) normalization of data. Discussions of other errors in CD estimates of protein secondary structure have been published by Hennessey and Johnson (1982), and Khan et al. (1989).

Protein Concentration

Different methods for determination of protein concentration can yield CD spectra that differ significantly. The preferred method for determination of membrane protein concentration is a modification of the Lowry method (Peterson, 1977). Studies of bacteriorhodopsin provide an example of how much confidence has been placed in these methods; normalization of results was proposed as a correction of incorrect determinations of concentration (Mao and Wallace, 1984). However, in light of the controversy over CD spectra of bacteriorhodopsin and normalization, discussed at the beginning of this chapter, Glaeser and Jap (1985) have suggested some alternative methods.

Since FTIR also shows low estimates of the helix content in bacteriorhodopsin (suggesting that there is something unusual about those helical structures), and because there is no compelling evidence that protein determinations for bacteriorhodopsin (and other proteins) are actually in error, normalization of CD results appears to be an arbitrary and cosmetic procedure. The anomalous results for bacteriorhodopsin may be due to an inadequately representative set of reference CD spectra, as discussed above for FTIR and Raman methods. Concentrations can also be determined gravimetrically in the case of synthetic peptides or when purified proteins are reconstituted into liposomes. It may be useful to show that at least two methods of protein concentration determination agree. Two recent papers discuss new ways to eliminate interferences from the Lowry method (Rodríguez-Vico et al., 1989; van Stokkum et al., 1990). Adsorption of proteins and liposomes onto glass surfaces can significantly affect protein concentrations. This problem can be minimized by using plastic or siliconized containers and by wetting cells before adding the membrane solution (Wu and Chen, 1989).

Absorption Flattening

Both CDAF and CDS are discussed by Tinoco et al. (1983), Wallace and Mao (1984), and Heyn (1989). Investigators who wish to perform CD measurements of membrane protein structure need to be familiar with these papers and many of the references cited therein.

CDAF arises from high localized concentrations of proteins in membranes. It appears to be the most significant artifact in CD spectra of membranes. Although membrane particles may be randomly distributed in solution, the protein molecules are not. The probability of photons being absorbed by protein molecules is lowered in this case, defeating the validity of the Beer-Lambert law:

$$A(\lambda) = -\log_{10} \frac{I}{I_0} = \epsilon l c$$

There are two methods for detecting and correcting for CDAF. Reconstitution of membrane proteins into small unilamellar vesicles (SUVs) effectively dilutes the local concentration of protein and decreases CDS as well (Mao and Wallace, 1984). "However, not all membrane proteins can be incorporated into SUVs in active forms." To solve this problem, Wallace and Mao (1984) have developed the flattening quotient method. The effects of absorption flattening are first measured using ultraviolet absorption measurements in the absence and presence of detergent. Solubilization in detergent dilutes the local protein concentration. Unpolarized ultraviolet spectra in the region of interest are relatively insensitive to protein conformation, so the difference between these measurements contains only the CDAF effects. This result can then be used to correct CD spectra computationally that have otherwise been corrected for CDS.

Differential Scattering

CDS arises from a differential scattering of left- and right-handed circularly polarized light, caused by long-range chiral arrangements of scattering particles. Much of the scattered light may not hit the detector. The CD spectrum is a combination of differentially absorbed and scattered light,

$$c[\Theta] = \epsilon_L - \epsilon_R = (a_L - a_R) + (s_L - s_R)$$

where the extinction coefficient is a sum of the absorption coefficient (a) and the scattering coefficient (s). Artifacts may occur in the spectrum if the difference in scattering between left and right circularly polarized light, $s_L - s_R$, is large relative to differential absorption.

There are two preferred ways to detect and correct for CDS. Moving the sample closer to the detector appears to reduce CDS to an acceptable level in the case of bacteriorhodopsin in purple membrane sheets (Wallace and Mao, 1984). However, this approach may also make CDS artifacts worse (Reich et al., 1980). The usefulness of this method should be established for each new system. Fluorescence-detected CD (FDCD) allows for collection of all of the scattered and transmitted light (Reich et al., 1980) by introducing a fluorescent probe molecule, whose excitation profile covers the range from 185 to 240 nm, directly into the sample solution. Fluorescence emitted by the probe is detected at right angles to the incident light. However, some concern has been expressed that the probe excitation and emission profiles may be changed as it partitions into lipid bilayers and that the probe may change the structure of the protein (Wallace and Mao, 1984).

Wavelength Limits

The dependence of conformation estimates on the lower wavelength limit available to the experimenter has been analyzed by Venyaminov et al. (1991). They compared CD and x-ray results for a number of reference proteins using lower wavelength limits that varied from 190 to 235 nm at 5 nm intervals. The results show that estimates of helix content are relatively accurate, even when only a small segment of the CD spectrum is analyzed. However, accurate estimates of β-sheet content appear to require data down to 190 nm, and estimates based on a limit of 205 nm can show large errors.

Normalization of Spectra

Many authors have used some form of normalization to obtain a sum of the fractions of secondary structure types that is equal to 1. It has been proposed, for example, that normalization of the results of CD calculations, by dividing each fraction by the sum of fractions of structure, may correct for inaccurate measurements of protein concentration (Mao et al., 1982; Mao and Wallace, 1984). Normalization brings the measured fraction of helix in bacteriorhodopsin into agreement with estimates from low-resolution x-ray diffraction results, but results that are not normalized give a fraction of helix that is nearly 30% lower (Glaeser and Jap, 1985). In another example, measurements from CD studies of the conformation of substance P bound to membranes are normalized in a dramatic way to yield an estimate of 40% helix (Rolka et al., 1986). However, an analysis without normalization indicates essentially no helix (Williams and Weaver, 1990), a result that is confirmed by Raman measurements. Authors who wish to continue the practice of normalizing CD results should be familiar with the paper of Glaeser and Jap (1985) and should provide a more convincing justification of normalization than has been provided previously.

Examples of the Use of Circular Dichroism Spectra for Membrane Protein Structure

CD has been used in a variety of studies on membrane proteins; some examples are cited below. Information about the orientation of secondary structure elements can be obtained from CD spectra (Bazzi and Woody, 1985). CD can also provide information about the state of aggregation of membrane proteins (Heyn, 1989). Measurements of secondary structure have been performed on apolipoprotein E (Mims et al., 1990), gap junction protein (Cascio et al., 1990), porin (Eisele and Rosenbusch, 1990), acetylcholine receptor (Mielke and Wallace, 1988), a membrane-bound peptide from lipophilin (Kahan et al., 1988), the main intrinsic polypeptide from lens plasma membranes (Horwitz and Bok, 1987), the human erythrocyte anion transport protein (Werner and Reithmeier, 1985), the fd phage gene 8 protein (Fodor et al., 1981), and cytochrome b_5 (Dailey and Strittmatter, 1978).

References

Bazzi, M., and Woody, R. W. (1985) Oriented secondary structure in integral membrane proteins. *Biophys. J.* 48: 957–966.

Berjot, M., Marx, J., and Alix, A.J.P. (1987) The determination of the secondary structure of proteins from the Raman amide I band: the reference intensity profiles method. *J. Raman Spec.* 18: 289–300.

Bolotina, I. A., Chekhov, V. O., Lugauskas, V. Y., and Ptitsyn, O. B. (1980) Determination of the secondary structure of proteins from the circular dichroism spectra. II. Consideration of the contribution of β-bends. *Mol. Biol.* (Mosc.) 14: 709–715.

Bolotina, I. A., Chekhov, V. O., Lugauskas, V. Y., and Ptitsyn, O. B. (1981) Determination of the secondary structure of proteins from the circular dichroism spectra. III. Protein-derived reference spectra for antiparallel and parallel β-structures. *Mol. Biol.* (Mosc.) 15: 130–137.

Brahms, S., and Brahms, J. (1980) Determination of protein secondary structure in solution by vacuum ultraviolet circular dichroism. *J. Mol. Biol.* 138: 149–178.

Braiman, M. S., Mogi, T., Marti, T., Stern, L. J., Hackett, N. R., Chao, B. H,. Khorana, H. G., and Rothschild, K. J. (1988a) Vibrational spectroscopy of bacteriorhodopsin mutants: I. Tyrosine-185 protonates and deprotonates during the photocycle. *Proteins Struct. Funct. Genet.* 3: 219–229.

Braiman, M. S., Mogi, T., Marti, T., Stern, L. J., Khorana, H. G., and Rothschild, K. J. (1988b) Vibrational spectroscopy of bacteriorhodopsin mutants: light-driven protein transport involves protonation changes of aspartic acid residues 85, 96, and 212. *Biochemistry* 27: 8516–8520.

Braiman, M. S. and Rothschild, K. J. (1988) Fourier transform infrared techniques for probing membrane protein structure. *Annu. Rev. Biophys. Biophys. Chem.* 17: 541–570.

Bussian, B. M., and Sander, C. (1989) How to determine protein secondary structure in solution by Raman spectroscopy: practical guide and test case DNase I. *Biochemistry* 28: 4271–4277.

Byler, M., and Susi, H. (1986) Examination of the secondary structure of proteins by deconvolved FTIR spectra. *Biopolymers* 25: 469–487.

Cascio, M., Gogol, E., and Wallace, B. A. (1990) The secondary structure of gap junctions. *J. Biol. Chem.* 265: 2358–2364.

Chang, C. T., Wu, C. S., and Yang, J. T. (1978) Circular dichroic analysis of protein conformation: inclusion of the β-turns. *Anal. Biochem.* 92: 13–31.

Chirgadze, Y. N., Shestopalov, B. V., and Venyaminov, S. Y. (1973) Intensities and other spectral parameters of infrared amide bands of polypeptides in the β- and random forms. *Biopolymers* 12: 1337–1351.

Chirgadze, Y. N., and Brazhnikov, E. V. (1974) Intensities and other spectral parameters of infrared amide bands of polypeptides in the α-helical form. *Biopolymers* 13: 1701–1712.

Compton, L. A., and Johnson, W. C. Jr. (1986) Analysis of protein circular dichroism spectra for secondary structure using a simple matrix multiplication. *Anal. Biochem.* 155: 155–167.

Dailey, H. A., and Strittmatter, P. (1978) Structural and functional properties of the membrane binding segment of cytochrome b_5. *J. Biol. Chem.* 253: 8203–8209.

Dong, A., Huang, P., and Caughey, W. S. (1990) Protein secondary structures in water from second-derivative amide I infrared spectra. *Biochemistry* 29: 3303–3308.

Dousseau, F., and Pézolet, M. (1990) Determination of the secondary structure content of proteins in aqueous solutions from their amide I and amide II infrared bands. Comparison between classical and partial least-squares methods. *Biochemistry* 29: 8771–8779.

Draheim, J. E., Gibson, N. J., and Cassim, J. Y. (1991) Dramatic in situ conformational dynamics of the transmembrane protein bacteriorhodopsin. *Biophys. J.* 60: 89–100.

Dunker, A. K., Fodor, S., and Williams, R. W. (1982) Lipid dependent structural changes of an amphomorphic membrane protein. *Biophys. J.* 37: 201–203.

Eisele, J. L., and Rosenbusch, J. P. (1990) In vitro folding and oligomerization of a membrane protein. *J. Biol. Chem.* 265: 10217–10220.

Eckert, K., Grosse, R., Malur, J., and Repke, K.R.H. (1977) Calculation and use of protein-derived conformation related spectra for the estimate of the secondary structure of proteins from their infrared spectra. *Biopolymers* 16: 2549–2563.

Earnest, T. N., Herzfeld, J., and Rothschild, K. J. (1990) Polarized FTIR of bacteriorhodopsin: transmembrane α-helices are resistant to hydrogen–deuterium exchange. *Biophys. J.* 58: 1539–1546.

Fodor, S.P.A., Dunker, A. K., Ng, Y. C., Carsten, D., and Williams, R. W. (1981) Lipid-tail group dependent structure of the fd gene 8 protein. In: *Bacteriophage Assembly.* New York: Alan R. Liss, Inc., pp. 441–455.

Fogarasi, G., and Pulay, P. (1985) Ab initio calculation of force fields and vibrational spectra. In: *Vibrational Spectra and Structure: a Series of Advances,* edited by J. R. Durig. New York: Elsevier, vol. 14, pp. 125–219.

Fong, T. M., and McNamee, M. G. (1987) Stabilization of acetylcholine receptor secondary structure by cholesterol and negatively charged phospholipids in membranes. *Biochemistry* 26: 3871–3880.

Frisch, M. J., Head-Gordon, M., Schlegel, H. B. Raghavachari, K., Binkley, J. S., Gonzalez, C., Defrees, D. J., Fox, D. J., Whiteside, R. A., Seeger, R. C., Melius, F., Baker, J., Martin, R. L., Kahn, L. R., Stewart, J.J.P., Fluder, E. M., Topiol, S., and Pople, J. A. (1989) *Gaussian 90.* Pittsburgh: Gaussian, Inc.

Glaeser, R. M., Downing, K. H., and Jap, B. K. (1991) What spectroscopy can still tell us about the secondary structure of bacteriorhodopsin. *Biophys. J.* 59: 934–938.

Glaeser, R. M., and Jap, B. K. (1985) Absorption flattening in the circular dichroism spectra of small membrane fragments. *Biochemistry* 24: 6398–6401.

Goormaghtigh, E., Cabiaux, V., and Ruysschaert, J. M. (1990) Secondary structure and dosage of soluble and membrane proteins by attenuated total reflection Fourier-transform infrared spectroscopy on hydrated films. *Eur. J. Biochem.* 193: 409–420.

Grosse, R., Malur, J., and Repke, K.R.H. (1972) Determination of secondary structures in isolated or membrane proteins by computer curve-fitting analysis of infrared and circular dichroic spectra. *FEBS Lett.* 25: 313–315.

Han, S., Ching, Y., Hammes, S. L., and Rousseau, D. L. (1991) Vibrational structure of the formyl group on heme A. *Biophys. J.* 60: 45–52.

He, W.-Z., Newell, W. R., Haris, P. I., Chapman, D. and Barber, J. (1991) Protein secondary structure of the isolated photosystem II reaction center and conformational changes studied by Fourier transform infrared spectroscopy. *Biochemistry* 30: 4552–4559.

Hennessey, J. P., Jr., and Johnson, W. C., Jr. (1981) Information content in the circular dichroism of proteins. *Biochemistry* 20: 1085–1094.

Hennessey, J. P., Jr., and Johnson, W. C., Jr. (1982) Experimental errors and their effect on analyzing circular dichroism spectra of proteins. *Anal. Biochem.* 125: 177–188.

Herzyk, E., Owen, J. S., and Chapman, D. (1988) The secondary structure of apolipoproteins in human HDL$_3$ particles after chemical modification of their tyrosine, lysine, cysteine or arginine residues. A Fourier transform infrared spectroscopy study. *Biochim. Biophys. Acta* 962: 131–142.

Heyn, M. P. (1989) Circular dichroism for determining secondary structure and state of aggregation of membrane proteins. *Methods Enzymol.* 172: 575–584.

Horwitz, J., and Bok, D. (1987) Conformational properties of the main intrinsic polypeptide (MIP26) isolated from lens plasma membranes. *Biochemistry* 26: 8092–8098.

Hunt, J. F., Earnest, T. N., Bousche, O., Engelman, D. M., and Rothschild, K. J. (1993) The origin of the anomalous amide I vibrational frequency of purple membrane. *Biophys. J.* 64: A293.

Jap, B. K., Maestre, M. F., Hayward, S. B., and Glaeser, R. M. (1983) Peptide-chain secondary structure of bacteriorhodopsin. *Biophys. J.* 43: 81–89.

Kahan, I., Epand, R. M., and Moscarello, M. A. (1988) The secondary structure of a membrane-embedded peptide from the carboxy terminus of lipophilin as revealed by circular dichroism. *Biochim. Biophys. Acta* 952: 230–237.

Kalnin, N. N., Baikalov, I. A., and Venyaminov, S. Y. (1990) Quantitative IR spectrophotometry of peptide compounds in water (H$_2$O) solutions. III. Estimation of the protein secondary structure. *Biopolymers* 30: 1273–1280.

Khan, M. Y., Villanueva, G., and Newman, S. A. (1989) On the origin of the positive band in the far-ultraviolet circular dichroic spectrum of fibronectin. *J. Biol. Chem.* 264: 2139–2142.

Kleffel, B., Garavito, R. M., and Baumeister, W. (1985) Secondary structure of a channel-forming protein: porin from *E. coli* outer membranes. *EMBO J.* 4: 1589–1592.

Krimm, S., and Bandekar, J. (1986) Vibrational spectroscopy and conformation of peptides, polypeptides, and proteins. in *Adv. Protein Chem.* 38: 183–364.

Krimm, S., and Dwivedi, A. M. (1982) Infrared spectrum of the purple membrane: clue to a proton conduction mechanism? *Science* 216: 407–408.

Lawson, C. L., and Hanson, F. J. (1974) *Solving Least Squares Problems.* Englewood Cliffs, NJ: Prentice-Hall, Inc.

Lee, D. C., Haris, P. I., Chapman, D., and Mitchell, R. C. (1990) Determination of protein secondary structure using factor analysis of infrared spectra. *Biochemistry* 29: 9185–9193.

Levitt, M., and Greer, J. (1977) Automatic identification of secondary structure in globular proteins. *J. Mol. Biol.* 114: 181–293.

Lippert, J. L., Tyminski, D., and Desmeules, P. J. (1976) Determination of the secondary structure of proteins by laser Raman spectroscopy. *J. Am. Chem. Soc.* 98: 7075–7080.

Manavalan, P., and Johnson, W. C. Jr. (1987) Variable selection method improves the prediction of protein secondary structure from circular dichroism spectra. *Anal. Biochem.* 167: 76–85.

Mao, D., and Wallace, B. A. (1984) Differential light scattering and absorption flattening optical effects are minimal in the circular dichroism spectra of small unilamellar vesicles. *Biochemistry* 23: 2667–2673.

Mao, D., Wachter, E., and Wallace, B. A. (1982) Folding of the mitochondrial proton adenosinetriphosphatase proteolipid channel in phospholipid vesicles. *Biochemistry* 21: 4960–4968.

Mielke, D. L., and Wallace, B. A. (1988) Secondary structural analyses of the nicotinic acetylcholine receptor as a test of molecular models. *J. Biol. Chem.* 263: 3177–3182.

Mims, M. P., Soma, M. R., and Morrisett, J. D. (1990) Effect of particle size and temperature on the conformation and physiological behavior of apolipoprotein E bound to model lipoprotein particles. *Biochemistry* 29: 6639–6647.

Mitchell, R. C., Haris, P. I., Fallowfield, C., Keeling, D. J., and Chapman, D. (1988) Fourier transform infrared spectroscopic studies on gastric H^+/K^+-ATPase. *Biochim. Biophys. Acta* 941: 31–38.

Nabedryk, E., Garavito, R. M., and Breton, J. (1988) The orientation of β-sheets in porin. A polarized Fourier transform infrared spectroscopic investigation. *Biophys. J.* 53: 671–676.

Palmö, K., Pietilä, L.-O, and Krimm, S. (1991) Construction of molecular mechanics energy functions by mathematical transformation of ab initio force fields and structures. *J. Comp. Chem.* 12: 385–390.

Pemberton, J. E., Sobocinski, R. L., Bryant, M. A., and Carter, D. A. (1990) Raman spectroscopy using charge-coupled device detection. *Spectroscopy* 5: 26–36.

Peterson, G. L. (1977) A simplification of the protein assay method of Lowry et al which is more generally applicable. *Anal. Biochem.* 83: 346–356.

Pézolet, M., Pigeon-Gosselin, M., and Coulombe, L. (1976) Laser Raman investigation of the conformation of human immunoglobulin G. *Biochim. Biophys. Acta* 453: 502–512.

Provencher, S. W., and Glöckner, J. (1981) Estimation of globular protein secondary structure from circular dichroism. *Biochemistry* 20: 33–37.

Rath, P., Bousché, O., Merril, A. R., Cramer, W. A., and Rothschild, K. J. (1991) Fourier transform infrared evidence for a predominantly alpha-helical structure of the membrane bound channel forming COOH-terminal peptide of colicin E1. *Biophys. J.* 59: 516–522.

Reich, C., Maestre, M. F., Edmondson, S., and Gray, D. M. (1980) Circular dichroism and fluorescence-detected circular dichroism of deoxyribonucleic acid and poly[d(A − C) · d(G − T)] in ethanolic solutions: a new method for estimating circular intensity differential scattering. *Biochemistry* 19: 5208–5213.

Rial, E., Muga, A., Valpuesta, J. M., Arrondo, J.L.R., and Goni, F. M. (1990) Infrared spectroscopic studies of detergent-solubilized uncoupling protein from brown-adipose-tissue mitochondria. *Eur. J. Biochem.* 188: 83–89.

Rodríguez-Vico, R., Martínez-Cayuela, M., García-Peregrín, E., and Ramírez, H. (1989) A procedure for eliminating interferences in the Lowry method of protein determination. *Anal. Biochem.* 183: 275–278.

Rolka, K., Erne, D., and Schwyzer, R. (1986) Membrane structure of substance P II. Secondary structure of substance P, [9-leucine]substance P, and shorter segments in 2,2,2-trifluoroethanol, methanol, and on liposomes studied by circular dichroism. *Helv. Chim. Acta* 69: 1798–1806.

Sarver Jr., R. W., and Krueger, W. C. (1991) Protein secondary structure from Fourier transform infrared spectroscopy: a data base analysis. *Anal. Biochem.* 194: 89–100.

Surewicz, W. K., and Mantsch, H. H. (1988) New insight into protein secondary structure from resolution-enhanced infrared spectra. *Biochim. Biophys. Acta* 952: 115–130.

Surewicz, W. K., Moscarello, M. A., and Mantsch, H. H. (1987) Fourier transform infrared spectroscopic investigation of the interaction between myelin basic protein and dimyristoylphosphatidylglycerol bilayers. *Biochemistry* 26: 3881–3886.

Susi, H., and Byler, M. (1983) Protein structure by Fourier transform infrared spectroscopy: second derivative spectra. *Biochem. Biophys. Res. Commun.* 115: 391–397.

Susi, H., and Byler, M. (1986) Resolution-enhanced Fourier transform infrared spectroscopy of enzymes. *Methods Enzymol.* 130: 290–311.

Susi, H., and Byler, M. (1987) Fourier transform infrared study of proteins with parallel β-chains. *Arch. Biochem. Biophys.* 258: 465–469.

Susi, H., and Byler, M. (1988) Fourier deconvolution of the amide I Raman band of proteins as related to conformation. *Appl. Spec.* 42: 819–826.

Thomas, G. J., Jr., and Agard, D. A. (1984) Quantitative analysis of nucleic acids, proteins, and viruses by Raman band deconvolution. *Biophys. J.* 46: 763–768.

Tinoco, I., Jr., Maestre, M. F., and Bustamante, C. (1983) Circular dichroism in samples which scatter light. *Trends Biochem. Sci.* 8: 41–44.

Torii, H., and Tasumi, M. (1992) Model calculations on the amide-I infrared bands of globular proteins. *J. Chem. Phys.* 96: 3379–3387.

van Stokkum, I.H.M., Spoelder, H.J.W., Bloemendal, M., van Grondelle, R., and Groen, F.C.A. (1990) Estimation of protein secondary structure and error analysis from circular dichroism spectra. *Anal. Biochem.* 191: 110–118.

Venyaminov, S. Y., Baikalov, I. A., Wu, C.-S.C., and Yang, J. T. (1991) Some problems of CD analyses of protein conformation. *Anal. Biochem.* 198: 250–255.

Venyaminov, S. Y., and Kalnin, N. N. (1990a) Quantitative IR spectrophotometry of peptide compounds in water (H₂O) solutions. I. Spectral parameters of amino acid residue absorption bands. *Biopolymers* 30: 1243–1257.

Venyaminov, S. Y., and Kalnin, N. N. (1990b) Quantitative IR spectrophotometry of peptide compounds in water (H₂O) solutions. II. Amide absorption bands of polypeptides and fibrous proteins in alpha-, beta-, and random coil conformations. *Biopolymers* 30: 1259–1271.

Vogel, H., and Jähnig, F. (1986a) Models for the structure of outer-membrane proteins of *Escherichia coli* derived from Raman spectroscopy and prediction methods. *J. Mol. Biol.* 190: 191–199.

Vogel, H., and Jähnig, F. (1986b) The structure of mellitin in membranes. *Biophys. J.* 50: 573–582.

Vogel, H., Wright, J. K., and Jähnig, F. (1985) The structure of the lactose permease derived from Raman spectroscopy and prediction methods. *EMBO J.* 4: 3625–3631.

Wallace, B. A., and Mao, D. (1984) Circular dichroism analyses of membrane proteins: an examination of differential light scattering and absorption flattening effects in large membrane vesicles and membrane sheets. *Anal. Biochem.* 142: 317–328.

Weaver, J., and Williams, R. W. (1990) Amide III frequencies for Ala-X peptides depend on the X amino acid size. *Biopolymers* 30: 593–598.

Werner, P. K., and Reithmeier, R.A.F. (1985) Molecular characterization of the human erythrocyte anion transport protein in octyl glucoside. *Biochemistry* 24: 6375–6381.

Williams, R. W., Cutrera, T., Dunker, A. K., and Peticolas, W. L. (1980a) The estimation of protein secondary structure by laser Raman spectroscopy from the amide III intensity distribution. *FEBS Lett.* 115: 306–308.

Williams, R. W., Dunker, A. K., and Peticolas, W. L. (1980b) A new method for determining protein secondary structure by laser Raman spectroscopy applied to fd phage. *Biophys. J.* 32: 232–234.

Williams, R. W., and Dunker, A. K. (1981) Determination of the secondary structure of proteins from the amide I band of the laser Raman spectrum. *J. Mol. Biol.* 152: 783–813.

Williams, R. W. (1983) Estimation of protein secondary structure from the laser Raman amide I spectrum. *J. Mol. Biol.* 166: 581–603.

Williams, R. W. (1986) Protein secondary structure analysis using Raman amide I and amide III spectra. *Methods Enzymol.* 130: 311–331.

Williams, R. W., Lowrey, A. H., and Weaver, J. (1990) Relation between calculated amide frequencies and solution structure in Ala-X peptides. *Biopolymers* 30: 599–608.

Williams, R. W., McIntyre, J. O., Gaber, B. P., and Fleischer, S. (1986) The secondary structure of calcium pump protein in light sarcoplasmic reticulum and reconstituted in a single lipid component as determined by Raman spectroscopy. *J. Biol. Chem.* 261: 14520–14524.

Williams, R. W., and Weaver, J. (1990) Secondary structure of substance P bound to liposomes, in organic solvents, and in solution from Raman and CD spectroscopy. *J. Biol. Chem.* 265: 2505–2513.

Williams, R. W., Starman, R., Taylor, K.M.P., Gable, K., Beeler, T. Zasloff, M., and Covell, D. (1990) Raman spectroscopy of synthetic antimicrobial frog peptides magainin 2a and PGLa. *Biochemistry* 29: 4490–4496.

Wu, C.-S.C., and Chen, G. C. (1989) Adsorption of proteins onto glass surfaces and its effect on the intensity of circular dichroism spectra. *Anal. Biochem.* 177: 178–182.

Wu, J. R., and Lentz, B. R. (1991) Fourier transform infrared spectroscopic study of Ca²⁺ and membrane-induced secondary structural changes in bovine prothrombin fragment 1. *Biophys. J.* 60: 70–80.

Yager, P., Chang, E. L., Williams, R. W., and Dalziel, A. W. (1984) The secondary structure of acetylcholine receptor reconstituted in a single lipid component as determined by Raman spectroscopy. *Biophys. J.* 45: 26–28.

Yang, J. T., Wu, C.S.C., and Martinez, H. M. (1986) Calculation of protein conformation from circulation dichroism. *Methods Enzymol.* 130: 208–269.

Yu, N.-T. (1977) Raman spectroscopy: a conformational probe in biochemistry. *CRC Crit. Rev. Biochem.* 4: 229–280.

9

High-Resolution Electron Crystallography of Membrane Proteins

WERNER KÜHLBRANDT

For the foreseeable future, progress in determining high-resolution structures of membrane proteins will depend on crystallographic techniques. Until recently, x-ray crystallography seemed to be the only promising method. Progress with this technique, however, has not been as rapid as originally hoped because it is difficult to grow large and sufficiently well-ordered three-dimensional crystals. Electron crystallography of two-dimensional crystals is now a viable alternative that is particularly suitable for structural studies of membrane proteins because of their natural propensity to form two-dimensional arrays.

A number of membrane proteins have already been studied with this method. Atomic models of bacteriorhodopsin (Henderson et al., 1990) and of plant light harvesting complex (LHC-II) (Kühlbrandt et al., 1994) have been proposed, based on three-dimensional maps at 3.5 Å resolution in the membrane plane (but of lower resolution in the perpendicular direction), determined by electron crystallography. The structure of the bacterial porin PhoE has been determined to a resolution of 6 Å in three dimensions (Jap et al., 1991) and to about 3.5 Å in projection (Jap et al., 1990). Thin three-dimensional crystals of calcium ATPase have thus far yielded a 6 Å projection map (Stokes and Green, 1990a). Work toward higher resolution is in progress.

Electron crystallography is an extension to high resolution of the image processing techniques that have long been used to study the structure of membrane proteins at low and moderate resolution (for review, see Amos et al., 1982). The quest for high resolution does, however, place special demands not only on the quality and size of two-dimensional crystals but also on specimen preparation techniques, the instruments used for recording electron micrographs, and the computer programs for image processing. These requirements will be discussed briefly in this chapter.

Crystals for Electron Crystallography

Crystals for high-resolution electron crystallography need to satisfy three conditions: they must be thin, large, and highly ordered. Two-dimensional crystals with a thickness of only one unit cell are ideal, but thin three-dimensional crystals may be acceptable.

Two-Dimensional Crystallization of Membrane Proteins

Methods for growing two-dimensional crystals of membrane proteins have recently been reviewed (Kühlbrandt, 1992). The most promising approach is to start with the purified membrane protein and a suitable lipid or a combination of lipids, both solubilized in detergent. The detergent is then removed by dialysis or absorption so that the protein ends up in a reconstituted lipid bilayer. Under these conditions many purified membrane proteins tend to form two-dimensional lattices. Alternatively, membranous arrays can be grown by a batch method (Kühlbrandt, 1992). Both approaches have yielded two-dimensional crystals of excellent quality (Fig. 9.1a).

Other methods of two-dimensional crystallization by rearrangement of components within isolated membranes tend not to produce crystals of similar size and quality. Bacteriorhodopsin forms particularly well-ordered two-dimensional crystals *in vivo* (Fig. 9.1b), but unfortunately this appears to be an isolated case.

The size of two-dimensional crystals can sometimes be increased by fusion of smaller arrays. For example, crystalline patches of bacteriorhodopsin measuring 1 μm in diameter can be fused into 20 μm sheets by incubation with detergent (Baldwin and Henderson, 1989). Two-dimensional crystals of LHC-II 1–2 μm in diameter merge into large continuous lattices as the temperature of the crystal suspension is raised (Wang and Kühlbrandt, 1991). A similar effect has been found for two-dimensional crystals of PhoE porin (Jap, personal communication). The degree of order of several different two-dimensional crystals has been improved by treatment with phospholipase A_2 (Mannella, 1984), which removes excess phospholipid, helping the protein molecules to move more closely together.

Thickness

Atomic scattering factors for electrons are about 10,000 times higher than for x-rays (Wang and Kühlbrandt, 1992) so that even very thin layers scatter electrons quite strongly. Therefore, only the thinnest crystals can be used for electron crystallography. As a rule, specimens for high-resolution work should be no thicker than approximately 10% of the mean free path of electrons, which is about 2,400 Å for elastic scattering of 100 kV electrons by unstained biological specimens, and goes up to 5,700 Å for 300 kV electrons. According to this rule of thumb, specimens of less than 240 Å thickness are required with a standard 100 kV instrument. The thickness of two-dimensional membrane protein crystals falls within a range of 45 to 200 Å, depending on the size of the extramembranous domains. This makes them particularly suitable for electron crystallography. Thin three-dimensional crystals can be used, provided that the number of unit cells in the third dimension is small. Even though no three-dimensional structure of a biological macromolecule has yet been determined by electron crystallography of three-dimensional crystals, several groups are working toward a solution, and the chances of success seem good.

At greater specimen thicknesses, multiple scattering needs to be taken into consideration. Multiple scattering means that the observed image or diffraction pattern

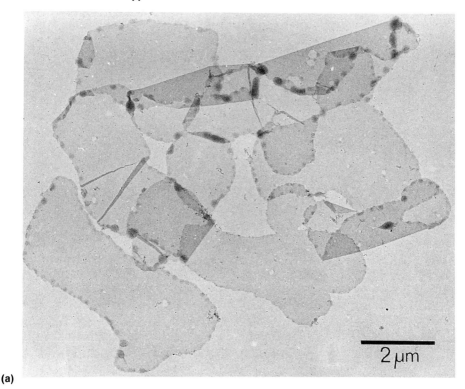

(a)

Fig. 9.1. Two-dimensional crystals of membrane proteins. *a*: Two-dimensional crystal of light harvesting complex grown in vitro from the purified membrane protein isolated from pea chloroplasts. Crystals are washed with a dilute buffered solution of tannin to preserve them for high-resolution electron diffraction and imaging. *b*: Purple membranes isolated from the

does not reflect structure of the specimen in a linear, straightforward way. Multiple (or dynamic) scattering can be demonstrated at 120 kV even for purple membrane, which has a thickness of 50 Å (Ceska and Glaeser, 1989) but is normally negligible for such thin biological specimens.

Order and Size

Initially, two-dimensional arrays in reconstituted lipid vesicles or membranes are most easily discovered by electron microscopy of negatively stained specimens. This is also the best method for monitoring the growth of larger and better two-dimensional crystals (see Kühlbrandt, 1992).

The only reliable way to assess the degree of order of two-dimensional and thin three-dimensional crystals is electron diffraction (see later under Electron Diffraction), which requires large, well-ordered arrays. For high-resolution work the criteria of order and size can therefore not be separated. Of course, large two-dimensional crystals are not necessarily well ordered. However, the diffraction pattern of a small crystal may be too weak for detection even if it is highly ordered. The mini-

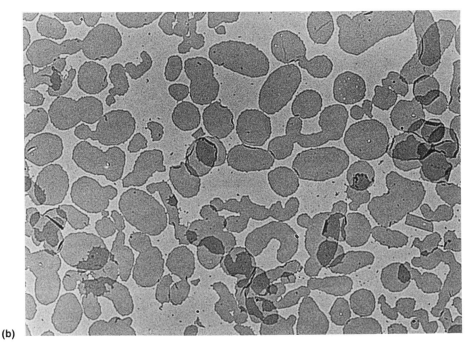

(b)

plasma membrane of *Halobacterium halobium*. Each patch of approximately 1 μm diameter is a perfect two-dimensional crystal. The membranes, supported on carbon film, are air dried in dilute glucose solution to preserve their crystallinity in the high vacuum of the electron microscope.

mum size for observing high-resolution diffraction peaks depends on the unit cell of the two-dimensional lattice and the packing density of the protein. For bacteriorhodopsin (small unit cell, high packing density), membranes as small as 0.5 μm in diameter yield reasonable diffraction patterns (Baldwin and Henderson, 1984). For LHC-II (large unit cell, low packing density), crystals of at least 2 μm diameter are needed.

Specimen Preparation

After two-dimensional crystallization, the development of a specimen preparation technique which preserves high-resolution detail in the high vacuum of the electron microscope is the next, critical stage. It is possible, and in some cases easy, to destroy or impair the order of two-dimensional crystals during specimen preparation. This step therefore requires particular care and attention.

For electron imaging and electron diffraction, crystals are deposited onto a thin carbon film, which in turn is supported by a metal (usually copper) grid. To find out if the crystals diffract to high resolution, it is best to prepare a vitrified specimen by rapid freezing of a thin film of aqueous crystal suspension in liquid ethane, followed by transfer into the electron microscope at liquid nitrogen temperature, as described by Dubochet et al. (1988). This procedure ensures minimal disturbance of the crystals. Even though conditions will not be ideal everywhere on the grid (e.g., due to varying thickness of vitrified buffer, specimen charging, and so forth), it should be possible to record diffraction patterns of at least some crystals if they are well ordered. Frequently, the diffraction peaks are too weak to be detected directly on the fluorescent screen, but they can easily be recorded on film.

Once the crystals have been shown to yield high-resolution diffraction patterns, the method of specimen preparation should be optimized. One approach is to replace the aqueous medium surrounding the crystals with a substance (such as a sugar or a sugar derivative) that mimics a liquid aqueous environment in the high vacuum of the electron microscope. Purple membrane, air-dried after washing with 1% aqueous glucose (Unwin and Henderson, 1975), diffracts electrons to 2.4 Å resolution (Ceska and Henderson, 1990). Glucose also works as an embedding medium for two-dimensional crystals of PhoE (Jap, 1988) and OmpF (Sass et al., 1989) and may be the most generally useful substance for this purpose. Trehalose was found to preserve two-dimensional crystals of PhoE somewhat better than glucose (Walian and Jap, 1990), but neither gave satisfactory results with two-dimensional crystals of LHC-II. These were, however, preserved very well by a wash with 0.5% tannin (Kühl-brandt and Downing, 1989). The reason for this is probably the higher detergent content of crystals of LHC-II compared to bacteriorhodopsin and PhoE. Tannin apparently prevents the re-equilibration of the detergent. This seems to occur upon washing with glucose or water and tends to disrupt the lattice (Wang and Kühl-brandt, 1991).

It should be emphasized that the use of these water-substituting media is largely a question of convenience. In most cases, rapidly frozen, vitrified specimens would give the same results, albeit with a lower success rate, partly because it is technically more difficult to prepare good vitrified specimens and to use them for high-resolution data collection, and partly because problems related to specimen charging and beam-induced movements are more severe with vitrified specimens (Henderson and Glaeser, 1985).

Electron Diffraction

Electron diffraction is not only a reliable test of crystallinity but also important as a technique of collecting diffraction data. The diffraction pattern is not sensitive to small object movements (since it measures the angle of diffraction from an array of molecules rather than their exact position) and hence is much easier to record than high-resolution electron micrographs, which are sensitive to such movements. The diffraction pattern is also unaffected by the contrast transfer function of the image-forming lens and therefore does not suffer from a loss of contrast at high resolution (see later under High-Resolution Imaging). Phase determination by electron diffraction of heavy metal isomorphous derivatives as in x-ray crystallography is, however, not feasible, due to the small increase in electron scattering factors with the atomic number and to the inherently lower signal to noise ratio of the data.

Electron diffraction patterns are collected by the procedure described by Unwin and Henderson (1975) for purple membrane, which has since been used with slight modification for other two-dimensional and thin three-dimensional crystals. Because the crystals are exposed to a fairly high dose of charged particles, each yields only one diffraction pattern and is destroyed in the process of recording it. It is therefore necessary to minimize preirradiation by searching for crystals at low magnification and low dose. An image-intensifying TV system is very helpful for localizing promising specimens at very low beam currents.

The critical electron dose (Unwin and Henderson, 1975) for a two-dimensional crystal at room temperature is about 0.5 electrons per $Å^2$ but roughly five times higher for specimens cooled with liquid nitrogen (International Experimental Study Group, 1986). At $4°$ $-20°$ K, temperatures reached by cooling the specimens with liquid helium, the critical dose increases by another factor of at least 2. By cooling the specimen to $-120°$ K or below, it is possible to record diffraction patterns (and images; see later under High-Resolution Imaging) with a much more favorable signal to noise ratio than at room temperature.

To obtain a three-dimensional set of diffraction data, the specimen is tilted relative to the incident electron beam. At this stage it is necessary for the crystal, and hence for the support film, to be as flat as possible; otherwise the diffraction spots in the direction perpendicular to the tilt axis are blurred (Baldwin and Henderson, 1984). This is particularly important for crystals that give diffraction patterns of a low signal to noise ratio, such as those of LHC-II. A method of making atomically flat carbon support films (Butt et. al., 1991) enabled collecting three-dimensional electron diffraction data of LHC-II (Fig. 9.2a). With purple membrane (Fig. 9.2b) and two-dimensional crystals of PhoE this problem is less serious, since the signal to noise ratio of diffraction peaks is higher due to the smaller unit cell (bacteriorhodopsin) or the higher packing density (PhoE) of the protein.

Diffraction patterns are processed and merged, using programs by Baldwin and Henderson (1984), into a three-dimensional set of diffraction data. For a two-dimensional crystal this consists of a set of lattice lines along which the structure factors are continuous. The number of diffraction patterns required to determine the structure factor amplitudes reliably along each lattice line depends on the resolution as well as the size and symmetry of the unit cell and can be estimated by the formula given by Klug and Crowther (1972). About 150 electron diffraction patterns of purple membrane (small unit cell, low symmetry) and about 85 of LHC-II (large unit cell, higher symmetry) were sufficient to determine amplitudes to resolutions of 3.0 Å and 3.2Å, respectively (Fig. 9.3). The average R-factor upon merging each diffraction pattern with the previously merged set provides a reliable indication of data quality. Merging R-factors in electron crystallography are typically 20%–30%, several times higher than the corresponding R-factors in x-ray crystallography. To a large extent, this difference is due to unfavorable counting statistics of electrons scattered by two-dimensional crystals, but other factors, still to be rigorously determined, may also play a role.

With standard, side entry specimen holders the tilt range is limited to $\pm 60°$ by the geometry of the microscope and the thickness of the holder. This means that a cone of 30° around the membrane normal (corresponding to about 13% of reciprocal space) is not accessible to measurement and that therefore the resolution of the resulting map is worse in this direction. According to the point spread function of an otherwise isotropic data set with a 30° missing cone, the resolution in the perpendicular

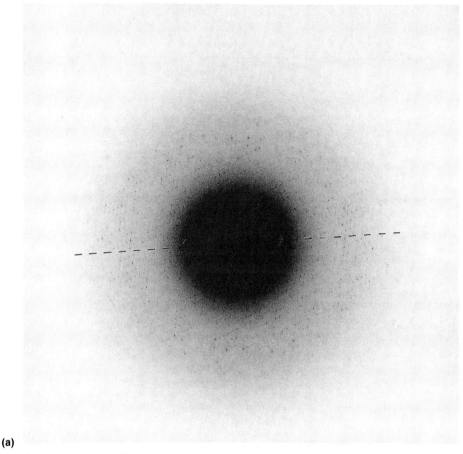

(a)

Fig. 9.2. Electron diffraction patterns of two-dimensional crystals tilted by 60 degrees relative to the incident electron beam. *a*: Two-dimensional crystal of light harvesting complex. Diffraction spots are visible to 3.3 Å resolution along the tilt axis *(dashed line)* and to 3.7 Å in the perpendicular direction. High-resolution spots need to be very sharp in all directions

direction is degraded only by a factor of about 1.3 (Glaeser et al., 1989). In practice, however, phase data at high tilt angles are more difficult to obtain, and therefore the resolution in this direction may be worse than is indicated by theory.

High-Resolution Imaging

High-resolution images are a prerequisite for the determination of phases. These are taken directly from the Fourier transforms of electron micrographs. Whereas it is fairly easy with most modern electron microscopes to achieve image resolutions better than 3 Å of nonbiological material, high-resolution images of radiation-sensitive biological specimens are rather more difficult to record. One major problem arises from the need to cool the specimen. This results in thermal gradients (since the electron

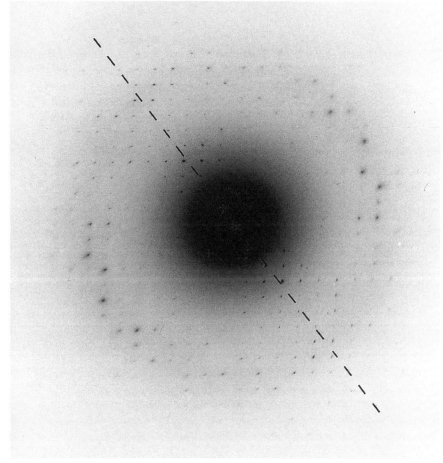

(b)

because their intensity is lower than in *b*. This is achieved by using atomically flat carbon support films (Butt et al., 1991). *b*: Purple membrane. Diffraction spots are visible to at least 3.5 Å resolution in all directions. High-resolution spots in the direction perpendicular to the tilt axis *(dashed line)* are blurred, but their intensity is measurable because it is relatively high.

microscope is operated at room temperature) that conflict with the essential requirement for mechanical stability of the specimen to within at least $\pm$ 1Å while the image is being recorded. This condition is most easily met with instruments that have been specially designed for this purpose (Hayward and Glaeser, 1980; LeFranc et al., 1982; Fujiyoshi et al., 1991).

A higher success rate than with standard, flood beam imaging can be achieved by recording images in spot-scan mode whereby successive small areas of the two-dimensional crystal are exposed in a stepwise manner (Fig. 9.4) rather than all at once (Downing and Glaeser, 1986; Bullough and Henderson, 1987; Downing, 1991). This minimizes the amount of beam-induced specimen movement, which is a major cause of poor image contrast at high resolution with biological specimens (Henderson and Glaeser, 1985). The stepwise recording of images also helps to

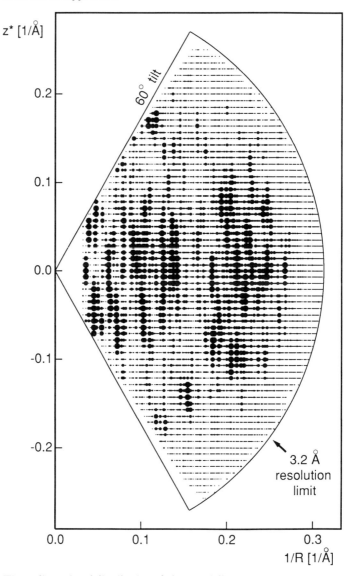

Fig. 9.3. Three-dimensional distribution of electron diffraction intensity of two-dimensional crystals of light harvesting complex. Intensities measured along 375 lattice lines to 3.2 Å resolution are projected onto the x–z^* plane. The geometry of the specimen holder means that tilt angles beyond 60 degrees are difficult to achieve so that there is a blind region around the tilt axis, corresponding to about 13% of reciprocal space. This effect limits the resolution in the perpendicular direction. (From Wang and Kühlbrandt, 1992).

reduce the effect of specimen drift since the exposure time for each spot is very much shorter than for a flood beam image. As a further advantage of the spot-scan procedure for imaging tilted crystals, the defocus of the objective lens may be adjusted between scan lines to that the defocus setting for every spot is optimal.

High-resolution images should be recorded on film with a magnification of about ×60,000. At lower magnifications, the emulsion does not reproduce structural detail

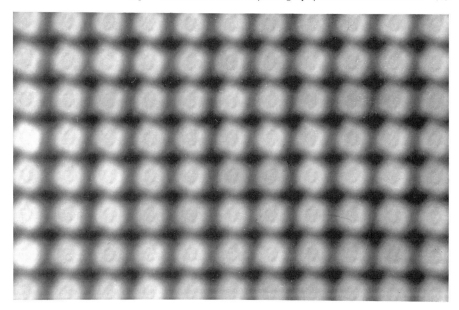

Fig. 9.4. Spot-scan image. A small illuminating spot of approximately 1,000 Å diameter is scanned across an area of the specimen to minimize beam-induced movements, which tend to limit the resolution obtainable with radiation-sensitive specimens. The structure of the specimen (a two-dimensional crystal of light harvesting complex) within the spots is not visible due to low contrast.

in the order of 3 Å sufficiently well. If the magnification is much higher, the electron dose at the specimen for an acceptable gray level on the film increases, while the usable area of the crystal on a sheet of film becomes too small.

Phase Determination by Crystallographic Image Processing

In electron crystallography the phases of structure factors are determined directly by image processing. Electron micrographs are processed in several stages, starting with the initial screening by optical diffraction, microdensitometry of selected areas, followed by computer processing and finally the merging of phase data.

Optical Diffusion

Electron micrographs of two-dimensional crystals are screened with a laser diffractometer (De Rosier and Klug, 1968). The resolution, sharpness, and, for untilted crystals, the symmetry of reflections are the best criteria for selecting images for processing. Frequently, only about 1%–2% of the recorded images meet the highest standards.

Optical diffraction even of the best images rarely reveals reflections beyond 7 Å resolution, because the lattice of two-dimensional crystals is always slightly distorted, either through interaction with the support film or, to a lesser extent, by the imaging lenses, which introduce spiral distortion. Lattice distortions can be corrected by computer processing (Henderson et al., 1986).

Microdensitometry

Areas giving the sharpest diffraction spots at the highest resolution by optical diffraction are marked on the negative and digitized on a flat-bed microdensitometer. The more usual rotating-drum scanners do not achieve the small stepsizes required for reproducing high-resolution features. The step size depends on the expected resolution and the image magnification and should correspond to about one-third of the smallest detail to be resolved (e.g., 6 μm for 3 Å resolution at an image magnification of $\times$60,000). The densitometered area should be as large as possible and may include the whole negative if the size and quality of the crystal permits it.

Computer Processing

A set of computer programs has been developed by Henderson and colleagues specifically for high-resolution image processing (see Henderson et al., 1986, 1990, for detailed discussion). For images of untilted crystals, the lattice distortions are first determined by cross-correlation with a central reference area and then reversed by reinterpolation of the densitometered image. This process is repeated with the distortion-corrected image as a reference until there is no significant improvement in the number and signal to noise ratio of diffraction peaks in the image transform. In this way it is frequently possible to double the image resolution. The exact amount of defocus is found by comparing the structure factor amplitudes calculated from the image (which are modulated by the defocus-dependent contrast transfer function of the objective lens) with the electron diffraction amplitudes (which are not). Next, the phases of symmetry-related reflections are examined. By minimizing the phase difference between these reflections, the phase origin is fixed to the position of a symmetry axis in the projected unit cell. The average phase deviation of symmetry-related reflections from their mean (or from their ideal values of 0 or 180 degrees for some crystal symmetries), referred to as the *phase residual*, is the most sensitive test of image quality. The average phase error is related to the signal to noise ratio of a reflection (Henderson et al., 1986). Accordingly, phase measurements for strong reflections are highly accurate, but weak spots have larger phase errors. Since the intensity of reflections in image transforms decreases with resolution, the phase error is resolution dependent. Loss of image contrast at high resolution is caused primarily by small specimen movements and the nonideal contrast transfer function of the objective lens (Henderson and Glaeser, 1985). For example, the mean phase error for purple membrane is less than 2° for reflections up to 7 Å but about 30° for reflections at 3.5 Å resolution (Henderson et al., 1986).

Small deviations of the incident electron beam from the optical axis of the objective lens, referred to as *beam tilt,* introduce a phase error that increases with the third power of the resolution. Even though the beam tilt is usually less than 1 mrad in a reasonably well-aligned microscope, the effect on the image phases cannot be neglected at a resolution of about 6 Å and above. In practical terms, beam tilt causes a resolution-dependent shift of the phase origin and can therefore be detected and compensated by image processing (Henderson et al., 1986).

With electron micrographs of tilted two-dimensional crystals, the focus gradient across the image adds a further complication. This can, however, be dealt with rather elegantly in the Fourier transform, provided that the direction of the tilt axis and the amount of defocus at a point in the centre of the image are known. Initially, the first two parameters are calculated from the lattice vectors. The defocus is first estimated by optical diffraction and then refined by a least-squares procedure that maximizes the signal to noise ratio of spots at lattice positions (Henderson et al., 1990). Again, processing micrographs of tilted crystals is an iterative procedure, with consecutive steps for unbending the crystal lattice and for correcting the focus gradient in each cycle. Since more parameters need to be determined and since these parameters are, to some extent, interdependent, four or five cycles are usually required. With the computers currently available in most laboratories, each cycle takes about 1 day, so the whole process tends to be rather slow. The net result is a set of amplitudes and phases of the observed reflections for each processed image.

Merging of Phase Data

Like the amplitudes, the phases of structure factors are merged to map out their variation along each lattice line (Fig. 9.5). Merging is done by comparing phases of tilted crystals with those from all previously merged images, starting with data from

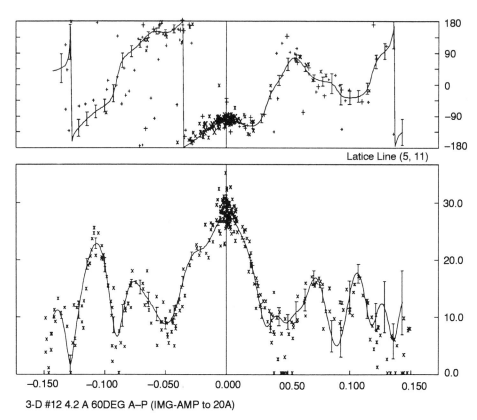

3-D #12 4.2 A 60DEG A–P (IMG-AMP to 20A)

Fig. 9.5. Lattice line (5,11) from the three-dimensional data set of plant light harvesting complex, showing the variation of amplitude *(lower panel)* and phase *(upper panel)* as a function of z^*, the distance from the x–y projection plane in Fourier space. Amplitudes and phases are measured to a resolution of 5.0 Å.

untilted crystals. An average phase error is calculated for each new image, which shows how well it agrees with those merged previously.

Crystal and beam tilt, defocus, and astigmatism of each processed image are then refined against the merged data set by minimizing the phase error. Finally, amplitudes and phases are combined into a single set of structure factors from which a three-dimensional map of the structure is calculated by standard crystallographic procedures.

Some Results

To date, the three-dimensional structures of bacteriorhodopsin (Henderson et al., 1990), plant LHC-II (Kühlbrandt et al., 1994), and PhoE porin (Jap et al., 1991), have been determined by these techniques at resolutions of 3.5, 3.4, and 6 Å, respectively. In all three cases, the resolution perpendicular to the membrane plane was less good but sufficient to recognize structural details important for biological function.

Bacteriorhodopsin

Figure 9.6*a* shows the structure of bacteriorhodopsin, a light-driven proton pump in the outer membrane of a halophilic archaebacterium. The structure and function of bacteriorhodopsin have been reviewed extensively, most recently by Tittor (1991). The map indicates the position of the covalently linked retinal in a cage formed by seven α-helices that run more or less perpendicular to the membrane plane. The membrane-spanning helices are particularly well resolved. Several distinct bulges protruding from the helices were identified as bulky amino acid side chains, which served as guide points for fitting the polypeptide sequence. The helices are connected

---

Fig. 9.6 (*opposite*). Three-dimensional structures of membrane proteins determined by high-resolution electron crystallography of two-dimensional crystals. *a*: Bacteriorhodopsin. The polypeptide sequence could be fitted to the three-dimensional map at a resolution of 3.5 Å in the *x–y* plane and roughly 9 Å in the perpendicular direction. Seven trans-membrane helices (labeled *A* to *G*) arranged in two layers surround a retinal molecule covalently attached to a lysine residue on helix G, roughly in the middle of the membrane. Charged amino acid side chains on helices C and G form a relay system along which protons are pumped out of the cell upon light-induced *cis-trans*-isomerization of the retinal pigment. *ct*, C terminus of the polypeptide; *nt*, N terminus of the polypeptide. (From Henderson et al., 1990.) *b*: Plant light harvesting complex. At a resolution of 6 Å in the *x–y* plane, the map shows three membrane-spanning helices, labeled *A*, *B*, and *C*. Regions of density thought to correspond to chlorophyll molecules are labeled *1* to *15*. The chlorophylls are arranged in two layers, corresponding roughly to the upper and lower leaflet of the lipid bilayer. At an average center-to-center distance of 12 Å, the chlorophylls are closely spaced for extremely rapid energy transfer by exciton coupling. (From Kühlbrandt and Wang, 1991.) *c*: PhoE porin from *E. coli* outer membrane. At an in-plane resolution of 6 Å, the three-dimensional map of the porin trimer shows three cylindrical walls of β-sheet, each belonging to one porin monomer and surrounding one pore. Loops and a short helix within the perimeter of the cylindrical wall define the size and substrate specificity of the pore. (From Jap et al., 1991.)

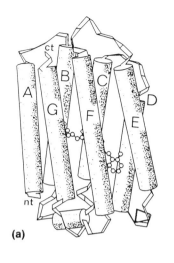

(a)

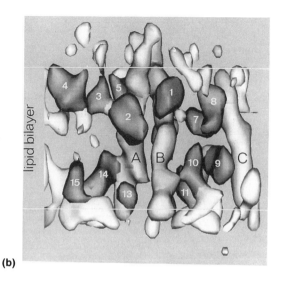

(b)

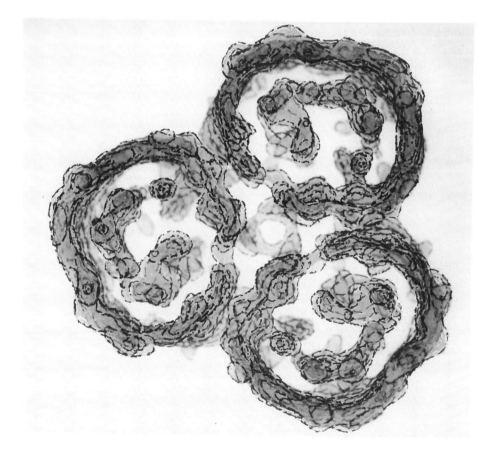

(c)

by short loops that are less clearly defined in the three-dimensional map but are nevertheless unambiguous. The light-induced *cis–trans* isomerization of the retinal is thought to affect the pK$_a$ values of nearby charged amino acid residues. These are buried in the membrane and line a channel through which protons are pumped from the inside to the outside of the cell. Even though the three-dimensional map only shows the resting state of bacteriorhodopsin at not quite atomic resolution, this detailed and plausible functional model could be proposed thanks to a wealth of biophysical and biochemical data, including extensive site-directed mutagenesis.

Plant Light-Harvesting Complex

The LHC-II from chlorophyll membranes is the major chlorophyll-binding protein in nature. It functions as a molecular antenna of solar energy. Photons are absorbed by the noncovalently bound pigment molecules and passed on to the reaction center complexes in the same membrane. These use the energy to transport electrons across the membrane, creating a biochemically useful, electrochemical membrane potential.

A three-dimensional map of the complex at 6 Å resolution (Fig. 9.6*b*) shows three membrane-spanning α-helices, two of which are inclined by 30° with respect to the membrane normal and related by noncrystallographic two fold symmetry (Kühlbrandt and Wang, 1991). Chlorophyll molecules (of which only the bulky tetrapyrrole ring systems of the head groups are visible at this resolution) are arranged in two layers, corresponding roughly to the position of the upper and lower leaflets of the lipid bilayer. The distance between adjacent chlorophyll molecules is close enough for energy transfer within 10^{-13} by strong coupling of delocalized electrons. The helices are connected by long loops that cannot yet be traced with certainty. More recently, a 3.4 Å map of this complex has been obtained which has yielded an atomic model showing the structure of the polypeptide and attached pigment molecules (Kühlbrandt et al., 1994).

PhoE Porin

Another structure determined by this method is that of PhoE porin (Jap et al., 1991). This protein forms channels in the outer membranes of *E. coli*. The 6 Å three-dimensional map (Fig. 9.6*c*) shows a trimer of three elliptical pores of about 38 by 28 Å. The walls of the pores consist of β-sheet, with strands apparently running at an average angle of 35 degrees relative to the membrane normal (Walian and Jap, 1990). Part of the polypeptide is found within the cylinder where it appears to control the permeability and selectivity of the pore.

The structures of these bacterial porins have now been solved by x-ray crystallography (Weiss et al., 1991; Cowan et al., 1993), including PhoE. The x-ray structure is in good agreement with that determined by electron microscopy at lower resolution.

Outlook

As a method of determining the structures of biological macromolecules at high resolution, electron crystallography is still in its infancy. Yet the results obtained thus far have already proven it to be invaluable, in particular for studying the structures of membrane proteins at high resolution. There can be no doubt that in the future there will be many more applications of this technique in structural biology.

An important advantage of electron crystallography is the direct determination of structure factor phases from image transforms. Phase data obtained in this way are of a much higher quality that those normally determined in x-ray crystallography by multiple isomorphous replacement. Other advantages over x-ray crystallography of membrane proteins include the tendency of these proteins to form two-dimensional crystals and the possibility of studying them in a membrane-like environment.

On the other hand, the method is still quite slow compared with other methods of structure analysis, and it is hard to achieve high resolution in the direction perpendicular to the membrane plane. Areas of further development of electron crystallographic techniques are, however, easily identified. First, significant improvements in electron microscope design and in techniques for recording high-resolution electron micrographs at high tilt angles are still possible and likely to be made in the near future. In addition, much faster and more powerful computers will soon be available for image processing. These two factors should make it possible to collect and process a full three-dimensional data set on a time scale comparable to x-ray crystallography.

Second, methods of refinement for protein structures solved by x-ray crystallography are being applied to three-dimensional maps determined by electron crystallography. These methods may also be useful for phase extension beyond the reach of image processing, in particular if the structure has noncrystallographic symmetry.

Third, the development of techniques for determining the three-dimensional structure of proteins by electron crystallography of thin three-dimensional crystals is still an unresolved challenge. For example, calcium ATPase (Stokes and Green, 1990b) forms such small, well-ordered three-dimensional crystals, as do other membrane proteins. A method for studying their molecular structure at high resolution is much needed.

Finally, methods for growing two-dimensional crystals need to be refined and applied to all available membrane proteins in order to produce more and better specimens for examination by this technique. These developments will certainly make electron crystallography even more important as a tool for structural biologists interested in the structure and function of membrane proteins.

References

Amos, L. A., Henderson, R., and Unwin, P.N.T. (1982) Three-dimensional structure determination by electron microscopy of two-dimensional crystals. *Prog. Biophys. Mol. Biol.* 39: 183–231.

Baldwin, J., and Henderson, R. (1984) Measurement and evaluation of electron diffraction patterns from two-dimensional crystals. *Ultramicroscopy* 14: 319–336.

Baldwin, J. M., Henderson, R., Beckmann, R., and Zemlin, F. (1988) Images of purple membrane at 2.8 Å resolution obtained by cryo-electron microscopy. *J. Mol. Biol.* 202: 585–591.

Bullough, P., and Henderson, R. (1987) Use of spot-scan procedure for recording low-dose micrographs of beam-sensitive specimens. *Ultramicroscopy* 21: 223–230.

Butt, H.-J., Wang, D. H., Hansma, P. K., and Kühlbrandt, W. (1991) Effect of surface roughness of carbon support films on high-resolution electron diffraction of two-dimensional protein crystals. *Ultramicroscopy* 36: 307–318.

Ceska, T., and Glaeser, R. M. (1989) High-voltage electron diffraction from bacteriorhodopsin (purple membrane) is measurably dynamical. *Acta Crystal.* A45: 620–628.

Ceska, T. A., and Henderson, R. (1990) Analysis of high-resolution electron diffraction patterns from purple membrane labelled with heavy-atoms. *J. Mol. Biol.* 213: 539–560.

De Rosier, D., and Klug, A. (1968). Reconstruction of three-dimensional structures from electron radiographs. *Nature* 217: 130–134.

Downing, K. H. (1991) Spot-scan imaging in transmission electron microscopy. *Science* 251: 53–59.

Downing, K. H., and Glaeser, R. M. (1986) Improvement in high resolution image quality of radiation-sensitive specimens achieved with reduced spot size of the electron beam. *Ultramicroscopy* 20: 269–278.

Dubochet, J., Adrian, M., Chang, J.-J., Homo, J.-C., Lepault, J., McDowall, A. W., and Schultz, P. (1988) Cryo-electron microscopy of vitrified specimens. *Q. Rev. Biophys.* 21: 129–228.

Fujiyoshi, Y., Mizusaki, T., Morikawa, K., Yamagishi, H., Aoki, Y., Kihara, H., and Harada, Y. (1991) Development of a superfluid helium stage for high-resolution electron microscopy. *Ultramicroscopy* 38: 241–251.

Glaeser, R. M., Tong, L., and Kim, S.-H. (1989) Three-dimensional reconstructions from incomplete data: interpretability of density maps at "atomic" resolution. *Ultramicroscopy* 27: 307–318.

Hayward, S. B., and Glaeser, R. M. (1980) High resolution cold stage for the JEOL 100B and 100C electron microscopes. *Ultramicroscopy* 5: 3–8.

Henderson, R., Baldwin, J. M., Ceska, T. A., Zemlin, F., Beckmann, E., and Downing, K. H. (1990) Model for the structure of bacteriorhodopsin based on high-resolution electron cryo-microscopy. *J. Mol. Biol.* 213: 899–929.

Henderson, R., Baldwin, J. M., Downing, K. H., Lepault, J., and Zemlin, F. (1986) Structure of purple membrane from *Halobacterium halobium:* recording, measurement and evaluation of electron micrographs at 3.5 Å resolution. *Ultramicroscopy* 19: 147–178.

Henderson, R., and Glaeser, R. M. (1985) Quantitative analysis of image contrast in electron micrographs of beam-sensitive crystals. *Ultramicroscopy* 16: 139–150.

International Experimental Study Group (1986) Cryoprotection in electron microscopy. *J. Microsc.* 141: 385–391.

Jap, B. K. (1988) High-resolution electron diffraction of reconstituted PhoE porin. *J. Mol. Biol.* 199: 229–231.

Jap, B. K., Downing, K. H., and Walian, P. J. (1990) Structure of PhoE porin in projection at 3.5 Å resolution. *J. Struct. Biol.* **103**: 57–63.

Jap, B. K., Walian, P. J., and Gehring, K. (1991) Structural architecture of an outer membrane channel as determined by electron crystallography. Nature 350: 167–170.

Klug, A., and Crowther, R. A. (1972) 3D image reconstruction from the viewpoint of information theory. *Nature* [*New Biol.*] 238: 435–440.

Kühlbrandt, W. (1992) Two-dimensional crystallization of membrane protein. *Q. Rev. Biophys.* 25: 1–49.

Kühlbrandt, W., and Downing, K. H. (1989) Two-dimensional structure of plant light-harvesting complex at 3.7 Å resolution by electron crystallography. *J. Mol. Biol.* 207: 823–828.

Kühlbrandt, W., and Wang, D. N. (1991) Three-dimensional structure of plant light-harvesting complex determined by electron crystallography. Nature 350: 130–134.

Kühlbrandt, W., Wang, D. N., and Fujiyoshi, Y. (1994) Atomic model of plant light-harvesting complex by electronic crystallography. *Nature* 367: 614–621.

LeFranc, G., Knapek, E., and Dietrich, I. (1982) Superconducting lens design. *Ultramicroscopy* 10: 111–124.

Mannella, C. A. (1984) Phospholipase-induced crystallization of channels in mitochondrial outer membranes. *Science* 224: 165–166.

Sass, H. J., Beckmann, E., Zemlin, F., van Heel, M., Zeitler, E., Rosenbusch, J. P., Dorset, D. L., and Massalski, A. (1989) Densely packed β-structure at the protein-lipid interface of porin is revealed by high-resolution cryo-electron microscopy. *J. Mol. Biol.* 209: 171–175.

Stokes, D. L., and Green, N. M. (1990a) Structure of CaATPase: electron microscopy of frozen-hydrated crystals at 6 Å resolution in projection. *J. Mol. Biol.* 213: 529–538.

Stokes, D. L., and Green, N. M. (1990b) Three-dimensional crystals of CaATPase from sacroplasmic reticulum. Symmetry and molecular packing. *Biophys. J.* 57: 1–14.

Tittor, J. (1991) A new view of an old pump: bacteriorhodopsin. *Curr. Top. Struct. Biol* 1: 534–538.

Unwin, P.N.T., and Henderson, R. (1975) Molecular structure determination by electron microscopy of unstained crystalline specimens. *J. Mol. Biol.* 94: 425–440.

Walian, P. J., and Jap, B. K. (1990) Three-dimensional electron diffraction of PhoE porin to 2.8 Å resolution. *J. Mol. Biol.* 215: 429–438.

Wang, D. N., and Kühlbrandt, W. (1991) High-resolution electron crystallography of light-harvesting chlorophyll a/b-protein complex in three different media. *J. Mol. Biol.* 217: 691–699.

Wang, D. N., and Kühlbrandt, W. (1992) 3D electron diffraction of plant light-harvesting complex. *Biophys. J.* 61: 287–297.

Weiss, M. S., Aebele, U., Weckesser, J., Welte, W., Schiltz, E., and Schulz, G. E. (1991) Molecular architecture and electron static properties of a bacterial porin. *Science* 254: 1627–1630.

10

Site-Directed Spin Labeling
of Membrane Proteins

WAYNE L. HUBBELL and CHRISTIAN ALTENBACH

Membrane-associated proteins present a particularly difficult problem for structure determination. Diffraction approaches are hampered by the lack of crystallization methods, and multidimensional nuclear magnetic resonance (NMR)-approaches are not generally applicable due to the lack of high-resolution spectra (but see Opella, Chapter 11). For this class of proteins, the technique of *spin labeling* offers an attractive alternative for obtaining structural information. In this method, a stable nitroxide-free radical (the "spin label") is attached at a specific site in the system of interest, and the electron paramagnetic resonance (EPR) spectrum is analyzed to yield information regarding the local environment around the label. Humphries and McConnell (1982) and Marsh (1981) have written excellent reviews of the technique and its capabilities. The two-volume series, *Spin Labeling: Theory and Application,* (Berliner, 1976, 1979) and Volume 8 of the series, *Biological Magnetic Resonance,* (Berliner and Reuben, 1990) provide a comprehensive treatment of continuous-wave EPR aspects of the subject. Two recent books, *EPR and Advanced EPR Studies of Biological Systems* (Dalton, 1985) and *Advanced EPR: Applications in Biology and Biochemistry* (Hoff, 1989), treat more advanced concepts and time-domain EPR.

Spin labeling has been highly successful in providing dynamic and structural information on lipids in membranes (see Marsh [1981], Hemminga [1983], and Volwerk and Griffith [1988] for reviews). It has had much less application to the study of protein structure, primarily due to technical difficulties in achieving site-selective labeling in these complex molecules. However, recent advances in molecular genetics have made it possible to introduce spin labels at arbitrarily chosen sites using site-directed mutagenesis. We will refer to this approach as *site-directed spin labeling* (SDSL).

The basic strategy of SDSL, as applied to structure determination, requires the substitution of a nitroxide-containing amino acid for the native residue at a number of positions in the protein sequence. Thus a *set* of spin-labeled proteins is prepared, each containing a single nitroxide amino acid and differing only by the position of that amino acid in the sequence. The number in the set and the sequence interval, if any, between the members are determined by the type of information sought.

Analysis of attached spin labels by EPR spectroscopy can be used to (*1*) determine topography of the polypeptide chain with respect to the bilayer interface, (*2*) determine the electrostatic potential at any surface site, (*3*) identify regions of regular secondary structure, (*4*) determine the orientation of the secondary structure in the protein, and (5) investigate the dynamics of the above characteristics. Additional information can be obtained by introducing *pairs* of spin labels in the protein, namely, the distance between the labels. With a sufficient number of pairs, the *proximity* of the secondary structural elements relative to each other can be deduced.

Thus, in principle, SDSL can provide a three-dimensional structure at the level of the backbone folding in domains of regular secondary organization. Since integral membrane proteins are expected to have a high content of regular secondary structure, a significant fraction of the structure can be determined. The sensitivity and response time of conventional EPR spectrometers also make it possible to monitor real-time changes in protein structure during function, and this is one of the potentially most useful capabilities of SDSL.

This chapter outlines the general strategies used to obtain the above information. Since a primary requirement for application of SDSL is the selective incorporation of a nitroxide in the sequence without disruption of the structure, the chemical aspects of site-directed incorporation of a nitroxide side chain and the problem of perturbation are presented first.

Site-Specific Introduction of Nitroxide Side Chains in Proteins

Direct Chemical Methods

A set of protein derivatives in which a spin label is located at different sites may be prepared by modification of existing residues with nitroxide reagents. In general, this leads to a large number of products since the reactive site is not unique. Resolution of the mixture into its components provides the required set. This method is not general because sites of labeling are limited to those containing reactive functions, and it is restricted to those cases in which product separation is possible. Nevertheless, it has been applied successfully to the peptide melittin (Altenbach and Hubbell, 1988; Altenbach et al., 1989a).

Nitroxide side chains may also be introduced at specific positions in a sequence by total synthesis of the polypeptide using nitroxide amino acids where desired. A number of nitroxide amino acids have been reported, and the structures of some are shown below (I–IV).

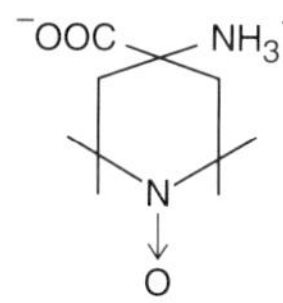

(Rassat and Rey, 1967)

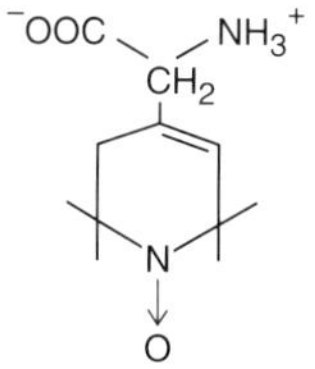

(Cseko et al., 1984)

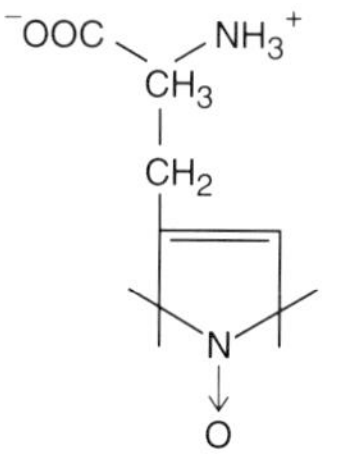

III
(Lex et al., 1982)

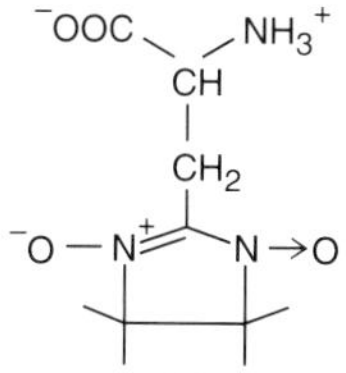

IV
(Weinkam and Jorgensen, 1971)

Amino acids I and IV have been incorporated into small peptides using solid-state methods (Nakaie et al., 1981; Weinkam and Jorgensen, 1971). The technical difficulties involved in total synthesis of hydrophobic membrane proteins make this approach currently practical only for low-molecular-weight peptides such as melittin, cercropins, and signal peptides.

Spin Labeling at Cysteine Introduced by Site-Directed Mutagenesis

To date, SDSL has relied primarily on site-directed mutagenesis to substitute cysteine for the native amino acid at the selected site. The reactive sulfhydryl group is then modified with a sulfhydryl-specific nitroxide spin label. Several choices for labels with essentially absolute specificity for the sulfhydryl group are shown below (V–XI):

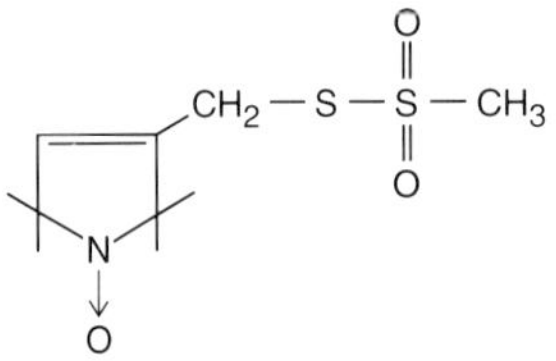

V
(Berliner etr al., 1982)

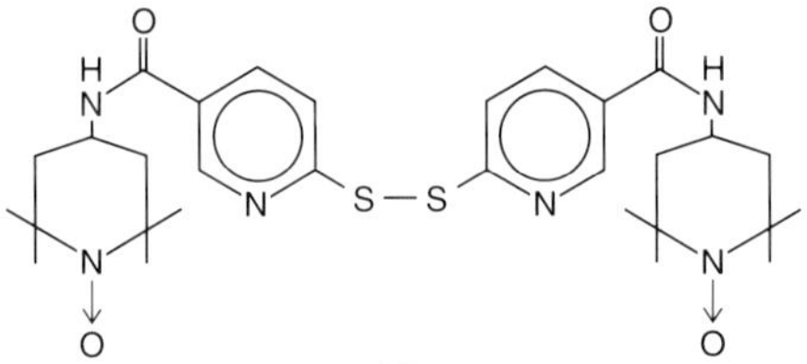

VI
(Todd et al., 1989)

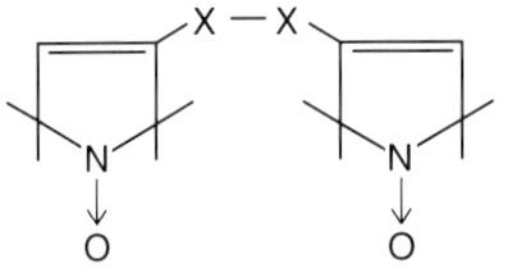

X = S   VII (Hideg et al., 1991)
X = Se VIII (Hideg et al., 1991)

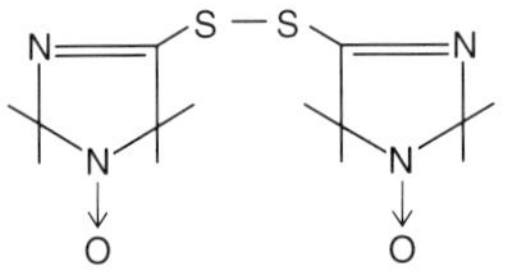

IX (Khramtsov et al., 1989)

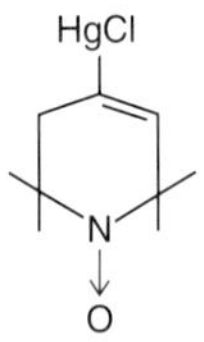

X
(Shapiro and Dmitnev, 1981)

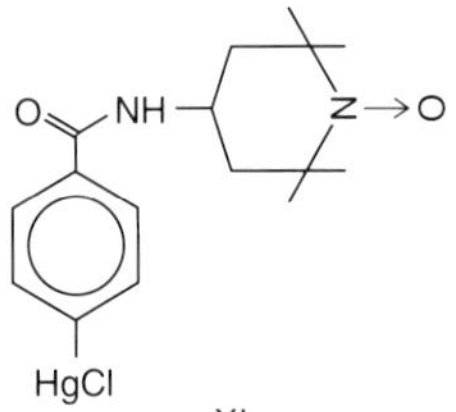

XI
(Boeyens and McConnell, 1966)

Of these, the methanethiosulfonate derivative V has been most extensively utilized because of its specificity, high reactivity, and relatively small molar volume of the group added to the cysteine side chain. Pyridine disulfide label VI has the useful property that the reaction progress can be followed by ultraviolet spectrophotometry (Grassetti and Murray, 1967). Reagent IX, an imidazoline nitroxide biradical, adds the smallest group to the cysteine side chain of any of the reagents, but has not yet been employed for chemical modification. Reagents X and XI are highly reactive and appear to have some selectivity for sulfhydryls located in a hydrophobic environment (Z. T. Farahbakhsh and W. L. Hubbell, unpublished data).

There are two potential problems regarding the substitution of cysteine. First, many proteins contain multiple cysteine residues, and the introduced cysteine is not unique in these cases. For some proteins, it has been found that the native cysteine residues can be replaced with nonreactive alternatives with no deleterious effect on protein function and presumably structure. Examples include the single native cysteine of colicin (Todd et al., 1989) and the six native cysteines of rhodopsin (Karnik and Khorana, 1990). Nevertheless, it is anticipated that in some cases essential native cysteine residues may present a problem. A second challenge to the cysteine substitution approach is that buried cysteines generally have low reactivity with spin-label reagents. In such cases the modification reaction is carried out in the unfolded state (Altenbach et al., 1989b, 1990). This, of course, requires that the denaturation be reversible.

Use of Nonsense Codons for Direct Incorporation of Nitroxide Amino Acids

Noren et al. (1989a,b) and Bain et al. (1989) have reported a general scheme for the incorporation of non-native amino acids at specific sites in a protein. The method involves the introduction of a nonsense codon at the desired position in the gene by site-directed mutagenesis. A suppressor tRNA is chemically acylated with the desired non-natural amino acid. Use of this tRNA together with the mutagenized DNA in an in vitro translation–transcription system provides a protein with the non-natural amino acid incorporated at the desired position. This method has not yet been used for nitroxide amino acid incorporation, but is currently under investigation (P. Schultz, personal communication).

Direct incorporation of nitroxide amino acids has some distinct advantages over the cysteine substitution approach. First, the size of the introduced side chain is smaller by the volume of the disulfide group, thus reducing potential steric perturbations. In addition, native cysteine residues need not be replaced, and unfolding of the protein for the purpose of introducing the nitroxide is unnecessary.

The Problem of Perturbation by the Nitroxide Side Chain

The introduction of a spin-label side chain in a protein must introduce a local perturbation in structure. As mentioned above, the resolution goal of the technique is secondary structure and topology of the backbone, and perturbations of side chain positions and minor backbone rearrangements are acceptable. Whether the introduction of a nitroxide side chain produces much larger perturbations inconsistent with structural stability is an important question. To what degree can a protein tolerate changes at a single site? Sauer and coworkers have carried out extensive studies to investigate this question in λ-repressor (Lim and Sauer, 1989; Pakula and Sauer, 1989; Bowie et al., 1990). Some relevant generalizations from these studies are (*1*) the identity of an individual amino acid is unimportant for either structure or activity for a large fraction of the residues in a protein; (*2*) for exposed (surface) residues, a wide range of substitutions is tolerated; and (*3*) there is less tolerance to substitution for buried residues. To maintain structure and activity in water-soluble proteins, the most important characteristic to conserve is the nonpolar nature of the buried residue. Next in order of importance are steric compatibility and residue volume.

The first point is certainly a favorable one from the point of view of application of SDSL and seems reasonable in view of the large number of interactions that determine the protein structure. The second point has been verified for a number of protein families, where it is found that surface residues are generally not conserved within the family (Dickerson, 1980; Lesk and Chothia, 1980, 1982; Bashford et al., 1987). This implies that no difficulties will be experienced in substituting spin-label side chains for surface residues. Fortunately, surface sites are interesting for membrane proteins, since a label at this position offers an opportunity to investigate solvation of the protein surface by the lipid bilayer.

With regard to the third generalization above, we note that the nitroxides most commonly applied in spin-label studies are amphoteric with respect to polarity. Although they have overall hydrophobicities similar to the valine side chain, the nitroxide function can participate in hydrogen bonding. Thus the nitroxide is a reasonable compromise for the substitution of nonpolar as well as polar residues, both of which are found frequently at buried sites in membrane proteins. Studies of λ-repressor suggest that the volume of the hydrophobic core can vary by as much as 10% in acceptable sequences, but changes at individual sites can be considerably larger. Apparently, local volume changes are accommodated by conformational changes in nearby side chains and subtle backbone movements. These often occur, however, with maintenance of the overall structure and activity. The molar volume of the nitroxide group is only about 25% larger than a tryptophan side chain and is not expected to be an intolerable steric load on the structure in view of the above findings.

SDSL is in its infancy, having been extensively applied to only colicin E1 (Todd et al., 1989) and bacteriorhodopsin (Altenbach et al., 1989b, 1990; Greenhalgh et al., 1991). Nevertheless, a sufficient number of nitroxide side chains have been introduced in these cases to permit some conclusions on the subject of perturbation. For bacteriorhodopsin, thirty-three mutants each containing a single cysteine have been prepared and the sulfhydryl derivatized with spin label V in the unfolded state in detergent solution. Following the addition of retinal, the protein was folded by the removal of detergent in the presence of lipid. If proper folding takes place, a pigment forms with an absorbance red-shifted from the free retinal. Thus pigment formation provides a convenient assay for assembly of a native-like structure. Of the thirty-three spin-labeled side chains in the different mutants, fourteen were buried residues. All of the external residues folded properly. Only one of the buried residues (No. 90) failed to fold. Two others (Nos. 96 and 141) folded, but were clearly less stable than wild type. From the point of view of structural analysis, it is not important if the modified structure is less stable than the wild type, but only that the analysis be done under stable conditions.

For colicin, twenty-two mutants containing a single cysteine substituted for the native amino acid have been prepared and the sulfhydryl group derivatized with spin labels V and VI. Thus far, nine of the spin labeled mutants have been examined for activity, and all show wild-type behavior with respect to cell killing. Of these, two are buried.

To the extent that they can be compared, these results are consistent with the generalizations enumerated above. That is, the protein structure and stability are not sensitive to changes of external residues, but are more sensitive to buried substitutions. Fortunately, the nitroxide properties appear to be compatible with the requirements for proper folding for most of the sites. In particular cases in which the nitroxide side chain may be too large, it is possible to compensate by reducing the volume of a nearby side chain (Lim and Sauer, 1989).

Interpretation of the Site-Directed Spin Labeling Experiment in Terms of Protein Structure

Table 10-1 lists some of the factors that determine the magnetic resonance properties of a nitroxide and the effects they produce. Many of these effects are understood at a fundamental level, and the factors that produce them can be quantitatively determined from experimental EPR spectra, as discussed below.

Given that a nitroxide side chain (or chains) can be introduced within a protein at any desired position, information regarding the factors shown in Table 10.1 can be determined for the nitroxide at the specific site in question. With this as primary experimental input, four specific types of structural information can be sought with SDSL at its present level of analysis: (*1*) chain topology; (*2*) electrostatic potential at a site; (*3*) secondary and tertiary structures; and (*4*) distance between two nitroxide side chains introduced at different sites. These points are discussed below with reference to Figure 10.1, which shows a hypothetical transmembrane protein to illustrate the main points of the method. The protein is shown as an α-helical bundle, a popular motif, but the methods discussed are quite general and applicable to any structure.

Table 10.1. Factors That Affect Magnetic Resonance Parameters of Nitroxides

Factor	Principal Parameters Used to Analyze Effects
Rotational correlation time, τ_r	
$10^{-11} < \tau_r < 10^{-7}$	Spectral lineshape, T_2[a]
$10^{-7} < \tau_r < 10^{-3}$	Spectral diffusion, T_2
Anisotropy of motion	Spectral lineshape
Orientation	Dependence of spectrum on orientation of magnetic field with respect to sample
Dielectric constant of medium	Spectral lineshape (through effects on g, A[b] tensor elements)
Collision rate with another radical	T_2, T_1[c], saturation transfer between radicals
Distance from other radicals	Spectral lineshape, T_1, T_2

[a] T_2 is the transverse relaxation time of the nitroxide.
[b] A and g are the hyperfine coupling and g tensors, respectively.
[c] T_1 is the spin-lattice relaxation time.

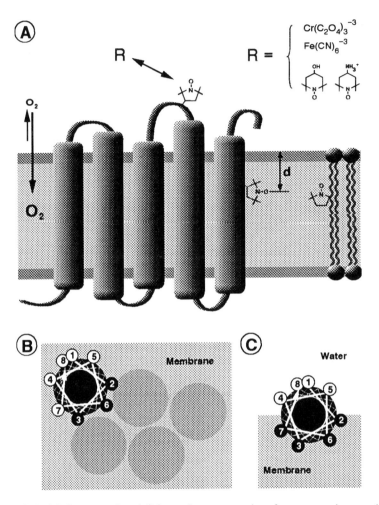

Fig. 10.1. Spin-label topography. *A*: Schematic representation of a transmembrane α-helical bundle showing the main topological features. Two nitroxide spin labels are shown attached to the protein, one facing the aqueous phase and the other the hydrophobic interior of the membrane. The substance *R* is a diffusible radical (an "exchange reagent") that may undergo collisions with the nitroxide radicals. Some examples of exchange reagents are shown. *B*: Views down the helical axes of the protein shown in *A*. On one helix, successive residues are numbered *1* to *8*. Nitroxide side chains on these positions would periodically experience two distinct environments, one on the interior of the protein (residues *2, 3, 6*) and the other on the external surface facing the chains of the lipids (*1, 4, 5, 7, 8*). *C*: View along the helical axis of an amphiphilic α-helix adsorbed to the surface of a bilayer. Successive residues along the helix are numbered *1* to *8*. Nitroxide side chains at these positions would periodically sample two distinct environments, one being the membrane interior (*1, 4, 5*) and the other the aqueous phase (*2, 3, 6, 7*).

Determination of Chain Topology and Surface Electrostatic Potential

For membrane proteins, the polypeptide chain may cross the solution–membrane interface multiple times, and the N- and C-terminal domains may be on the same or opposite side of the membrane. The chain topology is defined as a description of which residues are in the membrane or protein interior, which are water exposed, and, for the exposed residues, on which side of the membrane they are located.

This important information is available in a straightforward manner with SDSL. Consider a nitroxide side chain placed at an exposed site such as that in the inter-helical loop in Figure 10.1*A* and a diffusing radical *R* in the surrounding solution. Collisions between the nitroxide and *R* result in Heisenberg exchange (Eastman et al., 1969, 1970; Molin et al., 1980), and *the exchange rate is directly measurable from the nitroxide magnetic resonance* (see later under Experimental and Theoretical Methods of Analysis of Electron Paramagnetic Resonance Data). *R* is referred to as an *exchange reagent* and may be any paramagnetic substance, including another nitroxide. The exchange rate, W_{ex}, of the nitroxide with *R* can be written as (Shin and Hubbell, 1992)

$$W_{ex} = 4\pi gdD[C_R] \exp\left(-\frac{ZF\Phi}{RT}\right) \tag{1}$$

where d is the collision diameter; D is the relative diffusion coefficient of the nitroxide and R; g is a "steric factor"; $[C_R]$ and Z are the bulk concentration and valence of R, respectively; and ϕ is the local electrostatic potential at the site of the nitroxide. The steric factor takes into account environmental features that reduce the collision rate of the nitroxide more with a diffusing species than with a free solution and contains direct structural information on the local site on the protein surface.

To determine whether a side chain is water exposed, R is chosen such that it is water soluble, but completely insoluble in the membrane and protein interior. This is conveniently arranged, for example, if R bears a net charge or is zwitterionic. Chromium(III) oxalate (CROX) and ferricyanide ($Fe[CN]_6^{-3}$) ion are useful reagents for this purpose. If W_{ex} is finite with these reagents, the side chain may be concluded to be water exposed. For a given concentration of an exchange reagent, the magnitude of W_{ex} is a function of both g and ϕ. To obtain simple accessibility data, electrostatic effects can be reduced by using an uncharged reagent ($Z = 0$) or working at high salt concentration at which ϕ is greatly reduced.

If the nitroxide side chain is not water exposed, it may be located on an external surface of the protein, but in the bilayer interior phase. An example is shown for a nitroxide on the a transmembrane surface in Figure 10.1*A*. In this situation, the nitroxide group is solvated directly by the hydrocarbon chains of the bilayer. To determine whether this is the case, an exchange reagent soluble in the bilayer interior must be chosen. Molecular oxygen is an outstanding candidate. It has a higher solubility in a fluid bilayer interior than in the aqueous phase, a large diffusion coefficient, and a small size (Windrem and Plachy, 1980; Subczynski and Hyde, 1984; Hyde and Subczynski, 1990).

The topological location of a residue is most clearly displayed using the *contrast* in W_{ex} between the water- and lipid-soluble reagents. For example, a plot of W_{ex} with a water-soluble reagent versus that with a lipid-soluble reagent has distinct

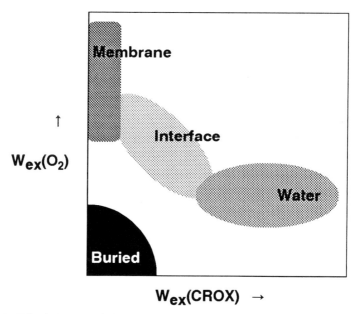

Fig. 10.2. Side chain accessibility plot of the exchange rate with a polar reagent (such as CROX) versus the exchange rate with a nonpolar reagent (such as O_2) reveals defined areas corresponding to the different topological domains for a membrane protein.

areas defining different topological locations as shown in Figure 10.2. Nitroxides facing the lipid bilayer will have high W_{ex} and O_2 and low W_{ex} with CROX and vice versa for water exposed groups. For buried nitroxides, low W_{ex} values are expected for both reagents.

Systematic application of the above ideas to a set of mutants in which the nitroxide is moved through the sequence will reveal the entrance and exit points of the polypeptide in the membrane as well as define the accessible–buried surfaces. The "inside–outside" orientation of a protein in a membrane may also be determined if the membrane is in a vesicular form with distinct inner and outer aqueous volumes. For example, a nitroxide at a particular site will undergo exchange with an impermeable reagent like CROX only if it is located on the membrane surface facing the phase to which the reagent was added. If the sample is heterogeneous with respect to orientation, the relative populations of the two orientations can be determined.

The above discussion has focused on the use of paramagnetic metal ion complexes and O_2 as exchange reagents. However, diffusible nitroxides may also be used for this purpose. In this case, the EPR spectrum of the exchange reagent must be distinguishable from that of the protein-attached nitroxide. This is readily accomplished using an ^{15}N-containing nitroxide as one species and an ^{14}N-containing nitroxide as the other. The use of nitroxides as exchange reagents has the advantage that the solubility behavior and electrical charge can be engineered by synthesis. One example in which this flexibility is employed is in the determination of the electrostatic potential at interfaces (Shin and Hubbell, 1992). For this purpose, W_{ex} for the water-exposed side chain is determined for the same concentration of both a neutral ($Z =$

0) and a charged nitroxide exchange reagent of similar size, such as the pair shown in Figure 10-1A. These have similar values of d and D. From Eq. 1, the ratio of these exchange rates is

$$\frac{W_{ex}}{W_{ex}^{o}} = \exp\left(-\frac{ZF\phi}{RT}\right) \qquad (2)$$

where W_{ex}^{o} is the exchange rate for the uncharged reagent. Thus the local electrostatic potential can be calculated from the experimentally determined exchange rates and constitutes a valuable piece of structural information. This method has been used to determine potentials at membrane, protein, and DNA surfaces (Shin and Hubbell, 1992).

Another use of a nitroxide as an exchange reagent is to determine the *depth* of an intramembrane, lipid-exposed nitroxide side chain from the aqueous interface. This depth is indicated as d in Figure 10.1A. The nitroxide exchange reagent is attached to a hydrocarbon chain of a phospholipid. The vertical position of the nitroxide on the hydrocarbon chain can be varied, and the position that gives maximal W_{ex} with the protein-fixed group defines the depth d. This method has been used to estimate the location of a nitroxide group on rhodopsin (Feix et al., 1989). Another approach to determine d utilizes the dipolar interaction of the protein-attached nitroxide with metal ions bound to the membrane surface. This approach was used by Dalton et al. (1987) to estimate the depth of a nitroxide on D-β-hydroxybutyrate dehydrogenase. Distance determination via dipolar interactions will be discussed below.

Determination of Secondary and Tertiary Structure: the Nitroxide Scanning Experiment

Consider a set of mutants in which the members differ only by the position of a single labeled cysteine *in sequence*. This will be referred to as a *nitroxide scanning* experiment. To appreciate the information content of such an experiment, consider the example shown in Figure 10.1b, which is a top view of a membrane protein with a helix bundle motif. Shown on one of the helices are the positions that might be occupied by a nitroxide in a scanning experiment through a helical region. All of the helices are characterized by an *asymmetric interaction,* i.e., one surface faces the bilayer and the other the protein interior. In this case, the nitroxides will *periodically* sample these two distinct molecular environments (surface and buried) as they are scanned through the helix. This periodicity is readily detected in a number of ways, for example, in the exchange rate of the attached nitroxide with a diffusable reagent. The contrast between the buried (g, D, and C_R in Eq. 1 all small) and surface-exposed locations (g, D, and C_R all large) is very high. For a helix embedded in a bilayer, O_2 or a hydrophobic nitroxide would be chosen as an exchange reagent. For a structure solvated by water, CROX or another water-soluble nitroxide would be necessary (Todd et al., 1989). *From the observed periodicity, one may deduce the class of secondary structure.* For example, a helix would give a period of 3.6 residues, a β-sheet a period of 2.0 residues, and so forth. The *orientation* of the secondary structure can be deduced from the *phase* of the periodic behavior, i.e., those residues with a high W_{ex} define the outer surface and vice versa.

The periodic data from a nitroxide scanning experiment in a helical segment can be displayed by representing the W_{ex} values as vectors originating at the helical axis and pointing to the appropriate residue with a length proportional to the magnitude of W_{ex}. The sum of such individual vectors can be viewed as an "accessibility moment" and points in the direction of the surface with greatest exposure to collision. The direction of the moment is a measure of the helix orientation and can be used to investigate helix rotations during protein function.

It is clear that any periodic structure can be identified by the above procedure if it has an asymmetric interaction with its surroundings. For example, a membrane surface bound amphiphilic α-helix fulfills the conditions, as shown in Figure 10.1C. In this case, a periodicity in W_{ex} with CROX would be observed 180° out of phase with W_{ex} for O_2.

For nitroxide side chains on exposed surfaces of helices, solvated by either water or fluid hydrocarbon chains, we have uniformly observed a relatively high degree of mobility relative to the protein rotational rate (Todd et al., 1989; Altenbach et al., 1990). This is consistent with molecular models that indicate that the side chains on helices do not sterically interfere with each other. Thus we conclude that *a slow motional spectrum for a nitroxide on a helix indicates that the residue is influenced by tertiary interactions with other parts of the protein.* Hence the periodicity of a regular structure in asymmetric interaction can also be detected by changes in mobility. However, this parameter is more difficult to quantitate since the spectra often contain multiple components and cannot be realistically simulated without more information. Nevertheless, changes in mobility during conformational changes provides a powerful means of investigating changes in *tertiary* organization. An example of this use will be given for the membrane binding of colicin E1 later under Examples of Applications.

Relative collision rates and hence accessibilities can also be measured using fluorescence quenching (Vaughan and Weber, 1970). However, collision frequencies must be comparable to the inverse of the fluorescence lifetime, which is generally on the order of 10^8 Hz for organic fluorophores. The "clock" for the Heisenberg exchange experiment is T_1, and collision frequencies must be comparable with $1/T_1$ or on the order of 10^6 Hz. Thus the EPR experiment is approximately 100-fold more sensitive in detecting collision frequencies. Consequently, a much lower concentration of quencher is needed.

Distance Determinations with Pairs of Nitroxides or a Nitroxide and a Paramagnetic Metal Ion

A pair of nitroxides can be introduced into a single protein structure in specific positions by any of the means discussed above. The determination of distance between such pairs in a folded protein is one of the most important capabilities of SDSL, since it is direct structural information. Having determined the segments of regular secondary structure by topological means as outlined above, a few critical distances would suffice to locate these segments relative to each other. In the absence of motion, dipole–dipole interactions between the nitroxides can be quantitatively analyzed by empirical or theoretical methods to give the interspin distance. The maximum interaction distance appears to be on the order of 35 Å (Kokorin et al., 1972).

To increase the range of distance that can be determined, nitroxide–paramagnetic ion pairs could be introduced rather than nitroxide pairs. In this case, measurable dipolar interactions can extend to 150 Å, depending on the metal (Kulikov and Likhtenstein, 1977). To introduce a nitroxide at one site and a metal at another, both a cysteine (or a nitroxide directly) and a metal ion–binding site could be engineered in the protein. Binding sites have already been engineered for purification of mutant proteins on metal ion columns. For example, introduction of a $-His-X_3-His-$ sequence in an α-helical segment of the peptide creates a binding site for Cu(II) (Arnold and Haymore, 1991).

Experimental and Theoretical Methods of Analysis of Electron Paramagnetic Resonance

Some of the molecular and environmental factors that influence the magnetic resonance parameters of a nitroxide are given in Table 10.1. While all of these factors reveal interesting features of the local environment in the protein, only those that have been exploited in SDSL to date will be discussed here. Of the most importance for the present purposes are the *apparent rotational correlation time* of the attached nitroxide, the *collision (exchange) frequency between radicals,* and the *dipolar interaction between radicals.* As discussed above, these factors have high structural information content when used in a nitroxide scanning experiment.

In the section below, a necessarily brief and selective description of these three relevant measurements will be given, along with specific literature references. A comprehensive review is beyond the scope of this chapter, and the interested reader is urged to consult the references given for a more complete analysis.

Determination of Rotational Correlation Time and Anisotropy

The incomplete averaging of the anisotropic interactions between a spin label and the magnetic field gives rise to spectral lineshapes that indicate the rotational rate of the nitroxide. As indicated in Table 10.1, lineshapes are most sensitive to motions with rotational correlations times in the range $10^{-7} < T_r < 10^{-11}$. Most membrane-bound proteins have rotational correlation times longer than this, and the motion of a surface nitroxide side chain is that *relative* to the protein, while that for a buried side chain reflects local structure fluctuations and protein rotary diffusion. The motional sensitivity can be extended down to the millisecond range using saturation transfer EPR spectroscopy (Hyde and Thomas, 1980). In principle, it is possible to determine the motional characteristics of an attached nitroxide by simulation of the spectrum using a variety of models (Schneider and Freed, 1989; Hyde and Thomas, 1980). However, in the most general case, the number of adjustable parameters is prohibitively large. Complications from orienting potentials, anisotropic motions, and heterogeneous populations of spins make unique simulation difficult. However, adequate approximations can usually be made and limits of motion set with simplified models assuming isotropic or simple anisotropic motions. For structural information of the type discussed here, it is generally sufficient to make coarse classifications from these simplified models in terms of mobile, intermediate, and immobile. A computer program for simulations is available, along with an excellent review of the state of the art (Schneider and Freed, 1989).

Determination of Collision Rates betweeen Radicals

Collision rates are determined through the Heisenberg exchange rate and its effect on the magnetic resonance parameters of the nitroxide. For the situations discussed in this chapter, the exchange is assumed to be "strong," i.e., collision rate and exchange rate are equal. A comprehensive treatment of Heisenberg exchange is given by Molin et al. (1980), and an excellent review slanted toward biological applications is that by Hyde et al. (1979). The method for determination of exchange rates depends on the nature of the exchange reagent undergoing collision with the nitroxide. One class of useful reagents consists of those with very short spin lattice relaxation times and the other of the nitroxides themselves. These are discussed separately below.

Collisions Between a Nitroxide and a Reagent with a Short Spin Lattice Relaxation Time. If the reagent has a spin lattice relaxation time T_{1R} such that $1/T_{1R} \gg W_{ex}$, Heisenberg exchange is effectively a spin lattice relaxation event for the nitroxide and produces changes in the relaxation rate equal to the exchange rate, i.e.,

$$\frac{1}{T_1} = \frac{1}{T_1^o} + 2W_{ex} \tag{3}$$

where T_1 and T_1^o are the nitroxide spin lattice relaxation times in the presence and absence of the exchange reagent, respectively. Thus methods that measure changes in T_1 can be used to study collision rates. An equivalent expression may be written for T_2, the effective spin–spin relaxation time, and W_{ex} may be estimated directly from the spectral linewidths, which are inversely related to T_2. However, for the relatively immobilized nitroxides bound to proteins, T_2 is much shorter than T_1, and proportionally larger exchange rates are required to observe an effect. Hence methods based on T_1 are more sensitive and are emphasized here.

Two methods have routinely been used to obtain T_1 or a value proportional to it: pulse saturation recovery EPR (SR-EPR) and continuous wave saturation EPR (CWS-EPR). SR-EPR determines the time course of recovery of magnetization following a saturating pulse of microwave radiation and hence measures T_1 directly. For a review of the basic instrumentation and principles, see Hyde (1979). This method of T_1 measurement was employed for the study of membrane-bound melittin (Altenbach et al., 1989a). A disadvantage at this time is the highly specialized equipment required.

CWS-EPR can be performed on a conventional EPR spectrometer, preferably fitted with a loop-gap resonator (LGR). The LGR is a recent development and is important in that it provides a sufficient microwave energy density to saturate a nitroxide resonance with any realistic T_1 (for review, see Hyde and Froncisz, 1989). A convenient experimental parameter determined from CWS-EPR is $P_{1/2}$, the microwave power required to saturate the signal to one-half the amplitude it would have if it did not saturate at all. Changes in $P_{1/2}$ are related to the exchange rate according to Subczynski and Hyde (1981) and Altenbach et al. (1989b):

$$\Delta P_{1/2} = P_{1/2} - P_{1/2}^o \propto \frac{1}{T_2 T_1} - \frac{1}{T_2^o T_1^o} \approx \frac{1}{T_2^o}\left(\frac{1}{T_1} - \frac{1}{T_1^o}\right) = \frac{2W_{ex}}{T_2^o} \quad (4)$$

where the superscript o refers to quantities in the absence of the exchange reagent, and T_2 is the effective spin–spin relaxation time of the nitroxide. As indicated, this relationship is approximate and assumes that T_2 is independent of the exchange rate. This is generally the case for a nitroxide on a membrane-bound protein where T_2 is much less than T_1 and where the concentration of exchange reagent is such that $W_{ex} \ll 1/T_2$.

Collision between Two Nitroxides. Collisions between two nitroxides give rise to Heisenberg exchange, but this is not a spin lattice relaxation event and does not lead to a change in T_1. However, collision rates between two nitroxides on the MHz time scale can be quantitated by electron–electron double resonance spectroscopy (ELDOR). The method was introduced by Hyde and is ideally suited to determination of Heisenberg exchange events (Hyde et al., 1968). An ELDOR spectrometer based on the LGR has a sensitivity roughly equal to a conventional spectrometer (Hyde et al., 1985), and double resonance techniques become a realistic consideration even for very limited samples.

The most useful implementation of the technique employs two nitroxide species, one containing ^{15}N and the other ^{14}N (Stetter et al., 1976). Under conditions where spectral resolution between the species is achieved, it is possible to saturate one species (the "pumped" species) with an intense microwave source and observe saturation transfer to the other ("observed") species via Heisenberg exchange. From the degree of saturation transfer, W_{ex} can be determined. For an excellent review of biological applications of the technique, see Hyde and Feix (1989).

Determination of Distances between Radicals

Nitroxide–Nitroxide Interspin Distances. In the absence of molecular motion, the dipolar interaction between two nitroxides separated by 10–35 Å may be quantitatively analyzed to obtain the interspin distance. Dipolar interactions give rise to splittings in the spectrum, and when these are well resolved the splitting may be used directly to obtain the interspin distance (see Eaton and Eaton, 1989, for a comprehensive review; Kokorin et al., 1972; Beth et al., 1984). When the distances are large and the dipolar interaction is small, the splittings are not resolved and appear as an increase in spectral linewidth. The linewidth increase is related to the strength of the interaction, and Kokorin et al. (1972) have proposed use of a very simple parameter, the ratio of two spectral intensities in frozen solution, as a sensitive measure of the linewidth increase. This parameter must be calibrated in terms of the interspin distance through the use of proper model compounds with known interspin distance and in the absence of exchange interaction (Eaton and Eaton, 1989). This method has been applied to hemoglobin (Kokorin et al., 1972), rhodopsin (Delmelle and Virmaux, 1977), melittin (Altenbach and Hubbell, 1988) and synthetic DNA binding peptides (Anthony-Cahill et al., 1991).

The dipolar splitting (and broadening) depends on the relative orientation of the nitroxides in the pair, and this is generally unknown. For nitroxide pairs in which one or both are located at the external surface of the protein, a random relative orientation may be assumed, and model systems in which a similar assumption can be made must be employed for calibration. Alternatively, spectral simulation may be utilized to extract distance information (Eaton et al., 1983; Beth et al., 1984). Nitroxide pairs introduced at the surface of proteins with accurately known structure provide an ideal system in which to evaluate critically the various strategies, and this is currently under study.

Nitroxide–Paramagnetic Ion Interspin Distances. The interaction between a nitroxide and a paramagnetic metal ion can be analyzed in terms of distance either by lineshape analysis or by direct determination of nitroxide relaxation times. Much of the relevant literature has been reviewed in the comprehensive series of reviews by Eaton and Eaton (1978, 1988, 1989). Most popular of the lineshape analyses is that of Leigh (1969). Eaton and Eaton (1988) discuss the rather restrictive conditions necessary for the Leigh theory to apply. The parametric approach of Kokorin and coworkers mentioned above has been extended to determine metal ion–nitroxide distances in immobilized systems (Kokorin and Formazyuk, 1981).

For fast-relaxing metal ions, the dipolar interaction results in changes in the nitroxide relaxation times. Kulikov (1976) has demonstrated that changes in T_1 due to the presence of fast-relaxing metals can be determined by CW saturation techniques and analytically related to interspin distance. Kulikov and Lichtenstein (1977) estimate that distances up to 150 Å can be determined. This is an extremely promising method for distance determination using SDSL.

Examples of Applications

The SDSL approach is very recent, and its full range of potential applications has not yet been explored. Nevertheless, two membrane proteins have been studied by the nitroxide scanning technique, and the results serve to illustrate most of the capabilities outlined in the preceding sections.

Bacteriorhodopsin

The most extensive application of SDSL reported to date has been on bacteriorhodopsin. This molecule is an excelllent choice for initial studies, since the main features of the structure are known from the electron diffraction studies of Henderson and Unwin (1975) and Henderson et al. (1990), yet many important details remain to be learned. The elegant work of Khorana and coworkers in which a synthetic bacteriorhodopsin gene was used in the expression of a large number of site-directed mutants also made the molecule a practical choice for study (Braiman et al., 1987; Nassal et al., 1987). In collaboration with the Khorana group, 33 spin-labeled cysteine mutants have been investigated (Altenbach et al., 1989b, 1990; Greenhalgh et al., 1991).

Figure 10.3 shows all of the spin-labeled sites on a representation of the structural model drawn according to the coordinates kindly provided by Richard Henderson. The data set did not include the coordinates of the loop atoms connecting the helices, and the loops were added in a somewhat arbitrary configuration to illustrate the positions of the spin labels in the sequence and the helix connectivity.

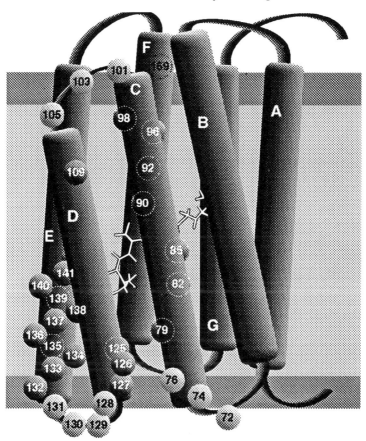

Fig. 10.3. Schematic structure of bacteriorhodopsin showing the positions of spin-labeled mutants. The cylindrical surfaces correspond to the helical transmembrane segments based on the coordinates determined by Henderson et al. (1990). The positions of all labeled mutants are shown. The loops are drawn arbitrarily to indicate helix connectivity. The lower part of helix E was extended according to data based on SDSL (Altenbach et al., 1990). The *dotted outlines* indicate spin-label positions hidden from view by the helical surfaces. The numbers in *black* indicate water-exposed residues as judged by CROX accessibility. The numbers in *white* are inaccessible to CROX. The boundaries between these two classes determine the positions at which the membrane surfaces intersect the protein. The retinal chromophore is shown in *white* between the helices.

The series from 125 to 142 constitutes a nitroxide scanning experiment and nicely illustrates secondary structure determination (Altenbach et al., 1990). According to the Henderson model (Henderson et al., 1990), some members of this series should be contained in the E helix, while others are in the D–E loop region or in the D helix itself. Collision frequency data in terms of $\Delta P_{1/2}$ for the nitroxide groups in this series with both O_2 and CROX are shown versus the sequence position in Figure 10-4A. The striking oscillation seen in $\Delta P_{1/2}$ for O_2 in the region 131–139 has a period of 3.6, corresponding to an α-helix. The orientation of the helical segment is readily determined from the phase of the periodic function: the residues with the highest

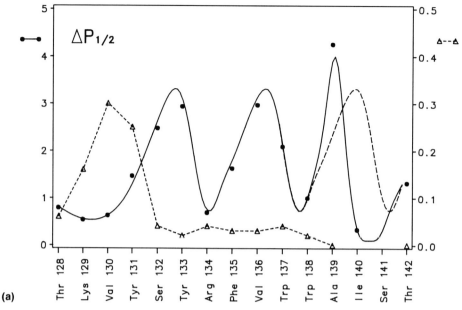

(a)

Fig. 10.4. The chromium oxalate and O_2 accessibility of the nitroxide side chains on spin-labeled bacteriorhodopsin mutants. *a*: Nitroxide scanning experiment for residues 128–142. Residues 129–131 are part of a water-exposed loop as shown by the CROX accessibility *(dotted line)*. Residues 132–139 show a periodic accessibility to O_2 with a period of 3.6 residues *(solid line)*, indicating an α-helical structure. This helix is within the membrane interior as

collision frequency with O_2 (largest $\Delta P_{1/2}$) define the outer (exposed) helical surface. The topological location of the helical segment is clearly revealed to be intramembrane by the low value of $\Delta P_{1/2}$ for CROX (dashed line, Fig. 10.4*A*). This is consistent with the large $\Delta P_{1/2}$ for O_2 for this region, since the O_2 solubility in the bilayer is high. The large values for $\Delta P_{1/2}$ for CROX in the region 129–132 define the loop between helices D and E in the aqueous phase.

Another experiment illustrates the capabilities of locating the membrane–solution boundaries relative to the protein structure (Greenhalgh et al., 1991). In this case, attention was directed to the C helix, which contains residues critical for proton pumping (82, 85, 96) and is believed to line a proton "channel" in the structure (Henderson et al., 1990) Figure 10-4*B* shows $\Delta P_{1/2}$ values for both CROX and O_2 plotted versus position through the sequence of helix C. Residues 82, 85, 96, and 98 are buried within the protein fold, judging by the low values of $\Delta P_{1/2}$ for both reagents and the low motional rate of the nitroxides (data now shown). The aqueous boundaries occur near Tyr[79] and Val[101] as shown by the abrupt increases in $\Delta P_{1/2}$ for CROX. Information of this type on the locations of the membrane interfaces is not available from the diffraction data.

Colicin E1

Colicin E1 is a member of a family of soluble proteins synthesized by bacteria as a cytotoxin (see Lazdunski et al., 1988, and Cramer et al., 1990, for recent reviews).

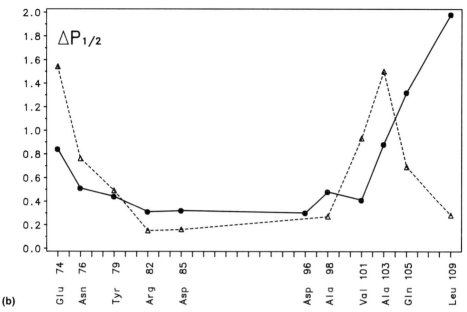

(b)

indicated by the low CROX accessibility for this entire region. *b*: Accessibility in helix C. The accessibility to CROX oxalate *(dotted line)* reveals the location of the membrane–solution interface to be near residues 76 and 101 in helix C. The O_2 accessibility is low in the membrane interior and not periodic *(solid line)*, since all of these mutations are on the *inner* surface of helix C (see Fig. 10.3).

Although synthesized as a soluble protein, it binds irreversibly to membranes of sensitive cells and forms a voltage-dependent ion channel. The C-terminal domain of the protein is responsible for channel formation. Recently, the structure of the water-soluble form of this domain was reported for the closely related colicin A (Parker et al., 1989). A suggested structure for the corresponding colicin E1 fragment generated by the programs HOMOLOGY and DISCOVER (Biosym, Inc. San Diego, CA) is shown in Figure 10.5*A*. The major sequence difference between colicins A and E1 is a deletion of 10 amino acids between the two central hydrophobic helices (numbered 8 and 9), and the model structure has a shorter connecting loop and slight rearrangements of some of the helices to overcome atomic overlap due to the differences in side chains. This is intended as a working model, but is likely to be reasonably close based on some recent two-dimensional NMR results (Wormald et al., 1990). The most striking feature of the water-soluble structure is the presence of a "helical hairpin" consisting of two completely hydrophobic helices buried within a cluster of surrounding amphiphilic helices. In collaboration with the Levinthal group at Columbia, nitroxide scanning experiments have been conducted in two domains: (*1*) 398–406 in the loop between helices 3 and 4 (Todd et al., 1989) and (*2*) 482–492 (Hayer-Hartl, M., Todd, P., Levinthal, F., Cong, J., Levinthal, C., Hubbell, W., work in progress) in the hydrophobic helices and interconnecting loop. The primary information sought is the structure of the membrane-bound fragment, and key aspects of this structure are clearly demonstrated by the application of SDSL using O_2 accessibility and *mobility* of the nitroxide.

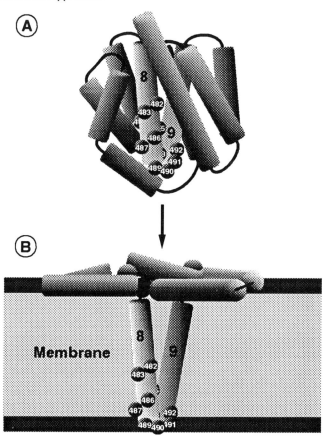

Fig. 10.5. Model for the C terminal fragment of colicin E1 and its membrane-bound form. *A*: A model for the solution structure of the water-soluble form of colicin E1 based on the known structure of the homologous colicin A. The helices 8 and 9 are hydrophobic and surrounded by eight other helices. The positions of a nitroxide scanning series in the helices 8 and 9 and the connecting loop are shown based on SDSL experiments described in the text. *B*: The structure of the membrane-bound form suggested by SDSL experiments.

Figure 10.6 shows data on the mobility of the side chains (in terms of correlation time) versus $\Delta P_{1/2}$ for O_2 in the interesting 482–492 sequence. Several regions can be identified on this plot. First, the area corresponding to long correlation times (slow motion) and low O_2 accessibility also corresponds to sites buried in the protein interior. Second, the area corresponding to short correlation times (fast motion) and high O_2 collision rates represents nitroxide side chains facing the fluid bilayer interior, where O_2 solubility is high. Finally, an area corresponding to short correlation times and low O_2 collision rates can be identified with water-exposed residues.

In Figure 10.6, data obtained with colicin E1 *in solution* are indicated with solid dots, and those obtained from the *membrane-bound* form are indicted with open circles. Residues 482, 484, 485, 487, and 492 are clearly buried within the fold in the soluble protein, as would be expected for the hydrophobic helices surrounded isotropically by amphiphilic helices (Fig. 10.5*A*). On the other hand, 488, 489, 490 and 491 are water exposed, strongly suggesting that this is the hairpin loop region in

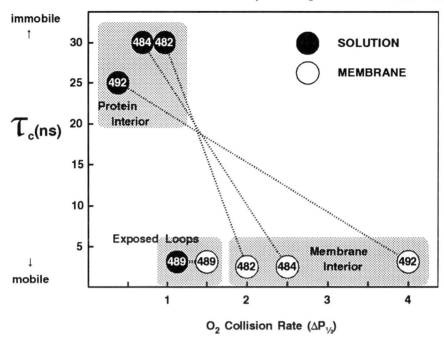

Fig. 10.6. A plot of nitroxide correlation time versus $\Delta P_{1/2}$ for O_2 for both the solution and the membrane-bound form of spin-labeled colicin E1. The *solid black dots* correspond to data obtained with the water-soluble form of colicin E1, while the *open circles* correspond to data obtained with the membrane-bound form. This plot defines different topological domains for the spin label, as indicated. Upon membrane binding, the nitroxides at 482, 484, and 492 move from the protein interior to a position facing the fluid hydrocarbon chains of the bilayer, while that at 489 undergoes no change. This result strongly supports the model in Figure 10.5.

Colicin E1, as indicated in the model. Figure 10.6 shows that a dramatic change occurs in membrane binding, namely, *residues 482, 484, and 492 move from the buried location to that facing the membrane interior.* The other members of the set have not yet been studied at the time of this writing, but this result clearly indicates the insertion of the hydrophobic hairpin into the bilayer to give a structure such as that shown in Figure 10.5B. Recent data obtained on fluorescent-labeled mutants of colicin A support a similar structure (Lakey et al., 1991a,b). Equally interesting is the lack of change at 489, in the loop. This suggests that the loop is inserted completely across the membrane, so it remains solvated before and after insertion. This example illustrates the combined use of nitroxide mobility and accessibility to monitor changes in tertiary interactions during conformational rearrangements.

Summary and Future Developments

Advantages of the SDSL Method

As stated in the beginning, and illustrated by the above examples, SDSL is capable of identifying regular secondary structural elements, their tertiary interactions, and their disposition relative to the membrane interfaces. Although a specific example was not provided, the surface electrostatic potential profile can also be determined. Many models of function for membrane proteins involve rigid-body motions of secondary structural elements, and in these instances this level of structural resolution is ideal to study mechanisms.

The major advantages of SDSL are (*1*) a crystalline array is not required; (*2*) proteins of any molecular weight or degree of mobility can be investigated; (*3*) useable data can be obtained from single-scan spectra using as little as 10–100 pmol quantities of labeled protein in an LGR; (*4*) it is possible to follow spectral changes in real time in the millisecond time domain, making direct investigation of conformational changes feasible; and (*5*) data need only be collected on the region of interest in a complex structure.

The last two points are of particular importance for high-molecular-weight membrane proteins whose functions are believed to involve rigid-body movements of only a small fraction of the molecule. The proposed motion of the S4 segment of the voltage-dependent sodium channel is an example (Guy and Seetharamulu, 1986; Catterall, 1988).

Future Developments

An important improvement in SDSL will be the use of suppressor RNAs for the direct incorporation of nitroxide amino acids. The many advantages were listed above, and the technology is already in place. Another rich area of exploration is the use of nitroxide pairs and nitroxide–metal ion pairs for distance determination in proteins. The long-range interaction of a metal ion with a nitroxide as detected by enhanced relaxation may be extremely useful in this context. Although the theory has been described, a careful test has yet to be made with proper model systems and time–domain measurements.

Perhaps the greatest strength of the SDSL method is its time resolution for detection of conformational changes. For example, it should be possible to time resolve the structural reorganization that occurs when colicin binds to membrane or when bacteriorhodopsin pumps protons. It is also obvious that protein folding could be studied. With nitroxides in different positions, it should be possible to determine in real time the rate and order in which domains assemble.

Acknowledgments

Research support was provided by NIH grant EY5216 and the Jules Stein Professor endowment.

References

Altenbach, C., and Hubbell, W. L. (1988) The aggregation state of spin-labeled melittin in solution and bound to phospholipid membranes: evidence that membrane bound melittin is monomeric. *Proteins: Struct. Funct. Genet.* 3: 230–242.

Altenbach, C., Froncisz, W., Hyde, J. S., and Hubbell, W. L. (1989a) Conformation of spin-labeled melittin at membrane surfaces investigated by pulse saturation recovery and continuous wave saturation ESR. *Biophys. J.* 56: 1183–1193.

Altenbach, C., Flitsch, S. L., Khorana, H. G., and Hubbell, W. L. (1989b) Structural studies on trans-membrane proteins. 2. Spin labeling of bacteriorhodopsin mutants at unique cysteines. *Biochemistry* 28: 7806–7812.

Altenbach, C., Marti, T., Khorana, H. G., and Hubbell, W. L. (1990) Transmembrane protein structure: spin labeling of bacteriorhodopsin mutants. *Science* 248: 1088–1092.

Anthony-Cahill, S., Benfield, P., Fairman, R., Wasserman, Z., Brenner, S., Altenbach, C., Hubbell, W., Stafford, W., DeGrado, W. (1992) Molecular characterization of helix-loop-helix peptides. *Science* 255:979–983.

Arnold, F. H., and Haymore, B. L. (1991) Engineered metal-binding proteins: purification to protein folding. *Science* 252: 1796–1797.

Bain, J. D., Diala, E. S., Glabe, C. G., Wacker, D. A., Lyttle, M. H., Dix, T. A., and Chamberlin, A. R. (1989) Site-specific incorporation of nonnatural residues during in vitro protein biosynthesis with semisynthetic aminoacyl-tRNAs. *Biochemistry* 30: 5411–5421.

Bashford, D., Chothia, C., and Lesk, A. M. (1987) Determinants of a protein fold. *J. Mol. Biol.* 196: 199–216.

Berliner, L. J. (1976) *Spin Labeling: Theory and Applications.* New York: Academic Press, 650 pp.

Berliner, L. J., Grinwald, J., Hankovszky, H. O., and Hideg, K. (1982) A novel reversible thiol-specific spin label-papain active-site labeling and inhibition. *Anal. Biochem.* 119: 450.

Berliner, L. J. (1979) *Spin Labeling II: Theory and Applications.* New York: Academic Press, 357 pp.

Berliner, L. J., and Reuben (1990) *Biological Magnetic Resonance, Vol. 8.* New York: Plenum Press, 650 pp.

Beth, A. H., Robinson, B. H., Cobb, C. E., Dalton, L. R., Trommer, W. E., Birktoft, J. J., and Park, J. H. (1984) Interactions and spatial arrangement of spin-labelled NAD^+ bound glyceraldehyde-3-phosphate dehydrogenase. *J. Biol. Chem.* 259: 9717–9728.

Boeyens, J.C.A., and McConnell, H. M. (1966) Spin labeled hemoglobin *Proc. Natl. Acad. Sci. USA* 56: 22–25.

Bowie, J. U., Reidhaar-Olson, J. F., Lim, W. A., and Sauer, R. T. (1990) Deciphering the message in protein sequences: tolerance to amino acid substitutions. *Science* 247: 1306–1310.

Braiman, M. S., Stern, L. J., Chao, B. H., and Khorana, H. G. (1987) Structure-function studies on bacteriorhodopsin IV. Purification and renaturation of bacterio-opsin polypeptide expressed in *Escherichia coli. J. Biol. Chem.* 262: 9271–9276.

Catterall, W. A. (1988) Structure and function of voltage-sensitive ion channels. *Science* 242: 50–61.

Cramer, W. A., Cohen, F. S., Merrill, A. R., and Song, H. Y. (1990) Structure and dynamics of the colicin E1 channel. *Mol. Microbiol.* 4: 519–526.

Cseko, J., Hankovszky, H. O., and Hideg, K. (1984) Synthesis of novel, highly reactive 1-oxyl-2,2,6,6-tetramethyl-1,2,5,6-tetrahydropyridine derivatives. *Can. J. Chem.* 63: 940–943.

Dalton, L. R. (1985) *Electron Paramagnetic Resonance.* Boca Raton, FL: CRC Press 314 pp.

Dalton, L. A., McIntyre, J. O., and Fleischer, S. (1987) Distance estimate of the active center of D-β-hydroxybutyrate dehydrogenase from the membrane surface. *Biochemistry* 26:2117–2130.

Delmelle, M., and Virmaux, N. (1977) Location of two sulfhydryl groups in the rhodopsin molecule by use of the spin label technique. *Biochim. Biophys. Acta* 464:370–377.

Dickerson, R. E. (1980) Cytochrome *c* and the evolution of energy metabolism. *Sci. Am.* 242: 136.

Eastman, M. P., Kooser, R. G., Das, M. R., and Freed, J. H. (1969) Studies of Heisenberg spin exchange in ESR spectra. I. Linewidth and saturation effects. *J. Chem. Phys.* 51: 2690–2709.

Eastman, M. P., Bruno, G. V., and Freed, J. H. (1970) ESR study of Heisenberg spin exchange. II. Effects of radial charge and size. *J. Chem. Phys.* 52: 2511–2522.

Eaton, G., and Eaton, S. (1989) Resolved electron-electron spin-spin splittings in EPR spectra. In: *Biological Magnetic Resonance,* edited by L. J. Berliner and J. Reuben. New York, Plenum, vol. 8, p. 340–397.

Eaton, S. S., and Eaton, G. R. (1978) Interaction of spin labels with transition metals. *Coord. Chem. Rev.* 26: 207–262.

Eaton, S., More, K. M., Sawant, B. M., Boymel, P. M., and Eaton, G. (1983) Metal-nitroxyl interations. 29. EPR studies of spin-labeled copper complexes in frozen solution. *J. Magn. Reson.* 52:435–449.

Eaton, S. S., and Eaton, G. R. (1988) Interaction of spin labels with transition metals: Part 2. *Coord. Chem. Rev.* 83: 29–72.

Feix, J., Hubbell, C., and Hubbell, W. L. (1989) Motional dynamics of steric acid spin labels and lipid protein interactions in bovine rod outer segment membranes as studied by ELDOR and saturation recovery EPR. *Biophys. J.* 55, 325a.

Grassetti, D. R., and Murray J. F. Jr. (1967) Determination of sulfhydryl groups with 2,2'-or 4,4'-dithio-pyridine. *Arch. Biochem. Biophys.* 119:41–49.

Greenhalgh, D., Altenbach, C., Hubbell, W. L., and Khorana, H. G. (1991) Locations of Arg-82, Asp-85 and Asp-96 in helix C of bacteriorhodopsin relative to the aqueous boundaries. *Proc. Natl. Acad. Sci. USA* 88, 8626–8630.

Guy, H. R., and Seetharamulu, P. (1986) Molecular model of the action potential sodium channel. *Proc. Natl. Acad. Sci. USA* 83: 508–512.

Henderson, R., and Unwin, P.N.T. (1975) Three-dimensional model of purple membrane obtained by electron microscopy. *Nature* 257: 28–32.

Henderson, R., Baldwin, J. M., Ceska, T. A., Zemlin, F., Beckmann, E., and Downing, K. H. (1990) A model of the structure of bacteriorhodopsin based on high resolution cryo-electron microscopy. *J. Mol. Biol.* 213: 899–929.

Hideg, K., Sar, C. P., Hankovszky, O. H., and Jerkovich, G. (1991) Allylic nitroxyl spin label reagents. *Synthesis* 615–620.

Hemminga, M. A. (1983) Interpretation of ESR and saturation transfer ESR spectra of spin labeled lipids and membranes. *Chem. Phys. Lipids* 32: 323–383.

Hoff, A. J. (1989) *Advanced EPR: Applications in Biology and Biochemistry.* New York: Elsevier, 918 pp.

Humphries, G.M.K., and McConnell, H. M. (1982) Nitroxide spin labels. In: *Methods of Experimental Physics*, edited by C. Marton. New York: Academic Press, vol. 20, p. 53–122.

Hyde, J. S., Chien, C. W., and Freed, J. H. (1968) Electron-electron double resonance of free radicals in solution. *J. Chem. Phys.* 48: 4211–4226.

Hyde, J. S. (1979) Saturation recovery methodology. In: *Time Domain Electron Spin Resonance,* edited by L. Kevan and R. N. Schwartz. New York: John Wiley and Sons, p. 1–29.

Hyde, J. S., Swartz, H. M., and Antholine, W. E. (1979) The spin-probe-spin-label method. In: *Spin Labeling*, edited by L. J. Berliner. New York: Academic Press, vol. 2, p. 71–113.

Hyde, J. S., and Thomas, D. D. (1980) Saturation transfer spectroscopy. *Annu. Rev. Phys. Chem.* 31: 293–317.

Hyde, J. S., Yin, J. J., Froncisz, W., and Feix, J. B. (1985) Electron-electron double resonance with a loop-gap resonator. *J. Magn. Reson.* 63: 142–150.

Hyde, J. S., and Froncisz, W. (1989) Loop-gap resonators. In: *Advanced EPR: Applications in Biology and Biochemistry*, edited by A. J. Hoff. Amsterdam: Elsevier, p. 277–305.

Hyde, J. S., and Feix, J. B. (1989) Electron-electron double resonance. In: *Biological Magnetic Resonance.* edited by L. J. Berliner and J. Reuben. New York: Plenum, vol. 8, p. 305–337.

Hyde, J. S., and Subszynski, W. K. (1990) Spin-label oximetry. In: *Biological Magnetic Resonance.* edited by L. J. Berliner and J. Reuben. New York: Plenum, p. 399–425.

Karnik, S. S., and Khorana, H. G. (1990) Assembly of functional rhodopsin requires a disulfide bond between residues 110 and 187. *J. Biol. Chem.* 265: 17520–17524.

Khramtsov, V. V., Yelinova, V. I., Weiner, L. M., Berezina, T. A., Martin, V. V. and Volodarsky, L. B. (1989) Quantitative determination of SH groups in low- and high-molecular-weight compounds by an electron spin resonance method. *Anal. Biochem.* 182:58–63.

Kokorin, A. I., Zamarayev, K. I., Grigoryan, G. L., Ivanov, V. P., and Rozantsex, E. G. (1972) Measurement of the distances between the paramagnetic centres in solid solutions of nitroxide radicals, biradicals and spin-labeled proteins. *Biofizika* 17: 34–41.

Kokorin, A. I., and Formazyuk, V. E. (1981) New method of measuring distances between spin label and paramagnetic metal ions in macromolecules. *Mol. Biol.* 15: 930–938.

Kulikov, A. V. (1976) Determination of distances between the spins of a label and a paramagnetic center in spin-labeled proteins from the parameters of the saturation curve of the ESR spectrum of the label at 77° K. *Mol. Biol.* 10: 132–141.

Kulikov, A. V., and Likhtenstein, G. I. (1977) The use of spin relaxation phenomena in the investigation of the structure of model and biological systems by the method of spin labels. *Adv. Mol. Relax. Interact. Processes* 10: 47–79.

Lakey, J. H., Baty, D., and Pattus, F. (1991a) Fluoresence energy transfer distance measurements using site-directed single cysteine mutants: the membrane insertion of colicin E1. *J. Mol. Biol.* 218: 639–653.

Lakey, J. H., Massotte, D., Heitz, F., Dasseux, J.-L., Faucon, J.-F., Parker, M. W., and Pattus, F. (199b) Membrane insertion of the pore forming domain of colicin A: a spectroscopic study. *Eur. J. Biochem.* 196: 599–607.

Lazdunski, C. J., Baty, D., Geli, V., Cavard, D., Morlon, J., Lloubes, R., Howard, S. P., Knibiehler, M., Chartier, M., Varenne, S., Frenette, M., Dasseux, J.-L., and Pattus, F. (1988) The membrane channel-forming colicin A: synthesis, secreation, structure, action and immunity. *Biochim. Biophys. Acta* 947: 445–464.

Leigh, J. S. (1969) ESR Rigid-lattice line shape in a system of two interacting spins. *J. Chem. Phys.* 52:2608–2612.

Lesk, A. M., and Chothia, C. (1980) How different amino acid sequences determine similar protein structures: the structure and evolutionary dynamics of the globins. *J. Mol. Biol.* 136: 225–270.

Lesk, A. M., and Chothia, C. (1982) Evolution of proteins formed by β-sheets. II. The core of the immunoglobulin domain. *J. Mol. Biol.* 160: 325–342.

Lex, L., Hideg, K., and Hankovszky, H. O. (1982) Nitroxide IX. Synthesis of nitroxide free radical α-amino acids. *Can. J. Chem.* 60: 1448–1451.

Lim, W. A., and Sauer, R. T. (1989) Alternative packing arrangements in the hydrophobic core of λ-repressor. *Nature* 339: 31–36.

Marsh, D. (1981) In: *Membrane Spectroscopy*, edited by E. Grell. Berlin: Springer-Verlag, p. 51–137.

Molin, Y. N., Salikhov, K. M., and Zamaraev, K. I. (1980) *Spin Exchange*. Berlin: Springer-Verlag.

Nakaie, C. R., Goissis, G., Schreier, S., and Paiva, A.C.M. (1981) pH dependence of EPR spectra of nitroxides containing ionizable groups. *Brazilian J. Med. Biol. Res.* 14: 173–180.

Nassal, M., Mogi, T., Karnik, S., and Khorana, H. G. (1987) Structure–function studies on bacterio-rhodopsin III. Total synthesis of a gene for bacterio-opsin and its expression in *Escherichia coli. J. Biol. Chem.* 262: 9264–9270.

Noren, C. J., Anthony-Cahill, S. J., Griffith, M. C., and Schultz, P. G. (1989a) A general method for site-specific incorporation of unnatural amino acids into proteins. *Science* 244: 182–188.

Noren, C. J., Anthony-Cahill, S. J., Suich, D. J., Noren, K. A., Griffith, M. C., and Schultz, P. G. (1989b) In vitro suppresion of an amber mutation by a chemically aminoacylated transfer RNA prepared by runoff transcription. *Nucleic Acids Res.* 18: 83–88.

Pakula, A. A., and Sauer, R. T. (1989) Genetic analysis of protein stability and function. *Annu. Rev. Genet.* 23: 289–310.

Parker, M. W., Pattus, F., Tucker, A. D., and Tsernoglou, D. (1989) Structure of the membrane-pore-forming fragment of colicin A. *Nature* 337: 93–96.

Rassat, A., and Rey, P. (1967) Nitroxides XXIII. Preparation d'aminoacides radicalaires et de leurs sels complexes. *Bull. Soc. Chim. Fr.* 3: 815–818.

Schneider, D. J., and Freed, J. H. (1989) Calculating slow motional magnetic resonance spectra: a user's guide. In: *Biological Magnetic Resonance*, edited by L. J. Berliner and J. Reuben. New York: Plenum, vol. 8, p. 1–76.

Shapiro, A. B., and Dmitriev, P. I. (1981) Organometallic nitroxyl radicals of piperidine. *Doklady Akad. Nauk SSSR* 257: 898–902.

Shin, Y.-K., and Hubbell, W. L. (1992) Determination of electrostatic potential at biological interfaces using electron-electron double resonance. *Biophys. J.* 61: 1443–1453.

Stetter, E., Vieth, E.-H., and Hausser, K. H. (1976) Eldor studies of nitroxide radicals: discrimination between rotational and translational correlation times in liquds. *J. Magn. Reson.* 23: 493–504.

Subczynski, W. K., and Hyde, J. S. (1981) The diffusion-concentration product of oxygen in lipid bilayers using the spin label T_1 method. *Biochim. Biophys. Acta* 643: 283–291.

Todd, A. P., Cong, J., Levinthal, F., Levinthal, C., and Hubbell, W. L. (1989) Site-directed mutagenesis of colicin E1 provides specific attachment sites for spin labels whose spectra are sensitive to local conformation. *Proteins Struct. Funct. Genet.* 6: 294.

Vaughan, W. M., and Weber, G. (1970) Oxygen quenching of pyrenebutyric acid fluorescence in water. A dynamic probe of the microenvironment. *Biochemistry* 9: 464–473.

Volwerk, J. J., and Griffith, O. H. (1988) In: *Magnetic Resonance Review.* London: Gordon and Breach, vol. 13, p. 135–178.

Weinkam, R. J., and Jorgensen, E. C. (1971) Angiotensin II analogs. VIII. The use of free radical containing peptides to indicate the conformation of the carboxyl terminal region of angiotensin II. *J. Am. Chem. Soc.* 93: 7033–7038.

Wormald, M. R., Merrill, A. R., Cramer, W. A., and Williams, R.J.P. (1990) Solution studies of colicin E1 C-terminal thermolytic peptide: structural comparison with colicin A and the effects of pH changes. *Eur. J. Biochem.* 191: 155–161.

11

Nuclear Magnetic Resonance Approaches to Membrane Protein Structure

STANLEY J. OPELLA

To understand the functions of membrane proteins requires the same high level of structural analysis that is now almost routinely applied to globular proteins by integrating results from the experimental methods of structural biology such as atomic resolution, x-ray crystallography, and multidimensional solution nuclear magnetic resonance (NMR) spectroscopy with those from molecular dynamics simulations and other calculations. Unfortunately, membrane proteins are problematic for the experimental and theoretical methods of structural biology, largely because these methods were developed with globular proteins in mind; as a result, both the breadth and depth of the structural analysis of membrane proteins lag far behind those of globular proteins. Structure determination by x-ray diffraction requires high-quality single crystals, and proteins associated with membranes are much more resistant to crystallization than water-soluble globular proteins; the multidimensional NMR methods that are so successful in determining the structures of globular proteins in solution are severely limited by the slow reorientation rates of proteins complexed with lipids; and molecular dynamics calculations of proteins were originally used with globular proteins in vacuum—including the effects of both lipid and solvent molecules in these calculations is an even more daunting task than for solvent molecules alone.

Developing generally applicable methods for determining the structures of membrane proteins is one of the most important challenges in the field of structural biology at present. The few structures of membrane proteins determined by diffraction (Deisenhofer et al., 1985; Rees et al., 1989; Weiss et al., 1991) and image reconstruction (Henderson et al., 1990; Kühlbrandt et al., 1994) methods required very favorable systems and extraordinary experimental efforts. These great triumphs of structural biology map out the basic secondary and tertiary structural features sure to be found in many membrane proteins. Even though NMR spectroscopy is at an earlier stage in its development as a method for determining the structures of membrane proteins than x-ray crystallography, it has played an important role in describing the dynamics of membrane proteins. Most of the NMR results on membrane peptides and proteins have come from solution NMR studies of relatively small helical polypeptides in mixed organic solvents or micelle samples (Hagen et al., 1978; Lauterwein et al., 1979; Cross and Opella, 1980; Brown et al., 1982; Braun et al., 1983;

Wilson and Dahlquist, 1985; Lee et al., 1987; Holak et al., 1988; Inagaki et al., 1989; Bruch et al., 1989; Mulvey et al., 1989; Henry and Sykes, 1990; Wennerberg et al., 1990; Shon et al., 1991a,b; Pervushin et al., 1991; Sobol et al., 1992). However, recent results show that many of the technical difficulties associated with conventional NMR studies of proteins in membrane environments can be overcome by utilizing a spectroscopic approach that combines the methods of high-resolution solid-state NMR spectroscopy on samples in phospholipid bilayers with those of multidimensional solution NMR spectroscopy on samples in detergent micelles (Shon et al., 1991a,b). Although high-resolution solid-state NMR spectroscopy (Cross and Opella, 1983; Opella et al., 1987; Opella and Stewart, 1989) and multidimensional solution NMR spectroscopy are independently capable of determining the backbone and side chain structures of peptides (Dyson and Wright, 1991) and proteins (Wuthrich, 1986; Clore and Gronenborn, 1989), and both methods are being developed toward that end for membrane proteins, at present it is necessary to derive some information from each in order to study the membrane proteins of interest.

This chapter is not a thorough review of the literature on NMR studies of membrane proteins; rather, it describes pertinent aspects of solid-state NMR spectroscopy and multidimensional solution NMR spectroscopy and several successful applications of NMR spectroscopy to membrane peptides and proteins. It will indicate the promise of NMR spectroscopy for this important class of polypeptides that is not amenable to investigation by current methods of structural biology.

Solid-state NMR spectroscopy is capable of characterizing immobile and noncrystalline proteins (Griffin, 1981; Oldfield et al., 1982; Opella, 1982; Torchia, 1984). Although the same few nuclear spin interactions (e.g., dipole–dipole, chemical shift, quadrupole) determine the spectral features and measurable parameters in solid-state NMR spectroscopy and in solution NMR spectroscopy, the experiments give quite different spectroscopic and molecular information because the averaging effects of rapid overall molecular reorientation are absent in immobile samples. In addition, solid-state NMR spectroscopy enables protein structure and dynamics to be described in a more integrated way than is possible in solution NMR spectroscopy, again because of the absence of the influence of overall reorientation on the timescales of the experiments. This is of substantial value, since the dynamic properties of backbone and side chain sites must be taken into account in order to approach a complete description of a protein. This is especially true for membrane proteins that characteristically have mobile loops and termini and rigid, structured helical regions (Keniry et al., 1984; Leo et al., 1987; Shon et al., 1991a,b).

Multidimensional solution NMR methods are applicable to peptides and proteins in micelles because the reorientation of the protein–micelle complex in solution averages the nuclear spin interactions to their isotropic values, enabling the indirect effects of their fluctuations through relaxation phenomena to monitor local dynamics as well as provide spatial information in the form of relative proximities. However, the broad lines and efficient spin diffusion that accompany the relatively slow reorientation of protein–micelle complexes in solution limit the effectiveness of multidimensional solution NMR experiments. These limitations can be reduced by optimizing the experimental conditions by using small micelles, isotopically labeled protein samples, and high-field spectrometers.

Nuclear Magnetic Resonance Spectroscopy of Membrane Proteins

Solid-State Nuclear Magnetic Resonance Spectroscopy of Membrane Proteins in Lipid Bilayers

Even the earliest NMR studies recognized the dominant role of molecular dynamics on the experiments and their results. Molecular motions strongly influence all NMR spectral features, directly through the motional averaging of lineshapes and indirectly through the induction of relaxation (Spiess, 1982). Only the indirect relaxation effects are available from solution experiments, since the lineshapes are completely averaged to their isotropic values by the overall motions of the molecules. When the overall molecular reorientation is slow compared with the timescales determined by the breadth of the lineshapes due to the underlying nuclear spin interactions, then local, internal molecular motions can be analyzed from their effects on the lineshapes. The slowest timescales available from the solid-state NMR experiments are around 10^{-4} Hz; when the molecule of interest reorients slower than this, even if the sample is a solution, the spectral properties of solids rather than solutions are observed in the spectra. This is the reason solid-state NMR methods are appropriate for many complexes of biopolymers that are not physically solids, such as virus particles in solution (Cross and Opella, 1983) or fully hydrated membrane bilayers. It is also the reason solid-state NMR spectroscopy gives such favorable opportunities for distinguishing mobile segments of membrane proteins against the background of their rigid regions of secondary structure (Bogusky et al., 1987). In studies of membrane proteins, the first step is to identify the structured regions both to simplify the structure determination and to assist in defining the boundaries of the regions of stable secondary structure. After the backbone structure of the protein is determined, it is essential to analyze the side chain dynamics along with their positions, since both aliphatic and aromatic side chains undergo large-amplitude, rapid motions. The results of solid-state NMR studies of protein dynamics have been reviewed (Torchia, 1984; Opella, 1985). This chapter is primarily concerned with structural studies on membrane proteins, although dynamics must be taken into account at all stages of experimental design, interpretation, and analysis of the protein structure itself.

Although solid-state NMR spectroscopy was established as an independent method for determining molecular structure at atomic resolution in 1948 (Pake, 1948), only recently has it become possible to obtain detailed structural information on proteins by utilizing high-field spectrometers; multiple-pulse, multiple-resonance, multidimensional experiments; and specific, selective, and uniform isotopic labeling schemes. The basic physical properties of the relevant nuclear spin interactions (Abragam, 1961) are so well understood that spectroscopic interpretations have not been a limiting factor in applying solid-state NMR spectroscopy to the study of proteins. The solid-state NMR approach that we are developing for determining the structures of proteins in oriented samples relies on the spectral simplifications that result from uniaxial sample orientation parallel to the direction of the applied magnetic field (Opella and Waugh, 1977). The spin interactions at individual sites yield single resonance lines characterized by their resonance frequencies or doublets (or triplets) characterized by the magnitudes (and asymmetry) of their splittings. The observed values of the frequencies and splittings depend on the orientations of the principal axes of the spin-interaction tensors present at each site relative to the direction of the applied magnetic field. Since the direction of sample orientation and the applied magnetic field of the NMR spectrometer is the same, it defines a frame of reference for the evaluation of the orientational information. The orientations of many spin-interaction tensors have been established in their molecular frames of reference, enabling angular factors to be determined from the experimental data. Molecular structures can be determined on the basis of angles alone, given standard bond lengths and geometries; therefore it is possible to determine the structure of a protein with a sufficient number of orientationally dependent spectroscopic measurements. Protein structures can also be determined from many short-range internuclear distance measurements, which can be made both with solution NMR experiments, through nuclear Overhauser enhancements (NOEs), and with several different solid-state NMR experiments. We have performed experiments that yield distance information on both oriented (Cross et al., 1983) and unoriented (Frey and Opella, 1984) samples and are currently working on several new dilute spin and abundant spin-exchange experiments. Other groups are now developing very sophisticated solid-state NMR methods of making quantitative distance measurements between isotopically labeled sites in unoriented samples (Raleigh et al., 1988; Gullion and Schaefer, 1989).

In principle, solid-state NMR spectroscopy is fully capable of determining the structures of immobile, oriented proteins (Opella et al., 1987; Opella and Stewart, 1989), including membrane proteins embedded in lipid bilayers oriented between glass plates (Bechinger et al., 1991; Shon et al., 1991a). A very high degree of orientation can be achieved when small amounts of lipids are placed between glass plates and partially dehydrated under controlled conditions. In the past this has been done by stacking rectangular plates within the cylinder of the coil (McLaughlin et al., 1975; Seelig and Niederberger, 1974). This sample arrangement compromises the orientation of the glass plates, gives large edge effects, and gives a poor filling factor, making the spectroscopic experiments inefficient. The feasibility of NMR experiments on oriented membrane samples is greatly improved by using a single pair of square glass plates (as large as 22×22 mm) with the rf coil wrapped directly around the plates. This unusual flat-coil arrangement, as shown in Figure 11.1, enables solid-state NMR spectra of oriented proteins to be obtained in a minimum amount of time (Bechinger and Opella, 1991).

Complete polypeptide backbone structures require several spectral parameters to be measured in order to characterize the angles between each of the peptide planes and the direction of sample orientation (Opella et al., 1987; Opella and Stewart, 1989; Chirlian and Opella, 1990). Fortunately, once the secondary structure of a membrane-bound form of a protein is established on the basis of NOE measurements in micelle samples, a single spectral parameter, for example, the ^{15}N chemical shift, is sufficient to establish the orientations of the helices relative to the plane of the bilayer (Bechinger et al., 1991; Shon et al., 1991a,b). Specific selective, and uniform labeling strategies are feasible for ^{15}N NMR studies of proteins, and solid-state ^{15}N NMR spectra or oriented peptides and protein in lipid bilayers can be simply and qualitatively interpreted by using the nearly axially symmetrical ^{15}N amide chemical shift tensor as a guide to the orientation of the peptide planes within the helices. The determination of helix orientations with respect to the normal of the lipid bilayer

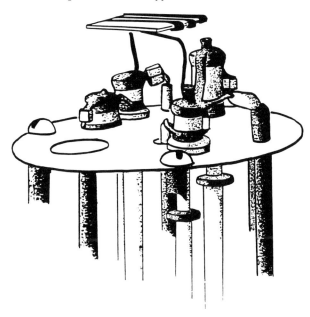

Fig. 11.1. Flat-coil probe for solid-state NMR experiments on peptides and proteins in lipid bilayers oriented between glass plates. Single pairs of plates as large as 22 × 22 mm have been used in these experiments. (From Bechinger and Opella, 1991.)

provides tertiary structural information that is essential for understanding the structure and function relationships of membrane proteins. For membrane proteins with structures dominated by α-helices, a description of the secondary structure of the backbone and its orientations is of great value and goes a long way toward determining the protein structure.

Multidimensional Solution Nuclear Magnetic Resonance Spectroscopy of Membrane Proteins in Micelles

The determination of protein structure by multidimensional NMR spectroscopy is straightforward in principle (Wuthrich, 1986; Clore and Gronenborn, 1989). For small globular proteins with less than 100 residues that are reasonably soluble and do not aggregate, the application of this approach is straightforward in practice as well, especially if uniformly ^{15}N- and/or ^{13}C-labeled protein samples are available (Ikura et al., 1990). Larger proteins are more difficult for two reasons: (*1*) they are more complex, so there are more resonances to resolve and assign, and (*2*) they reorient more slowly in solution, presenting the same problems as proteins in micelles due to broad lines and spin diffusion. There are three aspects to the basic multidimensional solution NMR approach to protein structure determination: (*1*) the resolution and assignment of backbone and side chain resonances based on both through-bond and through-space interactions observed in two- and three-dimensional NMR spectra; (*2*) the measurement of as many homonuclear ^{1}H/^{1}H NOEs as possible among the assigned resonances and supplementing these short-range distance constraints with other structural constraints, including spin–spin coupling constants; and (*3*) the interpretation of the distance and angular constraints in terms of secondary structure and then a family of three-dimensional protein structures using distance geometry, molecular dynamics, and other calculations (Braun, 1987; Havel, 1990; Borgias and James, 1988). The availability of high-field spectrometers, cloned proteins that can be expressed in organisms grown on chemically defined media, and software for data processing and protein structure determination have led to the widespread use of NMR in the structural biology of small globular proteins. However, a great deal of development needs to be performed in order to apply this approach to larger proteins (25–35 kD) and proteins in complexes with DNA and micelles. Both methods and instrumentation need to be developed so that a broader range of proteins can be investigated, including membrane proteins in micelles.

Multidimensional solution NMR studies of membrane proteins in micelles are deceptively difficult. The devastating effects of spin diffusion on homonuclear NOE measurements compound the sensitivity and resolution problems caused by the broad linewidths of the resonances and their limited chemical shift dispersion, especially from hydrogens bonded to α-carbons, in these slowly reorienting helical proteins. Our extensive efforts to optimize the samples, experiments, and instrumentation were motivated by absolute necessity. The starting point of the studies on filamentous bacteriophage coat proteins in micelles were spectra where essentially no cross-peaks could be observed in either conventional two-dimensional correlation (COSY) or NOESY spectra. Optimization of conditions and the implementation of heteronuclear experiments improved the situation to the point where complete resolution and assignment of all backbone ^{1}H and ^{15}N amide resonances of both Pf1 and fd coat proteins in micelles was possible (Schiksnis et al., 1987; Shon et al., 1991a,b). This led to descriptions of their backbone dynamics, secondary structure, and the incorporation of solid-state NMR into the analysis to establish the orientations of the helices in the membrane (Shon et al., 1991a,b).

Three major steps were required to make multidimensional NMR experiments work on coat proteins in micelles: (*1*) The experimental conditions for solubilizing these proteins in both perdeuterated dodecylphosphocholine (DPC) and sodium dodecyl sulfate (SDS) micelles were optimized. In favorable cases DPC yields narrower and more intense protein resonances than other detergents and eliminates the chemical nature of the headgroup as a potential source of criticism (Brown, 1979). However, in some cases SDS remains the detergent of choice because it gives the highest quality multidimensional NMR spectra. The optimization of the protein-containing micelle is at once the simplest and the most subtle aspect of the research. All aspects of the sample, including the choice of detergent, concentration of polypeptides and detergent, pH, temperature, and counterions, must be taken into account in order to prepare samples capable of yielding reproducible, resolved spectra that can be reliably interpreted. The chemical purity of the detergent has a significant role in determining the stability of the protein and the ultimate quality of the spectra. (*2*) We "tuned" the isotopic composition of the proteins to narrow the resonances, attenuate spin diffusion, and retain reasonable receptivity for the nuclear spin interactions that occur both through bonds and through space. The key experiments have been performed on proteins uniformly labeled with ^{15}N (98%), ^{2}H on all carbon sites (80%), and ^{2}H (50%) on amide nitrogen sites (Shon et al., 1991a,b). (*3*) Experiments were performed at the highest available magnetic field strengths (Shon and Opella, 1989).

Applications to Amphipathic Helical Peptides in Membranes

NMR studies of membrane peptides offer opportunities to develop and demonstrate the technology on well-defined and relatively small polypeptides in the membrane environments of micelles and bilayers that present all of the difficulties seen for larger proteins. The functional analysis of complex membrane proteins with peptides is particularly direct, since many peptide sequences can be identified as structural and functional entities as isolated molecules, oligomers, or domains of larger proteins. Hydrophobic helical peptides with 20–25 residues are generally found to cross the membrane bilayer, as found in membrane proteins like the photosynthetic reaction center and bacteriorhodopsin. Amphipathic helical peptides are thought to form transmembrane ion channels by aggregating in oligomeric bundles with their hydrophilic residues on the inside, forming a pore for ions, and their hydrophobic residues on the outside, interacting with the hydrocarbon chains of the lipids. Each of the peptides in these channels contributes a single membrane-spanning helix perpendicular to the plane of the bilayer. Amphipathic helical peptides also associate with the interface region of phospholipid bilayers in the plane of the bilayer, as found in membrane proteins. Multidimensional solution NMR methods have been successfully applied to peptides in solution in selected cases (Dyson and Wright, 1991), although sorting out conformational averaging of peptides in aqueous solution is typically a complex and difficult problem. The lipid environments provided by both micelles and bilayers enhance the opportunities for characterizing a stabilized peptide conformation by multidimensional solution NMR spectroscopy, and solid-state NMR spectroscopy overcomes many of the difficulties inherent in other methods by characterizing the conformation of peptides immobilized by their lipid environment. We are studying two classes of 20–25 residue amphipathic helical peptides in membrane environments, peptides derived from the pore-forming segments of ion channel proteins, and the magainin antibiotic peptides from frog skin. These peptides can be readily prepared by solid-phase peptide synthesis with stable isotopes placed at specific locations. After purification, samples for NMR experiments can be prepared as micelles or bilayers.

The major functional channels in membranes, such as the nicotinic acetylcholine receptor and cation channels, are large oligomeric proteins. Structural studies of these proteins are limited by their overall size and the difficulty in crystallizing them. A promising approach to their analysis is to synthesize and study peptide sequences corresponding to segments of the proteins (Montal, 1990). The peptide M2 was selected from the δ-subunit of the *Torpedo* acetylcholine receptor, because homology and model studies suggest that this sequence-specific motif is responsible for specific functions in the channel activity of the receptor (Oiki et al., 1988). The 23 residue M2δ peptide forms channels by self-association when added to membranes. This peptide lyses red blood cells (Kersh et al., 1989) and closely mimics the ion channel properties of the receptor in model membranes. M2δ and similar peptides have been shown to be helical by solution NMR spectroscopy (Brown et al., 1982; Braun et al., 1983; Lee et al., 1987; Mulvey et al., 1989; Wennerberg et al., 1990).

Antibiotic peptides are abundant in many organisms, forming a defense system exclusive of, or complementary to, the immune system (Boman, 1991). Magainins are a family of 21–26 residue peptides that protect frogs from infections (Zasloff, 1987). These peptides interact strongly with bacterial and model membranes. In contrast to the channel peptides, they do not lyse red blood cells even though they do interrupt the normal electrochemical gradient across cells, suggesting that they interact differently with normal vertebrate membranes than with bacterial membranes (Bevins and Zasloff, 1990). Multidimensional solution NMR experiments indicate that magainins are predominantly α-helical in detergent micelles (Gesell, J., Zasloff, M., and Opella, S. J., unpublished results) and trifluoroethanol–water solutions (Marion et al., 1989) and are unstructured in aqueous solution.

The secondary structure of both types of peptides is α-helix based on several physical measurements, including multidimensional solution NMR spectroscopy of representative peptides in micelles. The 23 residue M2δ peptide, EKMSTAISVLLAQ-AVFLLLTSQR, was synthesized with Ala^{12} specifically labeled with ^{15}N and the 23 residue magainin2 peptide GIGKFLHSAKKFGKAFVGEIMNS amide was synthesized with Ala^{15} specifically labeled with ^{15}N. Figure 11.2 compares experimental solid-state ^{15}N NMR spectra of the specifically labeled magainin2 and M2δ peptides in oriented phospholipid bilayers to a simulated ^{15}N amide chemical-shift powder pattern. The anisotropies of the chemical shift and dipole–dipole interactions, averaged out by rapid molecular reorientation in solution, are present in these immobile samples and serve as sources of structural and dynamic information. In the spectra presented in Figure 11.2, the heteronuclear (^{1}H/^{15}N) dipole–dipole interactions are decoupled by high-power irradiation of the ^{1}H resonances; therefore all spectral features reflect the ^{15}N chemical shift interaction of a specific ^{15}N-labeled site in each peptide sample. In other experiments we have actually measured these dipole–dipole splittings. The magnitudes and orientations in the molecular frame of the principal elements of the chemical shift tensor are prerequisites for interpretation of spectral features, and the ^{15}N chemical amide shift tensors of several model peptides have been described and analyzed for structural studies; an amide N–H bond approximately parallel to the direction of the applied magnetic field has a ^{15}N resonance frequency close to that of the principal element $\sigma_{\parallel}$ and an amide N–H bond perpendicular to the field has a ^{15}N resonance frequency close to that of the principal element $\sigma_{\perp}$ (Harbison et al., 1984; Hartzell et al., 1987; Teng and Cross, 1989).

Both spectra in Figure 11.2 have a relatively narrow single-line resonance from the one ^{15}N-labeled amide site in each peptide. The resonance frequencies observed in these two samples are quite different, indicating that the planes containing the labeled peptide groups have very different orientations relative to the direction of the applied magnetic field. To determine fully the orientation of a labeled peptide plane it would be necessary to measure at least one other spectral parameter associated with that site, such as the heteronuclear dipole–dipole splitting. However, since the secondary structure has been determined independently for both of the peptides, we can take advantage of the structural regularity of the α-helix to provide constraints on

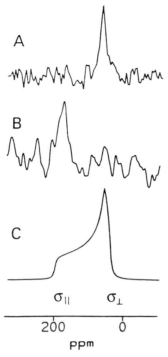

Fig. 11.2. Experimental solid-state ^{15}N NMR spectra of peptides oriented in lipid bilayers. A: ^{15}N-Ala$_{15}$-labeled magainin2. B: ^{15}N-Ala$_{12}$-labeled M2δ. C: Simulation of powder pattern for an immobile ^{15}N amide site. (From Bechinger et al., 1991.)

the orientations consistent with the data and to extend the results from the specifically labeled site to the entire polypeptide. Both qualitative and quantitative analyses of the ^{15}N resonance frequencies are in agreement in describing the orientations of these two helical peptides in lipid bilayers. Magainin2 is oriented approximately parallel to the plane of the bilayer while M2δ is clearly a transmembrane peptide oriented perpendicular to the plane of the bilayer. These orientations are illustrated in Figure 11.3. These results demonstrate that the combination of determining the secondary structure of proteins in micelles and the orientation of helices in bilayers is applicable to amphipathic helical peptides (Bechinger et al., 1991).

It was surprising to find that the magainin peptides lie parallel to the surface of membrane bilayers in contrast to genuine channel-forming peptides that span bilayers (Bechinger et al., 1991). Solid-state NMR spectroscopy has also been used to measure distances for structural studies of unoriented samples (Smith and Griffin, 1988), including magainins (Blazyk et al., 1991). Although a more refined structure of magainin awaits further experimental work, the alignment of the peptide helices parallel to the plane of the membrane and their striking biochemical and cell-biological properties suggest that these peptides disrupt membranes by an unusual mechanism. Many questions concerning their functional properties, including the detailed mechanism of membrane depolarization or the differentiation between vertebrate and prokaryotic membranes by these peptides, remain to be answered.

M2δ   Magainin2

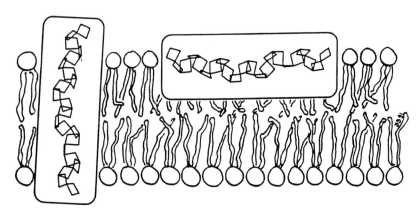

Fig. 11.3. Representation of orientations of transmembrane (M2δ) and in-plane (magainin2) 23 residue amphipathic helical peptides in membrane bilayers. (From Bechinger et al., 1991.)

Applications to Filamentous Bacteriophage Coat Proteins

The filamentous bacteriophage coat proteins present favorable opportunities for investigating membrane proteins, including the roles of leader sequences (Marvin and Hohn, 1969; Makowski, 1984). Bacterial cells infected with the filamentous bacteriophage fd (or its nearly identical relative M13) synthesize many copies of the protein encoded by viral gene 8 as the 73 residue procoat protein with a 23 residue N-terminal leader sequence (Chang et al., 1978). The product of gene 8 participates in a number of processes during the viral lifecycle, starting from its storage in the cell membrane after removal of the leader sequence. Although neutron (Nambudripad et al., 1991) and x-ray fiber (Marvin and Wachtel, 1975; Glucksman et al., 1992) diffraction has played an important role in describing the structure of the coat protein in the virus particles, despite substantial efforts in several laboratories none of the forms of coat protein have been crystallized. We obtain coat proteins by solid-phase peptide synthesis (Shon et al., 1989), isolation from virus particles (Cross and Opella, 1980), and expression in plasmid-containing bacteria. Procoat protein and coat protein can be reconstituted into phospholipid bilayers for solid-state NMR studies or detergent micelles for multidimensional solution NMR studies of their membrane-bound forms. Comparisons among all of the various coat protein species are of interest, especially between the structural form in the virus and the membrane-bound form, between the procoat protein and the mature coat protein, and between the proteins from class I bacteriophages (e.g., fd and M13) and class II bacteriophages (e.g., Pf1).

We have performed extensive NMR studies on the membrane-bound form of Pf1 coat protein in micelles and bilayers. The experiments on coat proteins in micelles were used to delineate the secondary structure of the protein, primarily on the basis of the short distances between hydrogens detected by homonuclear NOEs. The NOE cross-peaks between all amide correlation peaks from adjacent residues within α-

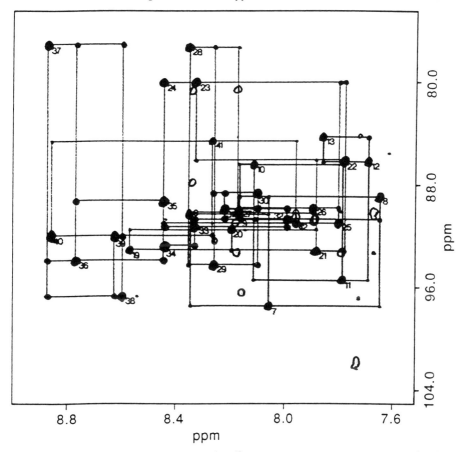

Fig. 11.4. Combined two-dimensional $^1H/^{15}N$ heteronuclear correlation and $^1H/^1H$ homonuclear NOE spectrum of uniformly ^2H- and ^{15}N-labeled Pf1 coat protein in dodecyl-phosphocholine micelles in 50% H_2O/50% D_2O solution. Each amide site in the protein gives rise to a single correlation peak. The lines connect the cross-peaks between correlation peaks from adjacent residues. The assignments of the correlation peaks are indicated with the number near them. (From Shon et al., 1991a.)

helices were observed in combined two- and three-dimensional $^1H/^{15}N$ heteronuclear correlation and $^1H/^1H$ NOE experiments on the multiply labeled samples of Pf1 coat protein (Shon and Opella, 1989; Shon et al., 1991a). The tracing of two continuous pathways of $^1H/^1H$ NOEs among the various amide hydrogen atoms shown in Figure 11.4 directly maps out the two stretches of α-helix in Pf1 coat protein. The existence of these two α-helices is strongly supported by the observation of many of the appropriate cross-peaks between amide ^1H and C_α^1H resonances in both two- and three-dimensional heteronuclear spectra. Importantly, the amide sites in the N- and C-terminal regions and the region between the two helices do not have $^1H/^1H$ NOE cross-peaks to other amide sites. These missing cross-peaks, which are structural data (albeit negative), are particularly relevant in the context of the dynamics data on this protein, which show these residues to be mobile.

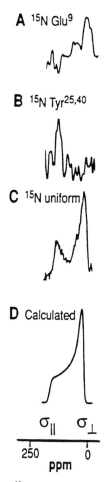

Fig. 11.5. Experimental solid-state ^{15}N NMR spectral of ^{15}N labeled Pf1 coat protein in oriented lipid bilayers. The experimental spectra are compared with a simulated powder pattern for an immobile ^{15}N amide site. (From Shon et al., 1991a.)

Since the secondary structure of the membrane-bound form of Pf1 coat protein is established by the homonuclear ^{1}H/^{1}H NOE cross-peaks, a single parameter from solid-state NMR spectra of oriented samples is sufficient to establish the orientations of the α-helices relative to the plane of the bilayer. By using a flat-coil probe, as shown in Figure 11.1, the ^{15}N chemical shift from selectively labeled amide sites in Pf1 coat protein in oriented lipid bilayers could be observed. This is shown in Figure 11.5. Since the orientation of this chemical shift tensor in the molecular frame is known, the orientations of individual residues could be determined. The N–H bond of Glu^9 and hence the amphipathic helix containing this residue is approximately parallel to the plane of the membrane bilayer. In contrast, the N–H bonds of Tyr^{25} and Tyr^{40} are approximately perpendicular to the plane of the bilayer, demonstrating that the hydrophobic helix spans the bilayer.

The dynamics of many backbone and side chain sites were described with the com-

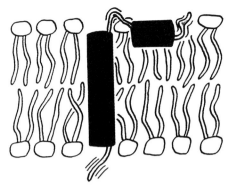

Fig. 11.6. Model of Pf1 coat protein in lipid bilayers based on the NMR data in Figures 10.4 and 10.5. The amphipathic helix is parallel to the plane of the bilayer, while the hydrophobic helix is transmembrane. The termini and internal loop between the helices are mobile on the NMR timescales. (From Shon et al., 1991a.)

bination of solid-state NMR measurements on bilayer samples and solution NMR measurements on micelle samples (Bogusky et al., 1987; Shon et al., 1991a). We have demonstrated that the ^{1}H/^{15}N heteronuclear NOE, along with the linewidths and T_1s of both ^{1}H and ^{15}N resonances, is an effective monitor of backbone dynamics (Bogusky et al., 1988). ^{13}C relaxation parameters can also be used to characterize the dynamics of these proteins. This detailed view of protein dynamics contributed to our confidence in interpreting the structural data in terms of a model of the protein. There is a strong synergistic effect to performing relaxation analysis and structural studies in parallel. They conclusively demonstrated the presence of the mobile loop region of the membrane-bound form of Pf1 coat protein (Shon et al., 1991a).

The results of the NMR experiments are summarized in the model shown in Figure 11.5. There are five distinct regions in this small 46 residue membrane protein. The protein has two α-helices, as defined by the observation of the appropriate homonuclear ^{1}H/^{1}H NOEs in micelles. The solid-state NMR data from oriented samples demonstrate that the short amphipathic helix is parallel to the plane of the bilayer and the long hydrophobic helix is perpendicular to the plane of the bilayer. The narrow isotropic resonance intensity observed in the spectra from unoriented samples indicates that the two rigid helices are connected by a mobile loop and that there are mobile residues at both the N and C termini of the membrane-bound form of the protein. Pf1 coat protein, like other membrane proteins, has both rigidly structured and mobile segments in its polypeptide backbone. Membrane proteins differ from soluble, globular proteins in having mobile internal loops as well as mobile N- and C-terminal regions. Since the structures of many membrane proteins are dominated by long hydrophobic helices spanning the bilayer and shorter amphipathic helices in the plane of the bilayer (Deisenhofer et al., 1985; Henderson et al., 1990), the mobile connecting loops are clearly key elements of their overall architecture. The juxtaposition of mobile and structured regions means that experimental and theoretical investigations of membrane protein dynamics are likely to be highly informative as part of structure determinations and other investigations.

The NMR results were supplemented with those from molecular dynamics calculations. The initial trials of molecular dynamics simulations on filamentous bacteriophage coat proteins (Sanders et al., 1991; Tobias et al., 1993) present opportunities to contribute to the development of new methodologies that may be generally useful for characterizing other membrane proteins. Our results for Pf1 coat protein show that vacuum molecular simulations can provide information directly relevant to the structure and dynamics of membrane-bound proteins, since they identified the mobile and structured segments of the polypeptide backbone of the membrane-bound form of Pf1 coat protein (Tobias et al., 1993).

We have also applied NMR spectroscopy to the study of fd coat protein and have now fully described the secondary structure and three-dimensional arrangement of the backbone of the membrane-bound form of fd coat protein (Shon et al., 1991b). Our NMR results differ from those of other groups (Henry and Sykes, 1990), especially in finding all spectral features to be consistent with the protein being a monomer in membrane environments and from those obtained with other techniques (Dunker et al., 1982; Spruijt et al., 1989), although they now seem to be agreeing with our findings of a predominantly helical structure with no β-sheet (Spruijt and Hemminga, 1991). Both fd and Pf1 coat proteins have long hydrophobic helices that span the membrane bilayer as well as a helix that is relatively short, distinctly amphipathic, and parallel to the plane of the bilayer, as expected for a helix with its hydrophobic side in contact with the lipid chains and with the hydrophilic side exposed to the lipid headgroups and solvent. The two helices are connected by a mobile loop that differs somewhat in frequencies of motion between the two proteins, but not in the presence of mobile internal backbone sites on slower timescales. fd Coat protein shows continuity of secondary structure through the bend between the helices parallel and perpendicular to the plane of the membrane bilayer. Both fd and Pf1 coat proteins have residues at both the N and C termini of the protein that are highly mobile.

Applications to Proteins with Seven Transmembrane Helices

A large and important class of membrane proteins has seven hydrophobic membrane-spanning helices as the major structural element (Dohlman et al., 1991). Bacteriorhodopsin is the best characterized of these proteins, based on both extensive biochemical studies and the structural studies that have been summarized in the model of Henderson and coworkers (1990). A major goal of a structure determination method for membrane proteins has to be the ability to deal with this class of proteins. Typical examples of these proteins have molecular weights around 30 kD. This size is near the upper limit of multidimensional solution NMR methods for well-behaved globular proteins. If the NMR techniques for studying membrane proteins in micelles and in bilayers continue to improve, especially with the implementation of very high field magnets, then structural studies of proteins of this size should become feasible.

Three different approaches have been used in NMR studies of bacteriorhodopsin. Significant work has been done in describing the dynamics of the protein in bilayers by solid-state NMR experiments, primarily with ^{2}H-labeled sites, on unoriented samples (Rice et al., 1981; Oldfield et al., 1982). Motional averaging of the ^{2}H powder pattern lineshapes has provided evidence of the internal motions of the aromatic and aliphatic side chains and, perhaps more importantly, some of the first evidence that membrane proteins have mobile segments (Keniry et al., 1984). A variant of this approach enabled structural conclusions to be drawn from the motional averaging of bacteriorhodopsin in lipid bilayers (Lewis et al., 1985). By isotopically labeling protein residues and the chromophore retinal, a variety of solid-state NMR measurements have led to models of the structure at the functional site and to the chemical transformations that accompany the photocycle (McDermott et al., 1991).

Bacteriorhodopsin can also be studied by multidimensional solution NMR methods by making samples in mixed organic solvents or micelles of portions of the protein (Pervushin et al., 1991; Sobol et al., 1992). In this way it has been possible to confirm the helical secondary structure of regions of the protein.

Summary and Conclusions

NMR structural studies of globular proteins are enjoying extraordinary success and acceptance, even though these studies, for the most part, are on the same proteins being studied by x-ray crystallography. The motivation for studying membrane proteins by NMR spectroscopy is clear, since it would be desirable to utilize noncrystalline samples of these proteins in membrane environments in structural studies.

This chapter describes the progress that has been made in adapting multidimensional solution NMR methods for studying membrane proteins in micelles and in developing solid-state NMR methods for studying membrane proteins in bilayers. The progress has been substantial, since several examples could be presented. The pace of technical improvements is increasing and should be greatly accelerated by the implementation of spectrometers with very high field magnets.

The structures of photosynthetic reaction centers, bacteriorhodopsin, Pf1 coat protein, and fd coat proteins are all dominated by long hydrophobic membrane-spanning helices connected by loops, some of which contain relatively short amphipathic bridging helices. Bacteriorhodopsin, Pf1 coat protein and fd coat proteins have all been shown to have mobile terminal and internal segments. NMR spectroscopy showed that the mobile N- and C-terminal regions as well as the mobile internal connecting loops are characteristic of membrane-bound proteins, as are the rigid hydrophobic bilayer-spanning helices and amphipathic bridging helices.

Acknowledgments

This chapter draws heavily on the research of my group in the Department of Chemistry at the University of Pennsylvania; recent results by B. Bechinger, J. Gesell, Y. Kim, P. McDonnell, and K. Shon have been especially important in developing and applying NMR spectroscopy for the study of membrane proteins. Several of the research projects benefit from substantial interactions and collaborations with L. Gierasch (University of Texas), M. Klein (University of Pennsylvania), L. Makowski (Boston University), M. Montal (University of California, San Diego), J. Richards (California Institute of Technology), J. Tomich (Children's Hospital of Los Angeles), and M. Zasloff (University of Pennsylvania).

My research program is supported by the National Institutes of Health through grants R37 GM24266, RO1 GM29754, RO1 AI20770, RO1 GM34343, and R24 RR05976.

References

Abragam, A. (1961) *The Principles of Nuclear Magnetism*. Oxford: Oxford University Press.

Bechinger, B., Kim, Y., Chirlian, L. E., Gesell, J., Neumann, J., Montal, M., Tomich, J., Zasloff, M., and Opella S. J. (1991) Orientations of amphipathic helical peptides in membrane bilayers determined by solid-state NMR spectroscopy. *J. Biomol. NMR* 1: 167–173.

Bechinger, B., and Opella, S. J. (1991) Flat coil probe for NMR spectroscopy of oriented membrane samples. *J. Magn. Reson.* 95: 585–588.

Bevins, C. and Zasloff, M. (1990) Peptides from Frog skin. *Annu. Rev. Biochem.* 59: 395–414.

Blazyk, J., Hing, A., Schaefer, J., and Ferguson, M. C. (1991) Rotational-echo double-resonance (REDOR) NMR spectroscopy of the antimicrobial peptide magainin 2. *J. Cell Biol. Suppl.* 15G, 73.

Bogusky, M. J., Schiksnis, R. A., Leo, G. C., and Opella, S. J. (1987) Protein backbone dynamics by solid state and solution ^{15}N NMR spectroscopy. *J. Magn. Reson.* 72: 186–190.

Bogusky, M. J., Leo, G. C., and Opella, S. J. (1988) Comparison of the dynamics of the membrane bound form of fd coat protein in micelles and in bilayers. *Proteins Struct. Funct. Genet.* 4: 123–130.

Boman, H. (1991) Developmental abnormalities in transgenic mice expressing a sialic acid-specific 9-O-acetylesterase. *Cell* 65: 205.

Borgias, B., and James, T. (1988) COMATOSE, a method for constrained refinement of macromolecular structure based on two-dimensional nuclear Overhauser effect spectra. *J. Magn. Reson.* 79: 493–512.

Braun, W. (1987) Distance geometry and related materials for protein structure determination from NMR data. *Q. Rev. Biophys.* 19: 115–157.

Braun, W., Wilder, G., Lee, K., and Wuthrich, K. (1983) Conformation of glucagon in lipid–water interphase by ^{1}H nuclear magnetic resonance. *J. Mol. Biol.* 169: 921–948.

Brown, L. (1979) Use of fully deuterated micelles for conformational studies of membrane proteins by high resolution ^{1}H nuclear magnetic resonance. *Biochim. Biophys. Acta* 557: 135–148.

Brown, L., Braun, W., Kumar, A., and Wuthrich, K. (1982) High resolution nuclear magnetic resonance studies of the conformation and orientation of melittin bound to a lipid–water interface. *Biophys. J.* 37: 319–328.

Bruch, M., Mcknight, C., and Gierasch, L. (1989) Helix formation and stability in a signal sequence. *Biochemistry* 28: 8554–8561.

Chang, C., Blobel, G., and Model, P. (1978) Detection of prokaryotic signal peptidase in an *Escherichia coli* membrane fraction: endoproteolytic cleavage of nascent f1 precoat protein. *Proc. Natl. Acad. Sci. USA* 75: 361–365.

Chirlian, L. E., and Opella, S. J. (1990) Molecular structure by solid-state NMR spectroscopy. *Adv. Magn. Reson.* (W. Warren, ed.), Acad. Press, NY, NY, 14: 183–202.

Clore, G., and Gronenborn, A. (1989) Determination of three-dimensional structures of proteins and nucleic acids in solution by nuclear magnetic resonance spectroscopy, *CRC Crit. Rev. Biochem. Mol. Biol.* 24: 479–564.

Cross, T. A., Frey, M. H., and Opella, S. J. (1983) ^{15}N spin exchange in a protein. *J. Am. Chem. Soc.* 105: 7741–7743.

Cross, T. A., and Opella, S. J. (1980) Structural properties of fd coat protein in sodium dodecyl sulfate micelles. *Biochem. Biophys. Res. Commun.* 92: 478–484.

Cross, T. A., and Opella, S. J. (1983) Protein structure by solid state NMR. *J. Am. Chem. Soc.* 105: 306–308.

Deisenhofer, J., Epp, O., Miki, K., Huber, R., and Michel, H. (1985) Structure of the protein subunits in the photosynthetic reaction centre of *Rhodopseudomonas viridis* at 3Å resolution. *Nature* 318: 618.

Dohlman, H., Thorner, J., Caron, M., and Lefkowitz, R. (1991) Model systems for the study of seven-transmembrane-segment receptors. *Annu. Rev. Biochem.* 60: 653–688.

Dunker, A., Fodor, S., and Williams, R. (1982) Lipid-dependent structural changes of an amphomorphic membrane protein. *Biophys. J.* 37: 201–203.

Dyson, H., and Wright, P. (1991) Defining solution conformations of small linear peptides. *Annu. Rev. Biophys. Biophys. Chem.* 20: 519–538.

Frey, M. H., and Opella, S. J. (1984) [13]C Spin exchange in amino acids and peptides. *J. Am. Chem. Soc.* 106: 4942–4945.

Gullion, T., and Schaefer, J. (1989) Rotational-echo double-resonance NMR. *J. Magn. Reson.* 81: 196–200.

Glucksman, M., Bhattacharjee, S., and Makowski, L. (1992) Three-dimensional structure of a cloning vector. *J. Mol. Biol.* 226: 455–470.

Griffin, R. (1981) Solid state nuclear magnetic resonance of lipid bilayers. *Methods Enzymol.* 72: 108–173.

Harbison, G., Jelinski, L., Stark, R., Torchia, D., Herzfeld, J., and Griffin, R. (1984) ^{15}N chemical shift and [15]N–[13]C dipolar tensors for the peptide bond in [1-^{13}C]Clycyl[^{15}N]glycine hydrochloride monohydrate. *J. Magn. Reson.* 60: 79–82.

Hagen, D., Weiner, J., and Sykes, B. (1978) Fluorotyrosine M13 coat protein: fluorine-19 nuclear magnetic resonance study of the motional properties of an integral membrane protein in phospholipid vesicles. *Biochemistry* 17: 3860–3866.

Hartzell, C., Whitfield, M., Oas, T., and Drobny, G. (1987) Determination of the ^{15}N and ^{13}C chemical shift tensors of L-[^{13}C]Alanyl-L-[^{15}N]alanine from the dipole-coupled powder patterns. *J. Am. Chem. Soc.* 109: 5966–5969.

Havel, T. (1990) The sampling properties of some distance geometry algorithms applied to unconstrained polypeptide chains: a study of 1830 independently computed conformations. *Biopolymers* 29: 1565–1585.

Henderson, R., Baldwin, J., Cesko, T., Zemlin, F., Beckmann, E., and Downing, K. (1990) Model for the structure of bacteriorhodopsin based on high-resolution electron cryo-microscopy. *J. Mol. Biol.* 213: 899–929.

Henry, G., and Sykes, B. (1990) Hydrogen exchange kinetics in a membrane protein determined by ^{15}N NMR spectroscopy: use of the INEPT experiment to follow individual amides in detergent-solubilized M13 coat protein. *Biochemistry* 29: 6303–6313.

Holak, T., Engstrom, A., Kraulis, P., Lindeberg, G., Bennich, H., Jones, T., Gronenborn, A., and Core, G. (1988) The solution conformation of the antibacterial peptide cecropin A: a nuclear magnetic resonance and dynamical simulated annealing study. *Biochemistry* 27: 7620–7629.

Ikura, M., Kay, L., and Bax A. (1990) A novel approach for sequential assignment of ^{1}H, ^{13}C and ^{15}N spectra of larger proteins: heteronuclear triple-resonance three-dimensional NMR spectroscopy. Application to calmodulin. *Biochemistry* 29: 4659–4667.

Inagaki, F., Shimada, I., Kawaguchi, K., Hirano, M., Terasawa, I., Ikura, T., and Go, N. (1989) Structure of melittin bound to perdeuterated dodecylphosphocholine micelles as studied by two-dimensional NMR and distance geometry calculations. *Biochemistry* 28: 5985–5991.

Keniry, M., Gutowsky, H., and Oldfield, E. (1984) Surface dynamics of the integral membrane protein bacteriorhodopsin. *Nature* 307: 383–386.

Kersh, J., Tomich, J., and Montal, M. (1989) The M2δ transmembrane domain of the nicotinic cholinergic receptor forms ion channels in human erythrocyte membranes. *Biochem. Biophys. Res. Commun.* 162: 352–356.

Kühlbrandt, W., Wang, D. N., and Fujiyoshi, Y. (1994) Atomic model of plant light-harvesting complex by electronic crystallography. *Nature* 367: 614–621.

Lauterwein, J., Bosch, C., Brown, L., and Wuthrich, K. (1979) Physiochemical studies of the protein-lipid interactions in melittin-containing micelles. *Biochim. Biophys. Acta* 556: 244–264.

Lee, K., Fitton, J., and Wuthrich, K. (1987) Nuclear magnetic resonance investigation of the conformation of *d*-haemolysin bound to dodecylphosphocholine micelles. *Biochim. Biophys. Acta.* 911: 144–153.

Leo, G. C., Conago, L. A., Valentine, K. G., and Opella, S. J. (1987) Dynamics of fd coat protein in lipid bilayers. *Biochemistry* 26: 854–862.

Lewis, B., Harbison, G., Herzfeld, J., and Griffin, R. (1985) NMR structural analysis of a membrane protein: bacteriorhodopsin peptide backbone orientation and motion. *Biochemistry* 24: 4671–4679.

Makowski, L. (1984) Structural diversity in filamentous bacteriophages. In: *Biological Macromolecules and Assemblies,* edited by A. McPherson. New York: Wiley, p. 202.

Marion, D., Ikura, M., Tshudin, R., and A. Bax (1989) Rapid recording of 2D NMR spectra without phase cycling. Application to the study of hydrogen exchange in proteins. *J. Magn. Reson.* 85: 393–399.

Marvin, D., and Hohn, B. (1969) Filamentous bacterial viruses. *Bacterial Rev.* 33: 172–209.

Marvin, D., and Wachtel, E. (1975) Structure and assembly of filamentous bacterial viruses. *Nature* 253: 19–23.

McDermott, A., Thompson, L., Winkler, C., Farrar, M., Pelletier, S., Lugtenburg, J., Herzfeld, J., and Griffin, R. (1991) Mechanism of proton pumping in bacteriorhodopsin by solid-state NMR: the protonation state of tyrosine in the light-adapted and M states. *Biochemistry* 30: 8366–8371.

McLaughlin, A., Cullis, P., Hemminga, M., Hoult, D., Redda, G., Ritchie, G., Seeley, P., and Richards, R. (1975) Application of ^{31}P NMR to model and biological membrane systems. *FEBS Lett.* 57: 213–218.

Montal, M. (1990) Molecular anatomy and molecular design of channel proteins. *FASEB J.* 9: 2623–2635.

Mulvey, D., King, G., Cooke, R., Doak, D., Harvey, T., and Campbell, I. (1989) High resolution ^{1}H NMR study of the solution structure of the S4 segment of the sodium channel protein. *FEBS Lett.* 257: 113–117.

Nambudripad, R., Stark, W., Opella, S. J., and Makowski, L. (1991) Membrane mediated assembly of filamentous bacteriophage Pf1. *Science* 252: 1305–1308.

Oiki, S., Danho, W., Madison, V., and Montal, M. (1988) M2δ, a candidate for the structure lining the ionic channel of the nicotinic cholinergic receptor. *Proc. Natl. Acad. Sci. USA* 85: 8703–8707.

Oldfield, E., Kinsey, R., and Kintanar, A. (1982) Recent advances in the study of bacteriorhodopsin dynamic structure using high-field solid-state nuclear magnetic resonance spectroscopy. *Methods Enzymol.* 88: 310–325.

Opella, S. J. (1982) Solid state NMR of biological systems. *Annu. Rev. Phys. Chem.* 33: 533–549.

Opella, S. J. (1985) Protein dynamics by solid state NMR. *Methods Enzymol.* 17: 327–361.

Opella, S. J., and Stewart, P. (1989) Solid-state nuclear magnetic resonance structural studies of proteins. *Method Enzymol.* 176: 242–275.

Opella, S. J., Stewart, P., and Valentine, K. (1987) Protein structure by solid-state NMR spectroscopy. *Q. Rev. Biophys.* 19: 7–49.

Opella, S. J., and Waugh, J. (1977) Two-dimensional ^{13}C NMR of highly oriented polyethylene. *J. Chem. Phys.* 66: 4919–4924.

Pake, G. (1948) Nuclear resonance absorption in hydrated crystals: fine structure of the proton line. *J. Chem. Phys.* 16: 327–339.

Pervushin, K., Arsenieu, A., Kozhich, A. and Ivanov, U. (1991) Two-dimensional NMR study of the conformation of (34–65) bacterioopsin polypeptide in SDS micelles. *J. Biomol. NMR* 1: 313–322.

Raleigh, D., Levitt, M., and Griffin, R. (1988) Rotational resonance in solid state NMR. *Chem. Phys. Lett.* 146: 71–76.

Rees, D., Komiga, H., Yeates, T., Allen, J., and Feher, G. (1989) The bacterial photosynthetic reaction center as a model for membrane proteins. *Annu. Rev. Biochem.* 58: 607–633.

Rice, D., Blume, A., Herzfeld, J., Wittebort, R., Huangi, T., Das Gupta, S., and Griffin, R. (1981) Solid state NMR investigations of lipid bilayers, peptides and proteins. *Biomol. Stereodynam.* II: 271.

Sanders, J., van Nuland, N., Edholm, O., and Hemminga, M. (1991) Conformation and aggregation of M13 coat protein studied by molecular dynamics. *Biophys. Chem.* 41: 193–202.

Schiksnis, R. A., Bogusky, M. J., Tsang, P., and Opella, S. J. (1987) Structure and dynamics of the Pf1 filamentous bacteriophage coat protein in micelles. *Biochemistry* 26: 1373–1381.

Seelig, J., and Niederberger, W. (1974) Deuterium-labeled lipids as structural probes in liquid crystalline bilayers. A deuterium magnetic resonance study. *J. Am. Chem. Soc.* 96: 2069–2072.

Shon, K., and Opella, S. J. (1989) Detection of ^{1}H homonuclear NOE between amide sites in proteins with ^{1}H/^{15}N heteronuclear correlation spectroscopy. *J. Magn. Reson.* 82: 193–197.

Shon, K., Kim, Y., Colnago, L. A., and Opella, S. J. (1991a) NMR studies of the structure and dynamics of membrane bound bacteriophage Pf1 coat protein. *Science* 252: 1303–1305.

Shon, K, Schrader, P., Kim, Y., Bechinger, B., Zasloff, M., and Opella, S. J. (1991) NMR structural studies of membrane bound peptides and proteins. In: *Biotechnology: Bridging Research and Applications*, edited by D. Kamely, A. Chakrabarty, and S. Kornguth. Dodrecht, the Netherlands: Kluwer, p. 109–124.

Shon, K., Schrader, P., Opella, S. J., Richards, J., and Tomich, J. (1989) NMR spectra of synthetic membrane bound coat protein species. In: *Frontiers of NMR in Molecular Biology: UCLA Symposia on Molecular and Cellular Biology, New Series*, edited by D. Live, I. Armitage, and D. Patel. New York: Alan R. Liss, p. 109–118.

Smith, S., and Griffin, R. (1988) High-resolution solid-state NMR of proteins. *Annu. Rev. Phys. Chem.* 39: 511–535.

Sobol, A., Arsenieu, A., Abdulaeva, G., Musina, L., and Bystrov, V. (1992) Sequence-specific resonance assignment and secondary structure of (1–71) bacterioopsin. *J. Biomol. NMR* 2: 161–171.

Spiess, H. (1982) Rotation of molecules and nuclear spin relaxation. In: *NMR Basic Principles and Progress,* edited by P. Diehl, E. Fluck, and R. Kosfeld. New York: Wiley, p. 55–214.

Spruijt, R., and Hemminga, M. (1991) The in situ aggregational and conformational state of the major coat protein of bacteriophage M13 in phospholipid bilayers mimicking the inner membrane of host *Escherichia coli. Biochemistry* 30: 11147–11154.

Spruijt, R., Wolfs, C., and Hemminga, M. (1989) Aggregation-related conformational changes of the membrane-associated coat protein of bacteriophage M13. *Biochemistry* 28: 9158–9165.

Teng, Q., and Cross, T. (1989) The in situ determination of the ^{15}N chemical-shift tensor orientation in a polypeptide. *J. Magn. Reson.* 85: 439–447.

Tobias, D., Klein, M., and Opella, S. J. (1993) Molecular dynamics simulation of Pf1 coat protein. *Biophys. J.* 64: 670–675.

Torchia, D. (1984) Solid-state NMR studies of protein internal dynamics. *Annu. Rev. Biophys. Bioeng.* 13: 125–144.

Weiss, M., Abele, U., Weckesser, J., Welte, W., Schiltz, E., and Schulz, G. (1991) Molecular architecture and electrostatic properties of a bacterial porin. *Science* 254: 1627–1630.

Wennerberg, A., Cooke, R., Carlquist, M., Rigler, R., and Campbell, J. (1990) A ^{1}H NMR study of the solution conformation of the neuropeptide galanin. *Biochem. Biophys. Res. Commun.* 166: 1102–1109.

Wuthrich, K. (1986) *NMR of Proteins and Nucleic Acids.* New York: Wiley.

Zasloff, M. (1987) Magainins, a class of antimicrobial peptides from *Xenopus* skin: isolation, characterization of two active forms, and partial cDNA sequence of a precursor. *Proc. Natl. Acad. Sci. USA* 84: 5449–5453.

12

Structure of Integral Membrane Proteins within Membranes via X-Ray and Neutron Diffraction: From Oriented Multilayers to a Single Monolayer

J. KENT BLASIE

One of the significant problems in membrane biology has concerned our understanding of the role of the interaction between an integral membrane protein and the host lipid bilayer in determining the structure and function of that protein in the biological membrane. As a result, it has been important to develop physical techniques capable of determining, initially, the structure of an integral membrane protein and the host lipid bilayer within the membrane in as much detail as possible and, ultimately, of determining the response of each of these structures to a perturbation (e.g., the physical state of the solvating lipid), including protein function.

Over roughly the past decade, x-ray and neutron diffraction have been successful in providing important information about the precise positioning of certain integral membrane proteins with respect to the host membrane lipid bilayer and their low-resolution structure within the biological membrane. In all cases, these techniques were applied to thick, oriented multilayers of isolated biological membranes containing essentially only one integral membrane protein possessing a unidirectional vectorial orientation; in most of these cases a symmetrical membrane pair was contained within the multilayer unit cell profile, the exceptions being for membranes isolated as single membrane sheets. Notable examples include rhodopsin within the isolated retinal rod disk membrane (Pascolini et al., 1984; Yeager, 1976; Chabre et al., 1976), bacteriorhodopsin within the isolated purple membrane (Henderson, 1975; Blaurock and King, 1977; Engelman and Zaccai, 1980; Trewhella et al., 1984), acetylcholine receptors within the isolated electroplax membrane (Kistler et al., 1982; Fairclough et al., 1986), "connexon" within isolated gap junctions (Caspar et al., 1977; Makowski et al., 1977), and Ca^{2+}-ATPase within isolated sarcoplasmic reticulum membranes (Herbette et al., 1985). For the Ca^{2+}-ATPase, neutron diffraction, coupled with selective deuteration of membrane molecular components, was critically employed to determine the separate contributions of ATPase protein, phospholipid, and water to the membrane profile structure and thereby define the moderate-resolution (~ 15 Å) Ca^{2+}-ATPase profile structure (as cylindrically averaged about the membrane normal), relative to that of the host, asymmetrical phospholipid bilayer profile structure within the sarcoplasmic reticulum membrane (Herbette et al., 1985). Also, resonance x-ray diffraction was recently used to identify the position of the high-affinity metal-binding sites involved in active calcium transport within this Ca^{2+}-ATPase profile structure to an accuracy of ± 2 Å (Asturias and Blasie, 1991). In the case of bacteriorhodopsin, neutron diffraction, coupled with the deuteration of selected amino acids and phase information from electron microscopy, has provided the distribution of polar versus nonpolar residues within the in-plane projection of its structure at ~ 10 Å resolution, resulting in its description as an "inside-out" protein (Engelman and Zaccai, 1980). However, since such thick, oriented membrane multilayers are generally not three-dimensional single crystals, this definitive, but therefore limited, structural information concerning the integral membrane protein in its natural environment must ultimately be coupled with a knowledge of its full three-dimensional structure at atomic resolution, as obtained by x-ray crystallography of three-dimensional single crystals (Deisenhofer et al., 1984, 1985; Allen et al., 1987), or by electron microscopy of two-dimensional single-crystals (Henderson and Unwin, 1975; Unwin and Henderson, 1975; Henderson et al., 1990; Kühlbrandt et al., 1994), of the detergent solubilized protein. Furthermore, the symmetry of the membrane stacking within such thick, oriented membrane multilayers generally precludes correlative structure–function studies of membrane protein-mediated transmembrane phenomena as detailed as could be achieved in single-monolayer or single-bilayer membrane systems (Schonfeld et al., 1979; Packham et al., 1980, 1982; Tiede et al., 1982; Popovic et al., 1986a,b; Alegria, 1989).

For integral membrane proteins that are not essentially the only protein within the biological membrane, x-ray and neutron diffraction have been similarly applied to thick, oriented multilayers of reconstituted vesicular membranes containing selected lipids and only the detergent-purified protein of interest. Examples include cytochrome oxidase from the mitochondrial inner membrane (Stamatoff et al., 1982; Blasie et al., 1982; Jayaraman et al., 1987), photosynthetic reaction centers from the bacterial chromatophore membrane (Pachence et al., 1979, 1981), as well as the Ca^{2+}-ATPase from the sarcoplasmic reticulum membrane (Herbette et al., 1981b, 1983). Such structural studies of integral membrane proteins in reconstituted vesicular membranes are usually problematical, due to the lack of a unique vectorial orientation for the membrane protein incorporated into the vesicle lipid bilayer (Blasie et al., 1982; Herbette et al., 1981b, 1983). The one notable exception concerned the photosynthetic reaction center from *Rhodopseudomonas sphaeroides* incorporated into unilamellar egg lecithin vesicles. In this case, neutron diffraction coupled with selective deuteration of membrane molecular components was critically employed to determine the separate profile structures of the reaction center at ~ 15 Å resolution (as cylindrically averaged about the membrane normal), relative to that of the host asymmetrical phospholipid bilayer within this particular reconstituted membrane. This work was extended to include the position of the peripheral membrane protein cytochrome c electron donor within the profile structure of the electrostatic reaction center–cytochrome c bimolecular complex within this reconstituted membrane formed subsequently to the reconstitution (Pachence et al., 1983). Resonance x-ray diffraction was then employed to determine the distance between the cytochrome c heme iron atom electron donor and the reaction center iron–quinone complex electron acceptor within this profile structure to an accuracy of ± 1–2 Å (Blasie et al., 1983). All of these structural results were in excellent agreement with the structure of the detergent-solubilized reaction center later determined to atomic resolution by x-ray crystallography (Deisenhofer et al., 1985; Allen et al., 1987).

Given the numerous results mentioned above, it seemed highly desirable to invent a means for the vectorial orientation of integral membrane proteins, especially those otherwise dilute in their natural membrane system, at an interface (e.g., solid–liquid) via their chemical and/or biochemical specificity, in order to form a two-dimensionally dense, vectorially oriented protein monolayer. With the availability of intense synchrotron x-ray sources, the structure of such a protein monolayer system could be determined, in principle, in at least as much detail as previously for thick, oriented multilayer systems, *and* the protein's transmonolayer functionality could be investigated in detail.

As will be discussed below, it is now indeed possible to fabricate such vectorially oriented protein monolayers, which can be used as templates for forming higher order vectorially oriented protein complexes, and their structures can be ascertained via high-resolution x-ray diffraction employing synchrotron sources. Furthermore, these protein monolayer systems maintain their biological functionality.

Methods

Engineering Biochemical Specificity at Interfaces

Biochemical specificity has already been extensively employed to self-assemble vectorially oriented monolayers of several *soluble* proteins at planar solid–liquid and liquid–gas interfaces (Uzgiris and Kornberg, 1983; Ribi et al., 1987; Ludwig et al., 1986; Darst et al., 1991). This work has generally utilized either Langmuir-Blodgett lipid monolayers on solid substrates or Langmuir lipid monolayers at the liquid–gas interface, where the binding specificity for a particular soluble protein was "engineered" into the lipid polar headgroup structure via synthetic or biosynthetic chemistry. However, both of these systems are attacked by the detergents used to solubilize *integral* membrane proteins.

Alternatively, biochemical specificity can be "engineered" on the surface of a solid substrate at the solid–liquid or solid–gas interface, employing bifunctional organic chain molecules to form self-assembled organic monolayers on the substrate surface (Ulman, 1991). These organic molecules are usually of the trichlorosilylalkyl-"protected endgroup" form; reaction with a hydrated silicon oxide surface, for example, results in the formation of a dense monolayer of siloxylalkyl-"protected endgroup" molecules *covalently bound* to the surface—subsequent chemical deprotection of the endgroup then provides the specificity required for the binding of a particular protein. Such self-assembled organic monolayers can therefore be resistant to attack by the detergents used to solubilize integral membrane proteins.

Requirements for X-Ray/Neutron Diffraction

The x-ray (or neutron) elastic scattering from a single monolayer of protein molecules specifically bound (or "tethered") to the planar surface of a *uniform* solid substrate, via a bifunctional organic self-assembled monolayer as described above, is rather weak, even utilizing intense synchrotron x-ray sources, focusing optics, and electronic position-sensitive detectors (Amador et al., 1989, 1993). However, this weak x-ray (or neutron) scattering from the protein monolayer can be dramatically enhanced through its interference with the strong x-ray (or neutron) diffraction from, instead, a *multilayer* solid substrate suitably tailored by magnetron sputtering or molecular beam epitaxy from two different "compatible" elements, while preserving the required surface chemistry, (e.g., silicon and germanium for the x-ray or neutron case). Given the ability to control the scattering contrast and widths of the features within the inorganic multilayer unit cell profile (especially via molecular beam epitaxy), together with the number of multilayer unit cells, this essential interference phenomenon can be made to occur effectively continuously over a broad-range momentum transfer (or reciprocal) space (Xu et al., 1991; Blasie et al., 1991). Furthermore, this multilayer substrate serves as a reference structure (Lesslauer and Blasie, 1971; Blasie et al., 1991), providing the phase information necessary to derive unambiguously the structure of the composite inorganic multilayer-tethered protein monolayer system from the diffraction data via interferometry and/or holography (Amador et al., 1989, 1993).

Results

Indirect Linking via Interaction with a Peripheral Membrane Protein

Cytochrome c is a peripheral membrane protein that binds electrostatically to two integral membrane proteins, cytochrome oxidase on the mitochondrial innermembrane surface and photosynthetic reaction centers lacking endogenous c-type heme groups on the chromatophore membrane surface, acting as the electron donor in both cases; it also binds electrostatically to the integral membrane protein cytochrome b/c_1, on the mitochondrial innermembrane surface, acting as the electron acceptor in this case. Yeast cytochrome c type VIII-A from *Saccharomyces cerevisiae* possesses a single surface cysteine residue 102. The sulfhydryl group of residue 102 has been utilized to form a covalent disulfide linkage with the sulfhydryl endgroup of an 11-siloxylundecylthiol self-assembled monolayer on a silicon oxide surface, following the deprotection of the thiol endgroup of the preformed 11-siloxylundecylthioacetate self-assembled monolayer via acid hydrolysis (Pachence et al., 1990; Pachence and Blasie, 1991; Amador et al., 1989, 1993). The fabrication of this two-dimensionally dense, covalently tethered monolayer of yeast cytochrome c has been ascertained, using optical absorption spectroscopy and optical linear dichroism with quartz substrates and meridional x-ray diffraction $[I(Q_{xy} = 0A^{-1}, Q_z)$, where z is normal to the substrate surface] with Ge–Si multilayer substrates fabricated by magnetron sputtering and molecular beam epitaxy. Results for the latter substrate are shown in Figure 12.1 (J. A. Chupa et al., in preparation).

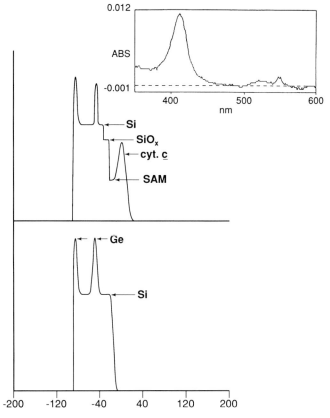

Fig. 12.1. Electron density profiles for the bare Ge–Si multilayer substrate *(bottom)* and for the yeast cytochrome *c* monolayer covalently bound to the 11-siloxylundecylthiol monolayer (*SAM*) on the surface of this substrate *(top)*. The spatial resolution (~7 Å) of these profiles, derived via x-ray interferometry/holography, is determined by the width (FWHM) of the Ge features in the substrate profile, as fabricated by molecular beam epitaxy. The optical absorption spectrum for the cytochrome *c* monolayer is shown in the *inset*.

These covalently tethered monolayers of yeast cytochrome *c* have been used as a template to self-assemble two-dimensionally dense monolayers of photosynthetic reaction centers from *Rhodopseudomonas sphaeroides* solubilized in the detergent LDAO (lauryldimethylamine oxide) via their electrostatic binding to the cytochrome *c* monolayer. The fabrication of this integral membrane protein monolayer on the tethered cytochrome *c* monolayer surface has been ascertained by optical absorption spectroscopy with quartz substrates and meridional x-ray diffraction with Ge–Si multilayer substrates fabricated by magnetron sputtering (Amador et al., 1989, 1993). It is especially important to note that these protein monolayer systems, thus fabricated, remain fully hydrated throughout, either via immersion in appropriate aqueous medium *or* via a controlled humidity helium atmosphere. As a result, both the covalent tethering of cytochrome *c* and the electrostatic binding of reaction centers are fully reversible, both proteins retain the spectral and redox properties of their prosthetic groups throughout, and light-induced oxidation of the reduced cytochrome

c by the photosynthetic reaction centers has been observed in the monolayer system. The tethered cytochrome c–photosynthetic reaction center monolayer thus fabricated is shown schematically in Figure 12.2.

Direct Linking via Electrostatic Interactions

Given that the positively charged residues of cytochrome c fringing the heme crevice opening (principally lysines) are thought to be responsible for its electrostatic binding to the photosynthetic reaction centers (lacking endogenous c-type heme groups) (Allen et al., 1987), one might expect that the detergent-solubilized reaction centers could also bind electrostatically to the amine endgroups of a ω-siloxylalkylamine self-assembled monolayer on a silicon oxide substrate. This result was recently obtained using the *Rhodop. sphaeroides* reaction centers in LDAO (lauryldimethylamine oxide) and an 11-siloxylundecylamine self-assembled monolayer, following removal of the t-butyl protecting group (J. A. Chupa et al., in preparation). The optical absorption spectrum is shown in Figure 12.3 in the near-infrared for such a two-dimensionally dense reaction center monolayer linked directly via electrostatic interactions to the organic self-assembled monolayer on a quartz substrate.

Future Prospects

With regard to the results described earlier under Indirect Linking via Interaction with a Peripheral Membrane Protein, the author's research group is currently investigating the degree of control of the vectorial orientation of the tethered cytochrome c monolayer via variation of the particular surface residue of the protein utilized for its covalent tethering to the organic self-assembled monolayer on the solid substrate. One could, in principle, "simply" move the single surface cysteine residue to different, minimally structure-perturbing positions on the protein's surface, using site-directed mutagenesis (Bowler et al., 1989). Alternatively, one could utilize the existing natural and site-directed mutants of cytochrome c possessing a single surface histidine residue (including residues 33, 39, and 62, in addition to the above-mentioned surface cysteine residue 102) and a 4-(ω-siloxylalkyl) pyridine as the organic tethering molecule, together with established ruthenium coordination chemistry (Gray and Malstrom, 1989; Therien et al., 1990; Bowler et al., 1989) to link the pyridyl moiety of the tethering molecule to the protein's surface histidine residue. This approach should provide a variety of very different vectorial orientations of the cytochrome c molecules within such tethered two-dimensionally dense monolayers, given these four residue locations on the cytochrome c surface.

Furthermore, clusters of positively charged residues of cytochrome c occur over most of its surface, and yeast cytochrome c covalently tethered via its cysteine residue 102 within a thiol-activated Sepharose column has already been utilized to bind selectively both detergent-solubilized cytochrome oxidase and cytochrome b/c_1 (Bill et al., 1980). Hence, such covalently tethered cytochrome c monolayers are expected also to bind these other two integral membrane protein ligands of cytochrome c electrostatically.

Finally, the extremely detailed profile features of Ge–Si multilayer substrates, as

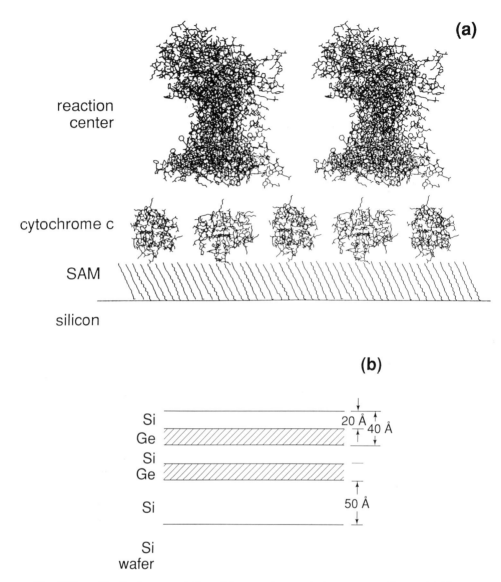

(a)

reaction
center

cytochrome c

SAM

silicon

(b)

Si

20 Å
40 Å

Ge

Si

Ge

Si

50 Å

Si
wafer

Fig. 12.2. *a*: Idealized representation of the monolayer cytochrome *c*–reaction center bimolecular complex. The 11-siloxylundecylthiol self-assembled monolayer (*SAM*) is covalently attached to a solid substrate, shown at *bottom*. Next, a monolayer of yeast cytochrome *c* is covalently attached to the *SAM*. The larger reaction center proteins bind electrostatically to the cytochrome *c* layer. The covalent disulfide linkage between the *SAM* and cytochrome *c* and the detergent solubilizing the reaction centers are not shown. *b*: Approximate structure of the synthetic inorganic multilayer substrate, showing the sequence of two unit cells of a Ge–Si bilayer deposited on a smoothed silicon substrate, as fabricated by magnetron sputtering.

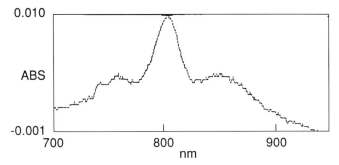

Fig. 12.3. Near-infrared absorption spectra of photosynthetic reaction centers electrostatically bound to the amine-terminated surface of an 11-siloxylundecylamine self-assembled monolayer covalently bound to the quartz substrate surface. The absorbance at ~800 nm indicates that the reaction centers have bound to within ~50% of that for a close-packed monolayer.

fabricated by molecular beam epitaxy, should permit more than sufficient spatial resolution in the electron density profiles, uniquely derived from the meridional x-ray diffraction from the composite inorganic multilayer-tethered protein monolayer system, to determine the vectorial orientation of the integral membrane protein molecules, as demonstrated in Figure 12.4 (J. A. Chupa et al., in preparation).

With regard to the results described earlier under Direct Linking Via Electrostatic Interactions, positively (e.g., NH_3^+) and/or negatively (e.g., CO_2^-) charged endgroups on the surface of the organic self-assembled monolayer on a silicon oxide solid substrate should permit the direct linking, and thereby vectorial orientation, of other integral membrane proteins, including cytochrome oxidase, cytochrome b/c_1, bacteriorhodopsin (given its putative structure and electrophoretic orientation [Trewhella et al., 1984]), and so forth.

Given a reasonable putative structure for an integral membrane protein, it may be possible to link directly the detergent-solubilized integral membrane protein to the endgroups of the organic self-assembled monolayers on a silicon oxide substrate via *covalent* interactions. In this case, site-directed mutagenesis could be utilized to place one (or more) cysteine or histidine residues at one (or more) strategic locations on the protein's putative surface for the covalent tethering of the protein to a solid substrate surface, utilizing either the disulfide or the ruthenium coordination chemistry as described above. This approach is being investigated in the author's research group, in collaboration with others, for the Ca^{2+}-ATPase of the sarcoplasm reticulum; its putative structure (Clark et al., 1989a,b) is based on its primary sequence and low-resolution structure derived by x-ray and neutron diffraction (Herbette et al., 1985) and electron microscopy (Taylor et al., 1986).

Finally, it may be possible in the systems described under Results above to effect a two-dimensional crystallization of the integral membrane protein of interest into micron-sized domains. Three-dimensional electron microscopic image-reconstruction methods could certainly be employed to determine the three-dimensional structure of the protein to possibly near-atomic resolution (Henderson et al., 1990). Alternatively, intense synchrotron x-radiation provided from the undulator sources at the Advanced Photon Source (under construction at Argonne National Laboratory), coupled with demagnifying x-ray optics and essential phase information from the

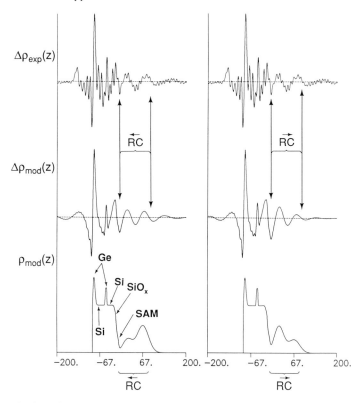

Fig. 12.4. Absolute electron density profile for a fully hydrated photosynthetic reaction center (*RC*) monolayer electrostatically tethered to the surface of an amine-terminated self-assembled monolayer (*SAM*) on the surface of a Ge–Si multilayer substrate (fabricated by MBE) derived and proven by x-ray interferometry/holography. The SAM amine groups were used to mimic the lysine and arginine residues of cytochrome *c* involved in the electrostatic reaction center–cytochrome *c* interaction. The spatial resolution of these profiles of <7 Å is more than adequate to establish the vectorial orientation of the reaction center molecules in this tethered monolayer. (The refined, absolute electron density model profiles for the Ge-Si multilayer substrate–amine-terminated SAM reaction center monolayer are shown at the bottom for the two opposite vectorial orientations of the reaction center; their corresponding relative electron density model profiles are shown immediately above as the middle two profiles. The top profile in each case is the experimental relative electron density profile determined and proven by x-ray interferometry/holography. Comparison of the two relative electron density model profiles with the experimentally determined relative electron density profile over the region occupied by the reaction centers clearly establishes the reaction center vectorial orientation as that shown in the absolute electron density model profile, *bottom left!*)

underlying multilayer substrate, may permit the determination of the full three-dimensional structure of the integral membrane protein via the x-ray crystallography of the micron-sized, two-dimensional crystalline domain. The anticipated reduction in radiation-induced sample damage for x-rays versus electrons might well facilitate the three-dimensional structure determination to near-atomic resolution.

Conclusions

Given the above, it now seems possible to fabricate vectorially oriented, densely packed monolayers of membrane proteins, including *integral* membrane proteins, tethered to the surface of a solid inorganic substrate via a bifunctional organic chain molecule. The approach described is based on the chemical and/or biochemical specificity of the protein's surface, which can be either natural or "engineered" via site-directed mutagenesis, coupled with clever synthetic organic chemistry. The "correctness" of the sequential fabrication can be ascertained by the spectroscopy of the protein's intrinsic prosthetic groups and x-ray diffraction employing selectively tailored multilayer inorganic solid substrates. The protein monolayer thus fabricated is maintained in a fully hydrated state and thereby retains its biological functionality. Such a protein monolayer is already in a form ideally suited for the detailed study of protein-mediated, transmonolayer electrochemical phenomena. [In this regard, it might ultimately be important to exchange the detergent for phospholipid within the tethered integral membrane protein monolayer, using the standard approach employed in membrane reconstitution (Herbette et al., 1981a, 1981b). This could be monitored, for example, utilizing perdeuterated phospholipids and meridional neutron diffraction from the composite multilayer substrate-tethered monolayer system.] Furthermore, when tethered to a suitable multilayer inorganic substrate, detailed structural studies, including time-resolved x-ray diffraction studies of the protein monolayer's response to a physical or chemical excitation including protein function, can be performed analogous to those performed previously on the Ca^{2+}-ATPase within thick, oriented multilayers of isolated sarcoplasmic reticulum membranes (Blasie et al., 1985; Pascolini et al., 1988). Hence, such a tethered protein monolayer system is well suited to detailed correlative structure–function studies. Finally, it remains to be seen whether well-ordered, two-dimensionally crystalline domains of the integral membrane protein of interest can be induced within such tethered protein monolayers suitable for three-dimensional structural studies of the protein via electron microscopic and/or x-ray crystallographic methods.

References

Alegria, G. (1989) *Use of the Langmuir-Blodgett Film Technique in Structural and Functional Studies of Photosynthetic Bacteria.* Ph.D. thesis, University of Pennsylvania.

Allen, J. P., Yeates, T. O., Komiya, H., and Rees, D. C. (1987) Structure of the reaction center from *Rhodobacter sphaeroides* R-26: the protein subunits. *Proc. Natl. Acad. Sci. U.S.A.* 84: 6162–6166.

Amador, S. M., Pachence, J. M., Fischetti, R., McCauley, J. P. Jr., Smith, A. B. III, Dutton, P. L., and Blasie, J. K. (1989) X-ray diffraction studies of protein monolayers bound to self-assembled monolayers. Materials Res. Soc. Symp. Proc. 177: 393–398.

Amador, S. M., Pachence, J. M., Fischetti, R., McCauley, J. P. Jr., Smith, A. B. III, Dutton, P. L., Blasie, J. K. (1993) Use of self-assembled monolayers to covalently tether protein monolayers to the surface of solid substrates. Langmuir, 9: 812–817.

Asturias, F. J., and Blasie, J. K. (1991) Location of high-affinity metal binding sites in the profile structure of the Ca^{2+}-ATPase in the sarcoplasmic reticulum by resonance X-ray diffraction. *Biophys. J.* 59: 488–502.

Bill, K., Casey, R. P., Broger, C., and Azzi, A. (1980) Affinity chromatography purification of cytochrome *c* oxidase: use of a yeast cytochrome *c*–thiol–Sepharose 4B column. *FEBS Lett* 120: 248–250.

Blasie, J. K., Herbette, L. G., Pascolini, D., Skita, V., Pierce, D., and Scarpa, A. (1985) Time-resolved x-ray diffraction studies of the sarcoplasmic reticulum membrane during active transport. *Biophys. J.* 48: 9–18.

Blasie, J. K., Xu, S., Murphy, M., Chupa, J., McCauley, J. P., Smith, A. B. III. Bean, J. C., and Peticolas, L. J. (1991) Profile structures of macromolecular monolayers on solid substrates by x-ray interferometry/halography. *Materials Res. Soc. Symp. Proc.* 237: 399–409.

Blasie, J. K., Pachence, J. M., Tavormina, A., Dutton, P. L., Stamatoff, J., Eisenberger, P., and Brown, G. (1983) The location of redox centers in the profile structure of a reconstituted membrane containing a photosynthetic reaction center-cytochrome *c* complex by resonance x-ray diffraction. *Biochim. Biophys. Acta* 723: 350–357.

Blasie, J. K., Pachence, J. M., Tavormina, A., Erecinska, M., Dutton, P. L., Stamatoff, J., Eisenberger, P., and Brown, G. (1982) The location of redox centers in biological membranes determined by resonance x-ray diffraction II. Analysis of the resonance diffraction data. *Biochim. Biophys. Acta* 679: 188–197.

Blaurock, A. E., and King, G. I. (1977) Asymmetric structure of the purple membrane. *Science* 196: 1101–1104.

Bowler, B. E., Meade, T. J., Mayo, S. L., Richards, J. H., and Gray H. B. (1989) Long-range electron transfer in structurally engineered pentaammineruthenium (histidine-62) cytochrome-*c*. *J. Am. Chem. Soc.* 111: 8757–8759.

Caspar, D.L.D., Goodenough, D. A., Makowski, L., and Phillips, W. C. (1977) Gap junction structures I. Correlated electron microscopy and x-ray diffraction. *J. Cell Biol.* 74: 605–628.

Chabre, M., Saibil, H., and Worcester, D. L. (1976) Neutron diffraction studies of oriented retinal rods. In: *Brookhaven Symposia in Biology, No. 27, Neutron Scattering for the Analysis of Biological Structures.* Upton, NY: Brookhaven National Laboratory, III, p. 77–85.

Chupa, J. A., McCauley, J. P., Strongin, R. M., Smith, A. B. III, Blasie, J. K., Peticolas, L. J., and Bean, J. C. Vectorially oriented membrane protein monolayers: Profile structures via x-ray interferometry/holography. In preparation.

Clarke, D. M., Loo, T. W., Inesi, G., and MacLennan, D. H 1989a) Location of high affinity Ca^{++}-binding sites within the predicted transmembrane domain of the sarcoplasmic reticulum Ca^{++}-ATPase. *Nature* 339: 476–478.

Clarke, D. M., Maruyama, K., Loo, T. W., Leberer, E., Inesi, G., and MacLennan D. H. (1989b) Functional consequences of glutamate, aspartate, glutamine, and asparagine mutations in the stalk sector of the Ca^{2+}-ATPase of sarcoplasmic reticulum. *J. Biol. Chem.* 264: 11246–11251.

Darst, S. A., Ahlers, M., Meller, P. H., Kubalek, E. W., Blankenberg, R., Ribi, H. O., Ringsdorf, H., and Kornberg, R. D. (1991) 2-Dimensional cyrstals of streptavidin on biotinylated lipid layers and their interactions with biotinylated macromolecules. *Biophys. J.* 59: 387–396.

Deisenhofer, J., Epp, O., Miki, K., Huber, R., and Michel, H. (1984) X-ray structure analysis of a membrane protein complex. Electron density map at 3 Å resolution and a model of the chromophores of the photosynthetic reaction center from *Rhodospeudomonas viridis. J. Mol. Biol.* 180: 385–398.

Deisenhofer, J., Epp, O., Miki, K., Huber, R., and Michel, H. (1985) Structure of the protein subunits in the photosynthetic reaction centre of *Rhodospeudomonas viridis* at 3 Å resolution. *Nature* 318: 618–624.

Engelman, D. M., and Zaccai, G. (1980) Bacteriorhodopsin is an inside-out protein. *Proc. Natl. Acad. Sci. USA* 77: 5894–5898.

Fairclough, R. H., Miake-Lye, R. C., Stroud, R. M., Hodgson, K. O., and Doniach, S. (1986) Location of terbium binding sites on acetycholine receptor–enriched membranes. *J. Mol. Biol.* 189: 673–680.

Gray, H. B., and Malmstrom, B. G. (1989) Long-range electron transfer in multisite metalloproteins. *Biochemistry* 28: 7499–7505.

Henderson, R. (1975) The structure of the purple membrane from *Halobacterium hallobium:* analysis of the x-ray diffraction pattern. *J. Mol. Biol.* 93: 123–138.

Henderson, R., Baldwin, J. M., Ceska, T. A., Zemlin, F., Beckmann, E., and Downing, K. H. (1990) Model for the structure of bacteriorhodopsin based on high-resolution electrol cryo-microscopy. *J. Mol. Biol.* 213: 899–929.

Henderson, R., and Unwin, P.N.T. (1975) Three-dimensional model of purple membrane obtained by electron microscopy. *Nature* 257: 28–32.

Herbette, L., DeFoor, P., Fleischer, S., Pascolini, D., Scarpa, A., and Blasie, J. K. (1985) The separate profile structures of the functional calcium pump protein and the phospholipid bilayer within isolated sarcoplasmic reticulum membranes determined by x-ray and neutron diffraction. *Biochim. Biophys. Acta* 817: 103–122.

Herbette, L., Scarpa, A., Blasie, J. K., Bauer, D. R., Wang, C. T., and Fleischer, S. (1981a) Functional characteristics of reconstituted sarcoplasmic reticulum membranes as a function of the lipid-to-protein ratio. *Biophys. J.* 36: 26–46.

Herbette, L., Scarpa, A., Blasie, J. K., Wang, C. T., Hymel, L., Seelig, J., and Fleischer, S. (1983) The determination of the separate Ca^{2+} pump protein and phospholipid profile structures within reconstituted sarcoplasmic reticulum membranes via x-ray and neutron diffraction. *Biochim. Biophys. Acta* 730: 369–378.

Herbette, L., Scarpa, A., Blasie, J. K., Wang, C. T., Saito, A., Fleischer, S. (1981b) Comparison of the profile structures of isolated and reconstituted sarcoplasmic reticulum membranes. *Biophys. J.* 36: 47–72.

Jayaraman, U., Chang, T., Frey, T. J., and Blasie, J. K. (1987) Electron density profile of two-dimensionally crystalline membranous cytochrome *c* oxidase at low resolution. *Biophys. J.* 51: 475–486.

Kistler, J., Stroud, R. M., Klymkowsky, W., Lalancette, R. A., and Fairclough, R. H. (1982) Structure and function of an acetylcholine receptor. *Biophys. J.* 37: 371–383.

Kühlbrandt, W., Wang, D. N., and Fujiyoshi, Y. (1994) Atomic model of plant light-harvesting complex by electronic crystallography. *Nature* 367: 614–621.

Lesslauer, W., and Blasie, J. K. (1971) X-ray holographic interferometry in the determination of planar multilayer structures. Theory and experimental observations. *Acta Crystallog. A* 27: 456–461.

Ludwig, D. S., Ribi, H. O., Schoolnik, G. K., and Kornberg, R. D. (1986) Two-dimensional crystals of cholera toxin β-subunit-receptor complexes: projected structure at 17 Å resolution. *Proc. Natl. Acad. Sci. USA* 83: 8585–8588.

Makowski, L., Caspar, D.L.D., Phillips, W. C., and Goodenough, D. A. (1977) Gap junction structures. II. Analysis of the x-ray diffraction data. *J. Cell. Biol.* 74: 629–645.

Pachence, J. M., Amador, S., Maniara, G., Vanderkooi, J., Dutton, P. L., and Blasie, J. K. (1990) Orientation and lateral mobility of cytochrome-*c* on the surface of ultrathin lipid multilayer films. *Biophys. J.* 58: 379–389.

Pachence, J. M., and Blasie, J. K. (1991) Structural investigation of the covalent and electrostatic binding of yeast cytochrome-*c* to the surface of various ultrathin lipid multilayers using x-ray diffraction. *Biophys. J.* 59: 894–900.

Pachence, J. M., Dutton, P. L., and Blasie, J. K. (1979) Structural studies on reconstituted reaction center–phosphatidylcholine membranes. *Biochim. Biophys. Acta* 548: 348–373.

Pachence, J. M., Dutton, P. L., and Blasie, J. K. (1981) The reaction center profile structure derived from neutron diffraction. *Biochim. Biophys. Acta* 635: 267–283.

Pachence, J. M., Dutton, P. L., and Blasie, J. K. (1983) A structural investigation of cytochrome c binding to photosynthectic reaction centers in reconstituted membranes. *Biochim. Biophys. Acta* 724: 6–19.

Packham, N. K., Dutton, P. L., and Mueller, P. (1982) Photoelectric currents across planar bilayer membranes containing bacterial reaction centers. Response under conditions of single electron turnover. *Biophys. J.* 37: 465–473.

Packham, N. K., Packham, C., Mueller, P., Tiede, D. M., and Dutton, P. L. (1980) Reconstitution of photochemically active reaction centers in planar phospholipid membranes. Light-induced electrical currents under voltage-clamp conditions. *FEBS Lett.* 110: 101–106.

Pascolini, D., Blasie, J. K., Gruner, S. M. (1984) A 12 Å resolution x-ray diffraction study of the profile structure of isolated bovine retinal rod outer segment disk membranes. *Biochim. Biophys. Acta* 777: 9–20.

Pascolini, D., Herbette, L. G., Skita, V., Asturias, F., Scarpa, A., and Blasie, J. K. (1988) Changes in the sarcoplasmic reticulum membrane profile induced by enzyme phosphorylation to E1-P at 16 Å resolution via time-resolved x-ray diffraction. *Biophys. J.* 54: 679–688.

Popovic, Z. D., Kovacs, G. J., Vincett, P. S., Allegria, G., and Dutton, P. L. (1986a) Electic-field dependence of the quantum yield in reaction centers of photosynthectic bacteria. *Biochim. Biophys. Acta* 851: 38–48.

Popovic, Z. D., Kovacs, G. J., Vincett, P. S., Allegria, G., and Dutton, P. L. (1986b) Electric-field dependence of recombination kinetics in reaction centers of photosynthetic bacteria. *Chem. Phys.* 110: 227–237.

Ribi, H. O., Reichard, P., and Kornberg, R. D. (1987) Two-dimensional crystals of enzyme–effector complexes: ribonucleotide reductase at 18 Å resolution. *Biochemistry* 26: 7974–7979.

Schonfeld, M., Montal, M., and Feher, G. (1979) Functional reconstitution of photosynthetic reaction centers in planar lipid bilayers. *Proc. Natl. Acad. Sci. USA* 76: 6351–6355.

Stamatoff, J., Eisenberger, P., Blasie, J. K., Pachence, J., Tavormina, A., Erecinska, M., Dutton, P. L., and Brown, G. T. (1982) The location of redox centers in biological membranes determined by resonance x-ray diffraction. Observation of the resonance effect. *Biochim. Biophys. Acta* 679: 177–187.

Taylor, K. A., Ho, M.-H., and Martonosi, A. (1986) Image analysis of the Ca^{2+}-ATPase from sarcoplasmic reticulum. *Ann. NY Acad. Sci.* 483: 31–43.

Therien, M. J., Selman, M. A., Gray, H. B., Chang, I.-J., and Winkler, J. R. (1990) Long-range electron transfer in ruthenium-modified cytochrome *c*: evaluation of porphyrin-ruthenium electronic couplings in the *Candida krusei* and horse heart proteins. *J. Am. Chem. Soc.* 112: 2420–2422.

Tiede, D. M., Mueller, P., and Dutton, P. L. (1982) Spectrophotometric and voltage clamp characterization of monolayers of bacterial photosynthetic reaction centers. *Biochim. Biophys. Acta* 681: 191–201.

Trewhella, J., Gogol, E., Zaccai, G., and Engelman, D. M. (1984) Neutron diffraction studies of bacteriorhodopsin structure. In *Neutrons in Biology,* edited by B. P. Schoenborn. New York: Plenum, p. 227–246.

Ulman, A. (1991) *Ultrathin Organic Films from Langmuir-Blodgett to Self-Assembly.* San Diego: Academic.

Unwin, P.N.T., and Henderson, R. (1975) Molecular structure determination by electron microscopy of unstained crystalline specimens. *J. Mol. Biol.* 94: 425–440.

Uzgiris, E. E., and Kornberg, R. D. (1983) Two-dimensional crystallization technique for imaging macromolecules, with application to antigen–antibody-complement complexes. *Nature* 301: 125–129.

Xu, S., Murphy, M. A., Amador, S. M., and Blasie, J. K. (1991) Proof of asymmetry in the Cd-arachidate bilayers of ultrathin Langmuir-Blodgett multilayer films via x-ray interferometry. *J. Phys. I* 1: 1131–1144.

Yeager, M. J. (1976) Neutron diffraction analysis of the structure of retinal photoreceptor membranes and rhodopsin. In: *Brookhaven Symposia in Biology, Vol. 27, Neutron Scattering for the Analysis of Biological Structures.* NY: Upton, Brookhaven National Laboratory, III, p. 3–36.

IV. Model and
Physicochemical Approaches

It should be apparent from the first three sections that membrane proteins yield their structural secrets grudgingly. As I emphasized in Chapter 4 on hydropathy plots, model and physicochemical approaches provide insights into the behavior of peptides in membrane environments that help us to test ideas about the architecture of membrane proteins. The first chapter in this section, by Lukas Tamm, reviews the large body of literature concerned with peptide–bilayer interactions. Such studies are important not only because they help us to understand basic issues related to protein folding in membranes; they provide basic information about the mechanisms of action of biologically active peptides as well. Some of these peptides, such as gramicidin, form ion channels and thus become useful for thinking about the organization and function of sodium, potassium, and other "big" ion channels. Andrew Woolley and Bonnie Wallace discuss the lessons we have learned from elegant structural and other biophysical studies of gramicidin. The chapter by Jim Lear and his colleagues is also concerned with channels formed by small peptides, but their focus is on engineering peptides from first principles. This "protein engineering" approach allows us to test our understanding of basic principles.

The main driving force for the folding of globular proteins is the burying of hydrophobic side chains in the protein interior to remove them from contact with water. The hydrophobic effect responsible for this phenomenon is also the major driving force for partitioning membrane proteins into bilayers. However, as discussed by Jean-Luc Popot and Douglas Rees and their colleagues in earlier chapters, once the hydrophobic transmembrane segments are inserted into the bilayer, the hydrophobic effect as we generally think of it is no longer applicable. What are the origins of the forces that cause the segments to form compact structures in the bilayer environment? One idea is that exceptionally favorable packing arrangements driven by van der Waals interactions are important. High-resolution crystallographic studies of small helical peptides provide information about that and other questions. In her chapter, Isabella Karl reviews her pioneering efforts in this area. Of particular interest is the fact that water molecules can participate in the backbone hydrogen bonds of hydrophobic helices.

13

Physical Studies of
Peptide–Bilayer Interactions

LUKAS K. TAMM

The biogenesis of biological membranes is one of the most important unresolved problems of biochemistry and cell biology. Although many proteins that accompany nascent polypeptide chains during their transfer from the ribosomes to the lipid bilayer and that catalyze the targeting of these polypeptides to the correct membrane in the cell have been identified and characterized in recent years, the actual process of polypeptide insertion and folding in biological and model membranes is still obscure. The fluid lipid bilayer of a membrane is a highly anisotropic and highly amphiphilic medium (see White, Cahpter 4). It is well structured and ordered in a liquid-crystalline fashion. Therefore, rules and principles that are different from those describing protein folding in solution are expected to govern the folding and insertion of proteins in membranes (see Rees et al., Chapter 1). Whether the insertion process is catalyzed by other proteins in vivo, the final product, i.e., the folded polypeptide in the membrane, must eventually attain a low energy state in the lipid bilayer. A thorough knowledge of the thermodynamic laws that describe the pertinent protein–lipid and protein–protein interactions will help us to understand and predict in more detail membrane protein structures.

Many algorithms (some of which are discussed in Chapters 2 and 4) have been developed to predict various structural features of membrane proteins. Most of them have focused on finding transmembrane α-helices and on determining the membrane topology (sidedness) of large membrane proteins. Usually, hydrophobic (and, in some methods, amphipathic) transmembrane α-helices of about 20–25 residues are the only structural elements that are considered and the membrane is generally modeled as a thin film of low dielectric constant; thus, these models neglect effects that different lipids with different polar headgroups and different fatty acyl chains might have on the structure of membrane proteins or on their folding pathway.

This chapter reviews experiments that have been conducted to characterize the thermodynamics and structural features of the interactions of synthetic and natural peptides with lipid bilayers. It concentrates on membrane-interactive peptides that comprise about 15–30 residues, i.e., peptides that are long enough to attain stable secondary structures and potentially to transverse a lipid bilayer in a single α-helix. This range includes peptide toxins, peptide hormones, synthetic transmembrane sequences of larger membrane proteins, segments of apolipoproteins, "hydrophobic" and "amphiphilic" signal sequences, fusogenic peptides, and some synthetic model peptides. Aspects of peptide structure are given more emphasis in this chapter than aspects of lipid structure and general membrane reorganization as a consequence of peptide–bilayer interactions. This bias emerges from the general theme of this book and does not mean that changes in lipid and membrane structure are less important than those of the polypeptides. The literature on peptide–bilayer interactions is very large, and reviews of various different aspects of this general problem are available (Kaiser and Kézdy, 1987; von Heijne, 1988; Gierasch, 1989; Segrest et al., 1990; Popot and Engelman, 1990; Tamm, 1991; Epand and Epand, 1992; White and Wimley, 1994).

Binding and Insertion of Peptides into Lipid Model Membranes

Theoretical Background

One of the keys to understanding peptide–bilayer interactions on a quantitative basis is to determine the relevant contributions to the total free energy of binding as a function of amino acid composition and sequence, when a peptide is transferred from an aqueous environment into the lipid bilayer of a membrane. To obtain such thermodynamic data, it is necessary to measure binding (or incorporation) isotherms and to find an appropriate binding–incorporation model that accurately fits the experimental curves. Many peptides contain charged and hydrophobic residues, and many biological lipids are also (usually negatively) charged. Therefore, it can be expected that hydrophobic and charge interactions are important in stabilizing peptide–membrane interactions. Changes in hydrogen bonding, conformational equilibria of lipid and peptide structures, dipole interactions, and entropy due to peptide immobilization can also contribute to the measured binding free energies, as will be discussed later in this section.

The binding of large peptides with a sufficient number of apolar residues to lipid membranes generally does not show saturation, and the lipids usually cannot be considered to constitute discrete binding sites for these peptides. Therefore, saturable Langmuir adsorption isotherms (and derived Scatchard plots) are often not the best choice for analyzing peptide–bilayer binding/incorporation isotherms. In contrast, partition models appear to be more adequate to describe peptide binding and insertion into membranes. The partition constant for the transfer of the peptide from the aqueous solution into the membrane (hydrophobic core or interface) is defined by

$$K_P = \frac{X_p^b}{C_p^f} = \frac{C_p^b}{C_p^f C_L^o} \, [M^{-1}] \tag{1}$$

where the mole fraction of bound peptide in the membrane, X_p^b, is the ratio between the bound peptide concentration, C_p^b, and the total lipid concentration, C_L^o, and C_p^f is the free peptide concentration. When there are reasons to believe that the peptide partitions only into the outer leaflet of closed vesicles or planar membranes, C_L^o in Eq. 1 has to be replaced with the effective total lipid concentration, $C_L^{o,eff}$, which is approximately $0.6 \times C_L^o$ for small unilamellar vesicles and $0.5 \times C_L^o$ for planar bilayers, respectively. In some literature, dimensionless partition coefficients/constants are given either in terms of bound peptide per total lipid volume, γ, or in terms of mole fraction of peptide–lipid divided by mole fraction of peptide–solvent (water), K_x. The two quantities are related to the partition constant defined in Eq. 1 by

$$K_P = \gamma \overline{V}_L = K_x/55.5 \tag{2}$$

where $\overline{V}_L$ is the partial molar volume of the lipid and 55.5 is the molarity of water.

Electrostatic interactions between charged peptides and charged lipids can in part be accounted for by combining the partition model with the Gouy-Chapman theory of the diffuse ionic double layer (for review, see McLaughlin, 1989). The basic assumptions of this approach are (1) that even under physiological salt conditions the electrostatic field dominates long-range interactions (≥ 10 Å from the membrane surface) and accumulates (or depletes) the local peptide concentration relative to the bulk concentration and (2) that the actual insertion process is driven by short range (<10 Å) interactions with the local peptide concentration at the membrane–water interface participating in the partition equilibrium. Despite a number of shortcomings, including these assumptions and those of a diffuse surface charge on the membrane and a concentrated point charge on the peptide, the Gouy-Chapman partition model has worked remarkably well for analyzing many peptide–bilayer (or peptide–monolayer) incorporation isotherms. In this framework, the partition constant becomes

$$K_P = \frac{X_p^b}{C_p^f} \exp(z_p e_o \psi_o / kT) \tag{3}$$

where z_p is the valence of the charge on the peptide, e_o the elementary charge, ψ_o the surface potential, k the Boltzmann constant, and T the absolute temperature. ψ_o can be calculated from the surface charge density, which in turn is a function of the mole fraction of bound peptide. Details of the theory, further references, and practical considerations for calculating isotherms with this model can be found in Tamm (1991).

The Gibbs free energies of peptide insertion may be derived from the measured partition constants with the familiar relation

$$\Delta G_{ins} = -RT \ln K_x = -RT \ln (55.5 K_P) \tag{4}$$

In this equation, all concentrations are expressed in units of mole fraction, which yields ΔG_{ins} relative to a standard state that is useful for further consideration of the hydrophobic effect (Reynolds et al., 1974). ΔG_{ins} is a sum of several contributions (Jähnig, 1983; Jacobs and White, 1989)

$$\Delta G_{ins} = \Delta G_H + \Delta G_F + \Delta G_D + \Delta G_C + \Delta G_I + \Delta G_L \tag{5}$$

namely, the hydrophobic effect (ΔG_H), hydrogen bonding, and other hydrophilic contributions (ΔG_F), interactions with the interfacial dipole potential (ΔG_D), conformational changes of the peptide (ΔG_C), the entropy changes due to the immobilization of the peptide in the membrane (ΔG_I), and lipid perturbation (ΔG_L). The contributions of ΔG_F, ΔG_C, and ΔG_L are probably smaller than those of ΔG_H and ΔG_I. The origin and magnitude of the interfacial dipole potential is not yet well understood. It has a pronounced effect on the distribution of hydrophobic ions in the membrane interface (Flewelling and Hubbell, 1986), but its contribution to the binding of the rather hydrophilic charged groups of polypeptides is likely to be small. For the binding of a peptide of a molecular weight of 3,000 Daltons to a liquid-crystalline bilayer, ΔG_I can be estimated to contribute roughly 16 kcal/mol (Janin and Chothia, 1978; Jähnig, 1983). The following equations are useful in order to obtain a rough empirical estimate of ΔG_I as a function of the relative mole mass, M_r, of the peptide

$$\Delta G_I = \tfrac{1}{3}\Delta G_t + \tfrac{2}{3}\Delta G_r \tag{6}$$

and at 20°C

$$\Delta G_I = 0.1933 \ln(8.90M_r^{3/2}) + 0.387 \ln(6.50 \times 10^5 M_r^{5/2}) \text{ [kcal/mol]} \tag{7}$$

Equation 6 incorporates the gain in energy due to the loss of one translational degree of freedom and two rotational degrees of freedom. Equations 6 and 7 were derived by Janin and Chothia (1978) for the entropy loss that is associated with the binding of a substrate to an enzyme. Strictly, the statistical–mechanical partition functions for two dimensional translational and one-dimensional rotational diffusion should have been calculated for the derivation of ΔG_I upon substrate binding to a membrane, but our simplistic approach of reducing the dimensionality seems to work quite well for practical purposes and produces similar values as more sophisticated calculations (Jähnig, 1983). With this estimate of ΔG_I, an estimate of ΔG_H can be calculated from Eq. 5. Since the driving force for the hydrophobic effect is largely a change of the entropy of water (and perhaps lipid) in contact with the hydrophobic surface, ΔG_H should be directly proportional to the hydrophobic contact area, A_C (Reynolds et al., 1974; Chothia, 1974)

$$\Delta G_H = -(20\text{–}25 \text{ cal/Å}^2)A_C \tag{8}$$

The experimental value of A_C may then be compared with predictions from the summed individual residue hydrophobic surface areas and from the summed hydrophobicity values of some common hydrophobicity scales (see later under Correlation of Thermodynamic Parameters of Peptide Insertion With Amino Acid Sequence).

Experimental Methods

Monolayers. A very simple method to measure membrane incorporation of peptides is to monitor the area increase in a lipid monolayer at constant surface pressure on a Langmuir film balance (Tamm, 1986). The surface pressure that produces lipid monolayers that most closely resemble lipid bilayers is called the *bilayer equivalence* pressure and is about 32 mN/m (Portlock et al., 1992). Since peptide incorporation into monolayers is strongly dependent on the chosen surface pressure, incorporation isotherms should be measured at the equivalence pressure, if the conclusions are to be extrapolated to lipid bilayers. Some examples of monolayer incorporation isotherms at 32 mN/m are shown in Figure 13.1. The incorporation of the amphiphilic signal peptide of the mannitol permease of the phosphoenol pyruvate-dependent sugar phosphotransferase system of *Escherichia coli* (mtl-23) and of some single site mutants of this peptide into monolayers of the zwitterionic phospholipid phosphatidylcholine has been measured in these experiments (Portlock et al., 1992). The solid lines are the best fits to Eq. 1, by assuming a peptide area in the monolayer of 420 Å^2 and a lipid area of 70 Å^2. In this case, the area per peptide in the monolayer could be estimated fairly accurately because the peptide was known to be about 80% α-

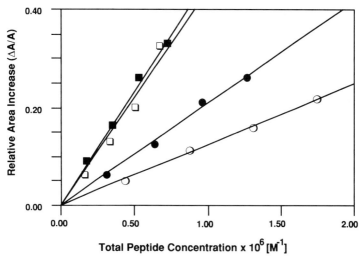

Fig. 13.1. Incorporation of wild-type and mutant signal peptides of the mannitol PTS permease of *E. coli* (mtl-23) into preformed monolayers of POPC. ■, Wild type; □, D4K; ●, S3P; ○, D4P. The relative area increases of the monolayers are plotted as a function of the total peptide concentration at a constant surface pressure of 32 mN/m. The *solid lines* represent the best fits to the partition equation (Eq. 1) and yield partition constants of 8.0×10^4 M^{-1} (■), 7.6×10^4 M^{-1} (□), 3.4×10^4 M^{-1} (●), and 2.1×10^4 M^{-1} (○). (From Portlock et al., 1992.)

helical in lipid model membranes (Portlock et al., 1992) with a preferential orientation of the α-helix long axis parallel to the plane of the membrane (Tamm and Tatulian, 1993). In other cases, peptide areas in the monolayer were measured independently by using a radioactive peptide and correlating the area increase with the radioactivity recovered from the surface of the Langmuir trough (Tamm, 1986).

Fluorescence. Binding isotherms are also conveniently measured with fluorescent peptides when they change their fluorescence properties upon interaction with lipid membranes. Intrinsic tryptophan fluorescence (Tamm et al., 1989; Portlock et al., 1992) or extrinsic fluorescence originating from a covalently attached label (Frey and Tamm, 1990) may be used. Since charge interactions often furnish important contributions to the peptide–lipid interactions, sulfhydro-reactive labels for cysteines rather than aminoreactive labels for lysines should be used. In these experiments, small unilamellar vesicles are titrated to a constant amount of fluorescent peptide, i.e., a reverse titration relative to the monolayer titration experiments. An example is given in Figure 13.2, which shows a strong effect of negatively charged lipids (phosphatidylglycerol) to bind the highly positively charged signal peptide of yeast cytochrome-*c* oxidase subunit IV (Frey and Tamm, 1990). The solid lines are best fits to the Gouy-Chapman partition model and yield a single partition constant, K_P = $(3.9 \pm 0.8) \times 10^3$ M^{-1} for all lipid compositions. The reverse titration with lipid vesicles can sometimes be a disadvantage, because much important information on the isotherm at high peptide-to-lipid ratios is contained in only the first few data points. A new method that uses single planar bilayers (SPBs) supported on solid sub-

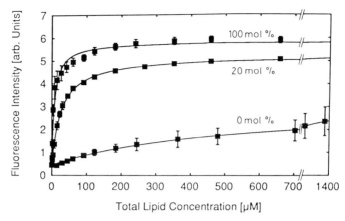

Fig. 13.2. Incorporation of the fluorescent-labeled mitochondrial signal peptide of yeast cyto-chrome-*c* oxidase subunit IV (coxIV-25) into charged and uncharged small unilamellar phos-pholipid vesicles. The nominal charge of this peptide is $+6$. Binding isotherms with vesicles of 0, 20, and 100 mol% negatively charged POPG in POPC are shown. The *solid lines* represent the best fits to the Gouy-Chapman partition equation (Eq. 3) and yield a partition constant of $(3.9 \pm 0.8) \times 10^3 \text{ M}^{-1}$ and an effective charge $z_p = 1.8 \pm 0.1$ for all three curves. (From Frey and Tamm, 1990.)

strates and total internal reflection fluorescence microscopy (TIRFM) may circumvent some of these problems (Kalb et al., 1990).

High-Sensitivity Titration Calorimetry. A third method for studying peptide–lipid binding is high-sensitivity titration calorimetry. The peptide is titrated to unilamellar vesicles, and the evolution (or absorption) of heat is measured. The total heat released (absorbed), Q, is equal to the enthalpy of binding, ΔH, multiplied by the number of moles of peptide bound (V = volume of the measuring cell)

$$Q = \Delta H \times V \times C_L^o \times X_p^b \qquad (9)$$

Combining Eq. 9 with Eq. 1 yields

$$Q = \Delta H V C_p^o \frac{K_P C_L^o}{1 + K_P C_L^o} \qquad (10)$$

where C_p^o is the total peptide concentration. ΔH and K_P can thus be obtained from fits of the experimental data to Eq. 10. This method has the further advantage that binding enthalpies *and* entropies can be obtained by recalling Eq. 4 and by using the fundamental thermodynamic relation

$$\Delta G = \Delta H + T \Delta S \qquad (11)$$

Partition Constants and Free Energies of Peptide Insertion

In this section, partition constants of various peptide sequences with model membranes and derived thermodynamic parameters are compared. Only studies in which the binding curves are analyzed with a partition equilibrium and, in the case of charged species, with the Gouy-Chapman theory are included here, because analyses with saturable binding sites or without explicitly accounting for charge effects are not directly comparable. Table 13.1 lists several peptide sequences with their experimental partition constants for partitioning into liquid-crystalline lipid membranes, Gibbs free energies of peptide insertion, estimated hydrophobic and immobilization contributions to ΔG_{ins}, and the derived hydrophobic contact areas. The partition constants of the peptides with 20 or more residues are in the range between 10^3 and 10^5 M^{-1}, yielding free energies of insertion between -6.5 and -9 kcal/mol. In general, the longer and more hydrophobic sequences exhibit larger partition constants than the smaller and more hydrophilic ones. However, as will be pointed out in the following sections, this simple rule is not strictly followed, and other factors such as peptide structure and depth of membrane penetration have to be considered as well. Using Eqs. 5, 7, and 8, hydrophobic binding free energies (ΔG_H) between -17 and -25 kcal/mol and hydrophobic contact areas (A_C) between 800 and 1,100 Å^2 were calculated from the experimental partition constants of the peptides of Table 13.1. These values are also included in Table 13.1.

Correlation of Thermodynamic Parameters of Peptide Insertion with Amino Acid Sequence

It is tempting to try to correlate the experimental thermodynamic data in Table 13.1 with parameters that are calculated directly from their sequences. Obviously, if such correlations are found to hold true for many different sequences, the reverse procedure, i.e., calculating thermodynamic parameters from the sequence, may be used to help make predictions on the insertion of protein sequences into membranes. Many different hydrophobicity scales have been proposed in the past to predict transmembrane α-helices. Some of these scales are based on thermodynamic data for the transfer of individual amino acyl side chains from water into an organic phase or into vacuum. Others are strictly correlated with the accessible surface areas of the different amino acyl side chains or are based on the statistical frequencies of particular residues buried in a hydrophobic pocket of proteins or exposed on their surface to the aqueous solvent, respectively. Values that are calculated based on two different representative scales are summarized in Table 13.2 for the same 9 peptides that are compared in Table 13.1. The second column of Table 13.2 lists the sums of the accessible surface areas of the apolar residues in the sequences. If the hydrophobic residues of these peptides were inserted into the membrane entirely and in an extended conformation, one might expect from Eq. 9 that the summed accessible hydrophobic surface areas of Table 13.2 correlate with the experimental hydrophobic binding energies and hydrophobic contact areas of Table 13.1. However, as can be seen from Figure 13.3A, this correlation is not particularly good ($r = 0.943$). Also, the calculated sums of accessible hydrophobic surface areas exceed the hydrophobic contact areas determined from the partition data by a factor of 2.1–2.5 (average 2.26). Substance P, an 11 residue peptide, has a calculated hydrophobic surface area 1.6 times larger than the measured contact area. A very similar effect has been previously noticed for the partitioning of small (three residue) model peptides at the membrane–water interface, and in this case the corresponding ratio was 1.8 (Jacobs and White, 1989). Therefore, the proportionality constant in Eq. 8 is likely to be overestimated for pep-

Table 13.1. Buffer–Membrane Partition Constants and Derived Thermodynamic Parameters of Various Amphiphilic Peptides

Peptide	Sequence[a]	M_r	Lipid	K_P, M^{-1}	ΔG_{ins}, kcal/mol[b]	ΔG_H, kcal/mol[c]	ΔG_I, kcal/mol[d]	A_G, Å²[e]	Ref[f]
Melittin	GIGAVLKVLTTGLPALISWIKRKPQQ	2,847	DOPC, POPC/POPG	$(4.5 \pm 0.6) \times 10^4$	−8.7	−24.3	15.6	1,105	1–4
CoxIV-25	MLSLRQSIRFFKPATRTLCSSRYLL	2,989	POPC/POPG	$(3.9 \pm 0.8) \times 10^3$	−7.1	−22.8	15.7	1,036	5
Mtl-23 (wt)	MSSDIKIKVQSFGRFLSNMVMPC	2,619	POPC	8.0×10^4	−8.9	−24.4	15.5	1,109	6
(S3P)	--P---------------------	2,629	POPC	3.5×10^4	−8.4	−23.9	15.5	1,086	6
(D4P)	---P--------------------	2,601	POPC	2.1×10^4	−8.1	−23.6	15.5	1,073	6
(D4K)	---K--------------------	2,632	POPC	7.6×10^4	−8.9	−24.4	15.5	1,109	6
Gut-22	MIETITHGAEWFIGLFQKGGEC	2,468	POPC	$(4.2 \pm 0.2) \times 10^4$	−8.5	−23.9	15.5	1,086	6
Alamethicin	Ac-αPαAααAQαVαGLαPVααQQ-phol	1,949	DOPC, eggPC	1.3×10^3	−6.5	−21.6	15.1	982	7–9
Substance P	RPKPQQFFGLM	1,349	POPC/POPG	~1	−2.3	−17.0	14.7	773	10

[a]One letter codes for amino acyl residues: α, α-aminoisobutyric acid; Ac, acetyl; phol, phenylalaninol.
[b]From Eq. 4.
[c]From Eq. 5.
[d]From Eq. 7.
[e]From Eq. 7; the constant of proportionality was taken to be 22 cal/Å² (Richards, 1977).
[f]1, Schwarz and Beschiaschvili (1989); 2, Kuchinka and Seelig (1989); 3, Beschiaschvili and Seelig (1990); 4, Stankowski et al. (1991); 5, Frey and Tamm (1990); 6, Portlock et al. (1992); 7, Schwarz et al. (1986); 8, Rizzo et al. (1987); 9, Archer et al. (1991); 10, Seelig and Macdonald (1989).

Table 13.2. Summed Accessible Surface Areas, Summed Hydrophobicities, and Helical Hydrophobic Moments of Various Amphiphilic Peptides

Peptide	Sum of Accessible Surface Areas of Hydrophobic Residues, $Å^2$[a]	Goldman-Engelman-Steitz Scale, kcal/mol[b]	Normalized Eisenberg Consensus Scale (Neg.)[c]	Number of Residues in α-Helical Conformation (n)[d]	Maximum Hydrophobic Moment of Segment of n Residues[e]
Melittin	2,558	−33.6	−14.2	20[f]	0.46 (3)
CoxIV-25	2,443	−30.6	−11.0	12[g]	0.85 (5)
Mtl-23 (wt)	2,321	−34.6	−11.2	14[h]	0.54 (9)
(S3P)	2,468	−34.4	−11.3	14[h]	0.54 (9)
(D4P)	2,468	−34.4	−11.3	14[h]	0.54 (9)
(D4K)	2,321	−34.6	−11.2	14[h]	0.54 (9)
Gut-22	2,268	−32.4	−11.9	14[i]	0.46 (5)
Alamethicin	2,493[j]	−29.1[j]	−13.2[j]	14[f]	0.33 (5)
Substance P	1,224	−14.2	−4.80	8[k]	0.35 (4)

[a] Rose et al. (1985); only hydrophobic residues (positive on normalized Eisenberg consensus scale) are summed.
[b] Engelman et al. (1986); only hydrophobic residues (positive on normalized Eisenberg consensus scale) are summed.
[c] Eisenberg et al. (1984); only hydrophobic residues (positive on normalized Eisenberg consensus scale) are summed.
[d] Estimates from circular dichroism experiments in bilayers.
[e] Eisenberg et al. (1984); the numbers in parentheses are the first residue of the n-residue segment on each peptide.
[f] Vogel (1987).
[g] Tamm and Bartoldus (1990).
[h] Portlock et al. (1992).
[i] Tamm et al. (1989).
[j] For α-aminoisobutyric acid, interpolated values between alanine and valine were used.
[k] Rolka et al. (1986) and Woolley and Deber (1987).

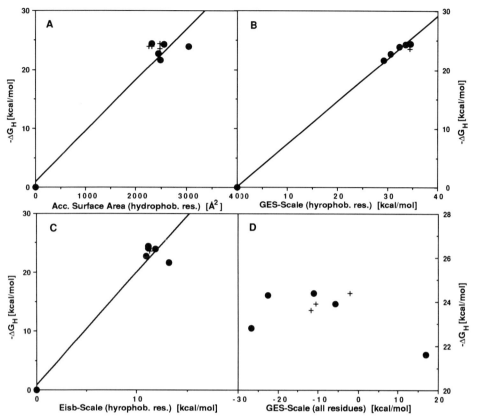

Fig. 13.3. Comparison of correlations of the experimental hydrophobic contributions to the free energies of peptide insertion into lipid model membranes with predictions from different hydrophobicity scales. The following peptides are included in these correlations: melittin, coxIV-25, mtl-23, gut-22, and alamethicin (●). The coordinates of the single site mutants of mtl-23 (S3P, D4P, and D4K) are also shown in the plots (+), but excluded from the correlations. The scales that are shown on the abscissas are A: the summed accessible surface areas of the apolar residues (Rose et al., 1985); B: the summed Goldman-Engelman-Steitz hydrophobicities of the apolar residues (Engelman et al., 1986); C: the summed normalized Eisenberg hydrophobicities of the apolar residues (Eisenberg et al., 1984); and D: the summed Goldman-Engelman-Steitz hydrophobicities of all residues. The slopes and correlation coefficients (including an arbitrary data point at 0,0) are, respectively, 8.7×10^{-3} and 0.943 (A), 0.73 and 0.997 (B), 1.92 and 0.934 (C).

tides that partition into a region of intermediate dielectric constant (i.e., near the membrane surface). A value of $20-25 \text{ cal}/\text{Å}^2$ is only adequate for residues that are transferred into the low dielectric center of the lipid bilayer where the full hydrophobic free energy can be satisfied, whereas $10-12 \text{ cal}/\text{Å}^2$ seems to be a better value for residues near the membrane–water interface.

Another factor contributing to the discrepancy between summed hydrophobicities (or surface areas) of individual residues and that of the whole polypeptide is the secondary structure of the peptide in the membrane. In the absence of aggregation, an induction of secondary structure is expected to cause a major contribution to an alteration of the hydrophobic contact area, because the polypeptide is much more compact in its folded than its unfolded state. (Evidence against extensive aggregation in the absence of an electric field across the membrane exists for melittin [Stankowski et al., 1991], alamethicin [Archer et al., 1991], and a mitochondrial signal peptide that is similar to coxIV-25 [Skerjanc et al., 1987].) Significantly, all peptides listed in Tables 13.1 and 13.2 are predominantly α-helical in membranes (column 5 of Table 13.2).

A popular scale for predicting transmembrane α-helices is the one of Goldman, Engelman, and Steitz (GES) (Engelman et al., 1986). In contrast to most other hydrophobicity scales, it is based on, among other factors, calculated residue surface areas *in the context of an α-helix*. Indeed, when the GES values of the hydrophobic residues are summed (Table 13.2, column 3) and compared with the experimental hydrophobic binding energies, a very good correlation ($r = 0.997$) between experiment and calculation can be found (Fig. 13.3B). However, the best proportionality factor between the summed GES and the experimental value is less than 1, leading to the following empirical relation for the eight listed peptides (substance P is excluded from this correlation because it is probably too short to express a stable secondary structure in the membrane):

$$\Delta G_H \approx 0.73 \ \Sigma \Delta G_{GES,hphob.res.} \tag{12}$$

Most other hydrophobicity scales do not take into account the induction of secondary structure, and, when we have tried, correlations with the experimental hydrophobic binding energies were worse than the correlation in Eq. 12. As an example, the correlation with the normalized Eisenberg consensus scale (Table 13.2, column 4) is shown in Figure 13.3C ($r = 0.934$). This scale emulates different features of many other scales in a single scale. When all, instead of only the hydrophobic, residues are summed on the GES scale, these values are scattered on a plot against ΔG_H (Fig. 13.3D), indicating (not surprisingly) that the hydrophilic residues are not in contact with the hydrophobic interior of the membrane, but rather face an aqueous environment.

A surface location of these peptides can also be predicted from their large hydrophobic moments calculated according to Eisenberg et al. (1984). Column 6 of Table 13.2 lists the maximal hydrophobic moments when a window of n residues is moved through the whole sequence. n is the number of residues in an α-helical conformation as estimated from circular dichroism experiments, and the numbers in parentheses in column 6 are the first residues of the n-residue segment with the maximal hydrophobic moment of each peptide.

Lipid-Dependent Structural Polymorphism of Polypeptides in Membranes

Experimental Methods

Circular Dichroism Spectroscopy. Far ultraviolet circular dichroism (CD) spectroscopy has been the most commonly used tool to study the secondary structure of peptides in membranes. Comprehensive reviews on various practical and theoretical aspects of CD spectroscopy and secondary structure analyses can be found in the literature (Yang et al., 1986; Johnson, 1988, 1990; see also the chapter by Williams in this volume). A common problem of extracting relative proportions of secondary structure from CD spectra is the spectral overlap of the far ultraviolet ellipticities of the different types of secondary structure and, as a consequence, the difficulty in defining the basic component spectra that are required for spectral decomposition. Reference spectra for individual secondary structures have been derived both from model polypeptides (Greenfield and Fasman, 1969; Brahms and Brahms, 1980) and proteins (Saxena and Wetlaufer, 1971; Grosse et al., 1974; Chen et al., 1974; Chang et al., 1978; Siegel et al., 1980, Bollotina et al., 1980). Alternatively, linear combinations of orthogonal spectra derived from proteins whose x-ray structures are known have been used as reference spectra (Provencher and Glöckner, 1981; Hennessey and Johnson, 1981; Manavalan and Johnson, 1987; Perczel et al., 1991). Two additional problems arise when CD spectra of *membrane* proteins are to be interpreted in terms of relative amounts of common secondary structures. First, reliable reference data are difficult to obtain, because x-ray structures of membrane proteins are still very scarce and because different folding patterns with other and/or additional basic CD spectral components may exist for membrane proteins and membrane-interactive polypeptides. Second, an experimental limitation is imposed by the light scattering of membrane vesicles. Even if well-sonicated, small unilamellar vesicles are used (Mao and Wallace, 1984), substantial distortions of the CD spectra can occur below 200 nm. Only the spectral component from α-helices can be reliably quantified from data above 200 nm. Most methods agree that a molar ellipicity at 222 nm of $\theta_{222} = -30{,}000$ deg $\cdot$ cm^2/dmol ($\Delta\epsilon = -9.1$ cm^{-1}M^{-1}) corresponds to roughly 100% α-helix (Chen et al., 1974). CD data to 190 nm or, preferably, to 184 nm (Johnson, 1990) are needed to extract the relative proportions of further spectral components.

Infrared Spectroscopy. With the advent of Fourier-transform infrared spectrometers, infrared spectroscopy of proteins in water (or D$_2$O) has become an additional valuable tool for secondary structure analysis of soluble and membrane-bound proteins (see Susi and Byler, 1986; Surewicz and Mantsch, 1988; Arrondo et al., 1993, for reviews). The amide I band at around 1,630–1,680 cm^{-1} is often used to determine relative proportions of secondary structure. Unfortunately, the spectral components arising from different secondary structures are not well resolved. The major exception is the β-strand conformation, which exhibits two characteristic vibrations at around 1,630 cm^{-1} and 1,670–1,690 cm^{-1}. Therefore, infrared spectroscopy can often yield data that is complementary to the CD data.

NMR Spectroscopy. NMR spectroscopy has been used thus far in only a few cases to determine the structure of polypeptides in membranes. High-resolution two-dimensional NMR techniques can only be applied to polypeptides in detergent micelles. The structure of a polypeptide obtained in detergent micelles cannot be extrapolated a priori to its structure in lipid bilayers. Because of their slow rates of rotational diffusion, membrane vesicles are not adequate for high-resolution NMR studies. However, solid-state NMR techniques have been applied successfully to determine structural features of a few polypeptides in lipid bilayers (Opella and Stewart, 1989; Nicholson and Cross, 1989; Shon et al., 1991).

Secondary Structures of Natural and Synthetic Peptides in Membranes

Table 13.3 lists natural and synthetic peptides whose secondary structures have been determined when bound to lipid membranes or detergent micelles. It is not the purpose of Table 13.3 to list comprehensively all peptide conformations that have been observed in lipid bilayers or membrane-mimetic environments. The list is rather to provide a broad overview of common conformations in membranes of amphiphilic and hydrophobic peptides, which are 15–30 residues long and originate from many different sources and serve many different biological functions. From an inspection of Table 13.3, it is obvious that α-helices are the preferred structural motifs of many of these peptides. Strong α-helix formers are melittin, alamethicin, and several hydrophobic and amphiphilic signal peptides. Most of these peptides in fact assume unordered structures in aqueous buffer, and the α-helices are only induced upon binding and insertion into lipid membranes. A significant contribution to the driving force of this conformational change is most likely a change in hydrogen bonding from peptide backbone–water hydrogen bonds in the unordered conformation to intramolecular peptide backbone hydrogen bonding in the α-helical structure. The α-helix is also the most commonly found structural motif in large integral membrane proteins (Deisenhofer et al., 1985; Allen et al., 1987; Henderson et al., 1990; Kühlbrandt and Wang, 1991).

Some peptides assume β-structures when bound to lipid membranes. These include some synthetic model peptides that have been designed to associate with membranes as β-strands, but also some few signal peptides under special conditions. For instance, the lamB-25 peptide has been found to be α-helical in supported monolayers that were transferred onto a solid substrate at low surface pressure, but assumed a β-structure when transferred at high surface pressure (Cornell et al., 1989). Similarly, phoE-21 was largely α-helical as determined by infrared spectroscopy in transferred monolayers of the zwitterionic lipid DOPC, but rather β-strand when associated with negatively charged DOPG (Demel et al., 1990). Interestingly, opposite conclusions were reached in a later CD study: phoE-21 was α-helical in negatively charged bilayers of DOPG or DOPS and β-strand in bilayers of DOPC (Keller et al., 1992). There is also at least one family of large integral membrane proteins, namely, the porins of the outer membranes of gram-negative bacteria, that contain predominantly β-structure (Weiss et al., 1991; Jap et al., 1991; Cowan et al., 1992).

Conformational flexibility, which depended on the charge on the phospholipid headgroup, was also found when the mitochondrial signal peptide coxIV-25 was bound to different phospholipid bilayers (Tamm and Bartoldus, 1990). In this case, the peptide was largely α-helical in negatively charged bilayers containing POPG (Fig. 13.4A) or cardiolipin, but assumed an unidentified (non-α, non-β, nonrandom) secondary structure in association with bilayers of POPC (Fig. 13.4B). These examples of the lamB, phoE, and coxIV signal peptides demonstrate that peptide conformations can critically depend on their lipid environment, such as headgroup charges, lipid packing density, and surface curvature, and that, perhaps, conformational flexibility is even a prerequisite for proper signal sequence function. The latter view is supported by the fact that both α-helix– and β-strand–preferring signal peptides can target and translocate proteins across mitochondrial membranes (Roise et al., 1988).

Table 13.3. Secondary Structures of Peptides in Lipid Bilayers and Detergent Micelles

Peptide	Sequence[a]	Lipid/Detergent[b]	Predominant Secondary Structure[c]	Ref.[d]
Peptide Toxins and Hormones				
Melittin	GIGAVLKVLTTGLPALISWIKRKPQQ	DTPC (Bil)	α (76)	1,2
		C$_{12}$-PC (Mic)	α	3
Alamethicin	Ac-αPαAαAQαVαGLαPVααEQ-phol	DTPC (Bil)	α (71)	2
Magainin 2	GIGKFLHSAKKFGKAFVGEIMNS	DPPG, DOPG, PS (Bil)	α (70–80)	4
Gramicidin A	VGALAVVWLWLWLW	DMPC, other PCs (Bil)	$\beta^{6.3}$-helix	5–7
Glucagon	HSQGTFTSDYSKYLDSRRAQDFVQWLMNT	DMPC (Bil)	α (35)	8–10
		C$_{12}$-PC (Mic)	α (40–50)	
"Hydrophobic" Signal Peptides				
LamB-25 (wt)	MMITLRKLPLAVAVAAGVMSAQAMA	POPE/POPG (Bil or low π monol)	α (60)	11, 12
		POPE/POPG (high π monol)	β	12
		SDS (Mic)	α (70)	11
(G17R)	----------R--------	SDS (Mic)	α (70)	11
(A13D)	--------D---------	SDS (Mic)	α (60)	11
LamB-21(Δ78)	MMITLRKLPVAAGVMSAQAMA	SDS (Mic)	α (35)	11
(Δ78r1)	-----------C-------	SDS (Mic)	α (40)	11
(Δ78r2)	--------L---------	SDS (Mic)	α (75)	11
LamB-16(wt)	-----RKLPLAVAVAAGVMSA----	SDS (Mic)	α (25)	13
PhoE-21	MKKSTLALVVMGIVASASVQA	SDS (Mic)	α (75)	14
		DOPC (Monol)	α	15
		DOPG (Monol)	β	15
		DOPC (Bil)	β (54)	27
		DOPG (Bil)	α (70)	27
		DOPS (Bil)	α (57)	27
		CL (Bil)	β (58)	27
(K2D/K3D)	-DD------------------	DOPG (Bil)	β (53)	27
PhoE-12	MKKSTLALVVMG	SDS (Mic)	α (41)	14
OmpA-25	MKKTAIAIAVALAGFATVAQAAPKD	POPE/POPG (Bil)	α (60)	28
(L6L8)	----L-L----------	POPE/POPG (Bil)	α (58)	28
(18N)	------N----------	POPE/POPG (Bil)	α (40)	28

(Δ6–9)	MKKTAVALAGFATVAQAAPKD	POPE/POPG (Bil)	α (17)	28
(Δ8)	MKKTAIAAVALAGFATVAQAAPKD	POPE/POPG (Bil)	α (60)	28
(Δ9)	MKKTAIAIVALAGFATVAQAAPKD	POPE/POPG (Bil)	α (55)	28

"Amphiphilic" Signal Peptides

CoxIV-25	MLSLRQSIRFFKPATRTLCSSRYLL	POPG (Bil)	α (49)	16
		POPC (Bil)	o	16
		lysoPC (Mic)	α (42)	16, 17
		C$_{12}$-PC (Mic)	α	18
Otc-27	MLSNLRILLNKAALRKAHTSMVRNFRY	DMPG (Bil)	β (63)	19
		DMPC (Bil)	β (58)	19
Adh-22	MLRAALSTARKGPRLSRLLSYA	SDS (Mic)	α (45)	20
		C$_{12}$-PC (Mic)	α (25)	21
F1β-20	MVLPRLYTATSRAAFKAAKQ	SDS (Mic)	α (45)	29
Gut-22	MIETITHGAEWFIGLFQKGGEC	POPC (Bil)	α (65)	22
Mtl-23	MSSDIKIKVQSFGRFLSNMVMPC	POPG (Bil)	α (63)	23
(S3P)	-----P-------------------	POPG (Bil)	α (76)	23
(D4P)	-------P----------------	POPG (Bil)	α (82)	23
(D4K)	-------K----------------	POPG (Bil)	α (77)	23

Some Model Peptides

Pept 4$_4$	Ac-LARLLARLLARLLARL	DPPC (Bil)	α (60)	24
Pept 1$_3$	Ac-SVKVSVKVSVKV	DPPC/DPPG (Bil)	β (80)	25
Syn A$_2$	MLSRLSLRLLSRLSLRLLSRYLL	SDS (Mic)	β (100)	17
SynC	MLSSLLRLRSLLRLRLSRYLL	SDS (Mic)	α (45)	17
K$_2$GL$_{24}$K$_2$A	KKGLLLLLLLLLLLLLLLLLLLLLLLLKKA	DPPC, eggPC (Bil)	α	26
		Ammonyx L$_o$ (Mic)	α (90)	26

[a] One letter code: α, α-aminoisobutyric acid; Ac, acetyl; phol, phenylalaninol.

[b] Mic, micelles; Bil, bilayer; Monol, monolayer.

[c] α, α-helix; β, β-strand; u, unordered; o, other (unidentified and turns), estimated percentages are in parentheses, where known.

[d] 1, Vogel and Jähnig (1986); 2, Vogel (1987); 3, Brown et al. (1982); 4, Matsuzaki et al. (1991); 5, Killian et al. (1988); 6, Nicholson and Cross (1989); 7, Smith et al. (1989), 8, Epand et al. (1977); 9, Bösch et al. (1980); 10, Braun et al. (1983); 11, McKnight et al. (1989); 12, Cornell et al. (1989); 13, Briggs and Gierasch (1984); 14, Batenburg et al. (1988); 15, Demel et al. (1990); 16, Tamm and Bartoldus (1990); 17, Roise et al. (1988); 18, Endo et al. (1989); 19, Epand et al. (1986); 20, Pak and Weiner, (1990); 21, Karslake et al. (1990); 22, Tamm et al. (1989); 23, Portlock et al. (1992); 24, Lee et al. (1986); 25, Ono et al. (1990); 26, Davis et al. (1983); 27, Keller et al. (1992); 28, Hoyt and Gierasch (1991); 29, Hoyt and Gierasch (1991).

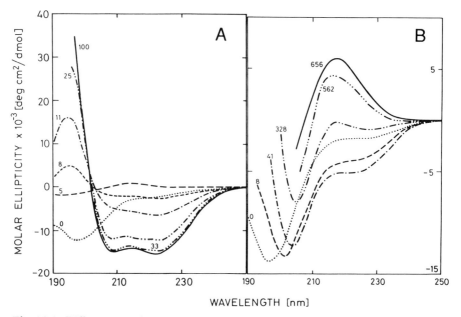

Fig. 13.4. Different secondary structures are induced in the mitochondrial signal peptide of yeast cytochrome-*c* oxidase subunit IV (coxIV-25) by different lipid environments. Circular dichroism spectra of the peptide in bilayers of POPG (*A*) and POPC (*B*) are shown at various lipid–peptide molar ratios as indicated. (From Tamm and Bartoldus, 1990.)

A special case is the channel-forming antibiotic gramicidin A. This peptide forms a $\beta^{6.3}$-helix in membranes with its residue side chains turned toward the inside of the helix. In the active channel form, two such helices are stacked on top of each other head to head, with both N termini oriented to the center plane of the membrane and the C termini exposed to the aqueous phases on either side of the bilayer (Urry, 1971; Smith et al., 1989; Nicholson and Cross, 1989).

Orientation of Polypeptide Segments of Defined Secondary Structure in Lipid Bilayers

Experimental Methods

Polarized Attenuated Total Reflection Infrared Spectroscopy. Polarized attenuated total reflection infrared spectroscopy is probably the most frequently used technique to determine peptide orientation in membranes. Several comprehensive reviews on Attenuated Total Reflection Infrared (ATR-IR) spectroscopy on oriented membranes are available (Fringeli and Günthardt, 1981; Goormaghtigh and Ruys-schaert, 1990; Fringeli, 1992). In this technique, the infrared beam is totally internally reflected many times in a multiple internal reflection element, i.e., usually a 50 × 20 × 1 mm³ germanium crystal. The membrane that is attached to the surface of this plate is illuminated by the evanescent wave. This experimental configuration has two advantages: (*1*) the membranes are oriented in a defined geometry relative to the electromagnetic radiation and (*2*) the membrane–water and therefore the signal–noise ratios are high in the thin volume that is illuminated by the evanescent wave.

Different techniques have been used to prepare lipid membranes with and without peptides on the surface of the germanium crystals. The lipids can be deposited on the surface from organic solvents. Multibilayer structures are formed spontaneously by this procedure. These multibilayers may be"reworked" with solvents to improve their coplanar structure, i.e., to minimize their "mosaic spread" (Fringeli and Günthardt, 1981). Alternatively, lipid monolayers can be deposited on the germanium crystals by the Langmuir-Blodgett technique. In some cases, peptides were incorporated into a monolayer before deposition, and ATR-IR spectroscopy was then performed on a dry single monolayer on germanium (e.g., by Cornell et al., 1989). However, it is also possible to use fully hydrated single supported phospholipid bilayers for ATR-IR spectroscopy of peptides in membranes. These are prepared either by two consecutive Langmuir-Blodgett steps (Tamm and McConnell, 1985) or by a single Langmuir-Blodgett deposition, followed by the fusion of small unilamellar vesicles to the supported monolayer (Kalb et al., 1992). The orientation of peptides in membranes can depend on the preparation technique and/or whether fully hydrated, partially hydrated, or dry membranes are used (see below).

Another important point is the mathematical procedure that is used to analyze the experimental data. Two factors should not be neglected. First, due to the special polarization properties of the evanescent field, perpendicular and parallel incident light intensities are generally not equal, which leads to dichroic ratios (R^{iso}) that differ from 1.0 for isotropically distributed absorption dipole moments. The magnitude of R^{iso} depends on the refractive indices of all materials near the solid–liquid interface. Second, like in many other spectroscopic techniques on liquid-crystalline materials, the spectroscopic signal, the dichroic ratio, depends on the order parameter

$$S = 3 < \cos^2\theta - 1 > /2 \tag{13}$$

and not directly on the angle θ between the molecular director and the membrane normal. The angle brackets in Eq. 13 denote the average of all possible angles at any time of the measurement, and because of this averaging it is not possible to extract a precisely defined orientation from such measurements. Both average orientation and the extent of fluctuation around this average contribute to the order parameter. However, the extreme values of $S = -0.5$ and $S = 1.0$ can be safely assigned to rigid orientations at $\theta = 90°$ and $\theta = 0°$, respectively.

Circular Dichroism Spectroscopy. CD spectroscopy on oriented samples has also been used to determine order parameters of peptides in membranes (Vogel, 1987; Huang and Wu, 1991). For sensitivity reasons, dry or partially hydrated multibilayers on quartz slides are used in these experiments.

NMR Spectroscopy. Two-dimensional high-resolution NMR spectroscopy has been used to solve the complete three-dimensional structure and relative orientation of glucagon on the surface of dodecylphosphocholine (Braun et al., 1983). Solid-state NMR techniques are now being used to determine the orientation and location of some peptides in oriented membrane samples (Shon et al., 1991; Bechinger et al., 1992). In this technique, isotopically labeled peptides are used for the determination of the order parameters of individual residues in peptides that are bound to stacks of coplanar oriented membranes. Unless many different residues are labeled in the peptide, other structural techniques such as CD spectroscopy (or high-resolution two-dimensional NMR spectroscopy, if the structures in micelles and bilayers are the same) are needed to extrapolate from the single residue orientation to the orientation of the whole peptide.

Orientational Distributions of Melittin and Some Other Peptides in Lipid Model Membranes

The most extensively studied peptide with respect to its orientation in membranes is the bee venom peptide melittin. Its crystal structure is known (Terwilliger et al., 1982), and its highly α-helical structure in its membrane-bound form is well established (Dawson et al., 1978; Knöppel et al., 1979; Brown et al., 1982; Vogel and Jähnig, 1986; Vogel, 1987). However, the orientation of the α-helix relative to the plane of the bilayer has been controversial. Accessibility measurements of spin-labeled melittin with chromium oxalate (Altenbach and Hubbell, 1988; Altenbach et al., 1989) and ^{13}C-NMR measurements in the presence of aqueous shift reagents (Stanislawski and Rüterjans, 1987) indicated a location of melittin on the membrane surface with only the hydrophobic residues buried in the lipid bilayer. In contrast, polarized infrared (Vogel et al., 1983; Brauner et al., 1987) and CD (Vogel, 1987) experiments on oriented bilayers yielded an α-helix orientation of melittin that was preferentially parallel to the bilayer normal. The magnetic resonance experiments were carried out with lipid vesicles in solution, and the infrared and CD experiments were performed with dry or partially hydrated multibilayers. A recent polarized ATR-IR study on the orientation of melittin in different membrane preparations resolved this discrepancy (Frey and Tamm, 1991). A positive order parameter, indicating a preferential orientation of the α-helix parallel to the fatty acyl chains, was found in dry multibilayers and a negative order parameter, indicating a preferential orientation of the α-helix parallel to the membrane surface, was found in fully hydrated single supported phospholipid bilayers.

Measurements on the orientation of the α-helix were also carried out with alamethicin. Dry and partially and fully hydrated multibilayers were used in an oriented infrared (Fringeli and Fringeli, 1979) and two oriented CD investigations (Vogel, 1987; Huang and Wu, 1991). A picture similar to the one with melittin seems to emerge from these studies; namely, the alamethicin α-helix is preferentially oriented parallel to the fatty acyl chains in the dry (or low rehydration) state and appears rather surface oriented at very high relative humidities or after the addition of bulk water. The orientation of the hydrophobic signal peptide lamB-25 was studied in transferred dry monolayers of POPE and POPG (Cornell et al., 1989). The orientation of the α-helix in the monolayers that were transferred at low surface pressure was predominantly parallel to the fatty acyl chains. The β-structure that was produced at high surface pressure was more likely aligned along the membrane surface. A similar result was found with the phoE-21 signal peptide (Demel et al., 1990). The α-helix in DOPC was preferentially perpendicular, and the β-strand in DOPG was preferentially parallel to the plane of the membrane. A polarized ATR-IR study on coxIV-25 found the α-helical segment preferentially aligned perpendicular to the plane of the membrane in dried bilayers of DOPC/cardiolipin (4:1) and parallel to the plane of the membrane in DOPC bilayers (Goormaghtigh et al., 1989). The orientation in DOPC may be questioned, because this peptide shows no

α-helix in bilayers of the very similar lipid POPC as determined from CD spectra (Tamm and Bartoldus, 1990).

A recent study on the orientation of the amphiphilic α-helix-forming mannitol and glucitol phosphoenol pyruvate-dependent phosphotransferase system (PTS) per-/ mease signal peptides and several single site mutants of the mannitol permease signal peptide revealed an orientation of the functional (wild-type) peptides parallel to the plane of the membrane and a more disordered orientation of the nonfunctional (mutant) signal peptides (Tamm and Tatulian, 1993).

Lateral and Rotational Diffusion of Polypeptides in Bilayers

Theoretical Background

Hydrodynamic studies should yield, in principle, information about the size, shape, and mode of insertion of polypeptides in membranes. It is well known that the diffusion of large macromolecules in membranes is mainly determined by the friction within the bilayers and that the domains exposed to the adjacent aqueous phases contribute only negligibly to the lateral and rotational diffusion coefficients (Saffmann and Delbrück, 1975; Hughes et al., 1982). The lateral diffusion coefficient, D_L, of large membrane-spanning proteins depends on the natural logarithm of the reciprocal radius, $1/a$, of the diffusing particle, whereas rotational diffusion responds much more sensitively to changes in a, namely, $D_R \sim 1/a^2$ (Saffmann and Delbrück, 1975):

$$D_L = \frac{kT}{4\pi\mu_M h} \ln \left(\frac{\mu_M h}{\mu_W a} - 0.5772 \right) \tag{14}$$

$$D_R = \frac{kT}{4\pi\mu_M a^2 h} \tag{15}$$

where k is the Boltzmann constant, T is the absolute temperature, h is the thickness of the bilayer, μ_M is the microviscosity of the bilayer, and μ_W is the viscosity of water. Equations 14 and 15 have been experimentally tested and have been proven to hold true for many membrane-spanning proteins of different sizes (Peters and Cherry, 1982; Vaz et al., 1984). The lateral self-diffusion of lipids is generally better modeled with free volume (or area) models (Galla et al., 1979; Peters and Beck, 1983; Vaz et al., 1984), which predict a logarithmic dependency of the diffusion coefficient on the lateral lipid packing density with a critical limiting lipid area (Peters and Beck, 1983) and insensitivity to the fatty acyl chain length (Vaz and Hallman, 1983). Rigorous diffusion models for peptides of sizes that are intermediate between lipids and proteins with multiple membrane-spanning sequences have not yet been developed. However, it has been suggested (Tamm, 1991) that an extension to the Saffmann-Delbrück theory with two different boundary fluids (with low and intermediate viscosities) in contact with the top and bottom of the diffusing particle (Evans and Sackmann, 1988) may also be used to describe the diffusion of peptides that are asymmetrically inserted into a lipid bilayer. As is shown in more detail by Tamm (1991), the Saffman-Delbrück Eqs. 14 and 15 can be reinterpreted for this case if the radius, a, of the diffusing particle is smaller than about 60 Å. Instead of being the membrane thickness, h becomes the depth of peptide penetration under these conditions. If a is greater than 60 Å, the explicit Evans-Sackmann equations (Evans and Sackmann, 1988) have to be used to determine the depth of membrane penetration of a cylindrical particle.

Lateral Diffusion of Gramicidins and a Mitochondrial Signal Peptide

Lateral diffusion coefficients of three peptides in lipid bilayers have been measured by fluorescence recovery after photobleaching (FRAP). They include gramicidin S, gramicidin A, and coxIV-25. The lateral diffusion coefficients of the two gramicidins were comparable with those of the lipids in the same membrane preparations, but that of coxIV-25 depended on the phospholipid headgroup charge. Gramicidin S is a cyclic decapeptide with a molecular weight of 1,141 daltons. Its exact mode of binding to phospholipid bilayers is unclear. The lateral diffusion coefficient of NBD-labeled gramacidin S in bilayers of DMPC was $1-2 \times 10^{-8}$ cm^2/s above the chain melting phase transition, T_c, of this lipid and $\leq 10^{-10}$ cm^2/s below T_c (Wu et al., 1978). Gramicidin A, which is the head-to-head dimer of two 15 residue $\beta^{6.3}$-helices (see section titled Secondary Structures of Natural and Synthetic Peptides in Membranes) exhibits a lateral diffusion coefficient of 3×10^{-8} cm^2/s in multibilayers of DMPC (25° C) and 4×10^{-8} cm^2/s in multibilayers of eggPC (25° C) (Tank et al., 1982); below the phase transition of DMPC, D_L was $< 10^{-10}$ cm^2/s. The lateral diffusion of the NBD-labeled mitochondrial signal peptide coxIV-25 depended on the charge of the headgroups of the phospholipids (Frey and Tamm, 1990). When bound to POPC bilayers in its unidentified nonhelical conformation (see section titled Secondary Structures of Natural and Synthetic Peptides in Membranes), the peptide diffused with a 50% larger lateral diffusion coefficient than the lipids themselves (D_L [peptide] $= 8.1 \times 10^{-8}$ cm^2/s; D_L [lipid] $= 5.2 \times 10^{-8}$ cm^2/s). Since 99% of all peptide was bound to the membrane under the conditions of the FRAP experiments, the lateral diffusion coefficient could safely be interpreted by diffusion of the peptide on the membrane surface, with the peptide interacting only with the polar headgroup region of the lipid bilayer. However, when bound to negatively charged bilayers of POPC/POPG (4:1) in its α-helical form, the lateral diffusion coefficient dropped to 2.8×10^{-8} cm^2/s, i.e., a value 1.8 times smaller than that of the lipids themselves, indicating an insertion of the peptide deeper into the hydrophobic part of the bilayer (Fig. 13.5). Since the orientation and state of aggregation of this peptide in the membrane is still uncertain, an application of Eq. 14 to determine molecular dimensions of the peptide in the membrane is premature. The same conclusion, namely, a deeper depth of membrane penetration of coxIV-25 in the presence of acidic lipids, was later reached by measurements of tryptophan quenching with brominated lipids (de Kroon et al., 1991).

Peptide–Lipid and Peptide–Peptide Proximity Measurements by Fluorescence Quenching and Resonance Energy Transfer

Experimental Methods

Tryptophan fluorescence is sensitive to the polarity of the environment of this residue. Generally, the quantum yield increases and the emission maximum shifts to

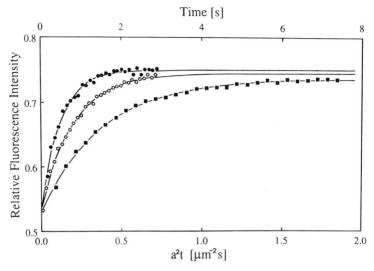

Fig. 13.5. Lateral diffusion of the fluorescent-labeled mitochondrial signal peptide of yeast cytochrome-c oxidase subunit IV (coxIV-25) in bilayers of different lipid composition. Fluorescence recovery (FRAP) curves are shown for the peptide bound to bilayers of POPC (●) and POPC:POPG (4:1) (■) and for the fluorescent lipid analog NBD–eggPE in POPC (O). The lateral diffusion coefficient of the depicted curves as derived from single-exponential fits (pattern photobleaching) are 8.2×10^{-8} cm^2/s (●), 5.0×10^{-8} cm^2/s (O), and 2.7×10^{-8} cm^2/s (■). (From Frey and Tamm, 1990.)

lower wavelengths as the hydrophobicity of the tryptophan environment increases (Lakowicz, 1983). This effect may be used to obtain a very rough idea of how deeply tryptophan residues penetrate into the lipid bilayer. However, caution is advised when spectral changes of tryptophan in larger peptides are interpreted, because local peptide environmental changes, such as adjacent residues or conformational changes, can also cause significant changes upon membrane insertion.

The accessibility of the tryptophans can be probed with water-soluble or membrane-bound quenchers. Useful water-soluble quenchers with little membrane permeability are iodide and acrylamide. Both are collisional quenchers, and their quenching efficiency can be described by the Stern-Volmer relation

$$F_o/F = K_{SV}[Q] + 1 \qquad (16)$$

where F_o is the fluorescence intensity in the absence of quencher, F is the fluorescence intensity at a given quencher concentration, $[Q]$, and K_{SV} is the Stern-Volmer quenching constant. A plot of F_o/F versus $[Q]$ yields a straight line with a slope of K_{SV}. Eq. 16 holds for a single tryptophan species in the system. If there are two environments with an accessible and an inaccessible tryptophan with a total fluorescence intensity F_o and an accessible fluorescence intensity $F_{o,a}$, respectively, Eq. 16 takes the form

$$\frac{F_o}{F_o - F} = \frac{1}{f_a K_{SV}[Q]} + \frac{1}{f_a} \qquad (17)$$

where $f_a = F_{o,a}/F_o$ is the fraction of the initial fluorescence that is accessible to the quencher. Again, caution is advised for the interpretation of the results when charged groups are located near the tryptophan residue(s), because these may accumulate or deplete local quencher concentrations.

To determine the depth of membrane penetration, quenchers may also be cova- lently bound to the lipid fatty acyl chains at different positions along the chains. Lip- ids that contain nitroxide spin labels (London, 1982) or bromines (Markello et al., 1985) in various chain positions have been prepared and demonstrated to be effective quenchers of tryptophan fluorescence. The brominated lipids are probably less bilayer perturbing than the nitroxide lipids, and the locations of the bromine atoms in the bilayer have been characterized by x-ray diffraction (McIntosh and Holloway, 1987; Wiener and White, 1991). By comparing the differences in fluorescence quenching of a given tryptophan residue by a homologous series of covalent lipid quenchers, a qualitative assessment of the depth of membrane penetration may be obtained. Unfortunately, relatively high mole fractions (10–100 mol%) of labeled lip- ids (spin label or bromine) have to be used to achieve significant quenching. The effect of a possible perturbation of the bilayer structure, especially by the bulky nitroxides, is not well studied.

Resonance energy transfer (RET) has been used to determine the aggregation behavior of peptides in membranes. If two fluorophors with sufficient overlap between the donor emission and acceptor adsorption spectra are in close ($<$100 Å) proximity, RET can occur. The transfer efficiency, E, can be measured either from the fluorescence intensities (F_o, F) or the fluorescence lifetimes (τ_o, τ_F) of the donor without and with the acceptor, respectively,

$$\frac{F}{F_o} = \frac{\tau_F}{\tau_o} = 1 - E \tag{18}$$

For the case of a fixed distance, r, between the donor and the acceptor (Förster, 1948),

$$E = \frac{R_o^6}{R_o^6 + r^6} \tag{19}$$

with the critical distance R_o (in Å)

$$R_o = 9.8 \times 10^3 (\kappa^2 n^{-4} Q_o J)^{1/6} \tag{20}$$

where κ is the orientation factor, n is the index of refraction between donor and accep- tor, Q_o = quantum yield in the absence of acceptor, and J is the spectral overlap integral. For the case of a two-dimensional random distribution of fluorophors, the relevant equations are (Fung and Stryer, 1978)

$$\tau_F = \int_0^\infty F(t)/F(0)\, dt \tag{21}$$

$$F(t) = F(0)e^{-(t/\tau_o)}e^{-\sigma S(t)} \tag{22}$$

$$S(t) = \int_a^\infty [1 - e^{-(t/\tau_o)(R_o/r)^6}]2\pi r\, dr \tag{23}$$

where a is the distance of closest approach and σ is the density of energy acceptors in the membrane. No closed form solution can be found for Eqs. 22 and 23, but values of E can be found by numerical integration of Eq. 23 and insertion into Eqs. 22, 21, and 18.

Depth of Bilayer Penetration

The embedding of tryptophan residues into lipid bilayers has been studied with two hydrophobic signal peptides, namely, phoE-21 (Killian et al., 1990) and lamB-25 (McKnight et al., 1991). The wild-type sequences of both peptides do not include any tryptophan residues. Therefore, variant peptides were synthesized that contained one tryptophan each, in different positions. In phoE, Val^{14}, which is part of the contiguous hydrophobic domain of this peptide, was replaced with a tryptophan (Killian et al., 1990). First, it was established that this substitution did not significantly affect the in vivo and in vitro translocation efficiencies of the entire protein precursor. Blue shifts and increased quantum yields of tryptophan emission were observed, when this peptide bound to phopholipid vesicles of phosphatidylcholine (PC), phosphatidylglycerol (PG), and cardiolipin (CL), respectively. The magnitude of both effects decreased on the order of CL > PG > PC, indicating a more hydrophobic environment and a deeper membrane penetration of this peptide in the negatively charged bilayers than in zwitterionic PC. The tryptophan was shielded from I^- in all three membranes, but acrylamide had limited access to the tryptophan in PC and very little access to the tryptophan in the negatively charged membranes. Finally, tryptophan quenching was observed with brominated lipids in PC or CL. Although there was a distinct difference of the quenching efficiency in PC and CL bilayers, the differences as a function of the position of the bromine atoms (C2 to C12) were barely significant. This relative positional insensitivity precluded a detailed determination of the position of the tryptophan in the bilayer.

Three different tryptophan-containing analogs of lamB-25 were synthesized in another study with a hydrophobic signal peptide (McKnight et al., 1991). Leu^5, Val^{18}, and Met^{24}, which represented positions in the N-terminal, the central, and the C-terminal parts of the peptide, respectively, were replaced by tryptophans. These substitutions did not significantly change the secondary structures of these peptides in bilayers, nor did they alter the export efficiency of the corresponding precursors in vivo. I^- had access to all three tryptophans in POPE–POPG bilayers. The apparent Stern-Volmer quenching constants decreased in the order $Trp^5 > Trp^{25} > Trp^{18}$, indicating that Trp^{18} was most buried in the bilayer. The somewhat better aqueous accessibilities of Trp^5 and Trp^{24} may be interpreted by a location of these tryptophans closer to either one of the membrane surfaces. These results are consistent with either a transmembrane or a bent orientation of the lamB signal peptide in the bilayer.

Quaternary Structure of Peptides in Bilayers

The oligomerization of peptides in bilayers and in solution has been investigated by fluorescence RET in a few cases. Again, the best studied case is the one of melittin. Melittin contains a single tryptophan residue in position 19. This tryptophan has been reacted with 2-hydroxy-5-nitrobenzylbromide (Habermann and Kowallek, 1970), and the product is called A-melittin. The ultraviolet absorption of A-melittin is strongly pH dependent. The absorption maximum ranges from 310 nm at pH 4.5 to 415 nm at pH 7.4. The modified tryptophan in A-melittin was then used as an energy acceptor for tryptophan in unmodified melittin at acidic and neutral pH

(Vogel and Jähnig, 1986; Schwarz and Beschiaschvili, 1989; John and Jähnig, 1991). Hermetter and Lakowicz (1986) prepared a *N*-methyl anthraniloyl-derivative of melittin, which also was a good energy acceptor for the tryptophan emission from melittin. Since this latter reaction involved the labeling of the ε-amino group of a lysine, the charge properties of this peptide derivative were altered. Intramolecular energy transfer could also occur in this molecule. A third derivative of melittin that can serve as an energy acceptor for tryptophan is oxiindole-melittin [O-melittin] (Talbot and Faucon, 1987). O-melittin has been prepared by reacting the tryptophan residue of melittin with *N*-bromosuccinimide. O-melittin is fluorescent and has a very broad absorption spectrum suitable for RET measurements with tryptophan as the energy donor. The picture that emerges from these collective studies is that melittin is monomeric in solution at low melittin and salt concentrations, tetrameric in solution at high salt concentration, and usually monomeric when bound to liquid-crystalline lipid bilayers. Only at a relatively high melittin–lipid molar ratio (1:200) and at high ionic strength, about 10% of all melittin was found to aggregate in the membrane (John and Jähnig, 1991). The number of subunits in each oligomer could not be obtained from these studies, but the observed power law as a function of peptide concentration in black lipid bilayer conductance measurements provides evidence for a heterogeneity in the number (n) of monomers per conducting channel. The average of n is about three to four subunits per conducting channel, but much higher oligomers may also be present in small numbers (Tosteson et al., 1990; Stankowski et al., 1991).

Two fluorescent derivatives of the amphiphilic mitochondrial signal peptide otc-27 were prepared, namely, bimane-otc-27 and NBD-otc-27 (Skerjanc et al., 1987). In both cases sulfhydro-reactive labels were used and reacted with a single cysteine in the sequence. Therefore, the charge distribution was preserved in these peptides. Efficient RET indicating aggregation was found when the two derivatives were mixed in solution, but no evidence for aggregation was observed when the peptide derivatives were bound simultaneously to vesicles of cardiolipin or eggPC–cardiolipin at peptide–lipid molar ratios of 1:200 (cardiolipin) or <1:330 (eggPC–cardiolipin).

Summary and Conclusions

Amphiphilic peptides, about 20–30 residues in length and with about 10 or more hydrophobic residues in their sequence, spontaneously bind and insert into lipid bilayers. Hydrophobic and electrostatic interactions are both found to be important contributors to the "affinity" of a given peptide for a membrane of a certain lipid composition. Hydrophobic and electrostatic interactions can be separated from each other by measuring binding–incorporation isotherms at different initial surface charge densities on the membrane and analyzing the data with a Gouy-Chapman partition model. After subtraction of the charge interactions, membrane–water partition coefficients on the order of 10^3–10^5 are typically found for these peptides. Taking further into account that the peptides become partially immobilized after binding to the membrane, one finds hydrophobic interaction energies of -21 to -25 kcal/

mol for a series of surface-seeking, strongly amphiphilic helical peptides. These values can be correlated with predictions from the summed hydrophobicity values of the individual amino acid residues, using the Goldman-Engelman-Steitz scale.

The predominant secondary structure of peptides in membranes is the α-helix, although β-strands and other forms are occasionally found. Structural polymorphism, i.e., an interconversion between different forms, which depends on the type and state of the phospholipids in the membrane, are commonly found in some signal peptides. Also, the orientations of α-helix– or β-strand–forming peptides appear to depend not only on the amino acid sequence, but also on the state of the membrane and, perhaps, on the lipids in the membrane. This may have interesting implications for the general mechanisms of protein folding in membranes, protein translocation across membranes, and protein-catalyzed membrane fusion. Much more remains to be learned about the determinants of peptide orientation and depth of penetration in lipid bilayers. This is also true for protein–protein interactions that eventually determine the tertiary and quaternary structures of membrane proteins.

Acknowledgments

I thank Dr. David Stokes for critically reading the manuscript and Ms. Jiki Pierson and Barbara Nordin for their word-processing help.

This work was supported by grants from the National Institutes of Health, the Life and Health Insurance Medical Research Fund, and the Swiss National Science Foundation.

References

Allen, J. P., Feher, G., Yeates, T. O., Komiya, H., and Rees, D. C. (1987) Structure of the reaction center from *Rhodobacter sphaeroides* R26: the protein subunits. *Proc. Natl. Acad. Sci. USA* 84: 6162–6166.

Altenbach, C., Froncisz, W., Hyde, J. S., and Hubbell, W. (1989) Conformation of spin-labeled melittin at membrane surfaces investigated by pulse saturation recovery and continuous wave power saturation electron paramagnetic resonance. *Biophys. J.* 56: 1183–1191.

Altenbach, C., and Hubbell, W. (1988) The aggregation state of spin-labeled melittin in solution and bound to phospholipid membranes: evidence that membrane-bound melittin is monomeric. *Proteins* 3: 230–242.

Archer, S. J., Ellena, J. F., and Cafiso, D. S. (1991) Dynamics and aggregation of the peptide ion channel, alamethicin. *Biophys. J.* 60: 389–398.

Arrondo, J.L.R., Muga, A., Castresana, J., and Goñi, F. M. (1993) Quantitative studies of the structure of proteins in solution by Fourier transform infrared spectroscopy. *Prog. Biophys. Molec. Biol.* 59: 23–56.

Batenburg, A. M., Brasseur, R., Ruysschaert, J.-M., Demel, R. A., and de Kruijff, B. (1988) Characterization of the interfacial behavior and structure of the signal sequence of *Escherichia coli* outer membrane pore protein *phoE*. *J. Biol. Chem.* 263: 4202–4207.

Bechinger, B., Zasloff, M., and Opella, S. J. (1992) Structure and interactions of magainin antibiotic peptides in lipid bilayers: a solid-state nuclear magnetic resonance investigation. *Biophys. J.* 62: 15–17.

Beschiaschvili, G., and Seelig, J. (1990) Peptide binding to lipid bilayers. Binding isotherms and ζ-potential of a cyclic somatostatin analogue. *Biochemistry* 29: 10995–11000.

Bollotina, I. A., Checkhov, V. O., Lugauskas, V., and Ptitsyn, O. B. (1980) Determination of the secondary structure of proteins from the circular dichroism spectra. A consideration of the contribution of β-bends. *Mol. Biol.* 14: 709–715.

Bösch, C., Brown, L. R., and Wüthrich, K. (1980) Physiochemical characterization of glucagon-containing lipid micelles. *Biochim. Biophys. Acta* 603: 298–312.

Brahms, S., and Brahms, J. (1980) Determination of protein secondary structure in solution by vacuum ultraviolet circular dichroism. *J. Mol. Biol.* 138: 149–178.

Braun, W., Wider, G., Lee, K. H., and Wüthrich, K. (1983) Conformation of glucagon in a lipid–water interphase by ¹H nuclear magnetic resonance. *J. Mol. Biol.* 169: 921–948.

Brauner, J. W., Mendelsohn, R., and Prendergast, F. G. (1987) Attenuated total reflectance Fourier transform infrared studies of the interaction of melittin, two fragments of melittin, and δ-hemolysin with phosphatidylcholines. *Biochemistry* 26: 8151–8158.

Briggs, M. S., and Gierasch, L. M. (1984) Exploring the conformation roles of signal sequences: synthesis and conformational analysis of *lamB* receptor protein wild-type and mutant signal peptides. *Biochemistry* 23: 3111–3114.

Brown, L. R., Braun, W., Kumar, A., and Wüthrich, K. (1982) High resolution nuclear magnetic resonance studies of the conformation and orientation of melittin bound to a lipid–water interface. *Biophys. J.* 37: 319–326.

Chang, C. T., Wu, C.-S.C., and Yang, J. T. (1978) Circular dichroic analysis of protein conformation: inclusion of the β-turns. *Anal. Biochem.* 91: 12–31.

Chen, Y.-H., Yang, J. T., and Chau, K. H. (1974) Determination of the helix and β-form of proteins in aqueous solution by circular dichroism. *Biochemistry* 13: 3350–3359.

Chothia, C. (1974) Hydrophobic bonding and accessible surface area in proteins. *Nature* 248: 338–339.

Cornell, D. G., Dluhy, R. A., Briggs, M. S., McKnight, C. J., and Gierasch, L. M. (1989) Conformations and orientations of a signal peptide interacting with phospholipid monolayers. *Biochemistry* 28: 2789–2797.

Cowan, S. W., Schirmer, T., Rummel, G., Steiert, M., Gosh, R., Pamptit, R. A., Jansonius, J. N., and Rosenbush, J. P. (1992) Crystal structures explain functional properties of two *E. coli* porins. *Nature* 358: 727–733.

Davis, J. H., Clare, D. M., Hodges, R. S., and Bloom, M. (1983) Interaction of a synthetic amphiphilic polypeptide and lipids in a bilayer structure. *Biochemistry* 22: 5298–5305.

Dawson, C. R., Drake, A. F., Helliwell, J., and Hider, R. C. (1978) The interaction of bee melittin with lipid bilayer membranes. *Biochim. Biophys. Acta* 510: 75–86.

Deisenhofer, J., Epp, O., Miki, K., Huber, R., and Michel, H. (1985) Structure of the protein subunits in the photosynthetic reaction centre of *Rhodopseudomonas viridis* at 3 Å resolution. *Nature* 312: 618–824.

de Kroon, A.I.P.M., de Gier, J., and de Krujff, B. (1991) The effect of a membrane potential on the interaction of mastoparan X, a mitochondrial presequence, and several regulatory peptides with phospholipid vesicles. *Biochim. Biophys. Acta* 1068: 111–124.

Demel, R. A., Goormaghtigh, E., and de Kruijff, B. (1990) Lipid and peptide specialities in signal peptide-lipid interactions in model membranes. *Biochim. Biophys. Acta* 1027: 155–162.

Eisenberg, D., Schwarz, E., Komaromy, M., and Wall, R. (1984) Analysis of membrane and surface protein sequences with the hydrophobic moment plot. *J. Mol. Biol.* 179: 125–142.

Endo, T., Shimada, I., Roise, D., and Inagaki, F. (1989) N-terminal half of a mitochondrial presequence peptide takes a helical conformation when bound to dodecylphosphocholine micelles: A proton nuclear magnetic resonance study. *J. Biochem.* 106: 396–400.

Engelman, D. M., Steitz, T. A., and Goldman, A. (1986) Identifying nonpolar transbilayer helices in amino acid sequences of membrane proteins. *Annu. Rev. Biophys. Chem.* 15: 321–353.

Epand, R. M., and Epand, R. F. (1992) Lipid-peptide interactions. In: *The Structure of Biological Membranes*, edited by P. Yeagle. Boca Raton, FL: CRC Press, p. 573–601.

Epand, R. M., Hui, S.-W., Argan, C., Gillespie, L. L., and Shore, G. (1986) Structural analysis and amphiphilic properties of a chemically synthesized mitochondrial signal peptide. *J. Biol. Chem.* 261: 10017–10020.

Epand, R. M., Jones, A.J.S., and Schreier, S. (1977) Interaction of glucagon with dimyristoyl glycerophosphocholine. *Biochim. Biophys. Acta* 481: 296–304.

Evans, E., and Sackmann, E. (1988) Translational and rotational drag coefficients for a disk moving in a liquid membrane associated with rigid structure. *J. Fluid Mech.* 194: 553–561.

Flewelling, R. F., and W. L. Hubbell. (1986) The membrane dipole potential in a total membrane potential model. Applications to hydrophobic ion interactions with membranes. *Biophys. J.* 49: 541–552.

Förster, T. (1948) Intermolecular energy migration and fluorescence. *Ann. Physiol. (Leipzig)* 2: 55–75.

Frey, S., and Tamm, L. K. (1990) Membrane insertion and lateral diffusion of fluorescence-labelled cytochrome *c* oxidase subunit IV signal peptide in charged and uncharged lipid bilayers. *Biochem. J.* 272: 713–719.

Frey, S., and Tamm, L. K. (1991) Orientation of melittin in phospholipid bilayers. A polarized attenuated total reflection infrared study. *Biophys. J.* 59: 922–930.

Fringeli, U. P., and Fringeli, M. (1979) Pore formation in lipid membranes by alamethicin. *Proc. Natl. Acad. Sci. USA* 76: 3852–3856.

Fringeli, U. P., and Günthardt, H. H. (1981) Infrared membrane spectroscopy. In: *Membrane Spectroscopy*, edited by E. Grell. Berlin: Springer, p. 270–332.

Fringeli, U. P. (1992) In situ infrared attenuated total reflection membrane spectroscopy. In *Internal Reflection Spectroscopy. Theory and Applications*, edited by F. M. Mirabella Jr. New York: Marcel Dekker, p. 255–324.

Fung, B. L., and Stryer, L. (1978) Surface density determination in membranes by fluorescence energy transfer. *Biochemistry* 17: 6241–5248.

Galla, H.-J., Hartmann, W., Theilen, V., and Sackmann, E. (1979) On two-dimensional passive random walk in lipid bilayers and fluid pathways in biomembranes. *J. Membrane Biol.* 48: 215–236.

Gierasch, L. M. (1989) Signal sequences. *Biochemistry* 28: 923–930.

Goormaghtigh, E., Martin, I., Vandenbranden, M., Brasseur, R., and Ruysschaert, J.-M. (1989) Secondary structure and orientation of a chemically synthesized mitochondrial signal sequence in phospholipid bilayers. *Biochem. Biophys. Res. Commun.* 158: 610–616.

Goormaghtigh, E., and Ruysschaert, J.-M. (1990) Polarized attenuated total reflection infrared spectroscopy as a tool to investigate the conformation and orientation of membrane components. In *Molecular Description of Biological Membranes by Computer-Aided Conformational Analysis*, edited by R. Brasseur. Boca Raton, FL: CRC Press, p. 285–329.

Greenfield, N., and Fasman, G. D. (1969) Computed dichroism spectra for the evaluation of protein conformation. *Biochemistry* 8: 4108–4116.

Grosse, R., Malur, J., Meiske, W., and Ripke, K.R.H. (1974) Statistical behaviour and suitability of protein-derived circular dichroic-basis spectra for the determination of globular protein conformation. *Biochim. Biophys. Acta* 359: 33–46.

Habermann, E., and Kowallek, H. (1970) Modifikation der Aminogruppen und des Tryptophans in Melittin als Mittel zur Erkennung der Struktur-Wirkungs-Beziehung. *Hoppe Seylers Z. Physiol. Chem.* 351: 884–880.

Henderson, R., Baldwin, J. M., Ceska, T. A., Zemlin, F., Beckmann, E., and Downing, K. H. (1990) Model for the structure of bacteriorhodopsin based on high-resolution electron cryo-microscopy. *J. Mol. Biol.* 213: 899–929.

Hennessey, J. P., and Johnson, W. C. (1981) Information content in the circular dichroism of proteins. *Biochemistry* 20: 1085–1094.

Hermetter, A., and Lakowicz, J. R. (1986) The aggregation state of mellitin in lipid bilayers. *J. Biol. Chem.* 261: 8243–8248.

Hoyt, D. W., Cyr, D. M., Gierasch, L. M., and Douglas, M. G. (1991) Interaction of peptides corresponding to mitochondrial presequences with membranes. *J. Biol. Chem.* 266: 21693–21699.

Hoyt, D. W., and Gierasch, L. M. (1991) Hydrophobic content and lipid interactions of wild-type and mutant ompA signal peptides correlate with their in vivo function. *Biochemistry* 30: 10155–10163.

Huang, H. W., and Wu, Y. (1991) Lipid–alamethicin interactions influence alamethicin orientation. *Biophys. J.* 60: 1079–1087.

Hughes, B. D., Pailthorpe, B. A., White, L. R., and Sawyer, W. H. (1982) Extraction of membrane microviscosity from translational and rotational diffusion coefficients. *Biophys. J.* 37: 673–676.

Jacobs, R. E., and White, S. E. (1989) The nature of the hydrophobic binding of small peptides at the bilayer, interface: Implications for the insertion of transbilayer helices. *Biochemistry* 28: 3421–3437.

Jähnig, F. (1983) Thermodynamics and kinetics of protein incorporation into membranes. *Proc. Natl. Acad. Sci. USA* 80: 3691–3695.

Janin, J., and Chothia, C. (1978) Role of hydrophobicity in the binding of co-enzymes. *Biochemistry* 17: 2943–2950.

Jap, B. K., Walian, P. J., and Gehring, K. (1991) Structural architecture of an outer membrane channel as determined by electron crystallography. *Nature* 350: 167–170.

John, E., and Jähnig, F. (1991) Aggregation state of melittin in lipid vesicle membranes. *Biophys.* 60: 319–328.

Johnson, W. C., Jr. (1988) Secondary structure of proteins through circular dichroism spectroscopy. *Annu. Rev. Biophys. Biophys. Chem.* 17: 145–166.

Johnson, W. C., Jr. (1990) Protein secondary structure and circular dichroism: a practical guide. *Proteins Struct. Funct. Genet.* 7: 205–214.

Kaiser, E. T., and Kézdy, F. J. (1987) Peptide with affinity for membranes. *Annu. Rev. Biophys. Biophys. Chem.* 16: 561–581.

Kalb, E., Engel, J., and Tamm, L. K. (1990) Binding of proteins to specific target sites in membranes measured by total internal reflection fluorescence microscopy. *Biochemistry* 29: 1607–1613.

Kalb, E., Frey, S., and Tamm, L. K. (1992) Formation of supported planar bilayers by fusion of vesicles to supported phospholipid monolayers. *Biochim. Biophys. Acta* 1103: 307–316.

Karslake, C., Piotto, M. E., Pak, Y. K., Weiner, H., and Gorenstein, D. G. (1990) 2D NMR and structure model for a mitochondrial signal peptide bound to a micelle. *Biochemistry* 29: 9872–9878.

Keller, R.C.A., Killian, J. A., and de Krujff, B. (1992) Anionic phospholipids are essential for α-helix formation of the signal peptide of pre PhoE upon interaction with phospholipid vesicles. *Biochemistry* 31: 1672–1677.

Killian, J. A., Prasad, K. U., Hains, D., and Urry, D. W. (1988) The membrane as an environment of minimal interconversion. A circular dichroism study on the solvent dependence of the conformational behavior of gramicidin in dioleoylphosphatidylcholine model membranes. *Biochemistry* 27: 4848–4855.

Killian, J. A., Keller, R.C.A. Struyve, M., de Kroon, A.J.P.M., Tommassen, J., and de Kruijff, B. (1990) Tryptophan fluorescence study on the interaction of the signal peptide of the *Escherichia coli* outer membrane protein *PhoE* with model membranes. *Biochemistry* 29: 8131–8137.

Knöppel, E., Eisenberg, D., and Wickner, W. (1979) Interactions of melittin, a preprotein model, with detergents. *Biochemistry* 28: 4177–4181.

Kuchinka, E., and Seelig, J. (1989) Interaction of melittin with phosphatidylcholine membranes. Binding isotherm and lipid head-group conformation. *Biochemistry* 28: 4216–4221.

Kühlbrandt, W., and Wang, D. W. (1991) Three-dimensional structure of plant light-harvesting complex determined by electron crystallography. *Nature* 350: 130–134.

Lakowicz, J. R. (1983) *Principles of Fluorescence Spectroscopy*. New York: Plenum.

Lee, S., Mihara, H., Aoyagi, H., Kato, T., Izumiya, N., and Yamasaki, N. (1986) Relationship between antimicrobial activity and amphiphilic property of basic model peptides. *Biochim. Biophys. Acta* 862: 211–219.

London, E. (1982) Investigation of membrane structure using fluorescence quenching by spin-labels (a review of recent studies). *Mol. Cell Biochem.* 45: 181–188.

Manavalan, P., and Johnson, W. C., Jr. (1987) Variable selection method improves the prediction of protein secondary structure from circular dichroism spectra. *Anal. Biochem.* 167: 76–85.

Mao, D., and Wallace, B. A. (1984) Differential light scattering and absorption flattening optical effects are minimal in the circular dichroism spectra of small unilamellar vesicles. *Biochemistry* 23: 2667–2673.

Markello, T., Zlotnick, A., Everett, J., Tennyson, J., and Holloway, P. W. (1985) Determination of the topography of cytochrome b₅ in lipid vesicles by fluorescence quenching. *Biochemistry* 24: 2895–2901.

Matsuzaki, K., Harada, M., Funakosh, S., Fujii, N., and Miyajima, K. (1991) Physiochemical determinants for the interactions of magainins 1 and 2 with acidic lipid bilayers. *Biochim. Biophys. Acta* 1063: 162–170.

McIntosh, T. J., and Holloway, P. W. (1987) Determination of the depth of bromine atoms in bilayers formed from bromolipid probes. *Biochemistry* 26: 1783–1788.

McKnight, C. J., Briggs, M. S., and Gierasch, L. M. (1989) Functional and nonfunctional LamB signal sequences can be distinguished by their biophysical properties. *J. Biol. Chem.* 264: 17293–17297.

McKnight, C. J., Rafalsky, M., and Gierasch, L. M. (1991) Fluorescence analysis of tryptophan-containing variants of the *lamB* signal sequence upon insertion into a lipid bilayer. *Biochemistry* 30: 6241–6246.

McLaughlin, S. H. (1989) The electrostatic properties of membranes. *Annu. Rev. Biophys. Biophys. Chem.* 18: 113–136.

Nicholson, L. K., and Cross, T. A. (1989) Gramacidin cation channel: an experimental determination of the right-handed helix sense and variation of β-type hydrogen bonding. *Biochemistry* 28: 9379–9385.

Ono, Lee, S., Mihara, H., Aoyagi, H., Kato, T., and Yamasaki, N. (1990) Design and synthesis of basic peptides having amphiphilic β-structure and their interaction with phospholipid membranes. *Biochim. Biophys. Acta* 1022: 237–244.

Opella, S. J., and Stewart, P. L. (1989) Solid-state nuclear magnetic resonance structural studies of proteins. *Methods Enzymol.* 176: 242–275.

Pak, Y. K., and Weiner, H. (1990) Import of chemically synthesized signal peptides into rat liver mitochondria. *J. Biol. Chem.* 265: 14298–14307.

Perczel, A. M., Hollósi, G., Tusnády, G., and Fasman, G. D. (1991) Convex constraint analysis: a natural deconvolution of circular dichroism curves of proteins. *Prot. Eng.* 4: 669–679.

Peters, R., and Beck, K. (1983) Translational diffusion in phospholipid monolayers measured by fluorescence microphotolysis. *Proc. Natl. Acad. Sci. USA* 80: 7183–7187.

Peters, R., and Cherry, R. J. (1982) Lateral and rotational diffusion of bacteriorhodopsin in lipid bilayers: experimental test of the Saffman-Delbrück equations. *Proc. Natl. Acad. Sci. USA* 79: 4317–4321.

Popot, J. L., and Engelman, P. M. (1990) Membrane protein folding and oligomerization: the two-stage model. *Biochemistry* 29: 4031–4037.

Portlock, S. H., Lee, Y., Tomich, J., and Tamm, L. K. (1992) Insertion and folding of the N-terminal amphiphilic signal sequence of the mannitol and glucitol permeases of *Escherichia coli J. Biol. Chem.* 267: 11017–11022.

Provencher, S. W., and Glöckner, J. (1981) Estimation of globular protein secondary structure from circular dichroism. *Biochemistry* 20: 33–37.

Reynolds, J. A., Gilbert, D. B., and Tanford, C. (1974) Empirical correlation between hydrophobic free energy and aqueous cavity surface area. *Proc. Natl. Acad. Sci. USA* 71: 2925–2927.

Richards, F. M. (1977) Areas, volumes, packing and protein structure. *Annu. Rev. Biophys. Bioeng.* 6: 151–176.

Rizzo, V., Stankowski, S., and Schwarz, G. (1987) Alamethicin incorporation in lipid bilayers: a thermodynamic study. *Biochemistry* 26: 2751–2759.

Roise, D., Theiler, F., Horvath, S. J., Tomich, J. M., Richards, J. H., Allison, D. S., and Schatz, G. (1988) Amphiphilicity is essential for mitochondrial presequence function. *EMBO J.* 7: 649–653.

Rolka, K., Erne, D., and Schwyzer, R. (1986) Membrane structure of substance P. I. Prediction of preferred conformation, orientation, and accumulation of substance P on lipid membranes. *Helv. Chim. Acta* 69: 1798–1806.

Rose, G. D., Geselowitz, A. R., Lesser, G. J., Lee, R. H., and Zehfus, M. H. (1985) Hydrophobicity of amino acid residues in globular proteins. *Science* 229: 834–838.

Saffman, P. G., and Delbrück, M. (1975) Brownian motion in biological membranes. *Proc. Natl. Acad. Sci. USA* 72: 3111–3113.

Saxena, V. P., and Wetlaufer, D. B. (1971) A new basis for interpreting circular dichroism spectra of proteins. *Proc. Natl. Acad. Sci. USA* 68: 969–972.

Schwarz, G., and Beschiaschvili, G. (1989) Thermodynamic and kinetic studies on the association of melittin with a phospholipid bilayer. *Biochim. Biophys. Acta* 979: 82–90.

Schwarz, G., Stankowski, S., and Rizzo, V. (1986) Thermodynamic analysis of incorporation and aggregation in a membrane: application to the pore-forming peptide alamethicin. *Biochim. Biophys. Acta* 861: 145–151.

Seelig, A., and Macdonald, P. M. (1989) Binding of a neuropeptide, substance P, to neutral and negatively charged lipids. *Biochemistry* 28: 2490–2496.

Segrest, J. P., DeLoof, H., Dohlman, J. G., Brouillette, C. G., and Anantharamariah, G. M. (1990) Amphipathic helix motif: Classes and properties. *Prot. Struct. Funct. Genet.* 8: 103–117.

Shon, K.-J., Kim, Y., Colnago, L., and Opella, S. J. (1991) NMR studies of the structure and dynamics of membrane-bound bacteriophage pf1 coat protein. *Science* 252: 1303–1305.

Siegel, J. B., Steinmetz, W. E., and Long, G. L. (1980) A computer-assisted model for estimating protein secondary structure from circular dichroic spectra: comparison of animal lactate dehydrogenases. *Anal. Biochem.* 104: 160–167.

Skerjanc, I. S., Shore, G. C., and Silvius, J. R. (1987) The interaction of a synthetic mitochondrial signal peptide with lipid membranes is dependent of the transbilayer potential. *EMBO J.* 6: 3117–3123.

Smith, R., Thomas, D. E., Separovic, F., Atkins, A. R., and Cornell, B. A. (1989) Determination of the structure of a membrane-incorporated ion channel. *Biophys. J.* 56: 307–314.

Stanislawski, R., and Rüterjans, H. (1987) C-NMR investigation of the insertion of bee venom melittin into lecithin vesicles. *Eur. Biophys. J.* 15: 1–12.

Stankowski, S., Pawlak, M., Kaisheva, E., Robert, C. H., and Schwarz, G. (1991) A combined study of aggregation, membrane affinity, and pore activity of natural and modified melittin. *Biochim. Biophys. Acta* 1069: 77–86.

Surewicz, W. K., and Mantsch, H. H. (1988) New insight into protein secondary structure from resolution enhanced infrared spectra. *Biochim. Biophys. Acta* 952: 115–130.

Susi, H., and Byler, D. M. (1986) Resolution-enhanced Fourier transform infrared spectroscopy of enzymes. *Methods Enzymol.* 130: 290–311.

Talbot, J. C., and Faucon, J. F. (1987) Different states of self-association of melittin in phospholipid bilayers. *Eur. Biophys. J.* 15: 147–157.

Tamm, L. K. (1986) Incorporation of a synthetic mitochondrial signal peptide into charged and uncharged phospholipid monolayers. *Biochemistry* 25: 7470–7476.

Tamm, L. K. (1991) Membrane insertion and lateral mobility of synthetic amphiphilic signal peptides in lipid model membranes. *Biochim. Biophys. Acta* 1071: 123–148.

Tamm, L. K., and Bartoldus, I. (1990) Secondary structure of a mitochondrial signal peptide in lipid bilayer membranes. *FEBS Lett.* 272: 29–33.

Tamm, L. K., and McConnell, H. M. (1985) Supported phospholipid bilayers. *Biophys. J.* 47: 105–113.

Tamm, L. K., and Tatulian, S. (1993) Orientation of functional and non-functional PTS permease signal sequences in lipid bilayers. A polarized attenuated total reflection infrared study. *Biochemistry* 32: 7720–7726.

Tamm, L. K., Tomich, J. M., and Saier, M. H., Jr. (1989) Membrane incorporation and induction of secondary structure of synthetic peptides corresponding to the N-terminal signal sequences of the glucitol and mannitol permeases of *E. coli. J. Biol. Chem.* 264: 2587–2592.

Tank, D. W., Wu, E. S., Meers, P. R., and Webb, W. W. (1982) Lateral diffusion of gramicidin c in phospholipid multibilayers. *Biophys. J.* 40: 129–135.

Terwilliger, T. C., Weissmann, L., and Eisenberg, D. (1982) The structure of melittin in the form I crystals and its implication for melittins lytic and surface activities. *Biophys. J.* 37: 353–361.

Tosteson, M. T., Alvarez, O., Hubbell, W., Beganski, R. M., Altenbach, C., Caporales, L. H., Levy, J. J., Nutt, R. F., Rosenblatt, M., and Tosteson, D. C. (1990) Primary structure of peptides and ion channels. Role of amino acid side chains in voltage gating of melittin channels. *Biophys. J.* 58: 1367–1375.

Urry, D. W. (1971) The gramicidin A transmembrane channel: a proposed $\pi_{(L,D)}$ helix. *Proc. Natl. Acad. Sci. USA* 68: 672–676.

Vaz, W.L.C., Goodsaid-Zalduondo, G., and Jacobson, K. (1984) Lateral diffusion of lipids and proteins in bilayer membranes. *FEBS Lett.* 174: 199–207.

Vaz, W.L.C., and Hallmann, D. (1983) Experimental evidence against the applicability of the Saffman-Delbrück model to the translational diffusion of lipids in phosphatidylcholine bilayer membranes. *FEBS Lett.* 152: 287–290.

Vogel, H. (1987) Comparison of the conformation and orientation of alamethicin and melittin in lipid membranes. *Biochemistry* 26: 4652–4672.

Vogel, H., and Jähnig, F. (1986) The structure of melittin in membranes. *Biophys. J.* 50: 573–582.

Vogel, H., Jähnig, F., Hoffmann, V., and Stümpel, J. (1983) The orientation of melittin in lipid membranes. A polarized infrared spectroscopic study. *Biochim. Biophys. Acta* 733: 201–209.

von Heijne, G. (1988) Transcending the impenetrable: how protein comes to terms with membranes. *Biochim. Biophys. Acta* 947: 307–333.

White, S. H. and Wimley, W. C. (1994) Peptides in bilayers: structural thermodynamic basis for partitioning and folding. *Cur. Opinion Struc. Biol.* 4: 79–86.

Weiss, M. S., Kreusch, A., Schiltz, E., Nestel, U., Welte, W., Weckesser, J., and Schulz, G. E. (1991) The structure of porin from *Rhodobacter capsulatus* at 1.8Å resolution. *FEBS Lett.* 280: 379–383.

Wiener, M. C., and White,. S. H. (1991) Transbilayer distribution of bromine in fluid bilayers containing a specifically brominated analogue of dioleoyl-phosphatidylcholine. *Biochemistry* 30: 697–7008.

Woolley, G. A., and Deber, C. M. (1987) Peptides in membranes: lipid-induced secondary structure of substance P. *Biopolymers* 26: 5109–5121.

Wu, E. S., Jacobson, K., Szoka, F., and Portis, A. (1978) Lateral diffusion of a hydrophobic peptide, 4-nitrobenzoxa-1,3-diazole gramicidin S, in phospholipid multibilayers. *Biochemistry* 16: 3936–3941.

Yang, J. T., Wu, C.-S.C., and Martiniez, H. M. (1986) Calculation of protein conformation from circular dichroism. *Methods Enzymol.* 130: 208–269.

14

Membrane Protein Structure:
Lessons from Gramicidin

G. ANDREW WOOLLEY and B. A. WALLACE

Gramicidin is an unusual membrane protein; it has a molecular weight of less than 2,000 daltons and contains D-amino acids, whereas most membrane proteins have molecular weights on the order of 100,000 daltons or more and contain L-amino acids exclusively. This small peptide, however, has the remarkable property of forming well-defined ion channels in lipid bilayer membranes. In fact, it is perhaps the best-characterized of all membrane ion channels. As a result of the many studies on gramicidin channels, a considerable amount of information on the structural and functional aspects of this molecule is available, and this information and the methods used to derive it are generally relevant to the study of other membrane protein structures.

Introduction

Gramicidins belong to a family of peptides produced by the bacterium *Bacillus brevis*. They were isolated by Rene Dubos and Rollin Hotchkiss at the Rockefeller Institute for Medical Research in 1939 (Hotchkiss, 1990). This was a time of discovery of many important antibiotics, and the initial interest in these molecules was for their antibiotic activity. Gramicidin was named for its activity against gram-positive bacteria, and, although it is not as useful today as some other antibiotics because of its toxicity in mammals, it still has importance as a topical bacteriostatic agent (Classen et al., 1991; Nash et al., 1991). The gramicidin isolated by Dubos (denoted gramicidin "D" for its discoverer) was shown by Sarges and Witkop (1965a) to be composed of a mixture of six different peptides. The primary sequence of the major component, Val-Gramicidin A, is shown below.

HCO-L-Val-Gly-L-Ala-D-Leu-L-Ala-D-Val-L-Val-D-Val-L-Trp

-D-Leu-L-Trp-D-Leu-L-Trp-D-Leu-L-Trp-NHCH₂CH₂OH

The Trp residue at position 11 may be substituted by Phe (called gramicidin "B") or Tyr (gramicidin "C"); about 20% of each of these species also has the Val in the first position substituted by Ile so that a total of six isomers are commonly found (Sarges and Witkop, 1965a,c,d). A minor component discovered more recently has been called gramicidin"K" and has a covalently attached fatty acid at the C terminus (Koeppe et al., 1985). *B. brevis* also produces gramicidin "S," but this is a cyclic peptide with little in common with the linear gramicidins (Izumiya et al., 1979). Experiments with the linear gramicidins have often been performed with a natural mixture that is predominantly (80%) gramicidin A.

Efficient chromatographic procedures have been developed for the separation of gramicidins A, B, and C from this mixture (e.g., Fields et al., 1989; Stankovic et al., 1990), and methods of complete synthesis have been described (e.g., Sarges and Witkop, 1965b; Prasad et al., 1982; Fields et al., 1989) so that pure isomers may be used when required. The basis of the antibacterial activity of gramicidin and the role of this peptide in the growth of *B. brevis* has been the subject of several studies (Sarkar et al., 1979; Bohg and Ristow, 1986). Sarkar et al. (1979) demonstrated an inhibitory interaction of gramicidin with RNA polymerase. Moreover, the ability of different gramicidin analogs to inhibit RNA polymerase correlates with their ability to restore normal sporulation behavior in gramicidin-negative mutants of *B. brevis*. In addition, Bohg and Ristow (1986) reported the effects of gramicidin on DNA supercoiling that may cause changes in DNA transcription, recombination, and replication processes. The focus of most of the interest in gramicidin, however, is the ability of this short peptide to form well-defined channels in lipid membranes.

Gramicidin forms channels that are selective for monovalent cations (for reviews, see Finkelstein and Andersen, 1981; Andersen, 1984; Hladky, 1987), and conductances on the order of 10^7 ions per second are typically observed. Divalent cations and anions are essentially impermeant, and the channel excludes all molecules with diameters greater than about 4.5 Å (Myers and Haydon, 1972; Urban et al., 1978). A continuous single file of water molecules is thought to be present in the channel and would account for the observed high permeability to protons.

The aim of this chapter is to present several broadly applicable lessons that have been learned over the course of about 50 years of work with gramicidin. The emphasis of course contains some personal bias and is very selective (for more general reviews on gramicidin, see Anderson, 1984; Cornell, 1987; Wallace, 1990). Gramicidin is one of the most thoroughly studied membrane proteins, and many aspects of its structure and function have been investigated in great detail. Because of the extensive knowledge about gramicidin, this molecule remains a testing ground for fundamental ideas about ion transport, peptide–lipid interactions, and membrane protein folding, as well as other subjects. It is quite likely there are several more lessons yet to be learned.

The Usefulness of Theoretical Models

As early as 1971, simple models of the three-dimensional structure of gramicidin were proposed based on primary sequence information and on knowledge about the peptide's activity. The presence of alternating D- and L-amino acid residues in gramicidin is rather unusual and produces some secondary structures not generally encountered with all-L-amino acid–containing peptides and proteins. Thus, while the specific conformations proposed for gramicidin are unlikely to be encountered in other membrane proteins, the process of model building is similar for full-sized pro-

tein systems. The criteria used for building models were as follows: (*1*) the conformations had to coincide with stereochemically allowed regions of peptide conformational space; (*2*) the structure had to be long enough to span a lipid bilayer since
the conductance was too high to be due to a carrier mechanism; (*3*) the molecularity
was probably two, although this was not firmly established in 1971; and (*4*) nonpolar faces should contact the lipid hydrocarbon region, while polar or hydrophilic
faces should contact water and ions. Stereochemically allowed regions for alternating
D/L peptides were calculated by Ramachandran and Chandrasekaran (1972). Helical structures in proteins may be described by the number of residues per turn and
the number of atoms contained in the ring formed by hydrogen bonds. For instance,
the common α-helix may be designated 3.6_{13} (3.6 residues per turn and 13 atoms
in the hydrogen-bonded ring). Stereochemically possible structures include 2.2_7 (rib-
bon), 3_{10}, 3.6_{13} (α), 4.3_{14}, and 4.4_{16} (π), 5.4_{17} (γ) helices. While none of these is a
particularly good model for the alternating D/L sequence of the gramicidin molecule,
a variant of the π helix was proposed by Urry (1971) in which consecutive peptide
carbonyl groups alternate direction with respect to the helix axis. This structure, designated a $\pi_{(L,D)}$ helix, results in a hybrid hydrogen-bonding pattern in which both 14
and 16 member rings are formed. It was soon recognized that a family of such structures was possible with even larger diameters (Urry et al., 1971). The $\pi_{(L,D)}$-helix
was consequently renamed the $\pi_{(L,D)}^4$-helix; and $\pi_{(L,D)}^6$-, $\pi_{(L,D)}^8$-, and $\pi_{(L,D)}^{10}$-helices
were described.

    The $\pi_{(L,D)}^6$ structure seemed particularly attractive as a model for the gramicidin
channel. Two of these helices placed end to end would be long enough to span the
membrane. A head-to-head dimer (the formyl ends joined) was favored over head-
to-tail or tail-to-tail arrangements because it is a symmetrical structure with little
disruption of hydrogen-bonding and because preliminary evidence indicated a sensitivity of channel formation to removal of the formyl group. Finally, and importantly, the $\pi_{(L,D)}^6$-helix has an internal cavity large enough to permit the passage of
water and small ions. The nomenclature of these structures was later changed to β-
helices to better reflect the type of hydrogen-bonding present, which is in fact the
same as that of β-sheets (Venkatachalam and Urry, 1983). Normally β-sheets have
consecutive side chains extending in alternating directions from the peptide backbone
but because of the sequence of alternating D and L residues in gramicidin all side
chains are on one side of the backbone, which then becomes the outside of the channel
when the sheet is rolled up into a helix (Fig. 14.1). The channel structure proposed
by Urry is referred to as the $\beta^{6.3}$-helical dimer (the superscript refers to the number
of residues per turn of the helix).

    Another set of potential structures for gramicidin was proposed by Will Veatch,
Eric Fossel, and Elkan Blout in 1974 (Veatch et al., 1974) based on spectroscopic
studies in organic solvents. Several other groups have extended and elaborated these
models (Lotz et al., 1976; Chandrasekaran and Prasad, 1978; Koeppe and Kimura,
1984). In the structures proposed by Veatch et al., hydrogen bonding is entirely intermolecular (between the two molecules forming the dimer) rather than largely intramolecular, as in Urry's model. If one imagines two gramicidin chains placed next to
one another in an extended conformation, a β-sheet-type bonding pattern may be
seen to be possible between the chains. It may be parallel or antiparallel and may
have different degrees of stagger (i.e., the number of unsatisfied hydrogen bonds at

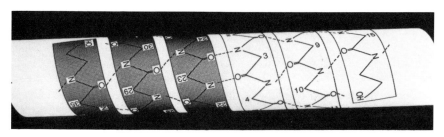

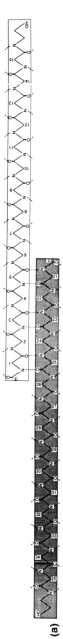

Fig. 14.1. *a*: The hydrogen-bonding motif of the right-handed helical dimer of gramicidin. Hydrogen-bonding is of the antiparallel β-type at the dimer junction and of the parallel β-type elsewhere. The residues in the two polypeptide chains are numbered from *1* to *15* and *21* to *35*, respectively. *b*: The model rolled up into a helix corresponding to the right-handed helical dimer.

the chain termini). Again these structures may be thought of as being rolled into helices with the side chains extending away from a central channel (Fig. 14.2). These structures have been referred to as *double helices* and have variously been designated $\pi\pi\uparrow\downarrow$ (antiparallel), $\pi\pi\uparrow\uparrow$ (parallel), or $\beta\beta$ structures in analogy with their single-stranded counterparts. Despite the differences in monomer association, these structures have rather similar overall dimensions and channel diameters that could accommodate ions below the known cutoff size of about 4.5 Å.

It turns out that both of these types of structures have been found to occur under different conditions. This constitutes something of a triumph for modeling. Even if these models had been incorrect, however, they were valuable in that they provided the impetus for a wide range of experimental studies. For instance, the relative dispositions of the N and C termini of gramicidin are predicted to be different in the different models, something that fueled a variety of studies aimed at determining the location of the N and C termini in membranes (e.g., Weinstein et al., 1979, 1985). Thus, in suggesting possible structures this modeling was extremely useful. Modeling alone, however, could not predict which of these families of structures would be the active channel in membranes. It remains a puzzle today why different forms are more stable under different conditions. Furthermore, modeling alone has been unable to predict side chain conformations, helical twist, stagger, or the handedness of the channel. Unlike all L or all D peptides, alternating D/L peptides have little intrinsic preference for right- or left-handed structures. The helical dimer proposed by Urry et al. (1971) is left handed, and energy calculations were presented to support this (Venkatachalam and Urry, 1983). The handedness of the channel, however, appears to be the sort of question that is difficult to resolve using energy calculations, since it involves a great variety of terms, including estimation of environmental influences, and the sum of these terms may not be vastly different for structures of opposite handedness (Etchebest and Pullman, 1988). Present experimental evidence favors a right-handed helix as predominant in membranes (see below), but this has not been an easy question to answer.

Another aspect of gramicidin structure that tends to be overstated in modeling studies is the conformation of the side chains. Because the motion of any particular side chain may be coupled with the motions of other side chains, the peptide backbone, and the lipid environment, accurate evaluations of the lifetimes of different side chain rotational states is not straightforward. This sort of problem is perhaps somewhat more tractable than evaluating the overall stability of different folding patterns, but it is an area in which experimental input from nuclear magnetic resonance (NMR) and fluorescence spectroscopic methods particularly will be needed.

On the other hand, theoretical methods have been very successful in describing motion around an established structure and for the refinement of experimental models (Langs, 1988; Wallace and Ravikumar, 1988). Thus gramicidin backbone dynamics and ion permeation have been investigated with the helical dimer as a starting point, and this has led to considerable insight into these aspects of channel behavior (e.g., Mackay et al., 1984; Jordan, 1987; Chiu et al., 1991; Roux and Karplus, 1991).

There are a number of factors that have made gramicidin a particularly simple case for modeling. First, only regular structures were considered, which greatly simplified the problem and may have worked well because of the unusual primary

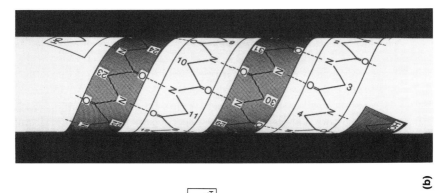

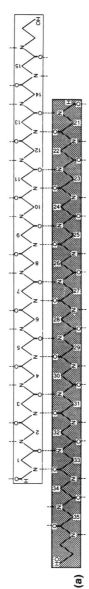

Fig. 14.2. *a*: The hydrogen-bonding motif of a left-handed, antiparallel double helix with a stagger of three residues. *b*: The model rolled up into a helix corresponding to the CsCl-bound form of the gramicidin pore.

sequence of gramicidin. Second, the observation that specific dimers formed further directed the modeling. Nevertheless, the usefulness and the limitations of modeling are expected to be broadly similar for other membrane proteins. Dealing with sections of aperiodic structure in proteins is problematical and of course the number of residues involved differs by orders of magnitude, but additional information is often available from homology studies. Modeling appears to be most useful for suggesting categories of structure. One is then able to pose questions to be addressed experimentally. As experimental data become available, theoretical methods are extremely useful in refining and adding detail to model structures.

The Use of Organic Solvents and Membrane Mimetics

The amino acid sequence of gramicidin is very hydrophobic and results in the peptide being virtually insoluble in water. Gramicidin is soluble, however, in the presence of detergents or lipid vesicles, behavior that is typical of membrane proteins. It is also soluble in a variety of organic solvents including ethanol, methanol, dimethylsulfoxide, trifluoroethanol, dimethylformamide, acetone, dioxane, and tetrahydrofuran, some of which may solubilize other membrane proteins. Working with organic solutions as opposed to membrane multibilayers or suspensions of lipid vesicles greatly simplifies the application of various spectroscopic techniques. Furthermore, it has been proposed that low dielectric organic solvents may mimic the environment of the membrane interior and thus provide a suitable medium for study of the native membrane–protein conformation.

In organic solvents it has been found that gramicidin can exist in a mixture of dimeric forms in equilibrium with monomers (Veatch and Blout, 1974). The relative fractions of dimers and monomers depend on the solvent type, temperature, and gramicidin concentration. These forms have been studied extensively using a variety of techniques (e.g., Veatch et al., 1974) of which perhaps multidimensional solution-state NMR has been the most effective (e.g., Bystrov et al., 1990). All of these forms appear to belong to the family of double helices originally proposed by Veatch et al. (1974). They vary in handedness and number of residues per turn, and parallel and antiparallel orientations appear to coexist. A predominant form is the antiparallel, left-handed $\beta^{5.6}$ double-helical dimer that has been crystallized and the crystal structure determined (Langs, 1988; Langs et al., 1991). The addition of ions to these solutions causes conformational changes that can be observed using circular dichroism (CD) (Wallace, 1984) and NMR (Arseniev et al., 1985) spectroscopy. The crystal structure of an ion-bound form has also been solved (the CsCl complex) (Wallace and Ravikumar, 1988). This is also a left-handed, antiparallel, double helix, although in this case the number of residues per turn is 6.4 and the overall length is 26 Å compared with 31 Å for the ion-free form; the ions are located in a central cavity formed by the double helix.

Although the crystallographically determined double-helical structures appear quite reasonable as ion channels, a variety of studies have essentially established the helical dimer model described above as the major form of the conducting channel in membranes. These studies have used either single planar bilayers [bilayer lipid membrane (BLM) or patch-clamp conductance experiments], lipid vesicles, oriented multibilayers, and, in some cases, detergent systems. We shall briefly review studies in each of these systems.

Measurement of gramicidin concentrations using O-dansyl tyrosine (fluorescent) gramicidin C analogs in combination with BLM conductance measurements (Veatch et al., 1975) confirmed that functional channels were dimers. Furthermore, gramicidin analogs with somewhat different single-channel conductances can be added to the same BLM lipid bilayer, and hybrid channels can be observed alongside pure channels of each analog, at a frequency predicted by the binomial distribution (Veatch and Stryer, 1977). If more than two monomers are required for an active channel, then such mixing experiments would be expected to result in a wider variety of hybrid channels than that observed.

The head-to-head association is supported by the observation that chemical modifications at the N terminus (e.g., pyromellityl [Bamberg et al., 1977]; des-formyl [Morrow et al., 1979]; and acetyl [Szabo and Urry, 1979]) drastically affect channel formation in BLM, whereas similar modifications to the C terminus do not. Charged analogs can be tolerated at the C terminus but not at the N terminus, where they would be required to be buried in the hydrocarbon region of the bilayer and also participate in the dimer junction. Covalent attachment of the N termini through a malonyl linkage (Bamberg and Janko, 1977) or a tartaric acid linkage (Stankovic et al., 1989) results in functional channels, in many ways similar to native gramicidin channels although with much longer lifetimes.

The CD spectrum of gramicidin in phospholipid vesicles is significantly different from the spectrum in solution and cannot be represented by any combination of the spectra of the different double-helical dimers or monomeric solution forms (Masotti et al., 1980; Wallace et al., 1981; Wallace, 1983) (Fig. 14.3). Furthermore, while the CD of the solution form changes upon the addition of ions, that of the membrane-bound form is relatively unaffected (Wallace, 1984). Veatch et al. (1975) were able to estimate the dimerization constant of gramicidin A in BLMs to be about 2×10^{13} $mol^{-1} cm^{-2}$. This means that at peptide concentrations generally employed for spectroscopic experiments the fraction of monomers is negligible. Channel formation by gramicidin in lipid vesicles has been observed (e.g., Hinton et al., 1988; Jyothi et al., 1990), but there are complexities not encountered with BLM systems and nonspecific leakage may occur when the peptide concentration is high. It is therefore difficult to simultaneously demonstrate ion channel activity and to perform spectroscopic measurements in vesicles. However, the observation that the far-ultraviolet CD spectrum of membrane-bound gramicidin is not sensitive to peptide–lipid ratio (Wallace, 1986) (at least for those ratios experimentally accessible) suggests that the conformation of gramicidin is approximately the same for conductance studies (low peptide–lipid ratios) and spectroscopic studies (high peptide–lipid ratios). The CD spectrum of the membrane-bound form has generally been taken as a "signature" evidencing the presence of active $\beta^{6.3}$-helical dimers.

The membrane-bound gramicidin structure has been investigated with vibrational spectroscopy, which confirms the β-type hydrogen-bonding pattern expected for the helical dimer (Naik and Krimm, 1986). Fluorescence energy transfer from gramicidin Trp residues to fluorescence acceptors covalently attached at different depths in the bilayer support the head-to-head topology (Boni et al., 1986) as do ^{13}C- and

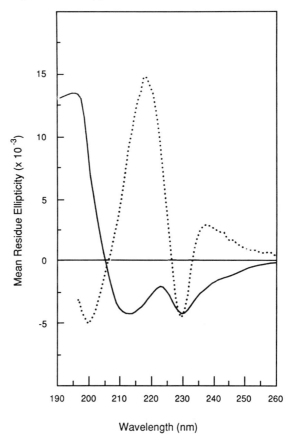

Fig. 14.3. Circular dichroism spectra of gramicidin in methanol *(solid line)*, and in phospholipid vesicles *(dotted line)*.

^{19}F-NMR studies with specifically labeled gramicidins in lipid vesicles (Weinstein et al., 1979, 1985). X-ray crystallography has been used to evaluate overall dimensions and the location of ion-binding sites (Olah et al., 1991) but, although co-crystals of gramicidin and lipid have recently been prepared (Wallace and Janes, 1991), a complete crystal structure for the membrane-bound form is not yet available. Solid-state NMR studies in oriented multibilayers using isotopically labeled (^{15}N, ^{2}H, ^{13}C) gramicidin have confirmed the $\beta^{6.3}$-helical fold oriented with the helix axis perpendicular to the membrane surface (Smith et al., 1989; Hing et al., 1990a,b; Nicholson et al., 1991; Prosser et al., 1991; Teng et al., 1991). A right-handed helical sense of the $\beta^{6.3}$-helix was found in dimyristoyl-phosphatidylcholine multibilayers (Nicholson et al., 1991; Prosser et al., 1991; Teng et al., 1991).

Use has also been made of micelle-forming detergents (particularly lysophosphatidylcholine (lyso-PC) and sodium dodecylsulfate (SDS)) as model membranes. These appear to act as better membrane mimetics than organic solutions for gramicidin, since the CD spectra in SDS or lyso-PC resemble those obtained in vesicles and not those obtained in solution. There are differences, however: the spectra are not identical to those in vesicles and change somewhat after addition of ions. A surprising finding (Killian et al., 1983; Spisni et al., 1983) was that, although lyso-PC alone forms micellar complexes, lyso-PC in the presence of gramicidin appears to organize into bilayer sheets. A tail-to-tail dimerization of gramicidin in lyso-PC has been suggested to be more consistent with the observed effects of the peptide on lipid morphology than a head-to-head arrangement (de Kruijff and Killian, 1987). The subtle differences between lyso-PC environments and phosphatidylcholine (vesicle) environments are highlighted by the finding that gramicidin B (the Phe[11] analog) shows a characteristic $\beta^{6.3}$ helical CD pattern in vesicles but not in lyso-PC sheets (Sawyer et al., 1990). Despite the added complexity, lyso-PC has proved useful for a series of NMR studies with specifically labeled ^{13}C gramicidin analogs designed to find ion-binding sites in the channel (Urry et al., 1983). Arseniev et al. (1985), Bystrov and Arseniev (1988), and Bystrov et al. (1990) have used gramicidin–SDS complexes to study gramicidin conformation by multidimensional NMR. These studies have indicated a right-handed $\beta^{6.3}$-helix conformation for gramicidin in this system.

The conformational behavior of gramicidin in organic solution was originally investigated because it was accessible and because it was thought that these solvents might mimic the hydrocarbon interior of lipid membranes. Indeed, the crystal structures obtained from these solvents appear quite reasonable as membrane ion channels. Although it has been suggested that double-helix forms may constitute a minor fraction of especially long-lived ion channels (Durkin and Andersen, 1987; Koeppe et al., 1991), there are various compelling reasons, as we have discussed, for believing that these do *not* correspond to the predominant structure of the active membrane-bound channel. This finding emphasizes the critical effect of environment on structure and the difficulty in using simple organic solvents as membrane mimetics. It does not, however, imply that studies in such solvents are without value; indeed, they have been indispensable for our current understanding of gramicidin structure and function, and indeed if situations may be found whereby there is evidence for a native conformation in an isotropic solution (e.g., by CD), then there are many technical advantages to using these systems. The CD spectrum appears to be a useful criterion generally for evaluating the degree to which a structure is native, since, although it is difficult to interpret quantitatively, it responds to often rather small changes in conformation. Of course, activity assays or specific binding assays may also be used to establish native structure for many membrane proteins. Detergents have been reasonably successful as membrane mimetics in the gramicidin case, but peculiarities exist (e.g., sheet formation) and their usefulness would appear to depend on the specific case and as with organic solvents some evidence for a "native-like," unperturbed structure would seem important.

These studies point out the rather special nature of the lipid bilayer in its juxtaposition of hydrophobic and hydrophilic groups of fairly well-defined dimension. The strong effect of environment on structure and presumably on function is an important general finding.

The Mutual Dependence of Peptide and Membrane Structures

Detailed effects of the lipid environment on protein structure are commonly ignored in membrane protein research. This is probably because the effects are usually complex, and only a few systems have been studied in any detail. Furthermore, the complementary problem—the effects of proteins on lipids—has been studied mainly by those interested in lipids (for a review, see Killian and de Kruijff, 1986). The mutual dependence of these effects is of course inescapable, and a thorough understanding of the effects of a membrane environment on protein structure and dynamics must include knowledge of the structure and dynamics of the membrane. While some of the effects of proteins on membranes may not be critical *in vivo*, they are often important for structural studies that employ nonphysiological protein–lipid concentrations and ratios, types of lipid, and conditions of temperature, pressure, hydration, and pH. We will briefly review the mutual dependence of gramicidin and lipid structures, because it is an extensively characterized system and gives an indication of what might be expected for membrane proteins generally.

Dependence of Gramicidin Structure and Dynamics on Membrane Properties

While the conductance of an open gramicidin channel appears on the whole to be little affected by membrane properties (Hladky and Haydon, 1972), the stability and dynamics of channels most definitely are. This is presumably because channel formation necessitates lipid rearrangement. The lifetime of gramicidin channels observed in conductance studies is directly related to the dynamics of peptide and lipid. Mean lifetimes of seconds are typically observed, but channel lifetimes are shorter in thicker membranes, which suggests that an energy of pinching the membrane may be required for channel formation (Hladky and Haydon, 1972; Elliott et al., 1983). The CD spectrum of gramicidin in lipid membranes also shows a sensitivity to bilayer thickness (Wallace et al., 1981). Calculations of the deformation energy of a lipid membrane surrounding a gramicidin channel suggest that thermal fluctuations in lipid thickness may play a role in the docking of monomers from each leaflet (Huang, 1986; Helfrich and Jakobsson, 1990).

Deuterium NMR of gramicidin with selectively deuterated Trp residues has been used to probe the rotational motion of the peptide in various lipid environments (Macdonald and Seelig, 1988). In phosphatidylcholine membranes, gramicidin was found to rotate axially at temperatures above the lipid phase transition; this motion ceased in the gel phase, although the channel is still active in gel-phase lipid (Krasne et al., 1971) and the structure does not seem to be much altered (Wallace et al., 1981; Cornell et al., 1988). Lateral diffusion of fluorescently labeled gramicidin C in the plane of the membrane at temperatures above the lipid phase transition has been measured using the technique of fluorescence photobleaching recovery in oriented multibilayers (Tank et al., 1982). A diffusion coefficient of 3×10^8 cm^2 s^{-1} was calculated, indicating rather rapid diffusion approximating that of lipid molecules themselves. This rate drops by more than a factor of 100 below the lipid phase transition temperature.

Besides the hydrocarbon length, the exact nature of the lipid tails does not seem to be critical. Channels form in both saturated and unsaturated lipids and in both solvent-free and solvent-containing membranes. Branched chain (diphytanoyl-phosphatidylcholine) membranes will also support channels. Some dependence on lipid headgroup has been reported (Neher and Eibl, 1977), although the reproducibility of these effects has been questioned (Ring, 1986). The chirality of the lipid headgroup does not seem to be a factor, since nonchiral, R, and S lipids can all support channels (e.g., Providence et al., 1991).

The dipolar potential of membranes seems to be little involved in gramicidin function in contrast to its effects on carriers such as valinomycin or nonactin. Bilayers formed from ether lipid and glycerol monooleate bilayers support channels in the same manner as ester lipid bilayers despite large (e.g. 150 mV) differences in the dipolar potentials (Bamberg and Benz, 1976). Jordan (1983) has discussed how the membrane dipole potential may be shielded in the gramicidin channel. Studies using CD spectroscopy (Woolley and Wallace, unpublished observations) and solid-state NMR (Cornell et al., 1988; Smith et al., 1989) have indicated a normal $\beta^{6.3}$ channel in bilayers of ether–lipids. Subtle changes may occur, however; for instance, a modeling study has indicated that a constriction of the mouth of the gramicidin channel due to a change in the interaction of Trp^{15} with lipid headgroups may occur when ester lipids are substituted by ether lipids (Meulendijks et al., 1989).

Effects of Gramicidin on Membrane Structure

The effects of gramicidin on membrane structure depend critically on the specific lipids involved and usually begin to occur at peptide concentrations of about 1,000-fold higher than those at which channel formation is observed (de Kruijff and Killian, 1987; de Kruijff et al., 1988). They are of particular importance for spectroscopic studies of channel structure using relatively high peptide concentrations, and some assessment of lipid morphology (e.g., [^{31}P]NMR, freeze-fracture electron microscopy, x-ray diffraction) is often necessary before such studies can begin. The membrane-modifying activities of gramicidin have been reviewed elsewhere (Killian and de Kruijff, 1986; Cornell, 1987; Killian & de Kruijff, 1988; Tournois et al., 1990).

Gramicidin has been found to induce lipid-chain ordering in fluid phase bilayers using infrared and Raman spectroscopy (Chapman et al., 1977; Lee et al., 1984; Davies and Mendelsohn, 1991). On the other hand, gramicidin is found to disorder gel-phase lipids. As discussed above, upon codispersion with lyso-PC, gramicidin induces a micelle to bilayer transition that is complete when a ratio of 1:4 (peptide:lipid) is reached (Killian et al., 1983). This transition occurs even with relatively low gramicidin concentrations. NMR and fluorescence studies indicate that gramicidin is largely self-associated in lyso-PC and has little rotational freedom (Macdonald and Seelig, 1988). Gramicidin has been found to promote H_{II} phase formation in phosphatidylethanolamines, phosphatidylserines, phosphatidylglycerols, and in phosphatidylcholines with an acyl chain length greater than 16 carbons (de Kruijff and Killian, 1987; de Kruijff et al., 1988). The formation of H_{II} phase can also be demonstrated in erythrocyte membranes (Tournois et al., 1987). Gramicidin may be self-associated in the H_{II} phase, and the extent of association appears to depend on lipid type (Tournois et al., 1989).

Gramicidin has been shown to enhance the rates of transbilayer flip-flop of lyso-PC and acylcarnitine in the erythrocyte membrane (Classen et al., 1987). This occurs at peptide:lipid ratios of 1:2,000, much lower than those required for H_{II} phase formation. Gramicidin can also induce fusion and aggregation of vesicles (Tournois et al., 1990). Both intervesicular lipid mixing and contents mixing were demonstrated with large unilamellar vesicles of dioleoyl-phosphatidylcholine. It has been suggested that gramicidin-induced vesicle fusion and H_{II} phase formation share common intermediates (e.g., Tournois et al., 1990).

All of these effects are thought to be due to the $\beta^{6.3}$-helical dimer conformation of gramicidin, since factors that affect the stability of this conformation (e.g., solvent history, formylation of Trp) also affect these lipid-modulating effects (Killian and de Kruijff, 1988; Killian and Urry, 1988; Tournois et al., 1990). CD and NMR studies are generally consistent with this interpretation. There are a few puzzles, however; for instance, O- and N-succinyl gramicidin analogs behave quite differently in conductance experiments, but their lipid-modulating abilities are similar (de Kruijff and Killian, 1987).

Unexpected and Long-Range Effects of Site-Directed Mutations

Mutating specific residues in order to probe structure and function is a common experimental approach in protein research. Gramicidin is synthesized nonribosomally in vivo; thus modifications must be performed using chemical rather than biochemical techniques [Kleinkauf and von Doehren, 1987]. Although chemical synthesis is less straightforward, it has the advantage that a wide range of specific mutations can be performed as one is not limited by the genetic code. In the absence of detailed structural information, the effects of mutations can be difficult to interpret. The study of structure–function relationships in gramicidin with this technique is thus facilitated by the knowledge of the structure of gramicidin in the membrane. We shall summarize two aspects of this work on gramicidin. The first is the sometimes surprisingly large effects of changes to specific residues on channel properties and general stability of the membrane-active form. The second is the effect of certain mutations on the structural dispersity, i.e., the relative populations of different conformational substates.

Despite the fact that the side chains of gramicidin are not directly involved in ion binding, they have been found to have significant effects on channel properties. The channel-forming properties of the naturally occurring analogs gramicidin B (Phe[11]) and gramicidin C (Tyr[11]) have been compared (Bamberg et al., 1976; Sawyer et al., 1990). Single channel conductances in 1 M NaCl at 25° C were 14.45 pS (gramicidin A), 9 pS (gramicidin B), and 13 pS (gramicidin C). Average lifetimes were 1 s (gramicidin A), 2 s (gramicidin B), and 0.9 s (gramicidin C). The ion selectivity changes somewhat as well. For instance, the ratio of single-channel conductances of Cs^+ to K^+ for gramicidin A is 1.8, whereas for gramicidin B it is 2.3 (glycerol monooleate membranes, 1 M ion concentration at 25°C). These channels were judged to be structurally equivalent by the criterion of hybrid formation when both are mixed in the same bilayer (Durkin et al., 1990; Sawyer et al., 1990). Tryptophan residues seem particularly important for channel function, since formylation of tryptophan (Killian et al., 1985) or tryptophan photolysis (Jones et al., 1986) results in inactive channels. Heitz et al. (1988) have reported the synthesis of a variety of analogs in which Trp residues have been substituted by tyrosine, tyrosine-O-benzyl, naphyla-lanine, and quinoleylalanine residues. Distinct effects on single-channel conductances, lifetimes, and channel voltage dependence were noted.

A further series of analogs has been used in the examination of the effects of replacing the amino acid at position one (usually Val^1) with either Phe, Trp, or Tyr for each of gramicidins A, B, and C (Mazet et al., 1984). These peptides again seemed to form structurally equivalent channels (i.e., $\beta^{6.3}$-dimers), as judged by hybrid formation, except perhaps for analogs with Tyr^1. Fairly large differences in single-channel properties were observed (e.g., the single-channel conductance of Trp^1–gramicidin A is sixfold larger than that of Tyr^1–gramicidin B in 1 M NaCl at 25°C) as well as altered selectivity ratios. Morrow et al. (1978, 1979) also prepared a series of analogs substituted at position one. They found a requirement for a nonpolar amino acid with L-chirality for this position. It was not clear whether these changes resulted from local conformational changes induced by the different side chains or from electrostatic effects (dipole or inductive) of different side chains on the energy profile an ion experiences. To address this point several isosteric analogs were prepared (e.g., valine, trifluorovaline, and hexafluorovaline at position one) (Barrett Russell et al., 1986), which had significantly different polarities and dipole moments. As the polarity of the side chains increased, the channel lifetimes and the single-channel conductances decreased. Interestingly, they decreased much more for sodium ion than for cesium. Further studies have implicated ion–dipole interactions as the dominant cause of the observed effects (Koeppe et al., 1988). These data can be incorporated into calculations of the energetics of ion transport and contribute to the detailed mathematical descriptions possible with this well-defined ion channel (e.g., Sancho and Martinez, 1991).

Another area in which side chain analogs have been used is in an investigation into the dispersity of single-channel conductances. It has been proposed that different subconductance states result from different side chain conformers. The three-dimensional fold of a $\beta^{6.3}$-helix results in residues six amino acids apart in the primary sequence being close together in space (Venkatachalam and Urry, 1983). Replacement of Ala^5 (residue i) by the bulkier Leu^5 was therefore expected to reduce the conformational space accessible to residue Trp^{11} (residue $i + 6$) (Urry et al., 1984). Thus, as expected, the Leu^5 analog was found to have a reduced dispersity of subconductance states. On the other hand, the Ala^7 (in place of Val^7) analog was synthesized, which might be expected to increase the conformational mobility of Trp^{13} and show an increased channel dispersity. Instead, a narrow range of channels with particularly high single-channel conductance was found (Prasad et al., 1986). It was suggested that this substitution created a new highly favorable orientation for Trp^{13}. A systematic analysis of such analogs in conjunction with molecular dynamics simulations (Brenneman et al., 1991) might prove revealing.

It is clear that chemical modifications to gramicidin can have unexpected effects, and even rather minor changes can have large effects on channel properties that are difficult to predict a priori. The side chains of gramicidin are not directly involved in ion transport so that alterations in side chains must affect channel properties at a distance through electrostatic or conformational effects on the peptide backbone or on the surrounding lipid. For most membrane proteins, however, side chains are often directly involved in active sites, so that, in addition to long-range effects of mutation, strong local effects will also occur and systematic studies on a range of analogs will often be required.

The Usefulness of Peptides as Models for Proteins

Perhaps the most obvious lesson to be learned from work with gramicidin is the usefulness of such a relatively simple peptide for understanding membrane protein and particularly ion channel structure and function. Gramicidin's utility as an antibiotic is rather minor, and its function in the host organism is not entirely clear; its usefulness as a model membrane protein, however, has generated a large literature and continues to provide a testing ground for ideas and experiments that would be impossible with more complex systems. It is easily obtained in large quantities, can be reconstituted in membranes in an active form, and can be manipulated chemically in far more varied ways than are possible with the techniques of site-directed mutagenesis. These properties are characteristic of peptides generally, and many peptides have been, and are being, used to address questions about membrane protein structure (White and Jacobs, 1989).

Peptides have been used to probe the influence of amino acid sequence and composition on conformation in membrane environments (e.g., Wallace and Blout, 1979; Wu and Yang, 1981; Wu et al., 1982; Deber and Behnam, 1984; Epand et al., 1986). Gramicidin has been used to study the process of membrane insertion and folding (Killian et al., 1988; LoGrasso et al., 1988; Bano et al., 1989, 1991). Peptides that comprise part of the bacteriorhodopsin sequence have been used to analyze the process of membrane assembly of bacteriorhodopsin (Engelman et al., 1989). Peptides have also been used to study the characteristics of the pores formed by ion channel proteins (e.g., the S4 peptide of the sodium channel [Tosteson et al., 1989] and the M2 peptide of the acetylcholine receptor [Montal, 1990]) and are being used as tools in the de novo design of membrane proteins (Lear et al., 1988).

Finally, because they are amenable to detailed spectroscopic analyses, the structure and dynamics of peptides can be studied at a molecular level. The pictures of molecular conformation thus obtained are an important conceptual tool: they make us think in ways that are much more realistic than the vaguely defined cubes and groups of cylinders that typically represent membrane protein structure in the literature.

Acknowledgments

The authors gratefully acknowledge financial support from the National Science Foundation (USA) (grant DMB-8816981) and the Medical Research Council of Canada (postdoctoral Fellowship to G.A.W.).

References

Andersen, O. S. (1984) Gramicidin channels. *Annu. Rev., Physiol.* 46: 531–548.
Arseniev, A. S., Barsukov, I. L., Bystrov, V. F., Lomize, A. L., and Ovchinnikov, Y. A. (1985) ^{1}H-NMR study of gramicidin A transmembrane ion channel. *FEBS Lett.* 186: 168–174.

Bamberg, E., Apell, J. H., and Alpes, H. (1977) Structure of the gramicidin A channel: discrimination between the $\pi_{(L,D)}$ and the β helix by electrical measurements with lipid bilayer membranes. *Proc. Natl. Acad. Sci. USA* 74: 2402–2406.

Bamberg, E., and Benz, R. (1976) Voltage-induced thickness changes of lipid bilayer membranes and the effect of an electric field on gramicidin A channel formation. *Biochim. Biophys. Acta* 426: 570–580.

Bamberg, E., and Janko, K. (1977) The action of a carbonsuboxide dimerized gramicidin A on lipid bilayer membranes. *Biochim. Biophys. Acta* 465: 486–499.

Bamberg, E., Noda, K., Gross, E., and Lauger, P. (1976) Single-channel parameters of gramicidin A, B, and C. *Biochim. Biophys. Acta* 419: 223–228.

Bano, M. C., Braco, L., and Abad, C. (1989) HPLC study of the "history" dependence of gramicidin A conformation in phospholipid model membranes. *FEBS Lett.* 250: 67–71.

Bano, M. C., Braco, L., and Abad, C. (1991) Conformational transitions of gramicidin A in phospholipid model membranes. A high-performance liquid chromatography assessment. *Biochemistry* 30: 886–894.

Barrett Russell, E. W., Weiss, L. B., Navetta, F. I., Koeppe, R. E. II and Andersen, O. S. (1986) Single-channel studies on linear gramicidins with altered amino acid side chains. Effects of altering the polarity of the side chain at position 1 in gramicidin A. *Biophys. J.* 49: 673–686.

Bohg, A., and Ristow, H. (1986) DNA-supercoiling is affected in vitro by the peptide antibiotics tyrocidine and gramicidin. *Eur. J. Biochem.* 160: 587–591.

Boni, L. T., Connolly, A. J., and Kleinfeld, A. M. (1986) Transmembrane distribution of gramicidin by tryptophan energy transfer. *Biophys. J.* 49: 122–123.

Brenneman, M., Chiu, S., and Jakobsson, E. (1991) Computational studies on the side chain conformations of gramicidin A. *Biophys. J.* 59: 320a.

Bystrov, V. F., and Arseniev, A. S. (1988) Diversity of the gramicidin A spatial structure: two-dimensional ^{1}H NMR study in solution. *Tetrahedron* 44: 925–940.

Bystrov, V. F., Arseniev, A. S., Barsukov, I. L., Golovanov, A. P., and Maslennikov, I. V. (1990) The structure of the transmembrane channel of gramicidin A: NMR study of its conformational stability and interaction with divalent cations. *Gazz. Chim. Ital* 120: 485–491.

Chandrasekaran, R., and Prasad, B.V.V. (1978) Conformations of polypeptides containing alternating L-amino and D-amino acids. *CRC Crit. Rev. Biochem.* 5: 125–161.

Chapman, D., Cornell, B. A., Eliasz, A. W., and Perry, A. (1977) Interactions of helical polypeptide segments which span the hydrocarbon region of lipid bilayers. Studies of the gramicidin A lipid–water system. *J. Mol. Biol.* 113: 517–538.

Chiu, S.-W., Jakobsson, E., Subramaniam, S., and McCammon, J. A. (1991). Time-correlation analysis of simulated water motion in flexible and rigid gramicidin channels. *Biophys. J.* 60: 273–285.

Classen, D. C., Larsen, R. A., Burke, J. P., Alling, D. W., and Stevens, L. E. (1991) Daily meatal care for prevention of catheter-associated bacteriuria: results using frequent applications of polyantibiotic cream. *Infect. Control Hosp. Epidemiol.* 12: 157–162.

Classen, J., Haest, C.W.M., Tournois, H., and Deuticke, B. (1987) Gramicidin-induced enhancement of transbilayer reorientation of lipids in the erythrocyte membrane. *Biochemistry* 26: 6604–6612.

Cornell, B. (1987) Gramicidin A—phospholipid model systems. *J. Bioenerg. Biomembrane* 19: 655–676.

Cornell, B. A., Separovic, F., Baldassi, A. J., and Smith, R. (1988) Conformation and orientation of gramicidin A in oriented phospholipid bilayers measured by solid state carbon-13 NMR. *Biophys. J.* 53: 67–76.

Davies, M. A., and Mendelsohn, R. (1991) Direct determination of the effect of gramicidin on DPPC conformational disorder by infrared spectroscopy. *Biophys. J.* 59: 321a.

de Kruijff, B., and Killian, J. A. (1987) Gramicidin: a modulator of lipid structure. In: *Ion Transport Through Membranes*, edited by K. Yagi and B. Pullman., Tokyo: Academic Press, p. 315–340.

de Kruijff, B., Killian, J. A., and Tournois, H. (1988) Influence of gramicidin on lipid organization and dynamics in membranes. In *Transport Through Membranes: Carriers, Channels, and Pumps*, edited by A. Pullman, J. Jortner, and B. Pullman, Dordrecht, Holland: Kluwer, p. 267–287.

Deber, C. M., and Behnam, B. A. (1984) Role of membrane lipids in peptide hormone function: binding of enkephalin to micelles. *Proc. Natl. Acad. Sci. USA* 81: 61–65.

Durkin, J. T., and Andersen, O. S. (1987) Linear gramicidins can form channels that do not have the $\beta^{6.3}$ structure. *Biophys. J.* 51: 451a.

Durkin, J. T., Koeppe, R. E. II, and Andersen, O. S. (1990) Energetics of gramicidin hybrid channel formation as a test for structural equivalence. Side-chain substitutions in the native sequence. *J. Mol. Biol.* 211: 221–234.

Elliott, J. R., Needham, D., Dilger, J. P., and Haydon, D. A. (1983) The effects of bilayer thickness and tension on gramicidin single-channel lifetime. *Biochim. Biophys. Acta* 735: 95–103.

Engelman, D. M., Adair, B. D., Hunt, J. F., Kahn, T. W. and Popot, J. L. (1989) Protein folding inside membrane bilayers. *Biophys. J.* 55: 398a.

Epand, R. M., Hui, S. W., Argan, C., Gillespie, L. L., and Shore, G. C. (1986) Structural analysis and amphiphilic properties of a chemically synthesized mitochondrial signal peptide. *J. Biol. Chem.* 261: 10017–10020.

Etchebest, C., and Pullman, A. (1988) The gramicidin A channel: left versus right-handed helix: In: *Transport Through Membranes: Carriers, Channels, and Pumps,* edited by A. Pullman, J. Jortner, and B. Pullman. Dordrecht, Holland: Kluwer, p. 167–185.

Fields, C. G., Fields, G. B., Noble, R. L., and Cross, T. A. (1989) Solid phase peptide synthesis of ^{15}N-gramicidins A, B, and C and high performance liquid chromatographic purification. *Int. J. Peptide Protein Res.* 33: 298–303.

Finkelstein, A., and Andersen, O. S. (1981) The gramicidin A channel: a review of its permeability characteristics with special reference to the single-file aspect of transport. *J. Membrane Biol.* 59: 155–171.

Heitz, F., Daumas, P., van Mau, N., Lazaro, R., Trudelle, Y., Etchebest, C., and Pullman, A. (1988) Linear gramicidins: influence of the nature of the aromatic side chains on the channel conductance. In: *Transport Through Membranes: Carriers, Channels, and Pumps,* edited by A. Pullman, J. Jortner, and B. Pullman. Dordrecht, Holland: Kluwer, p. 147–175.

Helfrich, P., and Jakobsson, E. (1990) Calculation of deformation energies and conformations in lipid membranes containing gramicidin channels. *Biophys. J.* 57: 1075–1084.

Hing, A. W., Adams, S. P., Silbert, D. F., and Norberg, R. E. (1990a) Deuterium NMR of [2]HCO-Val[1]-gramicidin A and [2]HCO-Val[1]-D-Leu[2]-gramicidin A in oriented DMPC bilayers. *Biochemistry* 29: 4156–4166.

Hing, A. W., Adams, S. P., Silbert, D. F., and Norberg, R. E. (1990b) Deuterium NMR of Val[1]-(2-^{2}H)Ala[3]-gramicidin A in oriented DMPC bilayers. *Biochemistry* 29: 4144–4156.

Hinton, J. F., Buster, D. C., Fernandez, J. Q., Privett, T. A., Easton, P. L., and Newkirk, D. K. (1988) Thermodynamics of cation binding and transport by gramicidin. In: *Transport Through Membranes: Carriers, Channels, and Pumps,* edited by A. Pullman, J. Jortner, and B. Pullman, Dordrecht: Holland: Kluwer, p. 203–218.

Hladky, S. B. (1987) Models for ion transport in gramicidin channels: how many sites? In: *Ion Transport Through Membranes,* edited by K. Yagi and B. Pullman. Tokyo: Academic Press, p. 213–232.

Hladky, S. B., and Haydon, D. A. (1972) Ion transfer across lipid membranes in the presence of gramicidin A. I. Studies of the unit conductance channel. *Biochim. Biophys. Acta* 274: 294–312.

Hotchkiss, R. D. (1990) From microbes to medicine: gramicidin, Rene Dubos, and the Rockefeller. In: *Launching the Antibiotic Era,* edited by C. L. Moberg and Z. A. Cohn. New York: The Rockefeller University Press, p. 1–18.

Huang, H. W. (1986) Deformation free energy of bilayer membrane and its effect on gramicidin channel lifetime. *Biophys. J.* 50: 1061–1070.

Izumiya, N., Kato, T., Aoyagi, H., Waki, M., and Kondo, M. (1979) *Synthetic Aspects of Biologically Active Cyclic Peptides—Gramicidin S and Tyrocidines.* New York: Halsted Press, John Wiley & Sons.

Jones, D., Hayon, E., and Busath, D. (1986) Tryptophan photolysis is responsible for gramicidin-channel inactivation by ultraviolet light. *Biochim. Biophys. Acta* 861: 62–66.

Jordan, P. C. (1983) Electrostatic modeling of ion pores. II. Effects attributable to the membrane dipole potential. *Biophys. J.* 41: 189–195.

Jordan, P. C. (1987) Microscopic approaches to ion transport through transmembrane channels. The model system gramicidin. *J. Phys. Chem.* 91: 6582–6591.

Jyothi, G., Mitra, C. K., and Krishnamoorthy, G. (1990) Studies on the kinetics of gramicidin channels in liposomes. Part I. *Bioelectrochem. Bioenerg.* 24: 297–304.

Killain, J. A., Timmermans, J. W., Keur, S., and de Kruijff, B. (1985) The tryptophans of gramicidin are essential for the lipid structure modulating effect of the peptide. *Biochim. Biophys. Acta* 820: 154–156.

Killian, J. A., and de Kruijff, B. (1986) The influence of proteins and peptides on the phase properties of lipids. *Chem. Phys. Lipids* 40: 259–284.

Killian, J. A., and de Kruijff, B. (1988) Proposed mechanism for H_{II} phase induction by gramicidin in model membranes and its relation to channel formation. *Biophys. J.* 53: 111–117.

Killian, J. A., de Kruijff, B., van Echteld, C.J.A., Verkleij, A. J., Leunissen-Bijvelt, J., and de Gier, J. (1983) Mixtures of gramicidin and lysophosphatidylcholine form lamellar structures. *Biochim. Biophys. Acta* 728: 141–144.

Killian, J. A., Prasad, K. U., Hains, D., and Urry, D. W. (1988) The membrane as an environment of minimal interconversion. A circular dichroism study on the solvent dependence of the conformational behavior of gramicidin in diacylphosphatidylcholine model membranes. *Biochemistry* 27: 4848–4855.

Killian, J. A., and Urry, D. W. (1988) Conformation of gramicidin in relation to its ability to form bilayers with lysophosphatidylcholine. *Biochemistry* 27: 7295–7301.

Kleinkauf, H., and von Doehren, H. (1987) Biosynthesis of peptide antibiotics. *Annu. Rev. Microbiol.* 41: 259–289.

Koeppe, R. E., II, Andersen, O. S., and Maddock, A. K. (1988) How do amino acid substitutions alter the function of gramicidin channels? In: *Transport Through Membranes: Carriers, Channels, and Pumps,* edited by A. Pullman, J. Jortner, and B. Pullman. Dordrecht, Holland: Kluwer, p. 133–145.

Koeppe, R. E., II, Greathouse, D. V., Providence, L. L., and Andersen, O. S. (1991)[L-Leu^9-D-Trp^{10}-L-Leu^{11}-D-Trp^{12}-L-Leu^{13}-D-Trp^{14}-L-Leu^{15}]-gramicidin forms both single- and double-helical channels. *Biophys. J.* 59: 319a.

Koeppe, R. E. II, and Kimura, M. (1984) Computer building of β-helical polypeptide models. *Biopolymers* 23: 23–38.

Koeppe, R. E. II, Paczkowski, J. A., and Whaley, W. L. (1985) Gramicidin K, a new linear channel-forming gramicidin from Bacillus brevis. *Biochemistry* 24: 2822–2826.

Krasne, S., Eisenman, G., and Szabo, G. (1971) Freezing and melting of lipid bilayers and the mode of action of nonactin, valinomycin, and gramicidin. *Science* 174: 412–415.

Langs, D. A. (1988) Three-dimensional structure at 0.86 Å of the uncomplexed form of the transmembrane ion channel peptide gramicidin A. *Science* 241: 188–191.

Langs, D. A., Smith, G. D., Courseille, C., Precigoux, G., and Hospital, M. (1991) Monoclinic uncomplexed double-stranded, antiparallel, left-handed $\beta^{5.6}$-helix ($\uparrow\downarrow\beta^{5.6}$) structure of gramicidin A: alternate patterns of helical association and deformation. *Proc. Natl. Acad. Sci. U.S.A.* 88: 5345–5349.

Lear, J. D., Wasserman, Z. R., and DeGrado, W. F. (1988) Synthetic amphiphilic peptide models for protein ion channels. *Science* 240: 1177–1181.

Lee, D. C., Durrani, A. A., and Chapman, D. (1984) A difference IR spectroscopic study of gramicidin A, alamethicin and bacteriorhodopsin in perdeuterated dimyristoylphosphatidylcholine. *Biochim. Biophys. Acta* 769: 49–56.

LoGrasso, P. V., Moll, F. III, and Cross, T. A. (1988) Solvent history dependence of gramicidin A conformations in hydrated lipid bilayers. *Biophys. J.* 54: 259–267.

Lotz, B., Colonna-Cesari, F., Heitz, F., and Spach, G. (1976) A family of double helices of alternating poly(γ-benzyl-D-L-glutamate), a stereochemical model for gramicidin A. *J. Mol. Biol.* 106: 915–942.

Macdonald, P. M., and Seelig, J. (1988) Dynamic properties of gramicidin A in phospholipid membranes. *Biochemistry* 27: 2357–2364.

Mackay, D.H.J., Berens, P. H., Wilson, K. R., and Hagler, A. T. (1984) Structure and dynamics of ion transport through gramicidin A. *Biophys. J.* 46: 229–248.

Masotti, L., Spisni, A., and Urry, D. W. (1980) Conformational studies on the gramicidin A transmembrane channel in lipid micelles and liposomes. *Cell Biophys.* 2: 241–251.

Mazet, J. L., Andersen, O. S., and Koeppe, R. E. II (1984) Single-channel studies on linear gramicidins with altered amino acid sequences. A comparison of phenylalanine, tryptophan, and tyrosine substitutions at positions 1 and 11. *Biophys. J.* 45: 263–276.

Meulendijks, G.H.W.M., Sonderkamp, T., Dubois, J. E., Nielen, R. J., Kremers, J. A., and Buck, H. M. (1989) The different influences of ether and ester phospholipids on the conformation of gramicidin A. A molecular modelling study. *Biochim. Biophys. Acta* 979: 321–330.

Montal, M. (1990) Molecular anatomy and molecular design of channel proteins. *FASEB J.* 4: 2623–2635.

Morrow, J. S., Veatch, W. R., and Stryer, L. (1978) Synthetic replacement of the N-terminal amino acid of gramicidin A: effect on transmembrane channel conductance. *Biophys. J.* 17: 26a.

Morrow, J. S., Veatch, W. R., and Stryer, L. (1979) Transmembrane channel activity of gramicidin A analogs: effects of modification and deletion of the amino-terminal residue. *J. Mol. Biol.* 132: 733–738.

Myers, V. B., and Haydon, D. A. (1972) Ion transfer across lipid membranes in the presence of gramicidin A. II. The ion selectivity. *Biochim. Biophys. Acta* 274: 313–322.

Naik, V. M., and Krimm, S. (1986) Vibrational analysis of the structure of gramicidin A. II. Vibrational spectra. *Biophys. J.* 49: 1147–1154.

Nash, R. W., Lindquist, T. D., and Kalina, R. E. (1991) An evaluation of saline irrigation and comparison of povidone-iodine and antibiotic in the surface decontamination of donor eyes. *Arch. Ophthalmol.* 109: 869–872.

Ncher, E., and Eibl, H. (1977) The influence of phospholipid polar groups on gramicidin channels. *Biochim. Biophys. Acta* 464: 37–44.

Nicholson, L. K., Teng, Q., and Cross, T. A. (1991) Solid-state nuclear magnetic resonance derived model for dynamics in the polypeptide backbone of the gramicidin A channel. *J. Mol. Biol.* 218: 621–637.

Olah, G. A., Huang, H. W., Liu, W., and Wu, Y. (1991) Location of ion-binding sites in the gramicidin channel by x-ray diffraction. *J. Mol. Biol.* 218: 847–858.

Prasad, K. U., Alonso-Romanowski, S., Venkatachalam, C. M., Trapane, T. L., and Urry, D. W. (1986) Synthesis, characterization, and black lipid membrane studies of [7-L-alanine] gramicidin A. *Biochemistry* 25: 456–463.

Prasad, K. U., Trapane, T. L., Busath, D., Szabo, G., and Urry, D. W. (1982) Synthesis and characterization of $1\text{-}^{13}\text{C-D-Leu}^{12,14}$ gramicidin A. *Int. J. Peptide Prot. Res.* 19: 162–171.

Prosser, R. S., Davis, J. H., Dahlquist, F. W., and Lindorfer, M. A. (1991) ^2H nuclear magnetic resonance of the gramicidin A backbone in a phospholipid bilayer. *Biochemistry* 30: 4687–4696.

Providence, L. L., Andersen, O. S., Bittman, R., and Koeppe, R. E. II (1991) Gramicidin channel function shows little dependence on phospholipid chirality. *Biophys. J.* 59: 321a.

Ramachandran, G. N., and Chandrasekaran, R. (1972) Conformation of peptide chains containing both L- and D-residues: Part I—helical structures with alternating L- and D-residues with special reference to the LD-ribbon and the LD-helices. *Ind. J. Biochem. Biophys.* 9: 1–11.

Ring, A. (1986) Brief closures of gramicidin A channels in lipid bilayer membranes. *Biochim. Biophys. Acta* 856: 646–653.

Roux, B., and Karplus, M. (1991) Ion transport in a model gramicidin channel. Structure and thermodynamics. *Biophys. J.* 59: 961–981.

Sancho, M., and Martinez, G. (1991) Electrostatic modeling of dipole–ion interactions in gramicidin-like channels. *Biophys. J.* 60: 81–88.

Sarges, R., and Witkop, B. (1965a) Gramicidin A. V. The structure of valine- and isoleucine-gramicidin A. *J. Am. Chem. Soc.* 87: 2011–2020.

Sarges, R., and Witkop, B. (1965b) Gramicidin A. VI. The synthesis of valine- and isoleucine-gramicidin A. *J. Am. Chem. Soc.* 87: 2020–2027.

Sarges, R., and Witkop, B. (1965c) Gramicidin. VII. The structure of valine- and isoleucine-gramicidin B. *J. Am. Chem. Soc.* 87: 2027–2030.

Sarges, R., and Witkop, B. (1965d) Gramicidin. VIII. The structure of valine- and isoleucine-gramicidin C. *Biochemistry* 4: 2491–2494.

Sarkar, N., Langley, D., and Paulus, H. (1979) Studies on the mechanism and specificity of inhibition of ribonucleic acid polymerase by linear gramicidin. *Biochemistry* 18: 4536–4541.

Sawyer, D. B., Williams, L. P., Whaley, W. L., Koeppe, R. E. II, and Andersen, O. S. (1990) Gramicidins A, B, and C form structurally equivalent ion channels. *Biophys. J.* 58: 1207–1212.

Smith, R., Thomas, D. E., Separovic, F., Atkins, A. R., and Cornell, B. A. (1989) Determination of the structure of a membrane-incorporated ion channel. Solid-state nuclear magnetic resonance studies of gramicidin A. *Biophys. J.* 56: 307–314.

Spisni, A., Pasquali-Ronchetti, I., Casali, E., Lindner, L., Cavatorta, P., Masotti, L., and Urry, D. W. (1983) Supramolecular organization of lysophosphatidylcholine-packaged gramicidin A'. *Biochim. Biophys. Acta* 732: 58–68.

Stankovic, C. J., Delfino, J. M., and Schreiber, S. L. (1990) Purification of gramicidin A. *Anal. Biochem.* 184: 100–103.

Stankovic, C. J., Heinemann, S. H., Delfino, J. M., Sigworth, F. J., and Schreiber, S. L. (1989) Trans-membrane channels based on tartaric acid–gramicidin A hybrids. *Science* 244: 813–817.

Szabo, G., and Urry, D. W. (1979) *N*-acetyl gramicidin: single-channel properties and implications for channel structure. *Science* 203: 55–57.

Tank, D. W., Wu, E. S., Meers, P. R., and Webb, W. W. (1982) Lateral diffusion of gramicidin C in phospholipid multibilayers. Effects of cholesterol and high gramicidin concentration. *Biophys. J.* 40: 129–135.

Teng, Q., Koeppe, R. E. II, and Scarlata, S. F. (1991) Effect of salt and membrane fluidity on fluorophore motions of a gramicidin C derivative. *Biochemistry* 30: 7984–7990.

Tosteson, M. T., Auld, D. S., and Tosteson, D. C. (1989) Voltage-gated channels formed in lipid bilayers by a positively charged segment of the Na-channel polypeptide. *Proc. Natl. Acad. Sci. USA* 86: 707–710.

Tournois, H., Fabrie, C.H.J.P., Burger, K.N.J., Mandersloot, J., Hilgers, P., van Dalen, H., de Gier, J., and de Kruijff, B. (1990) Gramicidin A induced fusion of large unilamellar dioleoylphosphatidylcholine vesicles and its relation to the induction of type II nonbilayer structures. *Biochemistry* 29: 8297–8307.

Tournois, H., Gieles, P., Demel, R., de Gier, J., and de Kruijff, B. (1989) Interfacial properties of gramicidin and gramicidin–lipid mixtures measured with static and dynamic monolayer techniques. *Biophys. J.* 55: 557–569.

Tournois, H., Leunissen-Bijvelt, J., Haest, C.W.M., de Gier, J., and de Kruijff, B. (1987) Gramicidin-induced hexagonal H_{II} phase formation in erythrocyte membranes. *Biochemistry* 26: 6613–6621.

Urban, B. W., Hladky, S. B., and Haydon, D. A. (1978) The kinetics of ion movements in the gramicidin channel. *Federation Proc.* 37: 2628–2632.

Urry, D. W. (1971) The gramicidin A transmembrane channel: a proposed $\pi_{(L,D)}$ helix. *Proc. Natl. Acad. Sci. USA* 68: 672–676.

Urry, D. W., Alonso-Romanowski, S., Venkatachalam, C. M., Harris, R. D., and Prasad, K. U. (1984) Dispersity of Des-L-Val[7]-D-Val[8]-gramicidin A single channel conductances argues for different side chain orientations as basis. *Biochem. Biophys. Res. Commun.* 118: 885–893.

Urry, D. W., Goodall, M. C., Glickson, J. D., and Mayers, D. F. (1971) The gramicidin A transmembrane channel: characteristics of head-to-head dimerized $\pi_{(L,D)}$ helices. *Proc. Natl. Acad. Sci. USA* 68: 1907–1911.

Urry, D. W., Trapane, T. L., and Prasad, K. U. (1983) Is the gramicidin A transmembrane channel single-stranded or double-stranded helix? A simple unequivocal determination. *Science* 221: 1064–1067.

Veatch, W. R., and Blout, E. R. (1974) The aggregation of gramicidin A in solution. *Biochemistry* 13: 5257–5263.

Veatch, W. R., Fossel, E. T., and Blout, E. R. (1974) The conformation of gramicidin A. *Biochemistry* 13: 5249–5256.

Veatch, W. R., Mathies, R., Eisenberg, M., and Stryer, L. (1975) Simultaneous fluorescence and conductance studies of planar bilayer membranes containing a highly active and fluorescent analog of gramicidin A. *J. Mol. Biol.* 99: 75–92.

Veatch, W. R., and Stryer, L. (1977) The dimeric nature of the gramicidin A transmembrane channel: conductance and fluorescence energy transfer studies of hybrid channels. *J. Mol. Biol.* 113: 89–102.

Venkatachalam, C. M., and Urry, D. W. (1983) Theoretical conformational analysis of the gramicidin A transmembrane channel. I. Helix sense and energetics of head-to-head dimerization. *J. Comput. Chem.* 4: 461–469.

Wallace, B. A. (1983) Gramicidin A adopts distinctly different conformations in membranes and in organic solvents. *Biopolymers* 22: 397–402.

Wallace, B. A. (1984) Ion-bound forms of the gramicidin A transmembrane channel. *Biophys. J.* 45: 114–116.

Wallace, B. A. (1986) Structure of gramicidin A. *Biophys. J.* 49: 295–306.

Wallace, B. A. (1990) Gramicidin channels and pores. *Annu. Rev. Biophys. Biophys. Chem.* 19: 127–157.

Wallace, B. A., and Blout, E. R. (1979) Conformation of an oligopeptide in phospholipid vesicles. *Proc. Natl. Acad. Sci USA* 76: 1175–1779.

Wallace, B. A., and Janes, R. W. (1991) Co-crystals of gramicidin A and phospholipid. A system for studying the structure of a transmembrane channel. *J. Mol. Biol.* 217: 625–627.

Wallace, B. A., and Ravikumar, K. (1988) The gramicidin pore: crystal structure of a cesium complex. *Science* 241: 182–187.

Wallace, B. A., Veatch, W. R., and Blout, E. R. (1981) Conformation of gramicidin A in phospholipid vesicles: circular dichroism studies of effects of ion binding, chemical modification, and lipid structure. *Biochemistry* 20: 5754–5760.

Weinstein, S., Durkin, J. T., Veatch, W. R., and Blout, E. R. (1985) Conformation of the gramicidin A channel in phospholipid vesicles: a fluorine-19 nuclear magnetic resonance study. *Biochemistry* 24: 4374–4382.

Weinstein, S., Wallace, B. A., Blout, E. R., Morrow, J. S., and Veatch, W. (1979) Conformation of the gramicidin A channel in phospholipid vesicles: A ^{13}C and ^{19}F nuclear magnetic resonance study. *Proc. Natl. Acad. Sci. USA* 76: 4230–4234.

White, S. H., and Jacobs, R. E. (1989) Interfacial hydrophobicity and the insertion of transbilayer helices into lipid bilayers. *Biophys. J.* 55: 399a.

Wu, C. C., Hachimori, A., and Yang, J. T. (1982) Lipid-induced ordered conformations of some peptide hormones and bioactive oligopeptides: predominance of helix over β form. *Biochemistry* 21: 4556–4562.

Wu, C. C., and Yang, J. T. (1981) Sequence-dependent conformations of short polypeptides in a hydrophobic environment. *Mol. Cell. Biochem.* 40: 109–122.

15

Use of Synthetic Peptides
for the Study of Membrane
Protein Structure

J. D. LEAR, Z. R. WASSERMAN, and W. F. DEGRADO

Living cells maintain tenfold or greater concentration gradients of Na^+, K^+, and Ca^{2+} across an ion-impermeant hydrocarbon layer approximately 30 Å thick in their lipid bilayer membranes. Protein "pumps" embedded in these membranes create the gradients, and protein ion channels modulate their discharge in response to various stimuli. Physiological processes involving ion channels range from the very elementary sensory systems of single-celled organisms such as *Escherichia coli* (e.g., Saimi et al., 1988) to the massively interconnected information-processing network of the mammalian brain (e.g., Nicoll, 1988). Historically, ion channels were proposed to be the elementary ion conduction elements in nerve impulse transmission (reviewed by Hille, 1984). Decades of study of nervous system and muscle physiology have since identified hundreds of functionally distinct ion channels. More recently, recombinant DNA technology has provided the amino acid sequences of many ion channel proteins. They appear to form a small number of "families" (Numa, 1989) characterized both by function and by associated, distinguishing features of their sequences. The apparent correlation of sequence features with channel functional type has prompted much curiosity and speculation concerning the three-dimensional structure and mechanisms of functioning of ion channel proteins (see, e.g., Montal, 1990). Most of these proteins, however, contain thousands of amino acid residues. Given our current level of understanding of protein folding, such proteins are far too large and complicated for molecular modeling to provide a satisfactory level of structural detail. With three-dimensional crystal structures, of course, one might hope to pinpoint the features relevant to channel function, but crystals of ion channel proteins have, so far, not provided sufficiently high-resolution diffraction information to resolve sequence-related details. Consequently, other ways are needed to obtain structure–function information from sequence data. Comparative studies of natural sequence variations within channel families (e.g., Butler et al., 1989), functional analysis of site-directed mutations (e.g., Imoto et al., 1988; Stühmer et al., 1989), and studies of synthetic peptides with sequences based on specific channel proteins (e.g., Oiki et al., 1988) are all being used.

In our work we study the ion channel properties of synthetic peptides with very simple, repetitive sequences designed to have some of the structural features thought to be important in the natural proteins (Lear et al., 1988). This approach offers the advantage that molecular models, to explain observed functional properties, have fewer structural possibilities (higher symmetry) than those generated with natural sequences. Also, the simpler sequence peptides can be expected to have somewhat simpler functional properties. The more complex functions of natural proteins might then be built up by introducing modifications and additions designed to test specific hypotheses. Here, we review what peptide studies, particularly the "minimalist approach" (DeGrado et al., 1989), are teaching us about ion channels.

Ion Channel Design Principles

Based on amino acid sequence hydrophobicity (Kyte and Doolittle, 1982) and "hydrophobic moment" (Eisenberg et al., 1984) analysis, many different structural models (e.g., Greenblatt et al., 1985; Guy and Seetharamulu, 1986) have been proposed to explain the particular ion channel characteristics of the different families. All such models contain aggregated, homologous subunits comprising multiple transmembrane segments, usually considered to be α-helical (Fig. 15.1). In their overall transmembrane topology, models such as these are probably correct. This judgement is based on the success of hydrophobicity analysis in predicting (Engleman et al., 1980) the multiple transmembrane α-helical structures of bacteriorhodopsin (Hen-

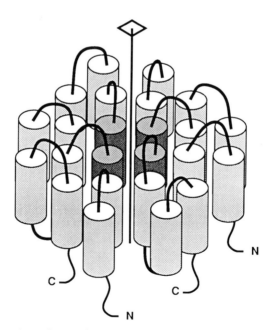

Fig. 15.1. A schematic rendering of proposed models for protein ion channels. Polypeptide subunits comprising multiple transmembrane α-helices with extra- and intracellular connecting segments are shown in a tetrameric aggregate with four central α-helices, presumably amphiphilic, forming an aqueous pore around the C_4 axis.

derson et al., 1990) and on the success of more sophisticated sequence analysis methods (Rees et al., 1989) in accounting for the observed transmembrane folding pattern of the photosynthetic reaction center (Diesenhoefer and Michel, 1989). The homologous subunit structure postulated in models is evident in the amino acid sequence of the single polypeptide sodium channel (Noda et al., 1984). Also, the homologous subunit aggregation structure ($\alpha\beta\alpha\gamma\delta$) of the five separate polypeptides of the nicotinic acetylcholine receptor can be seen in electron diffraction images obtained from two-dimensional crystals (Unwin et al., 1988). However, the following questions are much more difficult to answer on the basis of low-resolution models:

1. What are the underlying principles in the structural framework and arrangement of amino acid residues that allow for such rapid ($\sim 10^8$ s^{-1}) ion conduction through these proteins?
2. Are charged residues necessary for a channel to exhibit charge selectivity?
3. Is ion selectivity based on the channel lining residues or on structures near the channel ends?
4. Which features of the protein structure control the opening and closing kinetics of ion channels?

Synthetic peptides can be used to help answer these questions.

Synthetic Peptide Ion Channel Design

The most direct use of peptides to investigate protein ion channel structure is premised on models such as that shown in Figure 15.1 (Lear et al., 1988) in which the ion-permeant channel is formed by a specific subset of the α-helical segments surrounding the axis of symmetry. If these particular α-helices can exist in a transmembrane orientation independent of how the rest of the protein is structured, it is not unreasonable to expect that peptides with sequences chosen to represent those helices will be able at least partly to reproduce the ion channel function of the full protein. Synthetic peptides of at least 20 residues, and with sequences chosen from putative channel-forming segments of various ion channel proteins, have been made and investigated for their channel-forming properties. Peptides representing the cation-selective *Torpedo* acetylcholine receptor (Oiki et al., 1988), the anion-selective glycine receptor from rat spinal cord (Langosch et al., 1991), the voltage-gated, sodium-selective channel from rat brain (two different segments: S2 [Oiki et al., 1988] and S4 [Tosteson et al., 1989]), and the calcium-selective channel from skeletal muscle (Grove et al., 1991) all have been found to produce discrete ion channel conductance states. In the first and last cases cited above, control peptides of equal length, but from more hydrophobic segments, did not produce channel activity, supporting both the general premise of the work and the specific choice of segments. However, all of these peptides formed cation selective channels (although anion selectivity was seen in some of the channels formed by the glycine receptor M2 segment), and the channels from the sodium and potassium channel peptides were not particularly selective for their namesake ions. These differences between peptide and "parent" channel characteristics indicate a role for other segments of the protein in constraining peptide orientations and/or a need for longer segments to represent channel end structures better. Interestingly, however, the calcium channel peptides, prepared using

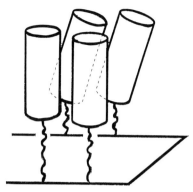

Fig. 15.2. Representation of the "template" strategy (Mütter et al., 1989) for making tetramer aggregates. The *lower line* represents a polypeptide chain containing lysine residues to which the α-helix-forming segments (cylinders) can be attached via short peptide branch segments *(wavy lines)*.

a"template" peptide (Mutter et al., 1989) to favor a tetrameric structure (diagrammed in Fig. 15.2), produced channels that responded to known calcium channel blockers much like the parent peptide, supporting the idea that the natural channel structure was being reproduced to an important extent.

Complementing the above-described approach, we are studying the physical chemistry underlying ion channel structure–function relationships using peptides not found in natural sequences, but rather designed de novo to contain only the essential features of proposed transmembrane ion channel models. Three criteria were considered in designing these peptides.

Secondary Structure

We chose the α-helix as a secondary structural framework because of its stability relative to other structures in a transmembrane environment. The physical reason for this is that the free energy difference between transferring hydrogen-bonded versus unbonded amide groups from water into a nonpolar solvent favors the bonded structure by nearly 5 kcal/mol per pair of amide groups (Roseman, 1988). Consequently, the intramolecular hydrogen bonds of the α-helix (as well as any formed by side chains; Jacobs and White, 1989) help to stabilize transmembrane segments. The geometry of the α-helix (length 1.5 Å per residue) and the thickness of the bilayer hydrocarbon (30 Å) together fix the minimum number of amino acid residues needed to cross the membrane interior at 20. It should be noted that only nine residues would be required for transmembrane β-strands (3.5 Å per residue) such as those observed in bacterial porins, large-diameter channels found in the outer wall of gram-negative bacteria (reviewed by Jap and Walian, 1990). Also, recent evidence from site-directed mutagenesis (Hartmann et al., 1991; Yellen et al., 1991; Yool et al., 1991) suggests that β-structures form at least part of the ion conduction pathway in voltage-gated potassium channels. However, our experience with α-helix design (Ho and DeGrado, 1987) and the difficulties others (Richardson and Richardson, 1989) have experienced with the design of water-soluble β-barrel structures, prompted us to begin with α-helices.

Amphiphilicity

The fundamental structural idea we wished to explore was whether ion channels can be formed by aggregated, amphiphilic transmembrane α-helices. To do this, a sequence of at least 20 amino acid residues is needed containing two different types of residues. One should be small and polar to provide a channel lining of sufficient diameter and polarity to accommodate ions such as potassium and chloride. The other should be apolar to favor exposure to the membrane hydrocarbon interior. Both residues should favor α-helix formation and should be uncharged to improve the chances for adopting an inserted, transmembrane configuration. Serine (small and polar) and leucine (large and apolar) satisfied these criteria. The hydoxyl groups of serine were also expected to provide ion solvation properties similar to water. This was considered to be important to avoid impeding the rate of ion passage by large energetic barriers or wells caused by differences in charge solvation along the ion permeation pathway.

Aggregate Structure

To improve the possibility for a stable, aggregated pore structure, the sequence (Fig. 15.3) was designed on the basis of a threefold repetitive heptad. The exact 3.5 residue periodicity allows the possibility of indefinitely long, straight coiled-coil aggregate structures (Cohen and Parry, 1990) with the large leucine residues involved in a "knobs-into-holes" packing arrangement such as that observed in coiled-coil proteins such as ROP (Banner et al., 1987) and the leucine "zipper" of GCN4 (O'Shea et al., 1991).

(LSSLLSL)₃–CONH₂: A Cation-Selective Channel Former

The first sequence designed on the above principles was based on the heptamer repeat LSSLLSL. Peptide synthesis and purification were accomplished by segment

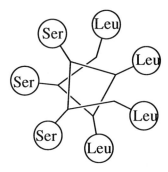

LSSLLSL Heptad Repeat

Fig. 15.3. Axial projection of a 3.5 repeat period α-helix of amino acid resides leucine (L) and serine (S) in the heptad sequence chosen for model ion channel studies.

condensation (DeGrado and Kaiser, 1980) of these heptad repeats. (In subsequent work, we have found that standard solid-phase synthesis, using quite different [BOC] chemistry, provides peptides with comparable channel-forming activity, eliminating the possibility of impurity-dominated channel effects, a significant concern in doing single-channel studies.) A 14 residue "control" peptide $(LSSLLSL)_2$–$CONH_2$ was also made (by condensation of two instead of three segments) to test the premise that at least 20 residues were necessary for stable transmembrane channel structures.

When incorporated into planar bilayers under conditions allowing single-channel conductance states to be detected in 0.5 M KCl, the 14 residue control peptide produced membrane perturbations similar to those reported (Tosteson et al., 1987) for the bee venom peptide melittin but did not produce the square wave currents characteristic of stable ion channel structures. However, the full 21 residue $(LSSLLSL)_3$–$CONH_2$ peptide did produce such currents. The distribution of conductance levels showed one predominant state that conducted cations smaller than approximately 8 Å. Chloride ion conductance was estimated from electrolyte substitution experiments to be less than one-tenth of the total ion conductance in 0.5 M or less KCl solutions. The "gating" properties were interesting in that greater numbers of channel openings per unit time were observed with voltages held negative on the side of the bilayer from which peptide had been incorporated, and the channel opening frequency increased quite sharply with voltage. The average time any channel stayed open, however, appeared to be independent of the voltage. These observations (Lear et al., 1988) provided a basis for a more detailed molecular modeling study.

Molecular Modeling the Possible Structures of Peptide Channels

Computer graphics and energy minimization were used to create molecular models for $(LSSLLSL)_3$–$CONH_2$. α-Helices were arranged in bundles with the polar side chains oriented toward the bundle center. The fact that channel activity was not symmetrical with voltage reversal across the bilayer suggested that the individual helices were oriented parallel to one another. Modeling aimed for local minimum energy conformations, allowing close packing of side chains between neighboring helices.

Various models of trimers, tetramers, pentamers, and hexamers of helical bundles were constructed. The best (those with the closest side chain packing and the lowest energies) all had C_n symmetry (n being the aggregation number). Two of these models, a tetramer and a hexamer, are shown in Figure 15.4. The tetramer model has a pore diameter of less than 1 Å, effectively precluding alkalai metal cation conduction. The hexamer model, however, has a pore diameter of 8 Å, consistent with the observed ion permeation cut-off between Tris and glucosammonium cations. An interesting feature of the hexamer model is the extensive hydrogen bonding between each serine hydroxyl hydrogen at residue i and the amide group carbonyl oxygen at residue i-4. Such an arrangement of hydrogen bonds is frequently observed in protein crystal structures (Baker and Hubbard, 1984) and could play a role in determining our peptide channel's charge selectivity, since it projects the lone pairs of the electronegative serine oxygen into the channel. This arrangement should create a negative electrostatic environment in the channel, favoring cation solvation.

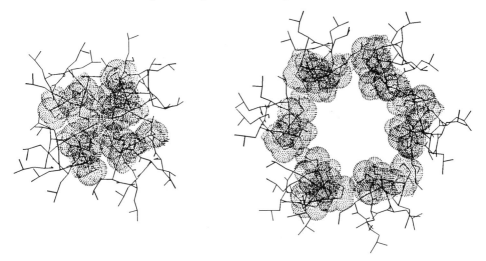

Fig. 15.4. Molecular models of parallel bundles of $(LSSLLSL)_3$–$CONH_2$ packed with C_4 *(left)* and C_6 *(right)* symmetry. Serine residues are shown with van der Walls surfaces to allow visual estimation of pore sizes.

$(LSLLLSL)_3$–$CONH_2$: A Proton-Selective Channel Former

Having established that $(LSSLLSL)_3$–$CONH_2$ makes channels, we next considered the question of how to change the amino acid arrangement to change the channel conduction properties. It is instructive to use single ion channel conductance values along with equivalent ionic conductances in bulk water to calculate the approximate physical dimensions of an equivalent-conductance, cylindrical, water-filled pore. The conductance of the $(LSSLLSL)_3$–$CONH_2$ channel as measured above was 70 pS in 0.5 M KCl. Using the known equivalent ionic conductance for potassium in aqueous 0.5 M KCl (0.074 S cm^2/M), the calculated area/length ratio for a simple water-filled pore of 70 pS conductance with 0.5 M potassium is approximately 0.2 Å. This translates into a diameter of 3 Å over the 30 Å length of the bilayer. Since the physical diameter of the channel was found to be much larger than 3 Å, this is a clear indication that the channel interior is different from bulk water. It also indicates considerable potential for varying the channel conductance properties simply by reducing the channel diameter. The effect of this on ionic conductance could exceed expectations based on hydrodynamic considerations (Eldridge and Morowitz, 1978). The reason is that the channel pore dimensions are of the same order of magnitude as atomic radii, introducing the possibility of selectivity arising both from "sieving" effects (Mullens, 1959) and from highly size-dependent differences in ion solvation energies (Eisenman, 1962; see discussion of both influences by Armstrong, 1989).

With the aggregated α-helices shown in Figure 15.4, pore diameter is determined both by the number of helices in the aggregate and by the size and spatial arrangement of amino acid side chains facing the aggregate axis of symmetry. Even without detailed molecular modeling, inspection of a tetrameric arrangement of a seven residue internal sequence in the $(LSSLLSL)_3$–$CONH_2$ peptide (SLLSSLL), viewed in

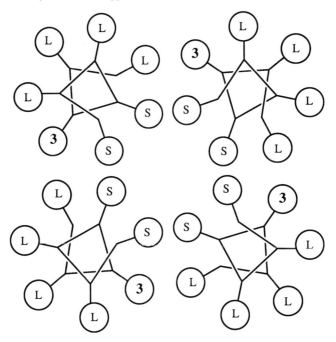

Fig. 15.5. A schematic representaion of a tetrameric aggregate of the internal sequence SLLS__LL showing the projection toward the helix–helix interface of the position 3 residue(__) in the channel peptide LS__LLSL heptad repeat.

an α-helical axial projection (Fig. 15.5), suggested replacing serine residue 3 in each heptad repeat by leucine. This would eliminate the potentially unfavorable placement of the polar serine group in the hydrophobic helix packing interface and leave a structure with a small, central pore lined with serines. Consequently, we made and characterized the channel properties of $(LSLLLSL)_3$–$CONH_2$. Discrete, millisecond time-scale single-channel openings and closings qualitatively similar to $(LSSLLSL)_3$–$CONH_2$ were found, but the channels could only be measured in relatively concentrated (>0.1 M) HCl. No alkali metal cation conductance could be measured. (Macroscopic current noise analysis measurements (unpublished data) made of $[LSLLLSL]_3$–$CONH_2$ channel conductance in 0.5 M HCl successively replaced with 1 M LiCl down to 0.016 M H^+ concentration have confirmed our earlier estimate that Li^+ conductance is <5% of the proton channel conductance.) This result is consistent with the difference in pore diameters calculated from molecular modeling.

Changing the Channel Lining Residues

Having succeeded in making the channel smaller, presumably by changing the aggregation number, we next considered changing the channel "lining" residues. One feature of particular interest in the $(LSSLLSL)_3$–$CONH_2$ channel is its cation selectivity. If, as previously mentioned, this arises from the serine intrahelical

hydrogen-bonding pattern, this channel might be made permeant to anions by changing the channel lining to provide a less negative dipolar electrical potential. This
might be done simply by making the channel larger so that it more closely resembles
water. The porins, for example (reviewed by Jap and Walian, 1990), although more
complex in structure, appear to be effectively larger than 8 Å cylindrical pores based
on their being permeable to mono-, di-, and trisaccharides, and they also readily con-
duct anions (Benz, 1984). We wished, however, to stay close to the properties of our
smaller diameter channels so we looked to the sequences of the naturally occurring
anion channels for clues. One modification we tried provides an instructive example
of the difficulties associated with these studies.

Examination of the hydrophobic sequences from the $GABA_A$ (Schofield et al.,
1987) and glycine (Grenningloh et al., 1987) receptors, both anion-selective channels, showed an XTT motif (X apolar) in the "M2" sequences thought to form the
channel lining. The resemblance to the LSSLLSL heptad sequence prompted us to
modify the $(LSSLLSL)_3$–$CONH_2$ hexamer model to accommodate threonine residues in place of the serines. The channel lining of the $(LTTLLTL)_3$–$CONH_2$ hexamer model (Fig. 15.6A) was significantly different; the 8 Å diameter is reduced to
about 5 Å by the threonine methyl groups. Since these groups projecting into the
channel interior are much less polar than the serine oxygens, we reasoned that they
could change the relative energetics of cation and anion solvation within the channel
and, therefore, the charge selectivity.

$(LTTLLTL)_3$–$CONH_2$ was made (L. A. Chung, unpublished data) and, after
N-terminal acetylation, ion channels were characterized as before in planar bilayers.
(Unpublished work in our laboratories by R. Mahlangu showed N-terminal acetylation to maintain the cationic charge selectivity of $(LSSLLSL)_3$–$CONH_2$ while
increasing the average open channel lifetime by over tenfold. Nonacetylated
$[LTTLLTL]_3$–$CONH_2$ produced very short (<1 ms) lifetime channels that could
not be resolved into a sufficiently narrow distribution of conductance states to char-

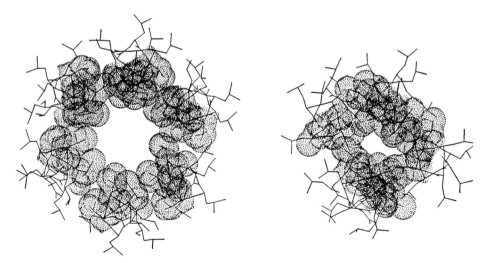

Fig. 15.6. Molecular models of $(LTTLLTL)_3$–$CONH_2$ aggregates. Threonine residues are
shown with van der Walls surfaces. *A*: hexamer model; *B*: tetramer model.

acterize channel selectivity. N-terminal acetylation increased the average lifetime to 10 ms, which allowed the protonic conductance to be characterized by measuring the effect of LiCl substitution [for HCl] on the conductance state distribution maximum [see Fig. 15.7].) Unexpectedly, we observed a proton-selective channel similar to that previously measured for the $(LSLLLSL)_3$–$CONH_2$ channel (Fig. 15.7). Modeling the threonine peptide as a tetramer instead of the hexamer (Fig. 15.6B) provided a reasonable explanation for this result; the threonine methyl group packs well into the helix–helix interface of the tetramer bundle, filling the void that would otherwise be present with serines in equivalent positions. As presumed for the $(LSLLLSL)_3$–$CONH_2$ structure, this packing could so stabilize the smaller aggregation number states that too few of the larger aggregation number states would form to be observed under our measurement conditions.

The above account underscores a problem facing not only peptide studies of channel function, but also directed mutagenesis studies of all proteins; amino acid residues can and frequently do play multiple roles in determining protein structure and specific substrate interactions (Knowles, 1987). This problem can be even more severe for small peptide studies because of the greater proportionate effect of any amino acid changes. Because of this problem, additional constraints on structure need to be introduced to make further progress in defining how channel lining might affect ion selectivity properties. The general approach of using peptides constrained to definite aggregation states (Mutter et al., 1989; Akerfeldt et al., 1992) appears promising because, in principle, it "decouples" peptide aggregation from amino acid sequence, allowing a wider range of sequence variabity to be explored.

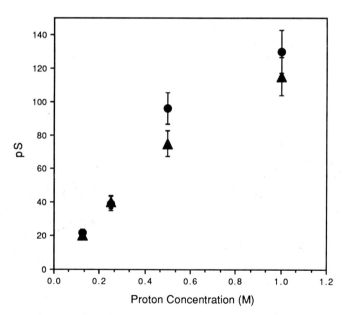

Fig. 15.7. Peptide channel conductances measured near 100 mY transmembrane potential in HCl/LiCl mixtures for $(LSLLLLSL)_3$–$CONH_2$ *(circles)* and Ac-$(LTTLLTL)_3$–$CONH_2$ *(triangles)*. Points at less than the highest noted proton concentrations were obtained by successive dilutions of HCl electrolyte with 1 M LiCl solutions.

Structural Aspects of the Opening and Closing of Channels

The gating kinetics of natural protein ion channels shows considerable diversity. Nerve sodium and potassium channels, for example, typically show a highly cooperative, voltage and voltage-history dependence of their open state probabilities, with wide ranging kinetic diversity among family subtypes. With some natural channels, gating kinetics is sufficiently complex that the lifetime distributions are more elegantly described using the mathematics of fractals rather than of equilibrium state transitions (Liebovitch et al., 1987). Also, changes in gating kinetics induced, for example, by protein phosphorylation (Greengard, 1976), can play an important regulatory role in cellular functions. Understanding the structural basis of channel gating is, therefore, of great scientific interest.

In considering possible relationships between peptide and protein channel gating mechanisms, it is important to realize that single-channel openings and closings are molecular scale events. In single-channel measurements, time resolution is limited to the microsecond or greater range, which is very long in comparison to molecular-scale vibration and rotation periods. Consequently, very different molecular processes connecting open and closed states can give identically appearing channel conductances. Detailed kinetic characterization of channel lifetimes is useful, but only to differentiate experimentally among broad classes of channel gating mechanisms because, for kinetics complex enough to require multiple open and closed states, many different mechanisms can produce the same kinetics (Kienker, 1989). However, an attractive aspect of the peptides we have been studying is that their kinetics appears to be relatively uncomplicated. This affords an opportunity to use channel lifetime data to propose and experimentally test, using other biophysical methods, specific gating mechanisms.

The gating kinetics of single channels is reflected in the statistics of their open and closed times. For large numbers of openings and closings that have no memory of previous state dwell times (Markovian processes), and that originate from transitions between only two possible states, single exponential functions can fully describe the distributions of both open and closed times (Colquhoun and Hawkes, 1983). The corresponding relaxation times are characteristic of the individual state transition probabilities, and the reciprocals of these times are the first order rate constants for the state changes. We might expect small, channel-forming peptides to have such simple kinetics because they have far fewer conformational possibilities than the larger ion channel proteins. In fact, the frequency distributions of both open times and times between openings for our peptide channels were found, to a first approximation, to be reasonably well described by single exponential distributions. (More sensitive methods for lifetime analysis [see Fig. 15.9] show that two exponential components provide better fits to the lifetime distributions, particularly to the closed time distributions. However, the statistical significance of the second exponential has not been rigorously established in our studies.) The average open times were relatively insensitive to the transmembrane voltage, but the closed times showed significant sensitivity both to voltage and to the amount of peptide incorporated into the bilayer. The voltage dependence was particularly interesting because some natural channels and peptides also show voltage-dependent opening kinetics. Consequently, we undertook to explain it in structural terms.

One possibility investigated (DeGrado and Lear, 1990) was that channel opening might involve a change of secondary structure. To test this, we used the peptide $(LSLBLSL)_3-CONH_2$, where B denotes α-aminoisobutyric acid, a residue that is sterically restricted to helical conformations (reviewed by Prasad and Balaram, 1984). Measured in diphytanoyl phosphatidylcholine vesicles in the absence of a membrane potential, this peptide gave a typical α-helical circular dichroism spectrum that was essentially identical to those similarly measured (L. A. Chung, unpublished data) for $(LSSLLSL)_3-CONH_2$ and $(LSLLLSL)_3-CONH_2$. Incorporated into planar bilayers, the peptide produced channels that, while shorter lived, showed voltage-dependent gating and proton conductance nearly the same as the $(LSLLLSL)_3-CONH_2$ peptide. This establishes with a fair degree of certainty that the peptides are helical in both open and closed channel states.

A possible three-state scheme (DeGrado and Lear, 1990) to account for the peptides' observed concentration- and voltage-dependent opening kinetics is

$$\text{Closed 1} \leftrightarrow \text{Closed 2} \leftrightarrow \text{Open}$$

where the equilibrium constant between closed states 1 and 2 depends on voltage. A geometric model of peptide–bilayer interactions that could underly such a mechanism is shown diagrammatically in Figure 15.8. Similar to models proposed for the antibiotic, channel-forming peptide alamethicin (reviewed by Hall et al., 1986), the voltage dependence of channel openings is related to a voltage-induced change in the relative proportions of the two different orientations of the peptide in the lipid membrane. In the absence of a transmembrane voltage, the horizontal orientation depicted in Figure 15.8a is expected to be more stable than the perpendicular orientation because the polar serine residues, on one side of the α-helix, can remain exposed to the aqueous exterior of the membrane while the apolar leucines on the other side can remain in the bilayer interior. However, because the α-helix has an electrical dipole moment, a transmembrane electrical potential can reduce the energy difference between the parallel and perpendicular orientations. Quantitatively, the difference will be equal to the energy of transferring one of the effective "end charges" to the different potential on the opposite side of the membrane. With our peptides, the N terminus has not only the $+0.6$ effective charge due to the α-helical dipole moment, but also has the formal $+1$ charge from protonation of the terminal amino group. (The value $+0.6$, higher than the generally accepted ± 0.5 e^- effective end charges for the α-helix dipole of aqueous proteins, was computed using Pethig's calculation (1979) of 5.3 ± 0.5 D for the limiting per residue dipole moment of a rigid, straight α-helix based on dielectric relaxation of poly[benzyl L-glutamate] in m-cresol.) The C terminus has only the effective α-helical dipole charge because it is blocked with a carboxamide group. We observe, for peptide added only to the membrane cis side, a preference for channel formation with a $trans$-positive potential. Presumably, this preference reflects a large energetic barrier associated with inserting the formally charged N terminus into the bilayer.

This general concept of dipole reorientation can be used to make a quantitative prediction of the steepness of the voltage dependence for single-channel closed time intervals. For measurement conditions in which the probability that any particular channel will open more than once is very small, the time between channel openings will depend on the fraction of peptide in the "active," perpendicular orientation. If this fraction is small enough so that only single-channel openings are seen, the aver-

A.

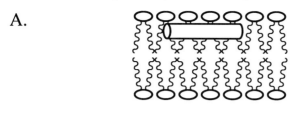

B.

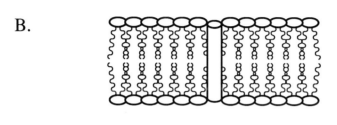

C.

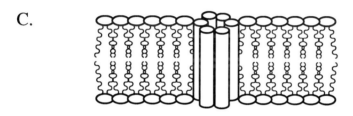

Fig. 15.8. Proposed model for the voltage-dependent frequency of channel openings. *A*: The predominant closed state. The peptide is oriented parallel to the plane of the bilayer in the lipid headgroup region of the membrane. *B*: The minor, voltage-dependent closed state fraction. The transmembrane orientation is made less energetically unfavorable by the alignment of the helical dipole moment with the electric field. *C*: An observable open state. Conducting ion channels are formed by aggregates of transmembrane-oriented peptide.

age time between openings (τ) should be proportional to the number of active peptides in the membrane. Based on Boltzmann statistics, the proportion of membrane-associated peptide in the transmembrane orientation should, as discussed above, increase exponentially with the transmembrane voltage. The steepness of this increase is conveniently expressed as the number of "gating charges" (z) transferred across the membrane potential difference. The equation used is

$$z = (RT/F)d(ln\,\tau)/dV = 25.4d(ln\,\tau/dV)$$

for V in mV at 20°C.

Single-channel open time and closed time interval distributions at three different transmembrane voltages, measured in an experiment with $(LSSLLSL)_3–CONH_2$ in 0.1 M HCl are shown in Figure 15.9. A logarithmic binning representation (Sigworth and Sine, 1987) is used that exhibits maxima at the exponential distribution

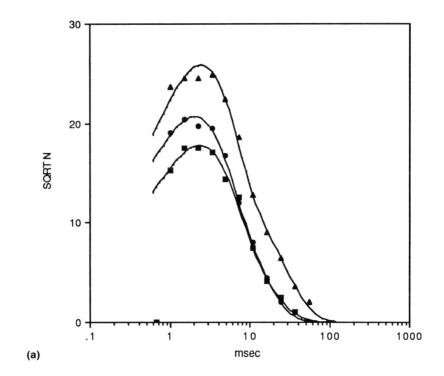

(a)

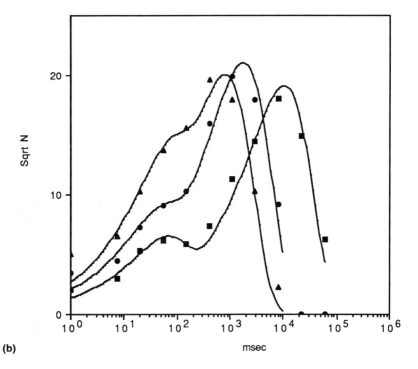

(b)

348

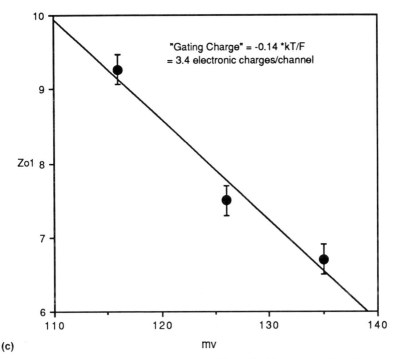

(c)

Fig. 15.9. Peptide channel gating data. A: Logarithmically binned open time histograms measured for $(LSSLLSL)_3$ channels in 0.1 M HCl at transmembrane potentials of 116 *(squares)*, 126 *(circles)*, and 135 *(triangles)* mV in an experiment with no other changes in bilayer conditions. The ordinate of the plots is the square root of the bin count (N). Solid lines are curve fits to the distribution function form: $N = \Sigma_i \{A_i \exp\{(z - z_{oi}) - \exp(z - z_{oi})\}$, where $z = Ln(t)$, $z_{oi} = Ln(t_{oi})$, t is the lower bin time, and t_{oi} is the *ith* exponential decay constant (Sigworth and Sine, 1983). Fits with two exponentials ($i = 1,2$) were used with parameter values:

Voltage	A_1	z_{o1}	A_2	z_{o2}
116	768 ± 93	0.8 ± 0.1	114 ± 97	1.7 ± 0.2
126	944 ± 107	0.6 ± 0.1	270 ± 114	1.4 ± 0.1
135	$1{,}638 \pm 87$	0.8 ± 0.1	293 ± 83	2.0 ± 0.1

B: Histograms as above except closed time distribution data and fits are shown. Data include only events with well-defined intervals between openings; closed time intervals containing any questionable intervening events (e.g., multiple openings or membrane noise bursts) were rejected from analysis. Parameter values from regression fitting were

Voltage	A_1	z_{o1}	A_2	z_{o2}
116	992 ± 77	9.3 ± 0.1	97 ± 27	4.1 ± 0.4
126	$1{,}200 \pm 83$	7.5 ± 0.1	137 ± 39	3.7 ± 0.4
135	$1{,}088 \pm 111$	6.7 ± 0.1	347 ± 83	4.1 ± 0.3

C: Values of z_{o1} (corresponding to the A_1 component in the closed time distribution fits) are plotted versus the transmembrane voltage to determine a value for gating charge. The least-squares-fit line has a slope of 0.14 ± 0.03 mV^{-1}, corresponding to a gating charge of 3.4 ± 0.7 electronic charge units.

average times. The open times (Fig. 15.9a) are, as mentioned, independent of the voltage. From the voltage-dependent component of the closed time distributions (Fig. 15.9b), we calculate (Fig. 15.9c) a gating charge of 3.4. This is within experimental error of the 3.6 charges expected for an open state comprising six aggregated, parallel-packed transmembrane α-helices, assuming that the majority of the peptide is in the nontransmembrane closed state depicted in Figure 15.8a and that the peptides insert primarily by translocating their C termini across the bilayer. The voltage-independent component of the closed time distributions in Figure 15.9b is of uncertain origin, but the presence of two exponential components in the distribution is consistent with a kinetics scheme involving two closed states (Colquhoun and Hawkes, 1983).

The predominant state of the (LSSLLSL)$_3$-CONH$_2$ peptide in our single-channel experiments most likely represents a closed state because the channels, presumably arising from very few molecules, are observed in the presence of billions of potentially channel-forming peptide molecules. To investigate the secondary structure and orientation of these closed state molecules using fluorescence techniques, a tryptophan substitution peptide study (O'Neil and DeGrado, 1987) was done. A series of seven (LSSLLSL)$_3$-CONH$_2$ variant peptides was made in which each variant contained a tryptophan substituted for each successive residue in the middle heptad (Chung et al., 1990). The peptides were incorporated into small, unilamellar, diphytanoyl phosphatidylcholine vesicles at peptide-lipid ratios of $<1:100$ to approximately represent the proportions of lipid and peptide used in the planar bilayer studies. Measurements were made of the peptides' circular dichroism and fluorescence spectra and of the quenching of their tryptophan fluorescence by both aqueous- and lipid hydrocarbon-associated quenchers. The circular dichroism spectra and the observed sequence periodicity of all fluorescence and fluorescence quenching data were consistent with an α-helical peptide located at a lipid–water interface. Static fluorescence quenching measurements, using the "parallax method" (Chattopadhyay and London, 1987) with a series of lipids bearing acyl chain-bound nitroxide group quenchers, showed the peptide's helical axis to be oriented parallel to the surface of the vesicle membrane and located a few angstroms below the polar headgroup–hydrocarbon boundary (Chung et al., 1992). This result supports the helical dipole reorientation model used to interpret the gating charge result.

It is, perhaps, important to reemphasize that the mechanism by which these small peptide channels open and close can be quite different from mechanisms involved in protein voltage-gated ion channels (see review by Catterall, 1988). The latter contain a conserved, repetitive motif (RXX)$_n$ where R represents a positively charged arginine (or lysine) and X is generally hydrophobic. It has been proposed that the (RXX)$_n$ segment forms a transmembrane helix that moves in a screw-like manner in response to membrane depolarization, the movement being coupled structurally to channel opening. Alternatively, the (RXX)$_n$ segment has been proposed (Lear, 1990) to form a charged, amphipathic helix oriented parallel to the bilayer surface, but with membrane depolarization-induced movements still coupled structurally to channel opening. In any case, the voltage-dependent opening kinetics observed for these protein channels (e.g., Quandt, 1987; Liman et al., 1991) is much more complex than that observed for peptide channels, most likely reflecting more complex structural rearrangements.

Summary

It is appropriate to ask at this point what has been learned from studying de novo designed and synthetic segments of ion channel proteins. Studies with peptides do seem to have demonstrated the general soundness of proposing that ion channels can be formed by aggregated, amphiphilic α-helices. We have shown that, for such structures, a sequence length greater than 14 residues is important, that amino acid sequence can affect channel conductance characteristics, and that significant cation selectivity can be attained without charged residues in the sequence. For anion selectivity, we do not yet know if charged residues are necessary or where they should be placed. We hope to make progress toward answering these questions by developing better channel characterization methods (e.g., voltage pulse methods for measuring single-channel current-voltage curves) and applying them to peptides of slightly different sequences designed to share a common structure. Regarding channel opening and closing, our work shows that highly complex protein "machinery" is not necessary to produce elementary, channel-like ion conduction through membranes. However, the "gating" kinetics we observe lacks many of the more complex features associated with natural protein channels. Their detailed gating features such as voltage and ligand-binding enhancement of opening probability and phosphorylation-modulated closing rates have important physiological functions, so there appears to be good reason for channel proteins to have evolved as such large structures.

Many different peptides, including some from natural sources other than the ion channels discussed here (see, e.g., reviews by Bernheimer and Rudy, 1986, and Sansom, 1991) are now known to form distinct conductance, ion channel states. We can surmise from this that the sequence requirements for making relatively stable, ion-conducting transmembrane aggregates of α-helices are not very stringent. However, we also know that peptides of different sequences can have different conduction properties. Even apparently minor sequence changes such as we made in changing $(LSSLLSL)_3$-$CONH_2$ to $(LSLLLSL)_3$-$CONH_2$ can have a very large effect. The unfortunate corollary of this is that efforts to modify the properties of a given structure by making sequence changes such as we attempted to do with the Ac-$(LTTLLTL)_3$-$CONH_2$ peptide are bound to encounter difficulties because the amino acid sequence influences both structure and functionality. Perhaps an important lesson from our experience is that these difficulties do not require very complex sequences to show up. Consequently, the design of even relatively small, simple functional proteins is a challenging exercise. The fact that this and related protein design endeavors (see review by Betz et al., 1993) have been at all successful does demonstrate that de novo design of functional polypeptides, including membrane proteins, is possible. We hope that continued efforts in this direction will complement the many other approaches being taken to increase our fundamental understanding of the structure–function relationships of natural membrane proteins.

Acknowledgments

We acknowledge with sincere appreciation the many coworkers who made essential contributions to this work: peptide synthesis, Ivan Turner, Arlene Rockwell, Sharon Jackson; peptide mass spectrometry analysis, Barbara Larsen; computer programming, John Kallal and Richard Hilmer; bilayer measurements, Dan Camac; computer graphics, James Krywko.

Special appreciation is extended to Howard E. Simmons Jr., Richard Quisenberry, Mark Pearson, and Stephen Brenner for their interest and support through Du Pont's Central Research and Development Department and to the Office of Naval Research for a postdoctoral program grant to W. F. DeGrado for support of Laura Ann Chung.

References

Akerfeldt, K. S., Kim, R. M., Camac, D., Groves, J. T., Lear, J. D., DeGrado, W. F. (1992) Tetraphilin: a four-helix proton channel built on a tetraphenylporphyrin framework. *J. Am. Chem. Soc.* 114: 9656–9657.

Armstrong, C. M. (1989) Reflections on selectivity. In: *Membrane Transport. People and Ideas,* edited by J. C. Tosteson. New York: Oxford University Press.

Baker, E. N., and Hubbard, R. E. (1984) Hydrogen bonding in globular proteins. *Prog. Biophys. Mol. Biol.* 44: 97–179.

Banner, D. W., Kokkinidis, M., and Tsernoglou, D. (1987) Structure of the ColE1 Rop protein at 1.7 Å resolution. *J. Mol. Biol.* 196: 657–675.

Benz, R. (1984) Structure and selectivity of porin channels. *Curr. Top. Membrane Transport* 21: 199–219.

Bernheimer, A. W., and Rudy, B. (1986) Interactions between membranes and cytolytic peptides. *Biochim. Biophys. Acta* 864: 123–141.

Betz, S. F., Raleigh, D. P., and DeGrado W. F. (1993) *De novo* protein design: from molten globules to native-like states. *Curr. Opinion Struct. Biol.* 3: 601–610.

Butler, A., Wei, A., Baker, K., and Salkoff, L. (1989) A family of putative potassium channel genes in *Drosophila. Science* 243: 943–947.

Catterall, W. A. (1988) Structure and function of voltage-sensitive ion channels. *Science* 242: 50–61.

Chattopadhyay, A., and London, E. (1987) Parallax method for direct measurement of membrane penetration depth utilizing fluorescence quenching by spin-labeled phospholipids. Biochemistry 26: 39–45.

Chung, L. A., DeGrado, W. F., and Lear, J. D. (1990) Orientation of a model ion channel peptide in lipid vesicles. *Biophys. J.* 57: 462a.

Chung, L. A., Lear, J. D., and DeGrado, W. F. (1992) Fluorescence study of the secondary structure and orientation of a model ion channel peptide in phospholipid vesicles. *Biochemistry* 31: 6608–6616.

Cohen, V., and Parry, D.A.D. (1990) α-Helical coils and bundles: how to design an α-helical protein. *Proteins* 7: 1–15.

Colquhoun, D., and Hawkes, A. G. (1983) The principles of the stochastic interpretation of ion-channel mechanisms. 135–175 In: *Single-Channel Recording,* edited by B. Sakmann and E. Neher. New York: Plenum.

DeGrado, W. F., and Kaiser, E. T. (1980) Polymer-based oxime esters as supports for solid-phase peptide synthesis. Preparation of protected fragments. *J. Org. Chem.* 45: 1295–1300.

DeGrado, W. F., and Lear, J. D. (1990) Conformationally constrained α-helical peptide models for protein ion channels. *Biopolymerization* 29: 209–213.

DeGrado, W. F., Wasserman, Z. R., and Lear, J. D. (1989) Protein design, a minimalist approach. *Science* 243: 622–628.

Diesenhoefer, J., and Michel, H. (1989) The photosynthetic reaction center from the purple bacterium *Rhodopseudomonas viridis. Science* 245: 1463–1473.

Eisenberg, D., Schwartz, E., Komaromy, M., and Wall, R. (1984) Analysis of membrane and surface protein sequences with the hydrophobic moment plot. *J. Mol. Biol.* 179: 125–142.

Eisenman, G. (1962) Cation selective glass electrodes and mode of operation. *Biophys. J.* 2(Suppl. 2): 259–323.

Eldridge, C., and Morowitz, H. J. (1978) A hydrodynamic theory for ion conduction through ohmic pores. *J. Theor. Biol.* 73: 539–548.

Engleman, D. M., Henderson, R., McLachlan, A. D., and Wallace, B. A. (1980) Path of the polypeptide in bacteriorhodopsin. *Proc. Natl. Acad. Sci. USA* 77: 2023–2027.

Greenblatt, R. E., Blatt, Y., and Montal, M. (1985) The structure of the voltage-sensitive sodium channel. *FEBS Lett.* 193(2): 125–134.

Greengard, P. (1976) Possible role for cyclic nucleotides and phosphorylated membrane proteins in postsynaptic actions of neurotransmitters. *Nature* 260: 101–108.

Grove, A., Tomich, J. M., and Montal, M. (1991) A molecular blueprint for the pore-forming structure of voltage-gated calcium channels. *Proc. Natl. Acad. Sci. USA* 88: 6418–6422.

Guy, H. R., and Hucho, F. (1987) The ion channel of the nicotinic acetylcholine receptor. *TINS* 10(8): 318–321.

Guy, H. R., and Seetharamulu, P. (1986) Molecular model of the action potential sodium channel. *Proc. Natl. Acad. Sci. USA* 83: 508–512.

Grenningloh, G., Rienitz, A., Schmidt, B., Methfessel, C., Zensen, M., Beyreuther, K., Gundelfinger, E. D., and Benz, H. (1987) The strychnine-binding subunit of the glycine receptor shows homology with nicotinic acetylcholine receptors. *Nature* 328: 215–220.

Hall, J. E., Vodyanoy, I., M.B.T., and Marshall, G. R. (1984) Alamethicin. A rich model for channel behavior. *Biophys. J.* 45: 233–247.

Hartmann, H. A., Kirsch, G. E., Drewe, J. A., Taglialatela, M., Joho, R. H., and Brown, A. M. (1991) Exchange of conduction pathways between two related K^+ channels. *Science* 251: 942–944.

Henderson, R., Baldwin, J. M., Ceska, T. A., Zemlin, F., Beckmann, E., and Downing, K. H. (1990) Model for the structure of bacteriorhodopsin based on high resolution electron cryo-microscopy. *J. Mol. Biol.* 213: 899–929.

Hille, B. (1984) *Ionic Channels of Excitable Membranes.* Sunderland, MA: Sinauer Associates Inc.

Ho, S. P., and DeGrado, W. F. (1987) Design of a 4-helix bundle protein: synthesis of peptides which self-associate into a helical protein. *J. Am. Chem. Soc.* 109: 6751–6758.

Imoto, K., Busch, C., Sakmann, B., Mishina, M., Konno, T., Nakai, J., Bujo, H., Mori, Y., and Fukuda, K. (1988) Rings of negatively charged amino acids determine the acetylcholine receptor channel conductance. *Nature* 335: 645–648.

Jacobs, R. E., and White, S. H. (1989) The nature of the hydrophobic binding of small peptides at the bilayer interface. Implications for the insertion of transbilayer helices. *Biochemistry* 28: 3421–3437.

Jap, B. K., and Walian, P. J. (1990) Biophysics of the structure and function of porins. *Q. Rev. Biophys.* 23: 367–403.

Kienker, P. (1989) Equivalence of aggregated Markov models of ion-channel gating. *Proc. R. Soc. Lond.* [*Biol.*] 236: 269–309.

Knowles, J. R. (1987) Tinkering with enzymes: what are we learning? *Science* 236: 1252–1256.

Kyte, J., and Doolittle, R. F. (1982) A simple method for displaying the hydropathic character of a protein. *J. Mol. Biol.* 157: 105–132.

Langosch, D., Hartung, K., Grell, E., Bamberg, E., and Bentz, H. (1991) Ion channel formation by synthetic transmembrane segments of the inhibitory glycine receptor—a model study. *Biochim. Biophys. Acta* 1063: 36–44.

Lear, J. D. (1990) Why did the voltage sensor cross the membrane? *Comments Theor. Biol.* 1(6): 329–340.

Lear, J. D., Wasserman, Z. R., and DeGrado, W. F. (1988) Synthetic amphiphilic peptide models for protein ion channels. *Science* 240: 1177–1181.

Liebovitch, L. S., Fischbarg, J., Koniarek, J. P., Todorova, I., and Wang, M. (1987) Fractal model of ion-channel kinetics. *Biochim. Biophys. Acta* 896: 173–180.

Liman, E. R., Hess, P., Weaver, F., and Koren, G. (1991) Voltage-sensing residues in the S4 region of a mammalian K^+ channel. *Nature* 353: 752–756.

Montal, M. (1990) Molecular anatomy and molecular design of channel proteins. *FASEB J.* 4: 2623–2635.

Mullens, L. J. (1959) An analysis of conductance changes in squid axon. *J. Gen. Physiol.* 42: 817–829.

Mutter, M., Hersperger, R., Gubernator, K., and Müller, K. (1989) The construction of new proteins: V. A template-assembled synthetic protein (TASP) containing both a 4-helix bundle and b-barrel-like structure. *Proteins Struct. Funct. Genet.* 5: 13–21.

Nicoll, R. (1988) The coupling of neurotransmitter receptors to ion channels in the brain. *Science* 241: 545–551.

Numa, S. (1989) A molecular view of neurotransmitter receptors and ion channels. 123–165 In: *The Harvey Lectures, Series 83.* New York: Alan R. Liss, Inc.

O'Shea, E. K., Klenner, J. D., King, P. S., and Alber, T. (1991) X-ray structure of the GCN4 leucine zipper, a two-stranded, parallel coiled coil. *Science* 254: 539–544.

Oiki, S., Danho, W., and Montal, M. (1988) Channel protein engineering: synthetic 22-mer peptide from the primary structure of the voltage-sensitive sodium channel forms ionic channels in lipid bilayers. *Proc. Natl. Acad. Sci. USA* 85: 2393–2397.

Pethig, R. (1979) *Dielectric and Electronic Properties of Biological Materials.* New York: John Wiley & Sons.

Prasad, B. V., and Balaram, P. (1984) The stereochemistry of peptides containing α-amino isobutyric acid. *CRC Crit. Rev. Biochem.* 16: 307–348.

Quandt, F. (1987) Burst kinetics of sodium channels which lack fast inactivation in mouse neuroblastoma cells. *J. Physiol.* 392: 563–585.

Rees, D. C., DeAntonio, L., and Eisenberg, D. (1989) Hydrophobic organization of membrane proteins. *Science* 245: 510–513.

Richardson, J. S., and Richardson, D. C. (1989) The de novo design of protein structures. *TIBS* 14: 304–309.

Roseman, M. A. (1988) Hydrophobicity of the peptide C $=$ O $\cdots$ H–N hydrogen bonded group. *J. Mol. Biol.* 201: 621–623.

Saimi, Y., Martinac, B., Gustin, M. C., Culbertson, M. R., Adler, J., and Kung, C. (1988) Ion channels in *Paramecium*, yeast, and *Eschericia coli. Cold Spring Harbor Symp. Quant. Biol.* 53: 667–673.

Sansom, M.S.P. (1991) The biophysics of peptide models of ion channels. *Prog. Biophys. Mol. Biol.* 55: 139–235.

Schofield, P. R., Darlison, M. G., Fujita, N., Burt, D. R., Stephenson, F. A., Rodriguez, H., Rhee, L. M., Ramachandran, J., Reale, V., Glencorse, T. A., Seeburg, P. H., and Barnard, E. A. (1987) Sequence and functional expression of the $GABA_A$ receptor shows a ligand-gated receptor superfamily. *Nature* 328: 221–227.

Sigworth, F. J., and Sine, S. M. (1987) Data transformation for improved display and fitting of single channel dwell time histograms. *Biophys. J.* 52: 1047–1054.

Stühmer, W. H., Conti, F., Suzuki, H., Wang, X., Noda, M., Yahagi, N., Kubo, H., and Numa, S. (1989) Structural parts involved in activation and inactivation of the sodium channel. *Nature* 339: 597–603.

Tosteson, M. T., Levy, J. J., Caporale, L. H., Rosenblatt, M., and Tosteson, D. C. (1987) Solid-phase synthesis of melittin: purification and functional characterization. *Biochemistry* 26: 6627–6631.

Tosteson, M. T., Auld, D. S., and Tosteson, D. C. (1989) Voltage-gated channels formed in lipid bilayers by a positively charged segment of the Na-channel polypeptide. *Proc. Natl. Acad. Sci. USA* 86: 707–710.

Unwin, R., Toyoshima, C., and Kubalek, E. (1988) Arrangement of the acetylcholine receptor subunits in the resting and desensitized states, determined by cryoelectron microscopy of crystallized *Torpedo* postsynaptic membranes. *J. Cell Biol.* 107: 1123–1138.

Yellen, G., Jurman, M. E., Abramson, T., and MacKinnon, R. (1991) Mutations affecting internal TEA blockade identify the probable pore-forming region of a K^+ channel. *Science* 251: 939–942.

Yool, A. J., and Schwartz, T. L. (1991) Alteration of ionic selectivity of a K^+ channel by mutation of the H5 region. *Nature* 349: 700–704.

16

Diffraction Studies of Model and Natural Helical Peptides

ISABELLA L. KARLE

The discovery of naturally occurring peptides that form voltage-gated ion channels in bilayer membranes has provided an impetus for the study of structural character-istics of this class of peptides (Mueller and Rudin, 1968; Mathew and Balaram, 1983). The relative difficulty of obtaining crystals of the natural peptides and deter-mining their structure has led to the synthesis of many apolar peptides that are frag-ments or analogs of the natural peptides. The naturally occurring peptides contain a number of α-aminoisobutyric acid (Aib) residues, (Fig. 16.1) which have proven to be strong helix formers (Marshall and Bosshard, 1972; Burgess and Leach, 1973; Balaram, 1984). A review of crystal structures of small linear peptides, containing up to five residues including at least one Aib residue, demonstrated that 28 out of 29 structures have an incipient 3_{10}-helix (Toniolo et al., 1983). Thirty-three crystal structures of 7–16 residue apolar peptides containing one or more Aib residues have shown completely helical conformations with a 3_{10}-helix, an α-helix, or a mixed $3_{10}/$ α-helix, depending mostly upon the length of the peptide and the number of Aib residues (Karle and Balaram, 1990).

This chapter will address the nature of apolar peptide helices, the motifs for asso-ciation of helices, the intrusion of water molecules into nonpolar cavities and into the backbone of helices, and, finally, structures of some naturally occurring channel for-mers and implications for ion transport. Each of the ionophores shown in Figure 16.1 contains at least one Gln residue and a Pro or Hyp (hydroxyproline) residue. The importance of these particular residues for channel formation and probably for gat-ing will be discussed.

Resolution

The findings discussed in this chapter are based on structures that have been derived from x-ray difraction analyses of single crystals. X-ray diffraction spots from crys-tals of peptides composed of 10–16 residues (there often is more than one independent peptide molecule per asymmetric unit of the crystal) have measurable intensities to much higher scattering angles than those produced by protein crystals. The higher the scattering angle obtained, the better the resolution of the structure and the more

5   10   15   20

I Ac-Aib-Pro-Aib-Ala-Aib-Ala-Gln-Aib-Val-Aib-Gly-Leu-Aib-Pro-Val-Aib-Aib-Glu-Gln-Phol
           (Aib)

5   10   15

II Ac-Phe-Aib-Aib-Aib-Iva-Gly-Leu-Aib-Aib-Hyp-Gln-Iva-Hyp-Aib-Pro-Phol
               (Pro)

5   10   15

III Ac-Phe-Aib-Aib-Aib-Val-Gly-Leu-Aib-Aib-Hyp-Gln-Iva-Hyp-Ala-Phol
               (Aib)

5   10   15

IV Ac-Trp-Ile-Gln-Iva-Ile-Thr-Aib-Leu-Aib-Hyp-Gln-Aib-Hyp-Aib-Pro-Phol
  (Leu)

Fig. 16.1. Sequences of some voltage-gated channel-forming peptides. *I*, alamethicin; *II*, antiamoebin; *III*, emerimicin; *IV*, zervamicin. The residues in *parentheses* represent the changes in related congeners. All residues except Gly and Aib have the L configuration. *Aib*, α-aminoisobutyric acid; *Iva*, isovaline; *Phol*, phenylalaninol; *Ac*, acetyl (Rinehart et al., 1981; Argoudelis and Johnson, 1974).

precise the geometric parameters of the molecule. An example of resolution is illustrated by the electron density map shown for a three residue fragment of Leu-zervamicin, a 16 residue peptide, in Figure 16.2 (Karle et al., 1991a). In Figure 16.2*a*, the map was calculated with data observed to 0.93 Å resolution (scattering angle $2\Theta_{max} = 112°$ for copper radiation) a typical value for most midsized peptides. Each atom is well resolved from adjoining atoms, and the electron density contours approximate the atomic number of the C, N, and O atoms quite well. In Figure 16.2*b*, the data have been truncated at a resolution of 2.0 Å (corresponding to a scattering angle $2\Theta_{max} = 45°$). All other parameters were the same as for the calculation in Figure 16.2*a*. The individual atoms are no longer resolved, but the envelope of the density for the molecule remains quite good. As the data are reduced further, by truncating at a resolution of 2.5 Å ($2\Theta_{max} = 36°$), the envelope of the density begins to shift away from the correct atomic positions and the pyrrolidine ring shows maximum density in the middle of the ring where a minimum should occur. (Fig. 16.2*c*). The attainment of 2.0 Å resolution for protein crystals is very good. Usually the resolution of reported structures is nearer to 2.5 Å or less. The lower resolution for proteins is due to the nature of the crystals, partly in that the large amount of water that cocrystallizes with the protein is most disordered and partly to the larger motion of individual atoms as compared with smaller molecules. For example, the very well-refined structure of staphylococcal nuclease at 1.7 Å resolution has an overall "thermal" value of 22.5 Å^2 (equivalent to an r.m.s. atomic amplitude of 0.53 Å) (Hynes and Fox, 1991), while the Leu-zervamicin structure used for Figure 16.2*a* has an overall "thermal" value of 7.0 Å^2 (r.m.s. atomic amplitude of 0.29 Å). Actually, the electron density maps as shown in Figure 16.2.*b,c* are enhanced in quality because the attenuation in the observed data was that obtained for 0.93 Å resolution. For crystals that scatter only to 2.0 or 2.5 Å resolution, additional attentuation would occur. Furthermore, the phase values used in the calculations also were those obtained at the 0.93 Å resolution.

The remarkable and useful results that are obtained from crystal structure analyses of proteins depend on compensation for lack of resolution in the form of model fitting of residues based on knowledge of their sequence and the known structures of small peptides or amino acids. In addition, considerable benefit is obtained from least-squares refinement using distance restraints between atoms (Konnert, 1975; Hendrickson and Konnert, 1980; Hendrickson, 1985) and, more recently, energy minimization and molecular dynamics techniques (Brunger et al., 1987; Brunger, 1988) before or during the application of distance restraints.

The greater resolution obtainable from crystals of peptides obviates the need for restraints or constraints because of the high ratio between the number of observed data to the number of unknown parameters (three coordinates and thermal values for each atom). The high resolution gives better precision in determining hydrogen bond lengths or nonbonded approaches between atoms, more reliability in the kinds of distortions observed in helices, more confidence in water molecules occurring in unusual places, and even the direct location of hydrogen atoms involved in hydrogen bonds in favorable cases.

The Helix

Helix Type

The introduction of Aib residues into a peptide sequence decreases the flexibility of the peptide chain and produces a helical backbone with rare exception. The replacement of the proton on the C^α atom in an alanine residue with another methyl group severely limits the possible rotations about the $N-C^\alpha$ and $C^\alpha-C'$ bonds. In calculating the allowable rotational space for ϕ (torsion about $N-C^\alpha$ bond) and ψ (torsion about $C^\alpha-C'$ bond), Marshall and Bosshard (1972) and Burgess and Leach (1973) demonstrated that the ϕ and ψ angles for Aib were restricted to a tight region near $+57°$, $+47°$ and $-57°$, $-47°$, respectively, which coincides with a left-handed or right-handed helix, respectively. An α-helical conformation was demonstrated for Boc-(Ala-Aib)$_2$-Ala-Glu(OBzℓ)-(Ala-Aib)$_2$-Ala-OMe (Butters et al., 1981) and a 3_{10}-helix for Boc-Aib-Pro-Val-Aib-Val-Ala-Aib-Ala-Aib-Aib-OMe (Francis et al., 1983), for example, by the design and synthesis of model peptides (Balaram, 1984), followed by crystallization and x-ray diffraction analysis. By this time a sufficient number of crystal structure analyses of longer peptides containing Aib residues have been obtained to indicate the important factor governing the type of helix formed. A plot indicating the type of helix, 3_{10}, α, or mixed $3_{10}/\alpha$, as a function of the length of the peptide and the number of Aib residues in the peptide is shown in Figure 16.3. It is an updated version of a similar plot appearing in an earlier article (Karle and Balaram, 1990) with 13 additional structures (Boc-LLLLULLLL-OBzℓ, Boc-LLLLULLLLU-OBzℓ [Okuyama et al., 1991], leucinostatin A [Cerrini et al., 1989], pBrBz-U$_{10}$-OtBu [Toniolo et al., 1991], Leu-zervamicin [Karle et al., 1991a], Boc-VALUVAL-Acp-VALUVAL-OMe [Karle et al., 1991b], Boc-ULU-ULLLULU-OMe [Karle et al., 1992a], Boc-dF-UUUUGLUU-OMe [Karle et al.,

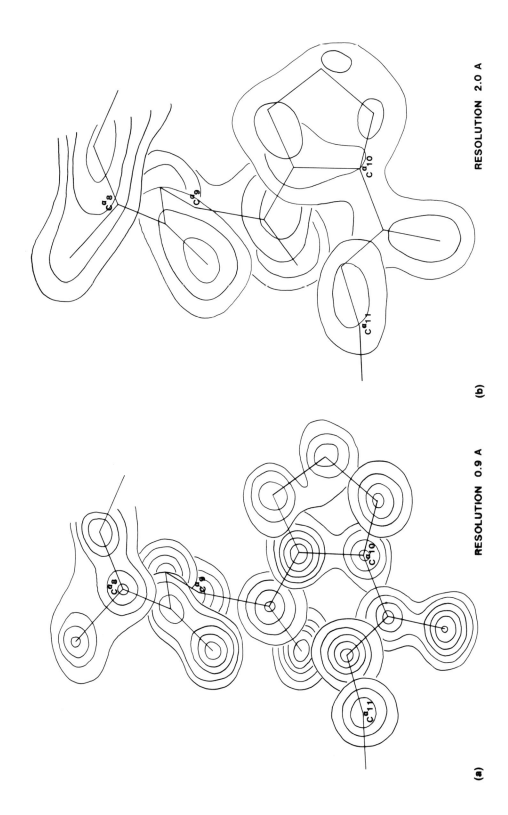

RESOLUTION 2.0 A

(b)

RESOLUTION 0.9 A

(a)

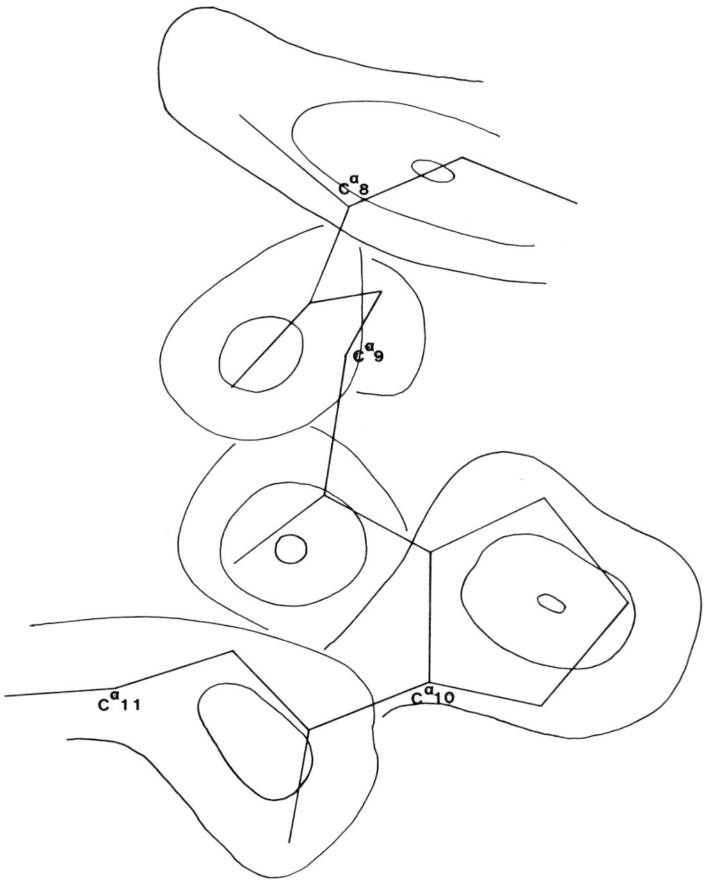

Fig. 16.2. *a*: An electron density map for a three-residue fragment in the crystal of Leu-zervamicin calculated from the final coordinates obtained from least-squares refinement. Number of observed data is $5,677$; $2\theta_{max} = 112°$; resolution 0.93 Å. Sections down the b axis are shown. Contours are at levels of $1, 3, 5, \ldots$ electrons/Å^3. The outermost contour is at the $/$electron/Å^3 level. *b*: Resolution reduced to 2.0 Å by truncating observed data at $2\theta_{max} = 45°$, $1,019$ reflections. Same coordinates and same phase values used as in *a*. Contours are at levels of $1, 2, 3 \ldots$ electrons/Å^3. At present, the best-determined protein structures are near 2.0 Å resolution. *c*: Resolution reduced to 2.5 Å by truncating observed data at $2\theta_{max} = 36°$, 541 reflections. Same coordinates and same phase values used as in *a*. Contours are at levels of $1, 2,$ and 3 electrons/Å^3. At present many protein structures are reported at $3.0-2.5$ Å.

RESOLUTION 2.5 Å

(c)

359

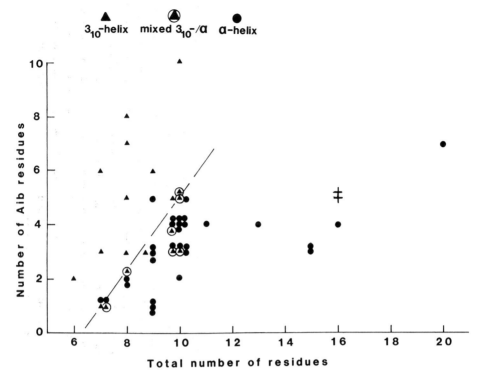

Fig. 16.3. Helix type as a function of total number of residues in peptide and total number of Aib residues. The *dashed line* separating the 3_{10}-helices from the α-helices has been placed arbitrarily. Aib-containing peptides with five or fewer total residues form 3_{10}-helices. This plot is an update with 12 new structures of a plot that was published in *Biochemistry* (Karle and Balaram, 1990). The *plus symbols* indicate the bent helical structures of zervamicin and an apolar analog that contain three Pro or Hyp residues.

1993a], Boc-VALUVALVALUVALU-OMe (polymorph) [Karle et al., 1992b], Boc-LUALUAPU-OMe,* Boc-WLUALUAPU-OMe,* Boc-UWLUALUAPU-OMe,* and Boc-VALPUVALP-OMe.* [Manuscripts describing the plots marked by asterisks are in preparation by Karle, Flippen-Anderson, Balaram and coworkers in Bangalore. The one-letter code for amino acid residues is used, where U = Aib; Acp = ϵ-aminocaproic acid; and d = D hand.]) There appear to be distinct regions for peptides with 3_{10}-helices and α-helices. The helices that are mixed $3_{10}/\alpha$ fall near the boundary between the two regions. Hence, the length of the peptide plus the number of Aib residues are major factors in determining helix type. In peptides of 9–20 residues, there can be a facile transition between 3_{10}- and α-type hydrogen bonds. Often the same peptide crystallized in different forms (polymorphs) will change from a mixed $3_{10}/\alpha$-helix to a completely α-helix. The positioning of Aib residues in a sequence seems to have little effect on helix-forming properties. Exchange of Aib and Ala or Aib and Leu, as well as replacement of Ala or Leu with Aib, or the reverse, seems to have little effect on the helical conformation. A large number of Aib residues will favor the formation of a 3_{10}-helix. As few as one Aib residue has produced an α-helix in three different nonapeptides. The Aib residue is not handed. In crystals of BrBz-U_{10}-OtBu (Toniolo et al., 1991) right-handed and left-handed 3_{10}-helices occur side by side. However, in conjunction with handed residues in a helix, the Aib residue will adopt the hand of the handed residue. In the peptides shown in Figure 16.3, the residues other than Aib have L-chirality; thus the Aib residues also adopt ϕ and ψ values and only right-handed helices are formed.

NonBonded NH in Helix

An α-helix forms $5 \rightarrow 1$ type hydrogen bonds between NH and CO moieties. In an isolated ideal α-helix segment the first three NH moieties and the last three CO moieties will be without hydrogen bonding. A similar situation exists in 3_{10}-helices. In crystals, helices assemble into continuous rods and form head-to-tail NH $\cdots$ O = C hydrogen bonds between the individual helices. When there is an ideal register between the top of one helix and the bottom of another, three NH $\cdots$ O = C bonds are formed (Karle et al., 1989a). When the helix termini are distorted, or the register between helical molecules is less than ideal, and there are no cocrystallized solvent molecules to mediate hydrogen bonding, the second or third NH moiety is found in a position such that there is no possibility for hydrogen bond formation (Karle et al., 1988a, 1989a).

Another common situation for the lack of a hydrogen bond acceptor for an NH moiety is in the transition area between a 3_{10}-helix and an α-helix. The example in Figure 16.4 shows N(4)H $\cdots$ O(1) as the last $4 \rightarrow 1$ type hydrogen bond and N(6)H $\cdots$ O(2) as the first $5 \rightarrow 1$ type hydrogen bond. The N(5)H moiety is bereft of any hydrogen bonding possibility. The lack of hydrogen bonding does not appear to affect the stability of the helix.

Helix Unfolding

Three stages of the unfolding of an α-helix have been captured in crystals of Boc-VALUVAL-OMe grown from MeOH/H$_2$O and DMSO/IprOH (Karle, et al.,

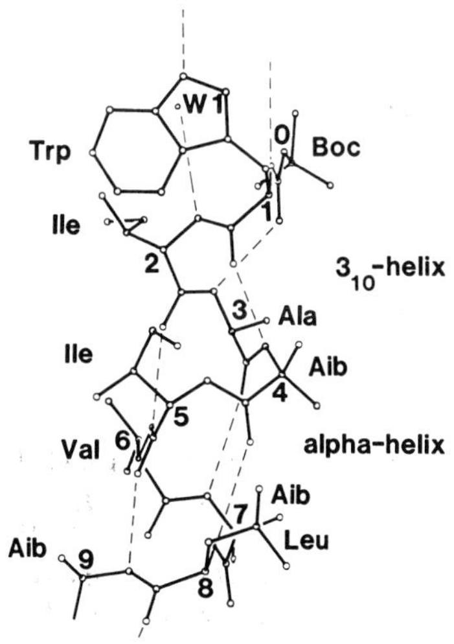

Fig. 16.4. Lack of a hydrogen bond for N(5)H. A fragment of the structure for the apolar analog of zervamicin is shown. The C$^\alpha$ atoms are numbered (Karle et al., 1987).

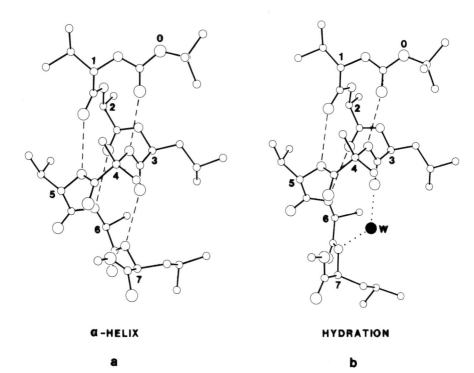

α-HELIX

a

HYDRATION

b

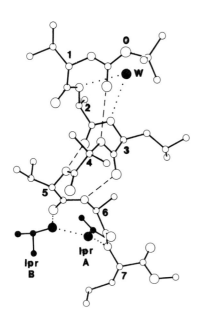

SOLVATION

c

Fig. 16.5. Unwinding of α-helix in Boc-VALUVAL-OMe by solvation. The Cα atoms are labeled *1–7*; *W*, water; *Ipr*, isopropanol. *Dashed lines* indicate NH··· O=C hydrogen bonds in helix; *dotted lines* indicate hydrogen bonds to solvent molecules (Karle et al., 1990a; 1993b).

1990a, 1993b). The molecule in an α-helical conformation is shown in Figure 16.5a. Side by side in the same crystal another conformation occurred in which a water molecule W had broken the N(7)H $\cdots$ O(3) hydrogen bond and two new hydrogen bonds were formed between N(7)H $\cdots$ W and W $\cdots$ O(3). (Figure 16.5.b). The process of inserting the W molecule into the backbone involved rotations only about the N(5)—C$^\alpha$(5) and C$^\alpha$(5)—C$'$(5) bonds by $-4°$ and $+13°$, respectively, so that the N(7) $\cdots$ O(3) separation increased to 4.13 Å. The remainder of the helix was unaffected. In a different crystal form, grown from DMSO containing some isopropanol, the helical backbone has been damaged considerably (Fig. 16.5c). Only the original N(4)H $\cdots$ O(0) hydrogen bond (O[0] from the Boc group) has been preserved. The central portion has become a 3_{10}-helix, and the lower portion is largely extended. The hydroxyl groups in two isopropanol molecules make hydrogen bonds with N(7) and O(5), as well as with each other. A symmetry equivalent of the water molecule W, shown near the top as an acceptor for hydrogen bonds from N(2) and N(3), also is a donor to hydrogen bonds with O(4) and O(6) (hydrogen bonds not shown). The progress of deterioration by solvating the backbone is reflected in rotations at C$^\alpha$(5), C$^\alpha$(6), and C$^\alpha$(7) and the large changes in the values of the torsional angles in this region.

The use of DMSO and/or isopropanol as a solvent has not been found to unfold other Aib-containing peptides. In general, most peptides have quite stable conformations in polymorphic crystals grown from a variety of solvents. However, the insertion of a water molecule into a helix backbone, similar to that in Figure 16.5b has also been found in crystals of Boc-U-(ALU)$_3$-OMe, (Figure 16.7), and Boc-(ALU)$_2$-OMe (Karle et al., 1988b, 1989b), as well as in protein crystals (Sundaralingam and Sekharudu, 1989). The implications of such hydration, which creates minipolar areas on nonpolar helices, is discussed in a later section.

Helix Association

Neighboring helices in proteins associate in an antiparallel or skewed motif (Richardson, 1981). The absence of parallel association of helices in proteins had been attributed by Hol (1981) to the presence of a significant dipole moment in a helix (Wada, 1976). Completely parallel association of helices, however, has occurred in more than one-third of the crystals of peptides with 10–16 residues. Furthermore, some of the peptides that crystallize in more than one crystal form will assemble in a completely parallel motif in one polymorph and an antiparallel motif in another polymorph, although the conformation of the peptide molecules is essentially the same in both. Some examples of such pairs are X-WIAUIVULUP-OMe (X = Boc or Ac) (Karle et al., 1990b), Boc-UALALULALU-OMe (Karle et al., 1990c) (Fig. 16.6), and Boc-VALUVALVALUVALU (Karle, et al., 1990d, 1992b). In another pair in which the residues are similar but not identical, Leu-zervamicin (Karle et al., 1991a) and its synthetic apolar analog Boc-WIAUIVULUPAUPUPF-OMe (Karle et al., 1987), the apolar analog packs in an all-parallel fashion, while the naturally occurring peptide with a small number of polar residues packs in an antiparallel fashion in several polymorphs. The conformation of the helix and the side chains that are in common are essentially identical in the two peptides.

The all-parallel assemblies have been found only in apolar peptides to date. There

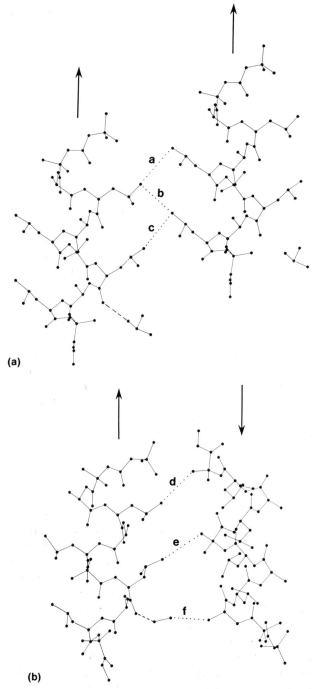

Fig. 16.6. Completely parallel (*a*) and antiparallel (*b*) association of helices in two different crystals of Boc-UALALULALU-OMe grown from isopropanol and methanol solutions, respectively. The arrows indicate the direction of the helix dipole., The letters *a–c* indicate van der Waal's approaches of 3.8–4.1 Å between Leu· · ·Leu side chains in the parallel packing mode. The letters *d* and *e* indicate approaches of 3.6–3.75 Å between Leu· · ·Aib side chains in the antiparallel packing (Karle et al., 1990c).

is no possibility for lateral hydrogen bonding between the apolar peptide helices. All the intermolecular contacts are between hydrophobic groups, usually with C · · · C separations in the range of 3.8–4.1 Å. In polymorphic crystals of the same peptide, there appear to be an equal number of intermolecular contacts in the van der Waals' range for the parallel and the antiparallel packing (Fig. 16.6). There does not appear to be a selective attractive process by the type of side chain, but rather by size and shape of the surface of the helices where knobs fit into holes.

The fairly common occurrence of all-parallel assemblies in crystals of nonpolar helical peptides indicates that factors other than the dipole moment have a major influence on the assembly of helix bundles. A discussion of several such factors can be found in a recent review by Sansom (1991) and elsewhere (Gilson and Honig, 1989). All-parallel packing has not been observed in the few helical peptides whose crystal structures have been reported that contain several polar side chains, such as zervamicin, melittin, and alamethicin. Furthermore, apolar peptides that have been rendered amphipathic by the insertion of a water molecule into the helix backbone have also been found to associate in an antiparallel fashion. Judging from the rather sparse structural information available at this time, antiparallel association of helices is favored if lateral hydrogen bonds can be made either between side chains or involving backbone carbonyl oxygens that protrude away from the helix (Fig. 16.7).

Alamethicin and Zervamicin

Pro and Hyp in Helices

The Pro and Hyp residues are generally considered strong helix breakers and occur often at the N terminus of a helix (Chou and Fasman, 1974; Richardson, 1981). In a number of membrane-active peptides the Pro and/or Hyp residues have been incorporated into the helix, with the result that the helix becomes significantly curved, as in melittin (Terwilliger and Eisenberg, 1982), alamethicin (Fox and Richards, 1982), and Leu-zervamicin (Karle et al., 1991a). The proline residue lacks an H atom on the N and therefore the carbonyl O at $i - 3$ or $i - 4$ remains free of intrahelical hydrogen bonding. The bulk of the pyrollidine ring causes the helix to bend with the pyrollidine ring on the convex side of the helix. Furthermore, the helix turns away from the carbonyl O at $i - 3$ and/or $i - 4$, which then extends into the surrounding environment and is available for hydrogen bonding with solvent molecules or neighboring helices (Fig. 16.8). The structure of a synthetic apolar analog of zervamicin (Karle et al., 1987) (Figs. 16.8, 16.9a) shows the helix bent at Pro[10] and the exposure of O7 to the outside environment. This peptide with a Pro-induced bend is an additional example to that shown in Figure 16.7 of a hydrophobic peptide acquiring amphipathic properties that may be important in considering potential ionic interactions in channel models.

Melittin and alamethicin have one Pro residue near the middle of the peptide. Zervamicin and its apolar analog have three Hyp or Pro residues near each other and still maintain a helical backbone, where the two additional Pro and Hyp residues are contained in an approximately 3_{10}-helix. A comparison of Leu[1]-zervamicin with the synthetic Trp analog in Figure 16.9 shows that the shape of the backbone is unaf-

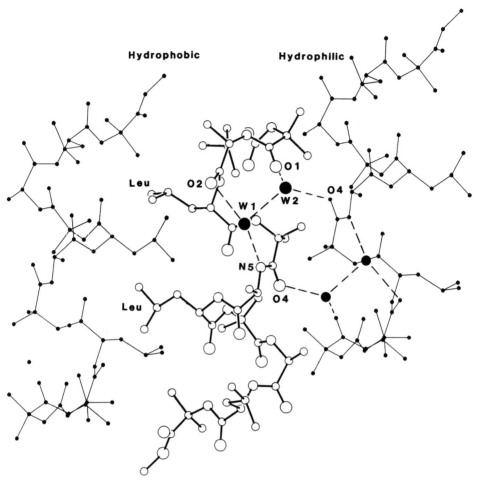

Hydrophobic   **Hydrophilic**

Fig. 16.7. Amphipathic behavior of the helical apolar peptide Boc-U-(ALU)₃-OMe and anti-parallel packing of three adjacent helices. The boundary between molecules on the left is entirely hydrophobic with Leu· · ·Leu contacts (compare with parallel Leu· · ·Leu contacts in Fig. 16.6). The boundary on the right is hydrophilic with water molecules (W(1), W(2), and symmetry-related molecules indicated by *large dark circles*) mediating lateral interhelical hydrogen bonds. Water molecule W(1) has broken the intrahelical N(5)· · ·O(2) hydrogen bond and formed two new hydrogen bonds, W(1)· · ·O(2) and N(5)· · ·W(1) Karle et al., 1988b).

fected by the removal of the polar function in five residues. Furthermore, Sansom (1991) has observed that the zervamicin analog backbone has a remarkable conformational resemblance to that of residues 5–20 of alamethicin.

Both alamethicin and Leu-zervamicin display a flexibility in the curvature of the helix. Three independent molecules of alamethicin had cocrystallized in the cell, that is, the three molecules were not related by symmetrical operations and the coordinates of each molecule had to be obtained from the diffraction data. Two of the alemethicin molecules had a similar bend in the helix, whereas the third molecule dis-

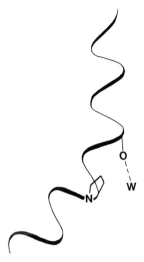

Fig. 16.8. Schematic diagram of the helical backbone of a 16 residue peptide with a proline residue at position 10. The bulk of the pyrrolidine ring caused the helix to curve. The carbonyl O at i-3, which lacks an NH donor to form an intrahelical hydrogen bond, protrudes into the solvent environment and attracts a water molecule.

played a much smaller bend (Fox and Richards, 1982). Leu-zervamicin has crystallized with only one molecule per asymmetric unit; however, several different crystal forms have been obtained with different cell dimensions and space groups. In the three forms that have been analyzed (Karle et al., 1991a, 1992c), the Leu-zer-vamicin molecule differs considerably in the amount of bend in the helix. Superposition of molecules from crystal A and crystal B are shown in Figure 16.10a, and superposition of molecules from crystal C and crystal B are shown in Figure 16.10b. The angles of bend are approximately 32 degrees for B, 42 degrees for A, and 51 degrees for C. The changes in the curvature do not occur at any one residue but take place by small increments in torsional angles in several residues between Pro^{10} and the C terminus. It is interesting to note that crystal forms A and B grew in the same crystallizing vial at the same time. Hence the changes in the curvature of the backbone require very little, if any, change in energy and attest to the flexibility of the bent helix.

Amphiphilicity

Alamethicin folds into a helix in such a manner that its three polar residues, Gln^7, Glu^{18}, and Gln^{19} have their side chains extended from the convex face. In addition, the presence of Pro^{14} causes carbonyl O10 and carbonyl O11 to be exposed on the convex face and to augment the polar spine. The curved helix results in a more amphiphilic helix than would be expected from an inspection of the residue sequence alone. Zervamicin has a shorter helix than alamethicin by four residues and contains a greater number of polar residues, all extended to the convex face. A comparison of residues and hydrogen bonding is shown in Figure 16.11. Antiamoebin, whose crystal structure is not available at this time, is also included for comparison since the

APOLAR ANALOG   **LEU-ZERVAMICIN**

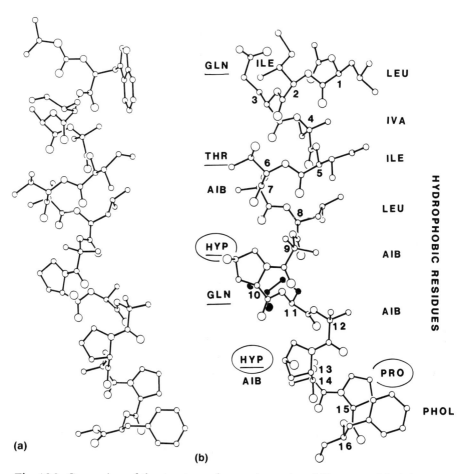

Fig. 16.9. Comparison of the structures of an apolar analog of Trp-zervamicin (*a*) and of Leu-zervamicin (*b*). The shape of the backbone is almost identical despite the presence of the five polar residues *(underlined)* in the naturally occurring peptide. Note that the Gln[11] side chain (emphasized by *heavy lines* and *filled circles*) is not extended away from the helix, but wraps around the helix so that its polar end is placed on the polar face.

gross features of the conformation can be inferred from the similarity of cell dimensions to those in the orthorhombic crystal form C of Leu-zervamicin, from the almost identical 10–16 sequence to Leu-zervamicin, and from the 3_{10}-helix found for the 1–9 fragment in a synthetic peptide (Karle, et al., 1993a). Although there are many similarities in the three ionophores shown in Figure 16.11, there is a difference in the type of helix before and after the Pro or Hyp residue shown in boldface type: (*1*) the helix sequence is $\alpha/3_{10}/\alpha$ in alamethicin; (*2*) the helix sequence is $\alpha/3_{10}$ in Leu-zervamicin; and (*3*) the helix is most probably all 3_{10} in antiamoebin.

The Leu-zervamicin and antiamoebin peptides are four residues shorter than alamethicin, and the question arises as to how the shorter peptides can span a lipid

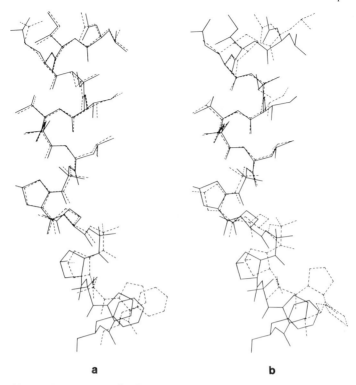

Fig. 16.10. Change in curvature of helix in Leu-zervamicin structures obtained from three different crystal polymorphs. (*a*) Superposition of crystal B *(solid line)* and crystal A *(dashed line)*. (*b*) Superposition of crystal B *(solid line)* and crystal C *(dashed line)*. The molecules were fitted with least-squares minimization of backbone distances in residues 2–10.

bilayer membrane to form an ion channel. The answer may lie with the presence of the two additional Pro and Hyp residues near the C terminus of zervamicin and antiamoebin. The Pro and Hyp residues form a β-ribbon that twists into a helix that approximates a 3_{10}-helix. Helices of the 3_{10}-type are slimmer and longer than helices of the α-type with the same number of residues. This possibility for elongation of zervamicin had been mentioned by Sansom (1991) and shown in a comparison diagram by Ballesteros and Weinstein (1992). A similar diagram in Figure 16.12 of a superposition of a 16 residue α-helix onto the 16 residue Leu-zervamicin molecule shows that the effective length of the Leu-zervamicin, even though it has a curved helix, is comparable to 19 or more residues in an α-helix, that is, Leu-zervamicin is almost as long as alamethicin.

Structural Characteristics of a Possible Ion Channel

The crystal structure analysis of alamethicin (Fox and Richards, 1982) provided valuable information about the molecule, such as the shape of the bent helix, the amphipathic nature, the role of Pro in exposing carbonyls to outside environment,

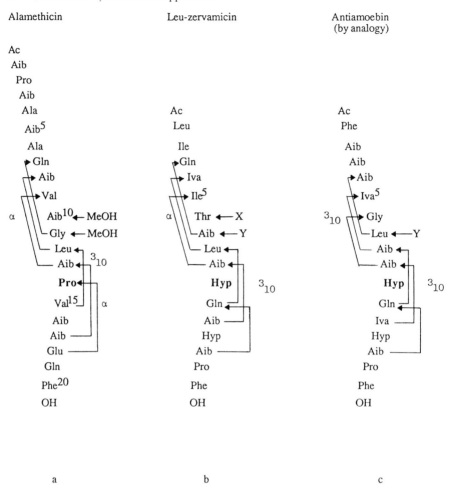

Fig. 16.11. Schematic comparison of bend in helix and hydrogen bonding in the midsection of the helix (*a*) alamethicin, (*b*) Leu-zervamicin (and apolar analog), (*c*) antiamoebin (by analogy; see text). Arrows indicate NH→O=C hydrogen bonds (except for *inter*molecular H bonds). *X*, polar side chain in neighboring peptide helix in Leu-zervamicin; no H bond in apolar analog; *Y*, polar side in neighboring peptide helix; H_2O in apolar analog.

and the type of intramolecular hydrogen bonding. However, the alamethicin molecules did not aggregate in the crystal in a manner that would suggest an ion channel. Fox and Richards (1982), as well as others (e.g., Mathew and Balaram, 1983; Hall et al., 1984; Menestrina et al., 1986), have proposed models for ion channels based on the structural characteristics of the alamethicin molecule. Currently, the results from crystal structure analyses show that in all four crystal forms of Leu-zervamicin the polar faces associate in a very similar antiparallel fashion and form water channels in which the water molecules have ample opportunity to make hydrogen bonds with the polar groups lining the channel and each other. The channels occurring in the crystal may provide a more direct model for ion transport.

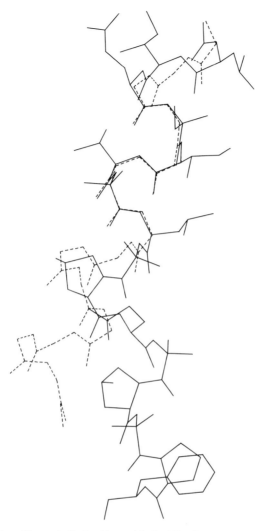

Fig. 16.12. A 16-residue α-helix backbone (*dashed lines*) superimposed on the $\alpha/3_{10}$-helix backbone of Leu-zervamicin (*solid lines*).

A number of striking structural similarities between alamethicin and zervamicin can be seen in Figure 16.11. An interesting and probably significant difference is the placement and conformation of Gln[11] in zervamicin (and antiamoebin). Usually side chains are extended to a large extent away from helix backbones. In zervamicin, if the Gln[11] side chain were extended, the polar end of the side chain would be located in the middle of an otherwise completely nonpolar face (Fig. 16.9). Rather, it wraps around the helix and places its polar end on the polar face of the helix. The torsion angles about the $C^{\alpha}-C^{\beta}$ and $C^{\beta}-C^{\gamma}$ bonds are near $-50°$ and $-55°$, respectively. In position 11, the Gln does not follow the $i + 3$ or $i + 4$ sequence motif of the other polar residues in positions 3, 6, 10, and 13 that fall on the same side of a helix.

In the crystalline state, Leu-zervamicin associates in an antiparallel fashion, as shown in Figure 16.13a,b, with the polar sides facing each other. The molecules are held together by lateral hydrogen bonds between helices that involve the $O^\delta H$ in Hyp^{10} (two hydrogen bonds) and the $N^\epsilon H_2$ in Gln^{11} (two hydrogen bonds). Acceptors are O6 and O7 in carbonyl groups that protrude away from the helix, owing to the bend caused by Hyp^{10}. There is no direct analogy to alamethicin because the comparable residues at the bend in alamethicin are Pro^{14} and Val^{15}, residues without the functional OH and NH_2 groups present in Hyp^{10} and Gln^{11} that are necessary for the interpeptide hydrogen bonding. The interrupted water channels made by association of Leu-zervamicin helices are shown in Figure 16.13a for the smallest bend in the helix (crystal B) and in Figure 16.13b for almost the largest bend (crystal C). The opening at the mouth, measured from N'3 of one molecule to O16 of the other molecule is 3.77 Å in Figure 16.13a and 10.3 Å in Figure 16.12b. The bend and mouth opening are intermediate in crystal A (not shown) and somewhat larger in crystal D than in crystal C. The number of water molecules in the channel increases with the increase of the bend in the helix. The water molecules have well-ordered positions in the narrow channel in Figure 16.13a and become much less ordered as the channel becomes wider. In each case there is a water molecule hydrogen bonded to carbonyl O10 near the constriction.

If the channels in the crystals have any resemblance to an ion channel in a bilayer lipid membrane, it is suggestive that a potassium ion could enter the channel at the mouth when it is in a wide position, that the mouth would constrict to capture the ion, and that the ion would displace water molecules or push them along the channel under the application of voltage. Without any application of potential, crystals C of Leu-zervamicin were soaked in a KCl solution. The volume of the crystal increased, but no potassium ion had been detected in the resulting crystal D.

The number of peptide helices required to form an ion channel in a bilayer lipid membrane and the parallel or antiparallel orientation of the helix bundle has been discussed by a number of investigators (e.g., Furois-Corbin and Pullman, 1986; Sansom, 1991). In a crystalline form, the adjacent helices are necessarily related by the symmetry operations of the crystal space group. Neighboring helices in Leu-zervamicin crystals A–D are related by a twofold screw operation. In Figure 16.13, the twofold screw is perpendicular to the page; in Figure 16.14 *(middle)*, the twofold screw is vertical. In Figure 16.14 three adjacent helices that form an interrupted water channel are shown. The two helices on the right are parallel to each other (related by a translation). The helix on the left is antiparallel to those on the right. Equivalently, two helices on the left and one on the right could have been chosen to describe the channel. In other words, the channel has no directional choice; it looks the same in a view from the top or from the bottom. Although the hydrophilic faces of the helices assemble only in an antiparallel mode to each other in all four crystal forms, the hydrophobic side of the helices make contact with other hydrophobic sides either in an antiparallel mode in crystals A and B (space group P2$_1$) or a parallel model in crystals C and D (space group P2$_1$2$_1$2$_1$) (Fig. 16.15). The nonspecificity for the nonpolar aggregation was discussed earlier (see Fig. 16.6). The implication of the nonspecificity of the nonpolar aggregation can be carried over to nonspecificity for the direction of Leu-zervamicin insertion into a membrane.

The three helices in crystals of Leu-zervamicin that form an interrupted water

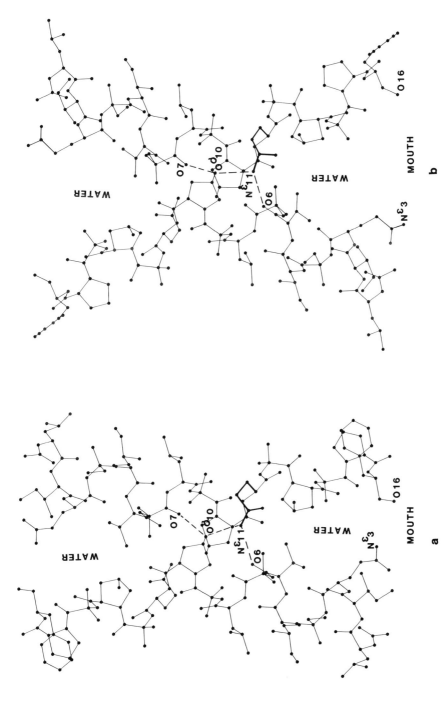

Fig. 16.13. Antiparallel association of polar faces of Leu-zervamicin. Interpeptide hydrogen bonds are indicated by *dashed lines*. *Bold lines* indicate the side chain of Gln^{11}. (*a*) Crystal form B with smallest bend in helix; (*b*) crystal form C with almost the largest bend in helix.

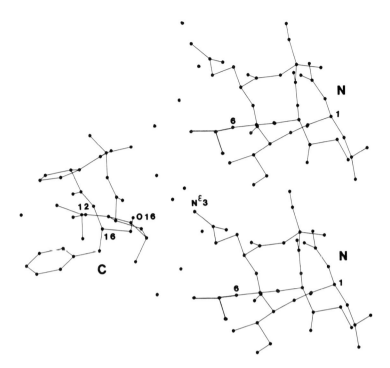

TOP

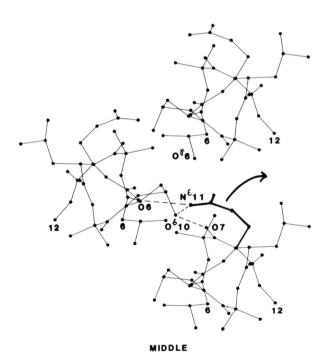

MIDDLE

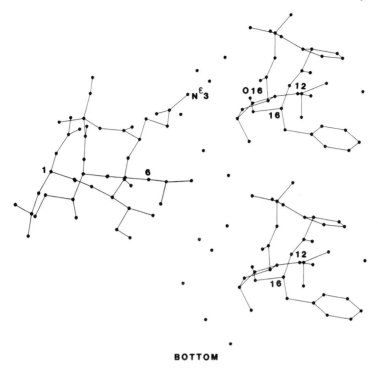

BOTTOM

Fig. 16.14. Three segments (opposite page and above) of Leu-zervamicin, 5–6 peptide residues each, in a view perpendicular to that in 16.13*a*, showing the water channel and interruption in the middle. An aggregation of three neighboring helices in the crystal is shown. The first and last C^α atoms in each segment are *numbered*. Water molecules are shown as *individual dots. Dashed lines* indicate interpeptide hydrogen bonds. A rotation of Gln^{11} side chain *(bold lines)* is suggested for a gating mechanism.

channel are, of course, surrounded by other helices. It is not in an environment that would be provided by a bilayer lipid membrane. Nevertheless, features found in the crystal may be suggestive for ion transport and for a gating mechanism. Figure 16.13*a,b* shows two bent molecules in an antiparallel mode with their polar (convex) sides facing each other and forming interpeptide hydrogen bonds in the middle. To form a three-helix channel another helix is needed, superimposed in this view either directly in front or back of the right or left helix. A view looking from the top into a three-helix channel is shown in Figure 16.14. For illustrative purposes the three-helix assembly has been cut into three slices, a top, middle, and bottom. The water molecules (individual dots) are found only in the top and bottom segments, and they form hydrogen bonds with the surrounding polar side groups, with each other, and with carbonyl O10 in the middle segment. The middle segment, shown with residues 6–11 and N12 and $C^\alpha12$, can form a channel large enough for passage of a water molecule, or a potassium ion, by a rotation of the Gln^{11} side chain about the $C^\beta - C^\gamma$ bond and/or the $C^\alpha - C^\beta$ bond to a more extended conformation. Either rotation will still accommodate the side chain without collision with other parts of the

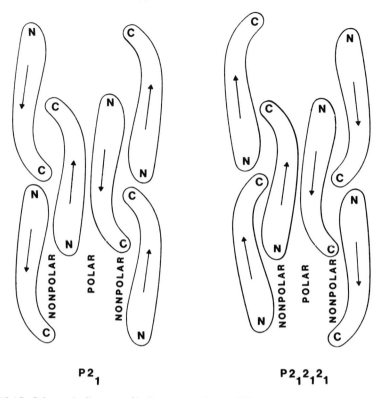

$$P2_1$$

$$P2_12_12_1$$

Fig. 16.15. Schematic diagram of helix aggregation in different crystal forms of Leu-zervamicin. The convex (polar) sides associate in an antiparallel mode and form interpeptide hydrogen bonds. The concave (nonpolar) sides associate in an antiparallel fashion in space group $P2_1$ and in a parallel fashion in space group $P2_12_12_1$. Hydrophobic contacts alone do not show a preference for parallel or antiparallel association.

three-helix assembly as found in the crystal. Such a rotation stimulated by an applied voltage would open the channel and serve as the gating mechanism (Karle et al., 1991a, 1992c). The zervamicins have been shown to form voltage-dependent multilevel ion channels in bilayer membranes (Balaram et al., 1992).

Several questions may arise about the suggested gating mechanism. One concerns the severing of several hydrogen bonds to $N^\epsilon 11$ and moving the long chain a considerable distance. An alternative gating mechanism for opening the channel may be the rotation of the Thr^6 side chain about the $C^\alpha - C^\beta$ bond so that the $C^\beta 6 - O^\gamma 6$ bond is brought into a vertical position. This alternative mechanism seems attractive in that it is closer to the concept of an on/off switch in that it leaves several strong interhelical hydrogen bonds intact and that the $O^\gamma 6$ atom is already hydrogen bonded to a water molecule (for which a ligand to a potassium ion can be substituted) that can be moved along with the rotation of the Thr^6 side chain. The drawback is that if the geometry as found in the crystal is held constant, the opening that would be formed in the constricted area may not be quite large enough for ion passage. Dynamic simulations of such motions for channel opening may provide further clues, such as distortions or motions of other parts of the helix that can be envisaged if the helices are inserted into a membrane.

Summary

The Aib residue is an important component of alamethicin, zervamicin, and other naturally occurring peptides that transport ions across lipid bilayer membranes. Crystal structure analyses of model synthetic peptides containing one to many Aib residues in various locations in the sequence show that helical backbones are formed almost without exception. The type of helix formed, α, 3_{10}, or mixed $\alpha/3_{10}$, is dependent on length of sequence and the ratio of Aib residues to total number of residues. α-Helical backbones are favored by longer sequences with proportionally fewer Aib residues. Helices in apolar, Aib-containing peptides associate in a completely parallel motif or in an antiparallel motif with equal ease; however, to date, no completely parallel association of helices has been found in crystals of peptides that contain some residues with polar side chains.

Naturally occurring ionophores like zervamicin and alamethicin have a helix that is curved at a Pro or Hyp residue. The bend in the curved helix of zervamicin changes by as much as 20° in different polymorphs of Leu-zervamicin, attesting to the easy flexibility of the helical backbone. The helices are more polar than the sequences would indicate. In addition to the polar side chains occurring on the convex face of the helix, the carbonyl oxygens at positions $i - 3$ and $i - 4$ above the Hyp or Pro bend extend away from the helix and augment the polarity of the convex face. In Leu-zervamicin, the Gln^{11} side chain wraps around the helix so that its polar endgroup also falls on the polar face of the helix. Interrupted water channels are formed in all polymorphs of Leu-zervamicin by antiparallel association of the polar convex faces. The Gln^{11} side chain that closes the channel in the middle may be the site of a gating mechanism that opens the channel dependent on the application of a potential. Furthermore, in Leu-zervamicin the mouth of the channel varies in size with the facile variation in the bend of the helix and the flexibility in the position of the Gln^3 side chain.

The insertion of a water molecule into a helix backbone of an apolar peptide (Fig. 16.7) imparts functional amphiphilic character to that peptide. Such hydration may play a role in ion transport by peptides with long hydrophobic sequences such as antiamoebin.

Investigations related to the molecular structures of ion channels are being pursued actively in a number of laboratories. More structural details should be forthcoming soon that will enable us to visualize the ion transfer process in a more precise fashion.

Acknowledgments

I am indebted to Prof. P. Balaram of the Indian Institute of Science, Bangalore, for his extensive collaborations in providing crystals of synthetic and natural peptides, for designing and synthesizing model peptides, and for his insights and the many discussions, all carried on by mail.

References

Argoudelis, A. D., and Johnson, L. E. (1974) Emerimicins II, III and IV, produced by *Emericellopsis microspora* in media supplemented with *trans*-4-*n*-propyl-L-proline. *J. Antibiot.* 27: 274–282.

Balaram, P. (1984) Peptides as bioorganic models. *Proc. Indian Acad. Sci.* 93: 703–717.

Balaram, P., Krishna, K., Sukumar, M., Mellor, I. R., and Sansom, M.S.P. (1992) The properties of ion channels formed by zervamicins. *Eur. Biophys. J.* 21: 117–128.

Ballesteros, J. A., and Weinstein, H. (1992) The role of Pro/Hyp-kinks in determining the transmembrane helix length and gating mechanism of a [Leu]zervamicin channel. *Biophys. Discussions* (submitted).

Brunger, A. T., Kuriyan, J., and Karplus, M. (1987) Crystallographic R factor refinement by molecular dynamics. *Science* 235: 458–460.

Brunger, A. T. (1988) Crystallographic refinement by simulated annealing. *J. Mol. Biol.* 203: 803–816.

Burgess, A. W., and Leach, S. J. (1973) An obligatory α-helical amino acid residue. *Biopolymers* 12: 2599–2605.

Butters, T., Hutter, P., Jung, G., Pauls, N., Schmitt, H., Sheldrick, G. M., and Winter, W. (1981) On the structure of the helical N-terminus in alamethicin: α-helix or 3_{10}-helix? *Angew. Chem. Int. Ed. Engl.* 20: 889–890.

Cerrini, S., Lamba, D., Scatturin, A., and Ughetto, G. (1989) The crystal and molecular structure of the α-helical nonapeptide antibiotic leucinostatin A. *Biopolymers* 28: 409–420.

Chou, P. Y., and Fasman, G. D. (1974) Prediction of protein conformation. *Biochemistry* 13: 222–245.

Fox, R. O., and Richards, F. M. (1982) A voltage-gated ion channel model inferred from the crystal structure of alamethicin at 1.5 Å resolution. *Nature* 300: 325–330.

Francis, A. K., Iqbal, M., Balaram, P., and Vijayan, M. (1983). The crystal structure of a 3_{10} helical decapeptide containing α-aminoisobutyric acid. *FEBS Lett.* 155: 230–232.

Furois-Corbin, S., and Pullman, A. (1987) Theoretical study of potential ion-channels formed by a bundle of α-helices: effect of the presence of polar residues along the channel inner wall. *J. Biomol. Struct. Dyn.* 4: 589–597.

Gilson, M. K., and Honig, B. (1989) Destabilization of an α-helix-bundle protein by helix dipoles. *Proc. Natl. Acad. Sci. USA* 86: 1524–1528.

Hall, J. E., Vodyanoy, I., Balasubramanian, T. M., and Marshall, G. R. (1984) Alamethicin: a rich model for channel behavior. *Biophys. J.* 45: 233–247.

Hendrickson, W. A., and Konnert, J. H. (1980) Incorporation of stereochemical information into crystallographic refinement. In:*Computing in Crystallography*, edited by R. Diamond, S. Ramaseshan, and K. Venkatesan. Bangalore, India: Indian Academy of Sciences, p. 9–13.

Hendrickson, W. A. (1985) Stereochemically restrained refinement of macromolecular structures. *Methods Enzymol.* 115: 252–270.

Hol, W.G.J., Halie, L. M., and Sander, C. (1981) Dipoles of the α-helix and β-sheet. Their role in protein folding. *Nature* 294: 532–536.

Hynes, T. R., and Fox, R. O. (1991) The crystal structure of staphylococcal nuclease refined at 1.7 Å resolution. *Prot. Struct. Funct. Genet.* 10: 92–105.

Karle, I. L., Flippen-Anderson, J. L., Sukumar, M., and Balaram, P. (1987) Conformation of a 16-residue zervamicin IIA analog peptide containing three different structural features: 3_{10}-helix, alpha helix and β-bend ribbon. *Proc. Natl. Acad. Sci. USA* 84: 5087–5091.

Karle, I. L., Flippen-Anderson, J. L., Sukumar, M., and Balaram, P. (1988a) Monoclinic polymorph of Boc-Trp-Ile-Ala-Aib-Ile-Val-Aib-Leu-Aib-Pro-OMe (anhydrous). *Int. J. Peptide Prot. Res.* 31: 567–576.

Karle, I. L., Flippen-Anderson, J. L., Uma, K., and Balaram, P. (1988b) Aqueous channels within apolar peptide aggregates: solvated helix of the α-aminoisobutyric acid (Aib)-containing peptide Boc-(Aib-Ala-Leu)$_3$-Aib-OMe · 2H$_2$O · CH$_3$OH in crystals. *Proc. Natl. Acad. Sci. USA* 85: 299–303.

Karle, I. L., Flippen-Anderson, J. L., Uma, K., and Balaram, H., and Balaram, P. (1989a) α-Helix and mixed $3_{10}/\alpha$-helix in cocrystallized conformers of Boc-Aib-Val-Aib-Aib-Val-Val-Val-Aib-Val-Aib-OMe. *Proc. Natl. Acad. Sci. USA* 86: 765–769.

Karle, I. L., Flippen-Anderson, J. L., Uma, K., and Balaram, P. (1989b) Solvated helical backbones: x-ray diffraction study of Boc-Ala-Leu-Aib-Ala-Leu-Aib-OMe · H$_2$O. *Biopolymers* 28: 773–781.

Karle, I. L., and Balaram, P. (1990) Structural characteristics of α-helical peptide molecules containing Aib residues. Biochemistry 29: 6747–6756.

Karle, I. L., Flippen-Anderson, J. L., Uma, K., and Balaram, P. (1990a) Apolar peptide models for conformational heterogeneity, hydration and packing of polypeptide helices: crystal structure of hepta- and octa-peptides containing α-aminoisobutyric acid. *Prot. Struct. Funct. Genet.* 7: 62–73.

Karle, I. L., Flippen-Anderson, J. L., Sukumar, M., and Balaram, P. (1990b) Parallel and antiparallel aggregation of α-helices. Crystal structures of two apolar decapeptides X-Trp-Ile-Ala-Aib-Ile-Val-Aib-Leu-Aib-Pro-OMe (X = Boc,Ac). *Int. J. Peptide Prot. Res.* 35: 518–526.

Karle, I. L., Flippen-Anderson, J. L., Uma, K., and Balaram, P. (1990c) Helix aggregation in peptide crystals: occurrence of either all parallel or antiparallel packing motifs for α-helices in polymorphs of Boc-Aib-Ala-Leu-Ala-Leu-Aib-Leu-Ala-Leu-Aib-OMe. *Biopolymers* 29: 1835–1845.

Karle, I. L., Flippen-Anderson, J. L., Uma, K., Sukumar, M., and Balaram, P. (1990d) Modular design of synthetic protein mimics. Crystal structures, assembly, and hydration of two 15- and 16-residue apolar, leucyl-rich helical peptides. *J. Am. Chem. Soc.* 112: 9350–9356.

Karle, I. L., Flippen-Anderson, J. L., Agarwalla, S., and Balaram, P. (1991a) Crystal structure of Leu-zervamicin, a membrane ion channel peptide. Implications for gating mechanisms. *Proc. Natl. Acad. Sci. USA* 88: 5307–5311.

Karle, I. L., Flippen-Anderson, J. L., Sukumar, M., Uma, K., and Balaram, P. (1991b) Modular design of synthetic protein mimics. Crystal structure of two seven-residue helical peptide segments linked by ϵ-aminocaproic acid. *J. Am. Chem. Soc.* 113: 3952–3956.

Karle, I. L., Flippen-Anderson, J. L., Sukumar, M., and Balaram, P. (1992a) Helix packing of leucine-rich peptides: a parallel leucine ladder in the structure of Boc-Aib-Leu-Aib-Aib-Leu-Leu-Leu-Aib-Leu-Aib-OMe. *Prot. Struct. Funct. Genet.* 12: 324–330.

Karle, I. L., Flippen-Anderson, J. L., Sukumar, M., and Balaram, P. (1992b) Differences in hydration and association of helical Boc-Val-Ala-Leu-Aib-Val-Ala-Leu-(Val-Ala-Leu-Aib)$_2$-OMe · H_2O in two crystalline polymorphs. *J. Med. Chem.* 35: 3885–3889.

Karle, I. L., Flippen-Anderson, J. L., Agarwalla, S., and Balaram, P. (1992c) Implications for an ion channel in Leu-zervamicin: crystal structure of polymorph B. In *Structure and Function: Proceedings of the 7th Conversation in Biomolecular Stereodynamics,* edited by R. H. Sarma and M. H. Sarma. New York: Adenine Press, vol. 2, p. 97–111.

Karle, I. L., Flippen-Anderson, J. L., Uma, K., and Balaram, P. (1993a) Accommodation of a D-Phe residue into a right-handed 3$_{10}$-helix: structure of Boc-D-Phe-(Aib)$_4$-Gly-L-Leu-(Aib)$_2$-OMe, an anlogue to the amino terminal segment of antiamoebins and emerimicins. *Biopolymers* 33: 401–407.

Karle, I. L., Flippen-Anderson, J. L., Uma, K., and Balaram, P. (1993b) Unfolding of an α-helix in peptide crystals by solvation: conformational fragility in a heptapeptide. *Biopolymers* 33: 827–837.

Konnert, J. H., Hendrickson, W. A., and Karle, J. (1975) *Proceedings of the Third East Coast Protein Crystallography Workshop.* Eastover, MA.

Marshall, G. R., and Bosshard, H. E. (1972) Angiotensin II. Biologically active conformation. *Circ. Res.* 30/31(Suppl II): 143–150.

Mathew, M. K., and Balaram, P. (1983) Alamethicin and related membrane channel forming polypeptides. *Mol. Cell Biochem.* 50: 47–64.

Menestrina, G., Voges, K.-P., Jung, G., and Boheim, G. (1986) Voltage dependent channel formation by rods of helical polypeptides. *J. Membrane Biol.* 93: 111–132.

Mueller, P., and Rudin, D. O. (1968) Action potentials induced in biomolecular lipid membranes. *Nature* 217: 713–719.

Okuyama, K., Saga, Y., Nakayama, M., and Narita, M. (1991) Molecular and crystal structures of Aib-containing oligopeptides Boc-Leu$_4$-Aib-Leu$_4$-OBzl and Boc-(Leu$_4$-Aib)$_2$-OBzl. *Biopolymers* 31: 975–985.

Prasad, B.V.V., and Balaram, P. (1984) The stereochemistry of peptides containing alpha-aminoisobutyric acid. *CRC Crit. Rev. Biochem.* 16: 307–348.

Richardson, J. S. (1981) The anatomy and toxonomy of protein structure. *Adv. Prot. Struct.* 34: 167–339.

Rinehart, K. L. Jr., Gaudioso, L. A., Moore, M. L., Pandey, R. C., Cook, J. C., Jr., Barber, M., Sedgwick, R. D., Bordoli, R. S., Tyler, A. N., and Green, B. N. (1981) Structures of eleven zervamicin and two emerimicin peptide antibiotics studied by fast atom bombardment mass spectroscopy. *J. Am. Chem. Soc.* 103: 6517–6520.

Sundaralingam, M., and Sekharudu, Y. C. (1989) Water-inserted α-helical segments implicate reverse turns as folding intermediates. Science 244: 1333–1337.

Sansom, M.S.P. (1991) The biophysics of peptide models of ion channels. *Prog. Biophys. Mol. Biol.* 55: 139–235.

Terwilliger, T. C., and Eisenberg, D. (1982): The structure of melittin. II. Interpretation of the structure. *J. Biol. Chem.* 257: 6016–6022.

Toniolo, C., Bonora, G. M., Bavoso, A., Benedetti, E., di Blasio, B., Pavone, V., and Pedone, C. (1983) Preferred conformations of peptides containing α,α-disubstituted α-amino acids. *Biopolymers* 22: 205–215.

Toniolo, C., Crisma, M., Bonora, G. M., Benedetti, E., di Blasio, B., Pavone, V., Pedone, C., and Santini, A. (1991) Preferred conformation of the terminally blocked $(Aib)_{10}$ homo-oligopeptide: a long regular 3_{10}-helix. *Biopolymers* 31: 129–138.

Wada, A. (1976) The alpha-helix as an electric macro-dipole. *Adv. Biophys.* 9: 1–63.

Index